Cognition & Occupation
Across the Life Span

Cognition & Occupation Across the Life Span

Models for Intervention in Occupational Therapy

2ND EDITION

Edited by Noomi Katz, PhD, OTR

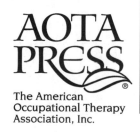

The American
Occupational Therapy
Association, Inc.

Vision Statement

AOTA advances occupational therapy as the pre-eminent profession in promoting the health, productivity, and quality of life of individuals and society through the therapeutic application of occupation.

Mission Statement

The American Occupational Therapy Association advances the quality, availability, use, and support of occupational therapy through standard-setting, advocacy, education, and research on behalf of its members and the public.

AOTA Staff

Frederick P. Somers, *Executive Director*
Christopher M. Bluhm, *Chief Operating Officer*
Audrey Rothstein, *Group Leader, Communications*
Chris Davis, *Managing Editor, AOTA Press*
Barbara Dickson, *Production Editor*
Robert A. Sacheli, *Manager, Creative Services*
Sarah E. Ely, *Book Production Coordinator*
Marge Wasson, *Marketing Manager*
Elizabeth Sarcia, *Marketing Specialist*

The American Occupational Therapy Association, Inc.
4720 Montgomery Lane
Bethesda, MD 20814
Phone: 301-652-AOTA (2682)
TDD: 800-377-8555
Fax: 301-652-7711
www.aota.org
To order: 1-877-404-AOTA (2682)

Disclaimers

This publication is designed to provide accurate and authoritative information in regard to the subject matter covered. It is sold or distributed with the understanding that the publisher is not engaged in rendering legal, accounting, or other professional service. If legal advice or other expert assistance is required, the services of a competent professional person should be sought.
—*From the Declaration of Principles jointly adopted by the American Bar Association and a Committee of Publishers and Associations*

It is the objective of the American Occupational Therapy Association to be a forum for free expression and interchange of ideas. The opinions expressed by the contributors to this work are their own and not necessarily those of either the editor or the American Occupational Therapy Association.

ISBN: 1-56900-198-7

Library of Congress Control Number: 2004116957

Cover design by Sarah E. Ely
Text design and composition by Circle Graphics, Columbia, MD
Printed by Victor Graphics, Baltimore MD

Contents

I PART
Introduction 1

II PART
Neurological Disabilities 27

III PART
Mental Health 167

v

List of Tables, Figures, Exhibits, Case Examples, and Appendixes

Foreword

When Adolph Meyer, a noted neurobiologist and physician, delivered the paper "The Philosophy of Occupation" to the Fifth Annual Meeting of the National Society for the Promotion of Occupational Therapy (now the American Occupational Therapy Association) in 1921, he challenged the occupational therapists of the day to provide opportunities for individuals to use their occupations to define their uniqueness and to promote health. His words reflected his interest in neurology and challenged the profession to build the science that would understand performance. As neuroscience began to link brain and behavior, much knowledge was generated that guided occupational therapists to understand the motor and sensory systems that support everyday life. It has been only over the past two decades when neuroscience has yielded an understanding of the brain and cognition that has guided our understanding of performance.

Cognition is central to everyday life. It is impossible to live independently without higher order functions of planning, organization, attention, memory, and awareness. Problems with these cognitive functions are seen in many of the clients treated by occupational therapists (e.g., learning disabilities, autism, attention-deficit/hyperactivity disorder [ADHD], developmental coordination disorders [DCDs], depression, schizophrenia, stroke, traumatic brain injury, Parkinson's disease, Alzheimer's disease, multiple sclerosis). Individuals with higher order cognitive impairments require specific strategies that are central to occupation-based,

client-centered care to maintain themselves, interact in families, work, go to school, and actively engage in community life. Occupational therapists' focus on cognition and learning as it supports everyday life is what defines the profession's uniqueness in its approach to care.

Noomi Katz has been a leader, mentor, and coach to occupational therapists all over the world and is the champion for cognition being central to occupational therapy practice. In this book, *Cognition and Occupation Across the Life Span: Models for Intervention in Occupational Therapy, 2nd Edition,* she has included the writings of many of those whom she has mentored. They are clinicians and scientists who have dedicated their professional efforts to develop and evaluate cognitive interventions, and with their work they have built a body of knowledge to support the profession of occupational therapy in this area of practice. This text is both a foundation book and a handbook for state-of-the-art knowledge to support occupational therapy interventions. Students and practitioners will be introduced to strategies for occupational therapy practice to support individuals with brain injury; individuals with mental health difficulties, including schizophrenia; children with ADHD and DCD; and older adults with normal changes of aging and dementia.

This is a must-have book for both the classroom and the clinic that will be used to help us understand behaviors, help us translate cognitive neuroscience into practice, and help us figure out how to tell parents and caregivers what has happened to their loved ones and how to best support their behaviors to achieve successful performance and participation in their daily lives. The authors have translated the latest cognitive neuroscience developments into interventions that occupational therapists can use to enhance the performance and quality of life of those they serve. For their efforts, we thank them. And for the gift of vision and knowledge and willingness to help us all understand the impor-tance of cognition to daily life, we thank Noomi Katz.

—*M. Carolyn Baum, PhD, OTR/L, FAOTA*
President, American Occupational Therapy
    Association
Professor, Occupational Therapy and
    Neurology at Washington University
    School of Medicine
Lifetime student of Noomi Katz

Preface

This work is a new and updated compilation of information on cognition and occupation spanning the life cycle, including a new section describing models of cognition developed and applied to pediatric populations. Since the publication of the first edition of this book in 1998, the literature on cognition and rehabilitation has expanded tremendously, with emerging evidence from brain imaging, neurobiological sciences, dynamic theories, and interdisciplinary works on cognition and the rehabilitation of cognitive disabilities. Recently, two publications of major importance related to rehabilitation and occupational therapy have been introduced—the *International Classification of Functioning, Disability, and Health* (*ICF*; World Health Organization, 2001) and the *Occupational Therapy Practice Framework: Domain and Process* (American Occupational Therapy Association, 2002)—both of which have had a significant impact on practice in all the rehabilitation professions, specifically on occupational therapy.

Cognitive components, which have been defined extensively according to *ICF* terminology, appear in that document within the category of body functions. This categorization also has been adopted by the *Framework* and, in addition, cognition is included within the occupational therapy professional domain of activity and participation, in which knowledge is applied to everyday tasks. The definitions in the box on the next page are from the *ICF,* and they show the major impact that these components have had on current conceptualizations of human functioning and their importance in occupational therapy intervention.

Within the *Framework,* in addition to its inclusion as a body function within the gamut of client factors, cognition also is incorporated as a major component within process, and communication/interaction, within performance skills. Thus, the focus of this book and the models for intervention described in it are of utmost importance for enabling individuals with cognitive disabilities to participate in daily activities to the best of their abilities at a given time. Arthanat, Nochajski, and Stone (2004) have provided an analysis and example of how to apply the *ICF* terminology to a person with cognitive dysfunctions. This approach can facilitate the development and use of a common language between interdisciplinary rehabilitation teams that will enable clearer communication among practitioners for the benefit of clients.

All cognitive models presented in this new edition are based on the most recent conceptualizations and research literature in their area. Some elaborate on previous writings, with recent findings, further developments on assessment and intervention methods, and illustrations of their use through case studies and group interventions. Most importantly, they provide research evidence supporting their practice that did not exist a few years ago. Some of the models are presented in this book for the first time, such as those appearing in Part IV on pediatrics, or are new altogether, such as the nonlinear approach by Lazzarini (see Chapter 8). All reflect the unique occupational therapy perspective with respect to the treatment and rehabilitation of children, adults, and elderly people with cognitive dysfunctions, namely that of cognitive reha-

ICF Definitions of Functions, Activity, and Participation Related to Cognition

BODY FUNCTIONS—MENTAL HEALTH

Attention functions: Specific mental functions of focusing on an external stimulus or internal experience for a required time. Includes functions of sustaining, shifting, dividing, and sharing attention; concentration; distractibility.

Memory functions: Specific mental functions of registering and storing information and retrieving it as needed. Includes functions of short- and long-term memory; immediate, recent, and remote memory; memory span; retrieval of memory; remembering; functions used in recalling and learning, such as in nominal, selective, and dissociative amnesia.

Higher level cognitive function: Specific mental functions especially dependent on the frontal lobes of the brain, including complex goal-directed behaviors such as decision making, abstract thinking, planning and carrying out plans, mental flexibility, and deciding which behaviors are appropriate under what circumstances; often called *executive functions.* Includes functions of abstraction and organization of ideas; time management, insight, and judgment; concept formation, categorization, and cognitive flexibility.

Insight: Mental functions of awareness and understanding of oneself and one's behavior.

Organization and planning: Mental functions of coordinating parts into a whole, of systematizing; the mental function involved in developing a method of proceeding or acting.

Problem-solving: Mental functions of identifying, analyzing, and integrating incongruent or conflicting information into a solution.

ACTIVITY AND PARTICIPATION—APPLYING KNOWLEDGE

Thinking: Formulating and manipulating ideas, concepts, and images, whether goal-oriented or not, either alone or with others, such as creating fiction, proving a theorem, playing with ideas, brainstorming, meditating, pondering, speculating, reflecting.

Solving problems: Finding solutions to questions or situations by identifying and analyzing issues; developing options and solutions; evaluating potential effects of solutions; executing a chosen solution, such as in resolving a dispute between two people.

Making decisions: Making a choice among options, implementing the choice, and evaluating the effects of the choice, such as selecting and purchasing a specific item, or deciding to undertake and undertaking one task from among several tasks that need to be done.

Note. Adapted from *International Classification of Functioning, Disability, and Health,* by the World Health Organization, 2001, Geneva, Switzerland: Author.

bilitation through occupation, with the ultimate goal being optimal occupational performance.

ORGANIZATION OF THIS BOOK

This book is organized into parts that focus, in one respect, on different client populations, such as Part II on neurological disabilities and Part III on mental health, and in another, on specific groups along the life span continuum, such as Part IV on children and Part V on elderly people.

In addition, Katz and Hartman-Maeir (Chapter 1) provide an introduction that focuses on *higher-level cognitive functions* (previously termed *metacognition*) that have implications for *all* populations. The main cognitive components of awareness and executive functions are then further presented in many of the chapters throughout the book, in which they emphasize their relevance to specific target populations. Chapter 1 provides the most recent major theories, assessment instruments, and intervention methods that may be used with various populations. Finally, Part VI includes a model by Hadas-Lidor and Weiss (see Chapter 15) that can be applied to a variety of populations.

Each cognitive model described in this book includes (a) the theoretical base; (b) intervention, including evaluation procedures, assessment instruments, and treatment methods; (c) case examples and group treatment illustrating the intervention process; and (d) research for evidence-based practice using the model or parts of it. The chapters start with learning objectives and finish with review questions to facilitate the learning process. *ICF* terminology and *Framework* concepts are incorporated by all authors.

As discussed in the past, two general approaches in cognitive rehabilitation were traditionally used, namely remedial versus functional/adaptive, with the recent emphasis being on strategy learning, remedial or compensatory. Severity of the dysfunctions and their underlying causes, the target populations and their ages, and environmental contexts are all major determinants of the approach taken. Hence, the focus of the various models presented in this book are similar in some aspects and differ in others along this remedial compensatory continuum. It is, however, important to stress that all models focus on the clients' occupational performance as the goal of intervention, which is what establishes them as occupational therapy cognitive models.

The order in which the chapters appear is of no major importance in itself. Each chapter is complete on its own, and thus chapters can be read in any sequence that readers choose. However, to choose a model for clinical intervention, an occupational therapist must consider the specific problems of the individual client and the context in which the client will have to function and read that particular chapter.

Part II: Neurological Disabilities

Part II relates to clients with neurological dysfunctions and includes four models of intervention by Toglia (Chapter 2), Abreu and Peloquin (Chapter 3), Averbuch and Katz (Chapter 4), and Giles (Chapter 5). These models were originally developed for clients with brain injuries but are applied now to clients with other neurological dysfunctions as well. Specifically, the application of Toglia's Dynamic Interactional Model is outlined in other parts of this book in two chapters by Josman, one for use with clients with schizophrenia (Chapter 6) and one for use with children with learning disabilities or traumatic brain injury (Chapter 10). These previous four chapters were included in the original edition, but the authors have updated, developed, and researched them extensively, providing new theoretical and clinical material.

Part III: Mental Health

The application of Toglia's Dynamic Interactional Model to clients with schizophrenia (Josman, Chapter 6) underwent a major update as the literature in these areas has grown extensively. Similarly, Duncombe (Chapter 7) further develops and updates the cognitive–behavioral model that is based on theories in mental health and their adaptation to occupational therapy. An additional new approach by Lazzarini (Chapter 8) focuses on a nonlinear approach to cognition and disability, which presents important new literature on dynamical systems and chaos theories and their application to occupational therapy in mental health.

Part IV: Pediatrics

As mentioned earlier, this part of the book is a new addition, included in response to an urgent need to introduce the work done with children who, on the one hand, do not have cognitive deficits per se but, on the other hand, can benefit from a cognitive intervention model, such as children with developmental coordination disorder. Polatajko and Mandich present the Cognitive Orientation to Daily Occupational Performance model for this population in Chapter 9, a model that has already extensive research evidence to support its use. For the first time, cognitive models also are presented that are to be used for intervention with children, such as Toglia's Dynamic Interactional Model, as applied to children with cognitive deficits such as those with learning disabilities and brain injuries (Josman, Chapter 10) and with children with attention-deficit/hyperactivity disorders (ADHD; Cermak, Chapter 11). Cermak provides a perspective to cognitive rehabilitation for children with ADHD, which is important to consider when working with children of different ages. These additions to the literature of occupational therapy for children is of utmost importance, as most of the existing models of intervention in pediatrics are designed for younger, preschool children and not for primary-school-age children and adolescents, in whom cognitive components have major ramifications for participation in daily functions.

Part V: Healthy Elderly People and Elderly People With Dementia

Dissemination of the updated literature on cognitive changes in later life, especially with respect to information processing, cognition, and memory (see Levy, Chapter 12), provides essential knowledge on a difficult issue that must always be considered when working with elderly individuals. Furthermore, the implication for occupational therapy practitioners, as also discussed by Levy (Chapter 13), is beneficial for the application of any model to the elderly population.

Following these two generally oriented chapters, Levy and Burns (Chapter 14) present a cognitive disabilities model adapted for use in the rehabilitation of older adults with dementia. This work is based on Allen's Cognitive Disabilities Model; however, the authors have further expanded its conceptualization, incorporating current thinking and research findings.

It is important to emphasize that, although this edition of the book does not include a chapter by Allen, her model and theory have had a major impact on the development of cognitive models for intervention in occupational therapy. Therefore, in Chapter 14, her work is extensively described as it can be applied by clinicians in the field of mental health, which represents the original focus of the model, as well as by clinicians who work with neurological populations.

Part VI: All Populations

Hadas-Lidor and Weiss in Chapter 15 describe the Dynamic Model for Cognitive Modifiability in occupational therapy, which is based on Feuerstein's Dynamic Theory for Cognitive Modifiability and Mediated Learning Experience. The authors have expanded the original approach for clinical use, especially within the community arena, applying it not only to clients with cognitive deficits but also to their caregivers and families, as well as to community workers who service these clients. As such, they have broadened the target populations with whom occupational therapists work and the capacity of their intervention.

SUMMARY

This book provides a broad knowledge base of the contribution of occupational therapy over the life span for children, adolescents, adults, and elderly people with cognitive and related dysfunctions, including in-depth discussions of clinical applications. The authors who collaborated to produce this book have made an important contribution to our knowledge on the interaction between cognition and occupation in influencing clients' state of health. They have provided a variety of ways to approach the problem of cognitive dysfunctions and to intervene with various populations. I am thankful for their collaboration and their thorough work, as it was a pleasure working with them. It is my hope that this book will inspire further study and intervention in the area of cognition and occupation in rehabilitation.

—*Noomi Katz, PhD, OTR*
School of Occupational Therapy
Hebrew University and Hadassah,
Jerusalem, Israel

REFERENCES

American Occupational Therapy Association. (2002). Occupational therapy practice framework: Domain and process. *American Journal of Occupational Therapy, 56,* 609–639.

Arthanat, S., Nochajski, S. M., & Stone, J. (2004). The International Classification of Functioning, Disability, and Health and its application to cognitive disorders. *Disability and Rehabilitation, 26,* 235–245.

World Health Organization. (2001). *International Classification of Functioning, Disability, and Health (ICF).* Geneva, Switzerland: Author.

Acknowledgment

I would like to thank the authors that participated in writing this new edition, some of whom worked on the previous one with me and some who have provided new chapters for this book. All are making great contributions to the topic of cognition and occupation and are a major force in developing and integrating cognitive aspects into theory and clinical application of occupational therapists, as well as contributing through research to the science of occupational therapy. I greatly appreciate the collaboration and efforts.

I also thank my colleagues and students (past and present) at the School of Occupational Therapy at Hebrew University and Hadassah Jerusalem for their many years of collaboration and mutual support; without them I would not be able to achieve any academic goals and enjoy my work at the same time.

—Noomi Katz, PhD, OTR

About the Contributors

Beatriz C. Abreu, PhD, OTR, FAOTA
Director, Occupational Therapy
Transitional Learning Center at Galveston
Clinical Professor, Graduate School of
    Biomedical Sciences
Department of Preventative Medicine &
    Community Health
University of Texas Medical Branch at
    Galveston

Sarah Averbuch, MA, OTR
Director, Department of Occupational
    Therapy
Loewenstein Rehabilitation Hospital
Rannana, Israel
Department of Occupational Therapy
Tel Aviv University
Tel Aviv, Israel

Theressa Burns, OTR
Minneapolis Geriatric Research, Education,
    and Clinical Center
Minneapolis

Sharon A. Cermak, EdD, OTR/L, FAOTA
Professor, Department of Occupational
    Therapy
Boston University, Sargent College
Boston

Linda Duncombe, PhD, OTR
Clinical Associate Professor, Department of
    Occupational Therapy
Boston University, Sargent College
Boston

Gordon Muir Giles, PhD, OTR, FAOTA
Director of Neurobehavioral Service,
    Crestwood Behavioral Health, Inc.
Associate Professor, Samuel Merritt College
Oakland, California

Naomi Josman, PhD, OTR
Senior Lecturer, Chairperson, Department of
    Occupational Therapy
Haifa University
Haifa Mount Carmel, Israel

Noomi Katz, PhD, OTR
Professor, School of Occupational Therapy
Hebrew University and Hadassah
Jerusalem, Israel

Naomi Hadas-Lidor, PhD, OTR
Senior Teacher, Department of
    Occupational Therapy
Tel Aviv University, Ramat Aviv
Tel Aviv, Israel

Adina Hartman-Maeir, PhD, OTR
Lecturer, School of Occupational Therapy
Hebrew University and Hadassah
Jerusalem, Israel

Ivelisse Lazzarini, OTD, OTR/L
Assistant Professor, Creighton University
School of Pharmacy and Health Professions
Omaha, Nebraska

Linda L. Levy, MA, OTR/L, FAOTA
Associate Professor, Department of
    Occupational Therapy
Temple University
Philadelphia

**Angie Mandich, PhD, OT Reg. (Ont.),
OT(C)**
Assistant Professor, School of Occupational
    Therapy
Director, The Kids Skills Clinic
University of Western Ontario
London, Ontario

Suzanne M. Peloquin, PhD, OTR, FAOTA
Professor, School of Allied Health Sciences
Department of Occupational Therapy
University of Texas Medical Branch at
    Galveston

**Helene J. Polatajko, PhD, OT Reg. (Ont.),
OT(C), FCAOT**
Professor and Chair
Department of Occupational Therapy
Rehabilitation Sciences Building
University of Toronto
Toronto, Ontario

Joan Pascale Toglia, PhD, OTR, FAOTA
Chairperson, Occupational Therapy
Program
Mercy College
Dobbs Ferry, New York

Penina Weiss, MSc, OTR
Department of Occupational Therapy
Tel Aviv University, Ramat Aviv
Tel Aviv, Israel

PART

Introduction

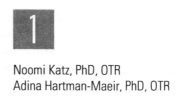

Noomi Katz, PhD, OTR
Adina Hartman-Maeir, PhD, OTR

Higher-Level Cognitive Functions

*Awareness and Executive Functions
Enabling Engagement in Occupation*

LEARNING OBJECTIVES

By the end of this chapter,
readers will
1. Be familiar with the concepts and theories of awareness and executive functions
2. Learn about methods and instruments for assessment and treatment approaches
3. Understand and appreciate the importance of higher-level cognitive functions in rehabilitation of clients with cognitive disabilities.

In this chapter we introduce the concepts of higher-level cognitive functions of awareness and executive functions and place them within the domain of rehabilitation of individuals with cognitive deficits. Traditionally, rehabilitation efforts have been aimed at restoring or compensating for basic cognitive deficits such as attention or memory, whereas the higher-level cognitive processes have not always been taken into consideration. In the past several years, the body of knowledge around these processes has grown significantly in the scientific world at large, and specifically within rehabilitation disciplines. Because these processes are essential for enabling occupation, it is important to include these concepts in occupational therapy models of intervention. Occupational therapy provides a unique contribution to the intervention of individuals with deficits in higher-level cognitive functions because these functions are highly integrative processes that are evident mainly in complex contexts of everyday living and cannot be fully understood nor treated with "laboratory-type" tools or settings. Because occupational therapists specialize in analysis of occupations, they have a unique opportunity to contribute to the assessment, treatment, and theoretical development in this area.

Higher-level cognitive functions are classified in the new *International Classification of Functioning, Disability, and Health* (*ICF*) terminology (World Health Organization,

2001) and the *Occupational Therapy Practice Framework* (American Occupational Therapy Association [AOTA], 2002), within the categories of *body functions* and *client factors* that affect activity and participation in occupation. Cognition is conceptualized as comprising basic cognitive skills (e.g., attention, memory, perception) and higher-level cognitive skills, which are also called *metacognitive skills* by some disciplines. The application of the ICF classification was recently discussed and exemplified with a case study providing a way to describe the status and performance of individuals with cognitive dysfunctions (Arthanat, Nochajski, & Stone, 2004).

The different terms for higher-level cognition found in various bodies of literature can be clustered into four general factors: (a) knowing about knowing and knowing how to know (Brown, 1987; Flavell, 1985); (b) metacognitive monitoring and metacognitive control (Jarman, Vavrik, & Walton, 1995); (c) metacognitive knowledge and metacognitive process (Butler, 1999); and (d) awareness and executive functions (Lezak, 1995; Prigatano, 1999; Sohlberg & Mateer, 2001a; Stuss, 1992). The first three classifications are used mainly in the developmental and educational psychology literature, whereas the fourth classification of awareness and executive functions are used in the neurological, neuropsychological, and rehabilitation literature.

The developmental educational definition of *metacognition* refers to "knowing about knowing"; this metacognitive knowledge includes knowledge about ourselves, the tasks we face, and the strategies we use (Flavell, 1985). Brown (1987) differentiated between "knowing about knowing" (i.e., declarative knowledge—e.g., knowing the name of a flower) and "knowing how to" (i.e., procedural knowledge—e.g., knowing how to ride a bike). The second cluster was developed by Nelson and Narrens (1994), who proposed a model of metacognition that distinguished between the components of monitoring and control. Jarman and colleagues (1995) elaborated on this model and denoted that these components correspond to those of knowledge and awareness of abilities and deficits—the monitoring aspect—and executive functions—the control aspect. More recently, Butler (1999), in a review of the concept of metacognition and its relation to learning disabilities, delineated the same components of *metacognitive knowledge* and *metacognitive process*. Butler focused on metacognition as a framework for understanding effective strategy use in learning and for understanding why students with learning disabilities may fail to coordinate use of knowledge. This literature is particularly relevant for interventions with pediatric populations addressed in Chapters 9 through 11.

This chapter is grounded in a neurorehabilitation perspective and its relation to occupational therapy process; therefore, we have adopted the terms *awareness* and *executive functions* to describe the main components of higher-level cognition. This perspective also reflects the important work of Stuss (1992) as presented in his hierarchical feedback–feedforward model of brain function that includes a sensory–perceptual component at the base, executive functions at the second level, and self-awareness at the top. Higher-level cognitive deficits have been identified in clients following traumatic brain injury (TBI), stroke, Parkinson's disease, dementia, and schizophrenia. Despite the relationships among these components, they also may be dissociated from each other. Therefore, to provide an in-depth review of these concepts, the following sections of the chapter deal with theoretical aspects, assessment, and treatment of awareness and executive function disorders separately.

AWARENESS

Definitions

Impaired awareness associated with neurological dysfunction encompasses a wide range of phenomena relating to the lack of knowledge or recognition of the disease or injury, the consequential deficits, and the functional disabilities. Prigatano and Schacter (1991) defined *awareness* as a highly integrated brain function, encompassing the ability to perceive oneself in relatively objective terms, maintaining a sense of subjectivity, and involving an interaction of thoughts and feelings. Unawareness may present itself in verbal and other behavioral forms: Clients with unawareness may demonstrate explicit verbal denial of their situation, underestimate the severity of deficits or disabilities, or fail to make appropriate behavioral accommodations to their situation (Berti, Ladavas, & Della Corte, 1996; Bisiach, Vallar, Perani, Papagno, & Berti, 1986). The terms *unawareness* and *anosognosia* (meaning lack of knowledge of disease) are used interchangeably in the literature and have been applied to unawareness of neurological or psychiatric disorders and unawareness of motor, sensory, and cognitive impairments and their consequences, such as anosognosia for hemiplegia (Cutting, 1978), anosognosia for hemianopia (Bisiach & Geminiani, 1991; Celesia, Brigell, & Vaphiades, 1997), anosognosia for aphasia (Rubens & Garrett, 1991), unawareness of cognitive deficits (Anderson & Tranel, 1989; Wagner & Cushman, 1994), and unawareness of disabilities (Prigatano, Altman, & O'Brien, 1990). The prevalence of awareness deficits is significant and has been shown to be a serious obstacle for successful rehabilitation in stroke (Appelros, Karlsson, Seiger, & Nydevik, 2002; Hartman-Maeir, Soroker, & Katz, 2001; Hartman-Maeir, Soroker, Oman, & Katz, 2003; Hartman-Maeir, Soroker, Ring, & Katz, 2002), TBI (Fleming & Strong, 1999; Prigatano, Altman, & O'Brien, 1990; Prigatano et al., 1998; Sherer, Bergloff, Boake, High, & Levin, 1998; Sherer, Bergloff, Levin, et al., 1998; Sherer et al., 2003), and schizophrenia (Amador, Strauss, Yale, & Gorman, 1991; Amador et al., 1994; McEvoy et al., 1996).

Crosson and colleagues (1989) and Barco, Crosson, Bolesta, Werts, and Stout (1991) developed a hierarchy of awareness levels observed in clinical practice. This model, called the *pyramid model of awareness,* describes a three-level hierarchy of awareness. Intellectual awareness is situated at the base of the hierarchy and denotes the knowledge of deficits subdivided into the following areas: basic knowledge pertaining to the existence of a deficit and knowledge of the functional implications of this deficit. At times, problems can be related to either component. For example, a client with intact intellectual awareness after brain injury involving a memory deficit acknowledges that he or she has a memory problem that interferes with shopping tasks. Another client may be unaware of memory loss or may be aware of memory problems but not of their functional implications and the need to overcome them.

The authors further described two additional higher levels, called *emergent awareness* and *anticipatory awareness,* that function to detect errors in performance, to anticipate problems, and to plan strategies for compensation. However, these two levels are in essence part of the executive functions. *Intellectual awareness* is the knowledge about deficits and how to compensate for them, and emergent and anticipatory awareness relate to the actual doing (i.e., planning and regulating performance). Thus, the use of the term awareness by Barco and colleagues (1991) combines the metacognitive aspects of knowledge and monitoring (awareness) and control (executive process and functions; Jarman et al., 1995) and appears not to be exclusively limited to awareness.

Models and Underlying Mechanisms

Toglia and Kirk (2000) developed a model of awareness for neurological rehabilitation that is based on the pyramid model but challenges the hierarchical relationship between the levels and proposes a dynamic process instead. They conceptualized two major components of awareness: *metacognitive knowledge* that exists prior to a task or situation (analogous to intellectual awareness) and *on-line awareness,* which includes self-monitoring and self-regulation processes that are activated within tasks and situations (analogous to anticipatory and emergent awareness). The model also accounts for additional influences on awareness, such as cognitive deficits, beliefs, affective states, task characteristics, and motivation. This model, like the pyramid model, essentially includes more than awareness as a knowledge factor and contains the second factor of metacognitive process as well. Thus, the literature on awareness in rehabilitation at times incorporates aspects of executive functions in their definitions and conceptualization of this construct.

The two main theoretical perspectives on unawareness address an essential neurological versus psychological origin of this deficit. The theories that emphasize the neurological underpinnings of unawareness propose that unawareness is a direct consequence of brain damage (Heilman, Barrett, & Adair, 1998). These theories hypothesize that unawareness is related to a breakdown of components in the neurological monitoring system and emphasize the role of various components of this system, such as feedback, feedforward, and comparative mechanisms.

The *discovery theory* (Cochini, Beschin, & Della Sala, 2002; Levine, 1990) claims that acquired deficits after brain injury are not immediately apparent to the individual but, rather, must be discovered by observation and inference. The discovery is dependent on intact sensory and attentional processes that provide feedback of deficits and on intellectual abilities that enable the integration of

this feedback. This theory does not link unawareness with a discrete neuroanatomical lesion location; however, it is associated with large, right-hemisphere lesions and concomitant left-hemisphere atrophy. There may be several clinical implications to the discovery theory: If the client with unawareness has sensory or attentional deficits, then the discovery process can be facilitated by compensations for these deficits in feedback mechanisms. For example, in the case of anosognosia for hemiplegia plus tactile and proprioceptive loss, the use of visual feedback (e.g., mirrors, videotape) can assist in providing accurate feedback about paralysis, and controlling for the density and display of stimuli can minimize the effect of the attention deficit. On the other hand, this theory suggests that the presence of coexisting cognitive deficits in the areas of reasoning and memory make it very difficult to enable any new discovery. These cognitive deficits prevent the client from understanding the cause-and-effect process and from updating preexisting personal schema. Therefore, these clients may not be able to benefit from a direct treatment for awareness and require functional–procedural training, bypassing unawareness (Sohlberg, Mateer, Penkman, Glang, & Todis, 1998).

The *feedforward theory* was presented to explain anosognosia for hemiplegia, and it emphasizes the role of the feedforward intentional component whereby a lack of intention prevents the setting of the monitor; hence, there is no detection of a mismatch between intention and failure, and awareness is precluded (Heilman, 1991; Heilman et al., 1998). The theory associates unawareness with damage to the motor–intentional system in dorsolateral and medial frontal lobe, inferior parietal lobe, thalamus, and basal ganglia. Furthermore, it is suggested that there is a right-hemisphere dominance for intentional systems manifested in bilateral control of the right hemisphere and unilateral control of the left one. The clinical implications of this theory suggest that clients do not become aware of deficits if they do not initiate activities that enable them to compare performance with expectations. Hence, an appropriate intervention method would focus on providing the framework of activities that would enable the required exploration and discovery. This was demonstrated in the research of Tham, Ginsburg, Fisher, and Tegner (2001) focusing on improving awareness of disabilities in individuals with right-hemisphere stroke and unilateral spatial neglect. The intervention program successfully used meaningful and purposeful occupations as therapeutic change agents in an in-depth qualitative stud .

The *model for impaired self-awareness* presented by Prigatano (1991, 1999) attempts to account for various types of unawareness depending on the location of the lesion. According to this model, awareness is localized in Mesulam's *heteromodal cortex* (Mesulam, 1985), which responds to multiple modalities and is responsible for integration of external feedback with internal signals received from the limbic areas. This localization coincides with the definition of awareness as involving an integration of thoughts and feelings. Within this model, individuals could have frontal, parietal, temporal, or occipital heteromodal disorders of self-awareness with different clinical manifestations and severity classified as complete or partial unawareness syndrome. For example, frontal damage could manifest itself in impaired awareness for planning or interpersonal deficits, parietal damage in impaired awareness for hemiplegia or unilateral inattention, temporal damage in impaired awareness for memory deficits or auditory perception, and occipital damage in impaired awareness for visual deficits. Regarding the severity of unawareness, complete unawareness syndrome is associated with bilateral damage to both hemispheres and manifested in early stages postinjury, and partial unawareness syndrome is associated with unilateral damage and a later stage in the recovery process, whereby psychological coping mechanisms may begin to come into play.

Prigatano's model is useful for understanding the implications of different lesions to unawareness and their specific manifestations and severity at different stages of the recovery process. Although this model focused on the neurological origins of unawareness, it emphasized that, in partial unawareness syndromes, psychological coping mechanisms come into play. On the other hand, the "purely" psychological perspective on unawareness (Lewis, 1991; Prigatano & Weinstein, 1996; Weinstein, 1991) asserted that the various forms of unawareness are a result of psychologically motivated denial, a coping mechanism created to protect the individual from a painful reality. According to this hypothesis, unawareness is conceptualized as a psychological phenomenon and the neurological damage as the specific circumstance under which the denial is elicited but unrelated to the essence of the mechanism. Despite the protective basis of this denial, Weinstein acknowledged that it has adaptive (protects from pain) and maladaptive (prevents acquisition of effective coping skills and limits functional participation) properties. The implications of this theory for treatment are that awareness training be conducted in the context of a nonthreatening, trusting, and safe environment and should be coupled with the provision of coping strategies that empower the client and reduce the need for denial. The issue of neurogenic versus psychogenic origin of unawareness may not be a dichotomous one, and both factors may contribute ei-

ther simultaneously or at different stages of the recovery process (Katz, Fleming, Keren, Lightbody, & Hartman-Maeir, 2002; Kortte, Wegener, & Chwalisz, 2003; Prigatano, 1999; Prigatano & Klonoff, 1998).

The above-proposed underlying mechanisms of unawareness are taken from the research on individuals with stroke and TBI. The research on clients with schizophrenia also has attempted to understand awareness deficits in this population, using the term *unawareness* as well as *impaired insight* to describe this issue. Unawareness is a central issue in schizophrenia and is included in the *Diagnostic and Statistical Manual of Mental Disorders* (4th ed., text rev.; *DSM–TR*): "A majority of individuals with schizophrenia have poor insight regarding the fact that they have a psychotic illness. Evidence suggests that poor insight is a manifestation of the illness itself rather than a coping strategy" (American Psychiatric Association, 2000, p. 304). Insight in schizophrenia is defined as a multidimensional concept that includes (a) awareness of mental disorder, (b) awareness of the social consequences of the disorder, (c) awareness of the need for treatment, (d) awareness of symptoms of disorder, and (e) attribution of symptoms to disorder (Amador & David, 1998).

The majority of the research on the theoretical origins of unawareness in schizophrenia has addressed the relationship of unawareness with disease symptomatology and with neuropsychological impairment. In a meta-analysis of this research, Mintz, Dobson, and Romney (2003) concluded that a small negative relationship exists between insight and global, positive and negative symptoms, implying that unawareness is associated with severity of disease. In recent studies it has been shown that different aspects of unawareness correlate with different symptom factors (Sevy, Nathanson, Visweswaraiah, & Amador, 2004) and that impaired insight in first-episode psychosis is associated with deficits in multiple cognitive domains (Keshevan, Rabinowitz, DeSmedt, Harvey, & Schooler, in press). In addition, researchers are acknowledging the multidimensional theoretical underpinnings of unawareness in schizophrenia, suggesting that, in some patients, unawareness may be accounted for by biological processes linked to the disease, whereas in others, unawareness may stem from psychological coping styles (Lysaker, Lancaster, Davis, & Clements, 2003). For a further discussion of unawareness in schizophrenia, see Chapter 6.

The literature on awareness in individuals with dementia documents a wide range of unawareness manifestations relating to disease, cognitive and behavioral symptoms, and their impact on daily living, supporting the complexity and heterogeneity of this issue in dementia as well other populations (Gil et al., 2001; Phiney, Wallhagen, & Sands, 2002). In early stages of dementia, most individuals acknowledge the presence of cognitive symptoms but not their functional consequences (Derouesne et al., 1999; Duke, Seltzer, Seltzer, & Vasterling, 2002).The presence of unawareness in dementia can result in delayed diagnosis, failure to get help, conflict with caregivers, and safety hazards (e.g., driving; Derouesne et al., 1999; Wild & Cotrell, 2003). Several researchers emphasized the biological origin of unawareness in dementia and have shown a relation of unawareness to disease severity (Migliorelli et al., 1995) and brain pathology such as hyperfusion of right frontal regions (Derouesne et al., 1999). However, others have stressed the central role of psychosocial factors, particularly in early-stage dementia, that underlie unawareness symptoms such as minimization and normalization (Clare, 2003). A recent approach acknowledges the complexity in awareness phenomena and advocates for an in-depth evaluation and subsequent treatment approach tailored to the specific awareness profile of clients with dementia (Phiney, Wallhagan, & Sands, 2002). For further discussion of unawareness in dementia, see Chapter 14.

In sum, unawareness is a complex phenomenon of multiple levels relating to disease and injury, symptoms, and their consequences. The origins of unawareness may be neurogenic, directly related to disease mechanisms, or psychogenic, related to coping mechanisms. Unawareness has been shown to be present in high percentages of individuals following stroke, TBI, schizophrenia, and dementia and has been shown an indicator of poor treatment outcome. Thus, unawareness has been placed in the realm of rehabilitation, and efforts to understand its underlying mechanisms are being conducted that will guide intervention in the future.

EXECUTIVE FUNCTIONS

Definitions

Godefroy (2003) recently defined *executive functions* as "high-order functions in non-routine situations such as novel, conflicting, or complex tasks" (p. 1). Elliot (2003) defined them as those "involved in complex cognitions, such as solving novel problems, modifying behavior in light of new information, generating strategies, or sequencing complex actions" (p. 50). Coordination, control, and goal orientation—including planning, shifting, and regulation—are fundamental to executive functions. Stuss (1992) originally defined the major role of execu-

tive functions as the conscious direction of behavior toward a selected goal. Similarly, Duncan (1995) emphasized the process of goal selection and adherence to goals in control of behavior in novel complex situations mediated by the frontal lobes.

Lezak (1995) adopted a broader and more comprehensive perspective, defining executive functions as those capacities inherent in directed, effective activity, including (a) volition, incorporating self-awareness, initiation, and motivation; (b) planning, comprising identification and organization of steps and elements needed to carry out the goal; requiring capacity for sustained attention, impulse control, reasonable intact memory; and being able to conceive of alternatives (flexibility) and choose among options (decision making); (c) purposive action, comprising self-regulation, namely the translation of an intention or plan into action requiring initiating, maintaining, switching, and stopping a sequence of action; and (d) effective performance and the ability to monitor, self-correct, and regulate the intensity, tempo, and other qualitative aspects of performance (Lezak, 1995). Finally, Ylvisaker, Szekeres, and Feneey (1998) suggested an operational definition of the executive functions on the basis of a clinical everyday perspective consisting of seven components: (a) self-awareness, (b) goal selection, (c) planning steps to achieve goals, (d) initiation of behavior toward implementing a plan, (e) inhibition of behavior that would interfere with goal achievement, (f) monitoring and evaluating performance in relation to the goals, and (g) strategic problem solving in the face of obstacles. It can be seen that, in both definitions, self-awareness is included as the first component, emphasizing the interconnections of both higher cognitive functions.

Traditionally, the term *frontal lobe function* was equated with executive function because of findings associating executive impairments in individuals with frontal-lobe pathology. However, today there is a preference to functional definitions such as executive functions or dysexecutive syndrome over anatomical definitions of frontal functions or frontal syndrome due to the multiple brain regions that have been implicated in these processes, including areas outside of the frontal lobes (Baddeley, 1996).

Theories, Models, and Neuroanatomical Network

Two major conceptualizations concerning the cognitive mechanisms of the executive functions have evolved following Luria's (1966) original approach of three functional brain systems distinguishing between controlled behavior manifested in novel complex tasks versus routine behavior in familiar tasks: (a) the supervisory attentional system (Norman & Shallice, 1986; Shallice & Burgess, 1991) and (b) the working memory model (Baddeley, 1996), which were proposed to explain the mechanisms of the executive functions. These two theories generated experimental paradigms and instruments for testing their theoretical contentions and bear significant influence on the rehabilitation literature.

The model developed by Norman and Shallice (1986) accounts for two types of control-to-action mechanisms. They suggested that lower levels of control are achieved by the contention programmer system, which responds to routine situations, supported by subcortical areas. However, a higher level of control is necessary to cope with planning, decision making, error correction, novel or difficult situations, and overcoming habitual responses. They propose the existence of the supervisory attentional system in the prefrontal lobes, which is a high-level attention mechanism to cope with these situations whose main function is inhibition, planning, and problem solving. This model generated the operational concept of *multitasking* that led to the development of ecological perspectives that capture this theoretical understanding of the executive functions (Alderman, Burgess, Knight, & Henman, 2003; Burgess, 2000; Burgess, Veitch, Lacy-Costello, & Schallice, 2000; Knight, Alderman, & Burgess, 2002; Shallice & Burgess, 1991).

The second theory advanced by Baddeley (1996) is the working memory model. *Working memory* is defined as storage and manipulation of incoming information on the basis of selective and divided attention. Working memory includes an attentional control system, the central executive (CE) that coordinates the operation of two slave systems, the phonological loop and the visuospatial scratchpad. CE is involved in reasoning, decision making, comprehension, and long- and short-term memory (Baddeley, Dela Salla, Papagno, & Spinnler, 1997). Intact function of the CE enables coordination between simultaneous tasks of the two slave systems operationalized in a dual-task paradigm. CE may be impaired following frontal lesions, but also may be impaired without frontal-lobe damage (Baddeley et al., 1997). Therefore, Baddeley argued against identification of CE exclusively with frontal-lobe damage and forwarded the functional definition of dysexecutive syndrome, not necessarily only following frontal lesions.

Hence, the argument is raised whether there is a central executive, or is there a need for a more multicomponent interpretation? This latter approach is suggested by

Stuss and Alexander (2000), who argued that the frontal lobes are responsible for differentiated processes under the concept of control functions. According to Stuss and Alexander, the executive mediation level is predominantly localized to ventrolateral and dorsolateral frontal regions. However, they and others argue for diversity of the frontal-lobe functions compared with a unified function as a supervisory system.

An alternative hypothesis is suggested by several authors "that executive functions are sustained by a distributed cortical neural network (prefrontal cortex and frontal–striatal structures; Andres, 2003; Burgess, 2000; Burgess & Shallice, 1996; Elliot, 2003; Royall et al., 2002; Stuss, 1992; Stuss & Alexander, 2000; Stuss & Levine, 2002). This idea of a diffuse neural network is particularly relevant in cases like Alzheimer's disease or schizophrenia in which no direct frontal damage is recorded. This suggests a functional as well as an anatomical connectivity between frontal cortex and striatum exemplified by basal ganglia disorders such as Parkinson's disease (Elliot, 2003). Executive functions depend not on prefrontal cortex in isolation but on corticostriatal circuitry mediated by dopaminergic neurotransmission (Elliot, 2003, p. 51). A network model also has implications to the processes of recovery and reorganization shown by functional imaging studies using PET and fMRI (Elliot, 2003; Royall et al., 2002). It also may explain the variety of patient populations that show executive dysfunctions. Sylvester and colleagues (2003) studied the issue of single versus multiple executive processes using fMRI looking at switching attention and resolving interference. They found multiple brain regions (such as bilateral parietal cortex and left dorsolateral prefrontal cortex) working across both tasks, and also some special regions for each task. Similarly, they concluded that separate cognitive processes in different brain regions underlie executive control.

Deficits in executive functions have been demonstrated in clients with TBI and stroke. These deficits have major ramifications for rehabilitation and everyday functioning of patients following TBI as demonstrated by numerous case examples and small group studies (Fortin, Godbout, & Braun, 2003; Levine et al., 2000; Manly, Hawkins, Evans, Woldt, & Robertson, 2002; Pachalska, Kurzbauer, Talar, & MacQueen, 2002; Sohlberg & Mateer, 2001b). Patients with ischemic stroke show high prevalence of executive dysfunctions, especially if lesions affect also the frontal–subcortical circuits (Vataja, Pohjasvaara, Mantyla, Ylikoski, Leppavuari, Leskala, et al., 2003). In a large study of 256 patients it was found that executive dysfunctions were prevalent in about 40% of patients 3 to

4 months post–ischemic stroke (Pohjasvaara, Leskela, Vataja, Kalska, Ylikoski, Hietanen, et al., 2002); these patients were also older, had lower education, and did worse on activities of daily living (ADL) and instrumental activities of daily living (IADL) tasks.

The study of executive functions has expanded extensively regarding additional populations in recent years. Executive deficits also have been demonstrated in different types of dementia (Binetti et al., 1996; Brugger, Monsch, Salmon, & Butters, 1996; Royall, Cordes, & Polk, 1998; Royall, Mahurin, & Gray, 1992; Swanberg, Tractenberg, Mohs, Thal, & Cummings, 2004), Parkinson's disease (Hanes, Andrews, Smith, & Pantelis, 1996; Pantelis et al., 1997), and schizophrenia (Elliot, 2003; Hutton et al., 1998; Pantelis et al., 1997, 1999; Stratta et al., 2003; Zakzanis & Heinrichs, 1999; Zalla, Joyce, Szoke, Schurhoff, Pillon, Komano, et al., 2004).

The relationship between executive dysfunctions and daily activity and self-care has been demonstrated in the population with Alzheimer's disease by Baum (1995). Her research acknowledges the major role that executive functions play in activity and self-care of elderly people afflicted with this disease and highlights the need to train caregivers in the accommodation of executive deficits to sustain higher levels of activity. (For further discussion, see Chapter 14.) Similarly, in schizophrenia, executive deficits have been shown to have significant relationships with functional outcomes (Green, Kern, Braff, & Mintz, 2000; Simon, Giacomini, Ferrero, & Mohr, 2003). (For further discussion, see Chapter 6.)

In sum, an increasing focus on the executive functions has led to clearer definitions and agreement on its central contribution in novel and complex task performance. Executive dysfunction is theoretically associated with damage and dysfunction to prefrontal regions but also is implicated in subcortical networks; therefore, the dysexecutive syndrome is prevalent in many populations with neurological involvement and has a negative impact on rehabilitation outcome. Hence, assessing and treating executive deficits is of primary concern to the rehabilitation professions.

ASSESSMENT

Awareness

Awareness assessment presents a unique challenge in that it is very difficult to measure directly and objectively and, therefore, awareness must be inferred. The most widely used method for measuring awareness is comparing the client's verbal report or rating of his or her illness,

deficits, or disabilities with a measure considered "more objective," such as therapist and caregiver ratings or test scores (e.g., cognitive, neurological). The discrepancies between the client's report and the "objective" measure represent the operational definition of unawareness, with larger discrepancies signifying more severe unawareness and overestimation of abilities.

The various interviews and questionnaires listed in Table 1.1 are examples of this method used in different population groups. Typically, the client is asked a series of questions probing his or her perception of his or her condition pertaining to the illness or injury and related deficits (e.g., motor, sensory, cognitive, or emotional) and difficulties encountered in daily living. Some measures address primarily the deficit level (e.g., Anosognosia Rating Scale, Awareness Interview [AI]), whereas others are more comprehensive, addressing both deficit and disability level (e.g., Self-Awareness of Deficit Interview [SADI], Prigatano Competency Rating Scale [PCRS], and Scale to Assess Unawareness of Mental Disorders [SUMD]). This method can be used with any functional rating scale by asking the clients to rate themselves in addition to the therapist's rating, as has been demonstrated in studies on awareness in dementia using the Physical Self-Maintenance Scale (DeBettignies, Mahurin, & Pirozzolo, 1990) and awareness in stroke using the Functional Independence Measure (Hartman-Maeir, Soroker, Oman, & Katz, 2003). Thus, a preliminary awareness assessment can easily be incorporated with the functional measures that are used in any setting by including the client's perspective.

The issue of the comparative "objective" criteria is not consistent between measures using this method. Some measures specifically delineate the objective criteria by providing parallel forms for therapist or caregiver (e.g., PCRS, Awareness Questionnaire), whereas others provide more general guidelines such as compare with information gathered from charts, family members, and so forth (e.g., SADI), or compare with neuropsychological tests, without specification (e.g., AI). The provision of specified, standard, comparative criteria contribute to the reliability of the assessment and, when not present, reliability between raters may be lower and may hinder comparisons between settings or studies. On the other hand, when the criteria are not specified, the therapist may gather information from multiple sources, which are potentially more valid than one specified criteria, such as caregiver rating.

A different method of assessment is linked to measurement of performance, in which clients are asked to predict their ability before performance or estimate their actual performance following completion of a specific task. The

TABLE 1.1. Assessment of Awareness

Instrument	Content (Awareness Component)	Scoring Method	Psychometric Data	Population	Reference
Rating Scales					
Anosognosia Rating Scale	Probing of awareness of motor and visual impairment	4-point scale from *0* (spontaneous report of deficit) to *3* (no acknowledgment of deficit)		Stroke	(Bisiach et al., 1986; Starkstein et al., 1992)
Awareness Interview	8 questions relating to presence and severity of disease, motor, and cognitive impairments	Awareness index: Sum of discrepancies between client response and test scores (each comparison rated on a 3-point scale: aware, mild unawareness, severe unawareness)	Interrater reliability, *r* = .92; significantly predicts functional outcomes at discharge from rehabilitation hospital	Stroke, Dementia, TBI	Anderson & Tranel, 1989; Hartman-Maeir et al., 2002; Labuda & Lichtenberg, 1999; Wagner & Cushman, 1994
Self-Awareness of Deficits Interview	Awareness of deficits, awareness of disabilities, and ability to set realistic goals	Each of the 3 awareness areas is scored on a 4-point scale (0–3); total awareness score (0–9)	Interrater ICC, *r* = .82; construct validity among groups using cluster analysis; prediction of outcomes 12 months post-TBI	TBI	Fleming and Strong, 1999; Fleming et al., 1996, 1998
Assessment of Awareness of Disabilities	Awareness of general, motor, and process aspects of performance of IADL task (from the Assessment of Motor and Process Skills)	5-point scale (0–4) that is rated based on comparing client's response with actual performance	Rasch model analysis showed acceptable reliability and validity	Stroke	Tham et al., 1999, 2001
Awareness Questionnaire	17 items assessing motor, sensory, cognitive, behavioral, affective; current functioning compared with pre-injury functional level	3 forms for client, clinician, and significant other; each item rated on a 5-point scale (*1* much worse, *5* much better) total score (range 17–85); awareness score: discrepancy between client and clinician or caregiver rating	Factor analysis identified 3 subscales: Motor–Sensory, Cognition, Behavioral–Affective prediction of functional outcome at discharge and employment status post-discharge	TBI	Sherer et al., 1998a, 1998b, 2003
Prigatano Competency Rating Scale	30 questions related to cognitive, physical, emotional, and social difficulties in daily activities	2 forms for client and relative; each item rated on a 5-point scale (*1* cannot do, *5* can do with ease); awareness score discrepancy between client and caregiver	Internal consistency of subscales ADL, Interpersonal–Social, Cognitive–Emotional; test–retest reliability within 1 week, *r* = .92–.97; extensive validity studies differentiating between groups with TBI, stroke, and control participants	TBI, Stroke	Prigatano, 1986; Prigatano et al., 1997, 1998
Impaired Self-Awareness (ISA) and Denial of Disability (DD) Clinicians Rating Scale	Differentiates between ISA of neurological origin and DD of psychological origin	10 items: yes–no; if yes, 1–10-point scale for severity (range 0–100)	Interrater reliability (no significant difference between raters); validity: ISA and DD scales correlated with different coping strategies in TBI	TBI	Kortte et al., 2003; Prigatano & Klonoff, 1998

(continued)

TABLE 1.1. Assessment of Awareness (*Continued*)

Instrument	Content (Awareness Component)	Scoring Method	Psychometric Data	Population	Reference
Scale to Assess Unawareness of Mental Disorder (SUMD)	Multidimensional scale, consists of 3 general items. Awareness of mental disorder, effects of medication, social consequences, and 14 specific symptoms (e.g. hallucinations, thought disorder). The symptoms are rated on 4 subscales: Awareness of Symptoms, Attribution of Symptoms to Mental Disorder, Past and Present	Scoring based on direct interview of client. Each item is rated on a 5-point scale (*1* aware, *5* unaware); the general items used for all clients with mental disorder and symptom items are rated based on the specific profile of each client (i.e., only symptoms that are clearly present are rated)	Interrater reliability correlations ranged from 0.56–0.98; convergent validity with other global measures of insight and significantly correlated with poorer compliance and course of illness	Schizophrenia, Mood Disorders	Amador et al., 1993, 1994; Dell'Osso et al., 2002
Beck Cognitive Insight Scale	Insight for distorted beliefs and misinterpretations, characteristic of psychotic states; clients rate their degree of agreement on 15 statements, which are divided into two subscales of Self-Reflectiveness (9 items) and Self-Certainty (6 items)	Self-report; 4-point scale for each item (*0* agree, *3* do not agree at all). Sub-scale scores comprise sum of ratings on individual items; composite score calculated by subtracting Self-Certainty from Self-Reflectiveness	Factor analysis confirmed two components; internal consistency of subscales 0.68, 0.60; convergent validity of Self-Reflectiveness subscale and composite score with SUMD; Self-Certainty subscale differentiated between depressed individuals with and without psychosis	Schizophrenia, Mood Disorders	Beck et al., 2004; Pedrelli et al., in press
Anosognosia Questionnaire–Dementia	30 questions on cognitive, emotional, and behavioral functioning	4-point scale; two forms for client with dementia and caregiver; awareness score discrepancy between client and caregiver rating	Test–retest reliability, $r = .90$ for client and care-giver; internal consistency, $\alpha = .91$; convergent validity with clinical judgment of awareness	Dementia	Migliorelli et al., 1995; Phinney et al., 2002

Performance-Based Measures: Online Awareness

Instrument	Content (Awareness Component)	Scoring Method	Psychometric Data	Population	Reference
Implicit Measure of Anosognosia for Hemiplegia	Clients with hemiplegia are required to choose between unimanual (e.g., stacking blocks) and bimanual tasks (e.g., zipping a zipper)	The number of correct choices (unimanual tasks) rated as implicit awareness	Implicit awareness was dissociated from explicit awareness measures (e.g., interview); significant predictor of safety at discharge from rehabilitation (Hartman-Maeir et al., 2001)	Stroke	Ramachandran, 1995; Ramachandran & Rogers-Ramachandran 1996
Awareness of errors in naturalistic action	Measures online awareness of errors (error detection and correction) during performance of the Multiple Level Action Test, including everyday tasks such as toast preparation and gift wrapping	Videotape analysis: Each error coded from 1–3—*1* corrected, *2* uncorrected but aware, *3* uncorrected and unaware; "Percent Aware" calculated by dividing the first two categories by the total number of errors	Interrater reliability, Cohen's $\kappa = 0.85$; awareness of errors significantly differentiated clients with neurological dysfunction from controls, was dissociated from explicit awareness measures (e.g., interview)	TBI, Dementia	Hart et al., 1998; Giovannetti et al., 2002

Note. TBI = traumatic brain injury; ICC = intraclass correlation; IADL = instrumental activities of daily living; ADL = activities of daily living.

TABLE 1.2. Assessment of Executive Functions (*Continued*)

Instrument	Content (EF Component)	Scoring Method	Psychometric Data	Population	Reference
Multiple Errands Test (MET)	The original task: 2 versions based on it				Shallice & Burgess, 1991
1. MET–SV simplified 2. MET–HV hospital	A multitask that has specific rules and a time frame, scored on inefficiencies, rule breaks, interpretation failure, task failures, total errors, and strategies used; a 10-point scale individual rating how well done the task, after exercise finished	1. Conducted in a shopping mall 2. Conducted in a large hospital	High interrater reliability, .81–1.00; internal consistency, .77; validity: Significant difference between brain-injured and control participants for both versions	Brain Injury	Alderman et al., 2003; Knight et al., 2002
Rating Scales					
Dysexecutive Questionnaire (DEX)	Questions related to difficulties experienced in everyday life associated with the dysexecutive syndrome; 2 versions for the subject and the carer–relative	20 questions scored on a 5-point scale (0–4)	Exploratory factor analysis showed 3 factors: Behavioral, Cogni-, tive and Emotional components; moderate significant correlations of the Behavioral factor with all BADS subtest; Cognitive factor with some and the profile score with all factors	Brain Injury, Schizophrenia Control participants	Wilson et al., 1996, 1998
Profile of Executive Control System	Observation on 7 components: goal selection, planning and sequencing, initiation, execution, time sense, awareness, and self-monitoring	Each component scored on a 7-point scale	Interrater reliability; weighted κ range .60–.90	Brain Injury	Braswell et al., 1993

Note. MS = multiple sclerosis; ADHD = attention-deficit/hyperactivity disorder; EF = executive function.

with a target destination, solving a physical–mechanical problem, or being able to move between task requirements within certain rules and time constraints (Modified Six Elements Test). The scoring comprises raw scores for each subtest and a profile score. The instrument underwent substantial research and is used in various countries and with different diagnostic groups such as TBI, schizophrenia, multiple sclerosis, and more (Evans, Chua, McKenna, & Wilson, 1997; Clark & O'Carroll, 1998; Norris & Tate, 2000; Wilson, Evans, Alderman, Burgess, & Emslie, 1997; Wilson, Evans, Emslie, Alderman, & Burgess, 1998).

An additional brief test, the Strategy Application Task (SAT; Levine et al., 1998), is based on the same concept as the Six Elements Test (Shallice & Burgess, 1991), using three paper-and-pencil exercises that require shifting between tasks within certain rules and in a 5-min time frame. Using the preferred strategy, adhering to the rules, and having the goal and time constraints in mind are abil-

ities considered important for multitasking and executive functions. The test was further studied and validated by Birnboim (2004), who showed significant differences between diagnostic groups.

Functional Tasks

The use of functional tasks is the preferred method of evaluation, as they have inherent ecological validity. The Woodrow Wilson Route-Finding Task (Boyd & Sautter, 1993; Sohlberg & Mateer, 2001c) is an open-ended performance task designed to assess executive functions in a relevant, real-world problem-solving activity of finding a destination (e.g., an office in a hospital, a class in a school). The task includes general instructions and hierarchical cueing procedures. Performance is scored according to a 4-point scale addressing areas of task comprehension, information seeking, direction retention, error detection, and on-task behavior. In addition, an overall total independent score is given, and a checklist of potentially contributing problems (in the emotional, interpersonal, communication, perceptual, and motoric domains) is suggested. Reliability and validity are high.

The Kitchen Task Assessment (KTA; Baum, 1995; Baum & Edwards, 1993) is a functional cooking task designed to measure executive function components. Initiation, organization, performance of all steps, sequencing, judgment, safety, and completion are scored on the following 4-point scale: independent, required verbal cues, required physical assistance, and not capable at all. Reliability and validity were established in people with dementia. However, the one cooking task of the KTA was not appropriate for all individuals; thus, the authors developed the Executive Function Performance Test (EFPT) that includes four tasks (cooking, phone use, taking medication, and paying bills). The same system of cuing is used, and a total score can be obtained over all tasks and executive function components. In a study with patients with schizophrenia (Katz et al., 2002) the EFPT was found to differentiate between stages of schizophrenia illness, as well as correlate significantly with the BADS scores and with the ADL and extended ADL functional status.

A more complex everyday IADL task, the Multiple Errands Test (MET), requiring multitasking was developed originally by Shallice and Burgess (1991) and further elaborated into two versions: the MET–HV hospital version (Knight et al., 2002) and MET–SV simplified version (Alderman et al, 2003). The MET was studied with clients following brain injury and was found to be reliable and valid (see Table 1.2). The MET requires higher-level functioning, and as such it provides a way to evaluate those individuals who have no problems in standard tests and in relatively simple and familiar tasks such as those in the EFPT, for example, but have difficulties in complex multitask situations with time constraints.

Rating Scales

Rating scales are based on self-report or proxy report such as the Dysexecutive Questionnaire (DEX; Wilson et al., 1996) or based on interview and clinical observation such as the Profile of Executive Control System (PRO-EX; Braswell et al., 1993). The DEX was developed with the BADS but also can be used independently. The DEX comprises 20 questions related to the frequency of executive dysfunction behaviors in everyday life (e.g., "I have trouble making decisions or deciding what I want to do"). It has two versions of self and relative, and as such it can

be used also as a measure of awareness, using the method of discrepancy between the person and a caregiver. The PRO-EX is unique in that it provides therapists with a detailed observational guide for rating each executive function component.

In summary, the unique properties of the executive functions require a combination of assessment methods to capture the complexity of this phenomenon. Royall and colleagues (1998) raised this issue when they stated that the problem of defining a "gold standard" to measure executive functions may not be attainable: "We may be searching for a frontal–executive battery, not an executive measure" (p. 381). This extensive report provides a major source for research related to executive functions and their measurement issues. Therefore, it is recommended that evaluators use a battery consisting of a combination of tabletop, functional, and observational measures such as the BADS, the MET, and the PRO-EX or any other combination of measures depending on the client situation and setting.

TREATMENT

Cognitive rehabilitation is traditionally divided into two major approaches. The first, remedial or process oriented, consists of direct retraining or restoration of impaired core areas of cognitive skills (bottom-up). The second, functional or compensatory substitution, teaches clients to use their assets to achieve successful performance despite the presence of underlying cognitive deficits (top-down) or suggests environmental modifications that will maximize participation (Mateer, 1999; Sohlberg & Mateer, 2001b). Some examples of both approaches are presented in the next section, which is divided into treatment of awareness deficits and executive dysfunctions, even though in most cases the two are interrelated and interdependent.

Awareness

The goal of the remedial approach for unawareness is to enhance the client's awareness of his or her condition, including the disease or injury and its consequences. Improved awareness is considered a prerequisite for the intensive effort that will be required in the rehabilitation process and for implementation of various strategies that can overcome deficits in a variety of areas. For example, learning to turn one's head to the right to compensate for a right visual field deficit requires the client be fully aware of this deficit and its functional significance in order to have the motivation to implement the strategy successfully in a variety of situations, such as finding food in the pantry and street crossing. On the other hand, the goal of the compensatory approach is to design an effective rehabilitation program that will improve participation in meaningful occupations despite the presence of various degrees of unawareness. For example, putting environmental supports in place will ensure safety during performance.

The remedial treatment of awareness is suitable for individuals with mild to moderate unawareness who have sufficient cognitive capacity to integrate information and experience (Sohlberg, 2000). This treatment targets the underlying mechanisms that may cause unawareness, both neurogenic and psychogenic (described earlier). To address the neurogenic feedback (discovery theory) and feedforward mechanisms that may cause unawareness, interventions are geared mainly toward facilitation of feedback on task performance and the process of integrating information that will enable the discovery of deficits and disabilities (Klonoff, O'Brien, Prigatano, Chiapello, & Cunningham, 1989; Schlund, 1999; Sohlberg, 2000; Tham, Ginsburg, Fisher, & Tegner, 2001). Because increased awareness also may lead to significant and threatening affective responses, it is essential for all interventions to carefully monitor client's emotional reactions.

According to Sohlberg (2000), awareness enhancement programs include educational and experiential approaches. The educational approach provides information regarding the illness or injury and its consequences coupled with active application of the information. The information may be provided verbally; visually with reading materials such as pamphlets, textbooks, and Web sites; or with videotapes, depending on the cognitive abilities of the client. This approach has been studied in adults with brain injury (Chittum, Johnson, Chittum, Guercio, & McMorrow, 1996; Zhou, Chittum, Johnson, Poppen, Guercio, & McMorrow, 1996), successfully using a game format with positive reinforcements for improving intellectual awareness, and in children (Beardmore, Tate, & Liddle, 1999), using one educational session, which did not show a positive effect on improving awareness. The success of the educational method may depend on the number of sessions, the way the information is delivered (e.g., visual or verbal game format), and the amount of information provided each time.

The experiential approach helps clients actually experience changes in their ability in order to increase their awareness, and this is achieved through linking awareness treatment with task performance (Berquist & Jacket, 1993), naturally placing this intervention within occupa-

tional therapy's domain. However, it requires expanding our view of activity to include prediction of performance, estimation of performance, and processing the discrepancies between expected and actual performance. Klonoff and colleagues (1989) described the use of cognitive retraining tasks, initially designed for cognitive remediation as a valuable setting for enhancing awareness. They describe several stages of the process:

1. Choosing appropriate tasks that target deficits such that clients can recognize problems without feeling overwhelmed (e.g., tasks that are not too easy and not too difficult); that allow clients to experience improvement with practice; and that allow the therapist and clients to explore strategies for improving performance once the client's level of performance has reached a plateau
2. Asking clients to analyze the required skills of the targeted task and predict their performance
3. Processing feedback after performance relating to discrepancies between expected and actual performance, the benefits and limitations of strategies they used, the variability in their performance, the degree of cuing they needed to complete the tasks, and the potential impact of residual difficulties on their everyday functioning.

Tham and colleagues (2001) developed an intervention program that emphasized choosing motivating training tasks that clients have a strong interest in performing, engaging the clients in discussion pre- and post-performance related to prediction, estimation, and compensatory strategies. Client's performance was reviewed with videotapes to enhance the feedback process. This program was shown to be effective in a single-subject research design for 4 clients after stroke with unawareness of unilateral neglect.

To address psychogenic denial that may be impeding awareness, one places a strong emphasis on the quality of the therapeutic alliance (Berquist & Jacket, 1993; Lewis, 1991); on choosing nonthreatening tasks and settings that may reduce resistance to awareness such as games and group settings (Chittum, Johnson, Chittum, Guercio, & McMorrow, 1996; Youngjohn & Altman, 1989); on using positive feedback for acknowledgment of problems (Rebman & Hannon, 1995); on facilitating self-discovery, and on coupling discovery of deficits with effective coping strategies (Toglia & Kirk, 2000). These recommendations are all designed to provide optimal conditions that facilitate recognition of problems and reduce the need for denial.

The compensatory approach for unawareness is suitable for rehabilitation of individuals with severe unawareness or severe cognitive deficits that are not able to benefit from direct awareness training. Beiman-Copland and Dywan (2000) argued against direct awareness training, claiming that the neurogenic mechanism of anosognosia is not amenable to change. They described a nonconfrontational approach bypassing unawareness, using behavioral methods to change maladaptive behavior in a case study of a young woman with severe TBI. Similarly, Flaharty and Wallat (1997) recommended modifying the physical and human environment of clients with severe anosognosia by adopting a nonconfrontational approach. The authors demonstrated with two case studies the use of environmental adaptations for improving safety and modifying caregiver interactions with clients for enabling them to improve performance in their natural context. Sohlberg and colleagues (Sohlberg, 2000; Sohlberg, Mateer, Penkman, Glang & Todis, 1998) further elaborated with the Procedural Training and Environmental Support (PTES) program, including functional training of tasks and routines and caregiver guidance concerning expectations from the client, achieving functional gains in spite of the presence of unawareness. The compensatory approach described by Crosson and colleagues (1989) and Barco and colleagues (1991) asserts that compensation is not uniform, but, rather, that different types of compensation (external, situational, and anticipatory) should be used depending on the highest level of awareness that the client demonstrates (based on the hierarchical model of awareness levels, described earlier).

In sum, recent advances in the literature on treatment of unawareness in neurological populations provide a variety of methods, guidelines, and techniques for managing awareness deficits. The choice of the treatment approach should be determined by the individual profile (sensory, cognitive, and emotional) of each client. Because unawareness is a major obstacle to the progress of therapy, it should be addressed in the initial stages of the rehabilitation process. Research on intervention provides preliminary support for the effectiveness of awareness intervention. Further studies are needed to establish the efficacy of different approaches and determine criteria for matching treatment methods with client characteristics.

Executive Functions

The main principle in the remediation of executive functions is to provide the person with opportunities for choice and selection, planning, and self-correction. The treatment goal is to attain independent problem solving (Lezak, 1995). Typically, remediation involves presenting the client with unfamiliar, unstructured open problems. In these situations the client is required to think of a plan of action, initiate it, implement it, and examine and regulate his or her own performance. Task demands should be graded according to the degree of structure and amount of feedback provided in order to enable gradual improvement (Sohlberg, Mateer, & Stuss, 1993). On the other hand, the main principles in the compensation of executive functions entail providing external support or strategies that enable performance of daily activities (Ylvisaker, Jacobs, & Feeney, 2003; Ylvisaker, Szekeres, & Feneey, 1998).

Sohlberg and Mateer (2001b) outlined four general management approaches on a continuum of functional to process specific:

1. *Environmental management* is a compensation method comprising two general categories: (a) organization of the physical space such as posting schedules to help with time management or reminders and pagers to help initiate activities and (b) manipulation of physiological factors such as nutrition, medication, and so forth, which assist in regulation of arousal and alertness, as is also demonstrated by the Auditory Alert method described below (Manly et al., 2002).
2. In *teaching task-specific routines,* certain behaviors are targeted that are adaptive for a specific setting; these are trained with behavioral techniques so they become automatic without a need for planning and self-regulation. (This approach is elaborated extensively by Giles in Chapter 5 of this book).
3. *Training the selection and execution of cognitive plans* is essentially a remedial approach that provides exercises targeting specific executive function components, such as planning or time management, that are expected to generalize to other tasks. Examples of this approach are the Process-Specific Methodology (PSM; Delahunty, Morice, & Frost, 1993) and the Brainwave–R module for Executive Functions (Malia, Bewick, Raymond, & Bennett, 1997), reviewed below.
4. *Metacognitve or self-instructional training* focuses on self-regulation of behavior through implementation of strategies. This method is based on Luria's concept that behavior is mediated by inner speech, as shown by Meichenbaum's techniques in developmental psychology, and then used successfully in remediation of acquired attention deficits in adults (Cicerone, 2002). Examples of self-instructional

training include self-talk, in which initially the plan of action is verbalized aloud, then whispered, and finally verbalized internally by the client (Cicerone & Giacino, 1992; Cicerone & Wood, 1987), and Goal Management Training (described in more detail below), in which steps to perform a task are explicitly delineated and practiced (Levine et al., 2000).

Manly and colleagues (2002) used *periodic auditory alerts* to interrupt a current action that patients became overly engaged in. The alert sound serves as a cue reminding the patient to consider his or her overall goal. This treatment triggers an underlying mechanism of alertness to refocus attention to the main goal of the task at hand. Individuals with executive dysfunction may show dissociation between their stated intentions and their actions as well as dissociation between knowledge of what they want to do and what they actually do. Shallice and Burgess (1991) proposed a marker hypothesis: Intentions set up a marker that will be triggered at a later time, interrupting current activity to express that plan. For example, "remembering to post a letter on the way home" would require an executive system to establish a marker that with any luck will interrupt other activity as we pass the postbox and activate the appropriate behavior" (p. 272). Manly and colleagues tested this idea using performance in a secretarial Hotel Task they developed on the basis of the original Six Elements test and the modified version from the BADS (Wilson et al., 1997) with TBI patients. The task included six activities that the individual had to alternate between (e.g., compiling individual bills, looking up telephone numbers). During performance, a short intense sound was heard in uneven intervals, the idea being that the sound interrupts the current activity and triggers returning to the overall goal and the steps to achieve it within a certain time frame. The patient's performance without the alert was significantly worse than the healthy control group. The patient's performance improved significantly with the alert and was not significantly different than the control group under this condition.

A neuropsychological remedial method of treatment called the Process Specific Methodology (PSM) was developed by Delahunty and colleagues (Delahunty, Morice, & Frost, 1993; Delahunty & Morice, 1996). It includes three modules—Cognitive Shift–Flexibility, Working Memory (A and B), and Planning (A and B)—consisting of mostly paper-and-pencil tasks with some construction items (Delahunty & Morice, 1996). Each module is graded in difficulty, and clients are directed to work in that order, providing practice until the person is able to do the task before moving on to the next one. The program was tested mainly with patients with schizophrenia and found to be effective in improving cognitive processing and self-esteem compared with an intensive occupational therapy traditional treatment (Wykes, Reeder, Corner, Williams, & Everitt, 1999); however, no change in symptoms or social functioning was attributed to the therapy.

The Executive Functions Module of the Brainwave–R rehabilitation program (Bewick, Raymond, Malia, & Bennett, 1995; Malia, Bewick, Raymond, & Bennett, 1997) includes exercises in the areas of self-organization, initiation and regulation, planning, strategy development, cognitive flexibility, and time management. Although this program designates the improvement of executive functions, it also explicitly combines metacognitive and awareness-training principles. Each exercise includes the use of comparative rating scales (e.g., therapist–client, prediction, estimation of task performance) to facilitate self-awareness in these areas. Prior to performance the individual is asked prediction questions, writing lists of steps, self-questioning about the nature of the task to accomplish, and speaking out loud (the method of verbal self-instruction mentioned earlier). Exercises range from paper-and-pencil tasks such as maze puzzles, through estimating time of various daily tasks, to planning daily activities. The program was used in a pilot study with 5 patients with schizophrenia in a residential treatment facility (Davalos, Green, & Rial, 2002). Four measures of executive functions were used pre- and posttreatment: Six Elements and Action Program from the BADS, Trail Making Test, and the DEX (see Table 1.2). Participants improved their performance on a composite executive score, showing that, for all participants, a shift occurred toward a normal range of functioning.

Goal management training (GMT) stems from Duncan's (1995) theory that states that the disorganized behavior of patients with frontal-lobe dysfunction can be attributed to impaired construction and use of goal lists. The purpose of goal lists is to impose coherence on behavior by controlling the activation or inhibition of actions that promote or oppose task completion and by selecting new actions when previously attempted actions failed to achieve the goal. Levine and colleagues (2000) developed a structured program comprising a five-stage process:

1. *Stop* (think, "What am I doing?")
2. *Define* (the main task)
3. *List* (the steps)
4. *Learn* (the steps: Encoding and retention of the goals and subgoals—"Do I know the steps?" If "No," go back to stage 3; if "Yes," go ahead [do it])

5. *Check* ("Am I doing what I planned to do?" If "Yes," go on to achieve the next step [subgoal] in stage 3; if "No," go back to stage 1. (Levine et al., Figure 1, p. 300).

Each of these stages corresponds to an important aspect of goal-directed behavior. Essentially it is a process of holding goals in mind, subgoal analysis, and monitoring. In Levine and colleagues' study comparing GMT (*n* = 15) with a Motor Skill Training program (*n* = 15) with TBI patients in the community a few years postinjury, they found improved performance of the GMT group on paper-and-pencil tasks such as proofreading. In a second investigation of GMT, they studied the case of a woman 5 months after an episode of meningoencephalitis. A more elaborate task of meal preparation was used, and GMT was found to be effective in improving performance on this task (Levine et al., 2000). The authors emphasized that the success of the intervention will depend on the level of awareness of the client to his or her problems, as was the case with this woman.

A similar approach is presented by Ylvisaker and colleagues (1998) under the concept of *environmental executive system intervention,* which targets improved everyday routine actions. They present an executive function map with the following steps:

1. *Goal:* What do you want to accomplish?
2. *Plan:* How will I accomplish my goal? (material and steps)
3. *Prediction:* How well will I do?
4. *Do:* What problems can arise? What are the solutions?
5. *Review:* How did I do? In self- and other ratings, what worked and didn't work? What will I try next time? (Figure 12-5, p. 244).

The method of Goal–Plan–Do–Review is suggested for children and adolescents following TBI and attention-deficit/hyperactivity disorder (Ylvisaker & DeBonis, 2000) but can apply to adults as well. The next stage in the treatment process is to discuss with the person the available options if the predicted level was not achieved, such as change the prediction; practice; modify the environment, the task, or the manner in which to perform it; ask for help; and increase the reward for achieving the goal. In this way, awareness is increased as well, which is one of the important objectives for long-term rehabilitation. Measurable objectives (executive function components) of the intervention are self-awareness, goal setting, planning, organizing, self-initiating, self-monitoring, self-evaluating, and problem solving. For each of these objectives, graded descriptions are provided to enable an ordinal scale for measuring changes following intervention (Ylvisaker et al., 1998, p. 246).

All of the intervention methods mentioned do not have enough supporting evidence; however, judging by the data in initial studies, they seem to be promising, and additional extensive research is required. To obtain meaningful findings, evidence from research in this area may be a compilation of many single-subject studies and small group clinical trials, as the variance in the target populations is large and groups are very heterogeneous. Toward this end, a small controlled randomized trial with clients with schizophrenia in a day treatment is currently under way. The study compares the PSM program with the Occupational Goals Intervention (OGI), which is based on the GMT program. The OGI program uses the same five-stage process as in the GMT but in a variety of graded occupational tasks in three areas (meal planning and preparing food; money management; reading, writing, and computer use; additional tasks are included depending on the preference of the clients). The study includes 10 clients in each of four groups, two experimental groups (OGI and PSM), and two control groups (attention training and emotional–social treatment). Treatment outcome is measured in terms of executive functions as well as in daily functional outcomes. It is hypothesized that the OGI program will be effective in improving executive functions similarly to the PSM but will be more effective in improving functional performance. Both executive functioning programs are hypothesized to be more effective on all measures than are the two control groups.

CONCLUSION AND RECOMMENDATIONS FOR THE FUTURE

This chapter provided a review of the theory and intervention of higher-level cognitive functions, required for any comprehensive rehabilitation approach to individuals with cognitive dysfunction. A review of the literature on the functional outcomes of individuals with awareness deficits and executive dysfunction clearly demonstrates the significance of these problems in rehabilitation. Current occupational therapy practice guidelines are steering the profession to a broad understanding of occupational participation, including full community integration (AOTA, 2002; Fleming, Doig, & Katz, 2000). Unawareness and executive dysfunction are significant barriers in the path toward full participation, particularly in the more complex and integrated activities of daily life. Therefore, any intervention for individuals with demonstrated or suspected cognitive deficits will not be complete without addressing these higher-level components.

To implement this recommendation, it is essential to begin this process with an explicit and comprehensive evaluation, including interviews, tests, and observations of task performance (see Tables 1.1 and 1.2). The need for observation of task performance in naturalistic environments is widely acknowledged in the neurorehabilitation literature today. This provides the foundation and rationale for occupational therapy's essential input in the evaluation process. Likewise, in the treatment process, meaningful and purposeful activities are powerful change agents for the problems of unawareness and executive deficits and place occupational therapists in a unique position to make a meaningful contribution. The profession of occupational therapy is moving in this direction, as can be seen in the inclusion of higher-level cognitive functions within the theoretical developments and updates of the models presented in this volume.

The body of research evidence in this area has grown immensely in the past few years. The evidence is well established concerning the functional significance of higher-level cognitive deficits in rehabilitation. In addition, many assessments have been developed with varied levels of evidence regarding their psychometric properties. Finally, theoretically driven interventions are being suggested with beginning stages of effectiveness research to provide evidence-based practice. This process of gathering the evidence and planning future studies is of utmost importance to neurorehabilitation, and the discipline of occupational therapy is well equipped to be a major participant in this research path.

REVIEW QUESTIONS

1. Why is understanding higher-level cognitive functions significant for rehabilitation?
2. What are the main concepts and theoretical underpinnings of awareness and executive functions?
3. What are the methods and instruments for assessment of awareness and executive functions?
4. What are the treatment methods that exist for awareness and executive functions?
5. What is the unique contribution of occupational therapy to assessment and treatment of individuals with deficits in higher-level cognitive functions?
6. How strong is the evidence for the effectiveness of intervention?

REFERENCES

Abreu, B. C., Seale, G., Scheibel, R. S., Huddleston, N., Zhang, L., & Ottenbacher, K. J. (2001). Levels of self-awareness after acute brain injury: How patients' and rehabilitation specialists' perception compare. *Archives of Physical Medicine Rehabilitation, 82,* 49–56.

Alderman, N., Burgess, P. W., Knight, C., & Henman, C. (2003). Ecological validity of a simplified version of the Multiple Errands Shopping Test. *Journal of the International Neuropsychological Society, 9,* 31–44.

Amador, X. F., & David, A. S. (Eds.). (1998). *Insight and psychosis.* New York: Oxford University Press.

Amador, X. V., Flaum, M., Andreason, N. C., Strauss, D. H., Yale, S. A., Clark, S. C., et al. (1994). Awareness of illness in schizophrenia and schizoaffective and mood disorders. *Archives of General Psychiatry, 51,* 826–836.

Amador, X. V., Strauss, D. H., Yale, S. A., Flaum, M. M., Endicott, J., & Gorman, J. M. (1993). Assessment of insight in psychosis. *American Journal of Psychiatry, 150,* 873–879.

Amador, X. F., Strauss, S. A., Yale, S. A., & Gorman, J. M. (1991). Awareness of illness in schizophrenia. *Schizophrenia Bulletin, 17,* 113–132.

American Occupational Therapy Association. (2002). Occupational therapy practice framework: Domain and process. *American Journal of Occupational Therapy, 56,* 609–639.

American Psychiatric Association. (2000). *Diagnostic and statistical manual of mental disorders* (4th ed., text rev.). Washington, DC: Author.

Anderson, S. W., & Tranel, D. (1989). Awareness of disease states following cerebral infarction, dementia and head trauma: Standardized assessment. *Clinical Neuropsychologist, 3,* 327–339.

Andres, P. (2003). Frontal cortex as the central executive of working memory: Time to revise our view. *Cortex, 39,* 871–895.

Appeleros, P., Karlsson, G. M., Seiger, A., & Nydevik, I. (2002). Neglect and anosognosia after first ever stroke: Incidence and relationship to disability. *Journal of Rehabilitation Medicine, 34,* 215–220.

Arthanat, S., Nochajski, S. M., & Stone, J. (2004). The International Classification of Functioning, Disability and Health and its application to cognitive disorders. *Disability and Rehabilitation, 26,* 235–245.

Baddeley, A. (1996). Exploring the central executive. *Quarterly Journal of Experimental Psychology, 49A,* 5–28.

Baddeley, A., Della Sala, S., Papagno, C., & Spinnler, H. (1997). Dual task performance in dysexecutive and nondysexecutive patients with frontal lesion. *Neuropsychology, 11,* 187–194.

Barco, P. P., Crosson, B., Bolesta, M. M., Werts, D., & Stout, R. (1991). Training awareness and compensation on postacute head injury rehabilitation. In S. J. Kreutzer & P. H. Wehman (Eds.), *Cognitive rehabilitation for persons with TBI* (pp. 129–146). Baltimore: Brookes.

Baum, C. (1995). The contribution of occupation to function in persons with Alzheimer's disease. *Journal of Occupational Science: Australia, 2,* 59–67.

Baum, C., & Edwards, D. F. (1993). Cognitive performance in senile dementia of the Alzheimer's type: The Kitchen Task Assessment. *American Journal of Occupational Therapy, 47,* 431–438.

Beardmore, S., Tate, R., & Liddle, B. (1999). Does information and feedback improve children's knowledge of awareness of deficits after traumatic brain injury? *Neuropyschological Rehabilitation, 9,* 45–62.

Beck, A. T., Baruch, E., Balter, J., Steer, R. A., & Warman, D. M. (2004). A new instrument for measuring insight: The Beck Cognitive Insight Scale. *Schizophrenia Research, 68,* 319–329.

Beiman-Copland, S., & Dywan, J. (2000). Achieving rehabilitation gains in anosognosia after TBI. *Brain and Cognition, 44,* 1–8.

Berquist, T. F., & Jacket, M. P. (1993). Programme methodology: Awareness and goal setting with the traumatically brain injured. *Brain Injury, 7,* 275–282.

Berti, A., Ladavas, E., & Della Corte, M. (1996). Anosognosia for hemiplegia, neglect dyslexia, and drawing neglect: Clinical findings and theoretical considerations. *Journal of International Neuropsychological Society, 2,* 426–440.

Bewick, K. C., Raymond, M. J., Malia, K. B., & Bennett, T. L. (1995). Metacognition as the ultimate executive: Techniques and tasks to facilitate executive functions. *Neurorehabilitation, 5,* 367–375.

Binetti, G., Magni, E., Padovani, A., Cappa, S. F., Bianchetti, A., & Trabucchi, M. (1996). Executive dysfunction in early Alzheimer's disease. *Journal of Neurology, Neurosurgery, and Psychiatry, 60,* 91–93.

Birnboim, S. (2004). Strategy Application Task (SAT). *Canadian Journal of Occupational Therapy, 71,* 47–56.

Bisiach, E., & Geminiani, G. (1991). Anosognosia related to hemiplegia and hemianopsia. In G. P. Prigatano & D. L. Schacter (Eds.), *Awareness of deficit after brain injury* (pp. 17–39). New York: Oxford University Press.

Bisiach, E., Vallar, G., Perani, D., Papagno, C., & Berti, A. (1986). Unawareness of disease following lesions of right hemisphere: Anosognosia for hemiplegia and anosognosia for hemianopia. *Neuropsychologia, 24,* 471–482.

Boyd, T. M., & Sautter, S. W. (1993). Route-finding: A measure of everyday executive functioning in the head-injured adult. *Applied Cognitive Psychology, 7,* 171–181.

Bozikas, V. P., Kosmidis, M. H., Gamvrula, K., Hatzigeoriadou, M., Kourtis, A., & Karavatos, A. (2004). Clock drawing test in patients with schizophrenia. *Psychiatry Research, 121,* 229–238.

Braswell, M. S., Hartry, A., Hoornbeek, S., Johansen, A., Johnson, L., Schultz, J., et al. (1993). *Profile of Executive Control System: Instruction manual and assessment.* Wake Forest, NC: Lash & Associates Publishing/Training.

Brown, A. L. (1987). Metacognition, executive control, self-regulation, and other more mysterious mechanisms. In F. E. Weinert & R. H. Kluwe (Eds.), *Metacognition, motivation, and understanding* (pp. 65–116). Hillsdale, NJ: Erlbaum.

Brugger, P., Monsch, A. U., Salmon, D. P., & Butters, N. (1996). Random number generation in dementia of the Alzheimer type: A test of frontal executive functions. *Neuropsychologia, 34,* 97–103.

Burgess, P. W. (2000). Strategy application disorder: The role of the frontal lobe in human multitasking. *Psychological Research, 63,* 279–288.

Burgess, P. W., & Shallice, T. (1996). Response suppression, initiation and strategy use following frontal lobe lesions. *Neuropsychologia, 34,* 263–273.

Burgess, P. W., Veitch, E., Lacy-Costello, A., & Shallice, T. (2000). The cognitive and neuroanatomical correlates of multitasking. *Neuropsychologia, 38,* 848–863.

Butler, D. L. (1999). Metacognition and learning disabilities. In B. Y. L. Wong (Ed.), *learning about learning disabilities* (pp. 277–307). New York: Academic Press.

Celesia, G. G., Brigell, M. G., & Vaphiades, M. S. (1997). Hemianopic anosognosia. *Neurology, 49,* 88–97.

Chittum, W. R., Johnson, K., Chittum, J. M., Guercio, J. M., & McMorrow, M. J. (1996). Road to awareness: An individualized training package for increasing knowledge and comprehension of personal deficits in persons with acquired brain injury. *Brain Injury, 10,* 763–776.

Cicerone, K. D. (2002). Remediation of "working attention" in mild traumatic brain injury. *Brain Injury, 16,* 185–195.

Cicerone, K. D., & Giacino, J. T. (1992). Remediation of executive function deficits after traumatic brain injury. *Neurorehabilitation, 2,* 12–22.

Cicerone, K. D., & Wood, J. W. (1987). Planning disorder after closed head injury: A case study. *Archives of Physical Medicine and Rehabilitation, 68,* 111–115.

Clare, L. (2003). Managing threats to self: Awareness in early stage Alzheimer's disease. *Social Science and Medicine, 57,* 1017–1029.

Clark, O., & O'Carrol, R. E. (1998). An examination of the relationship between executive function, memory, and rehabilitation status schizophrenia. *Neuropsychological Rehabilitation, 8,* 229–241.

Cochini, G., Beschin, N., & Della Sala, S. (2002). Chronic anosognosia: A case report and theoretical account. *Neuropsychologia, 40,* 2030–2038.

Crosson, B., Barco, P. P., Velozo, C. A., Bolesta, M. M., Cooper, P. V., Werts, D., et al. (1989). Awareness and compensation in postacute head injury rehabilitation. *Journal of Head Trauma Rehabilitation, 4,* 46–54.

Cutting, J. (1978). Study of anosognosia. *Journal of Neurology, Neurosurgery, and Psychiatry, 41,* 548–555.

Davalos, D. B., Green, M., & Rial, D. (2002). Enhancement of executive functioning skills: An additional tier in the treatment of schizophrenia. *Community Mental Health Journal, 38,* 403–412.

DeBettignies, B. H., Mahurin, R. K., & Pirozzolo, F. J. (1990). Insight for impairment in independent living skills in Alzheimer's disease and multi-infarct dementia. *Journal of Clinical and Experimental Neuropsychology, 12,* 355–363.

Delahunty, A., & Morice, R. (1996). Rehabilitation of frontal/executive impairments schizophrenia. *Australian and New Zealand Journal of Psychiatry, 30,* 760–767.

Delahunty, A., Morice, R., & Frost, B. (1993). Specific cognitive flexibility rehabilitation in schizophrenia. *Psychological Medicine, 23,* 221–227.

Dell'Osso L., Pini, S., Cassano, G. B., Mastrocinque, C., Seckinger, R. A., Saettani, M., et al. (2002). Insight into illness in patients with mania, bipolar depression and major depression with psychotic features. *Bipolar Disorders, 4,* 315–322

Derouesne, C., Thibault, S., Lagha-Pierucci, S., Baudouin-Madec, V., Ancri, D., & Lancombez, L. (1999). Decreased awareness of cognitive deficits in patients with mild dementia of the Alzheimer type. *International Journal of Geriatric Psychiatry, 14,* 1019–1030.

Duke, L. M., Seltzer, B., Seltzer, J. E., & Vasterling, J. J. (2002). Cognitive components of deficit awareness in Alzheimer's disease. *Neuropsychology, 16,* 359–369.

Duncan, J. (1995). Attention, intelligence and the frontal lobes. In M. S. Gazzanniga (Ed.), *The cognitive neurosciences* (pp. 721–734). Cambridge, MA: MIT Press.

Elliott, R. (2003). Executive functions and their disorders. *British Medical Bulletin, 65,* 49–59.

Evans, J. J., Chua, S. E., McKenna, P. J., & Wilson, B. A. (1997). Assessment of the dysexecutive syndrome in schizophrenia. *Psychological Medicine, 27,* 635–646.

Flavell, J. H. (1985). *Cognitive development.* Englewood Cliffs, NJ: Prentice Hall.

Fleming, J. M., Doig, E., & Katz, N. (2000). Beyond dressing and driving: Using occupation to facilitate community integration in neurorehabilitation. *Brain Impairment, 1,* 141–150.

Fleming, J. M., & Strong, J. (1999). A longitudinal study of self-awareness: Functional deficits underestimated by persons with brain injury. *Occupational Therapy Journal of Research, 19,* 3–17.

Fleming, J. M., Strong, J., & Ashton, R. (1996). Self-awareness of deficits in adults with traumatic brain injury: How best to measure? *Brain Injury, 10,* 1–15.

Fleming, J. M., Strong, J., & Ashton, R. (1998). Cluster analysis of self-awareness levels in adults with traumatic brain injury and relationship to outcome. *Journal of Head Trauma Rehabilitation, 13,* 39–51.

Flaharty, G., & Wallat, C. (1997). Modifying the environment to optimize outcome for people with behavior disorders associated with anosognosia. *Neurorehabilitation, 9,* 221–225.

Fortin, S., Godbout, L., & Braun, M. J. (2003). Cognitive structure of executive deficits in frontally lesioned head trauma

patients performing activities of daily living. *Cortex, 39,* 273–291.

Gil, R., Arroyo-Anllo, E. M., Ingrand, P., Gil, M., Neau, J. P., Ornon, C., & Bonnaud, V. (2001). Self-consciousness and Alzheimer's disease. *Acta Neurologica Scandinavica, 104,* 296–300.

Giovannetti, T., Libon, D., & Hart, T. (2002). Awareness of naturalistic action errors in dementia. *Journal of the International Neurological Society, 8,* 633–644.

Godefroy, O. (2003). Frontal syndrome and disorders of executive functions. *Journal Neurology, 250,* 1–6.

Green, F. M., Kern, R. S., Braff, D. L., & Mintz, J. (2000). Neurocognitive deficits and functional outcome in schizophrenia: Are we measuring the "right stuff"? *Schizophrenia Bulletin, 26,* 119–136.

Hanes, K. R., Andrews, D. G., Smith, D. J., & Pantelis, C. (1996). A brief assessment of executive control dysfunction: Discriminate validity and homogeneity of planning, set shift, and fluency measures. *Archives of Clinical Neuropsychology, 11,* 185–191.

Hart, T., Giovanetti, T., Montgomery, M. W., & Schwartz, M. F. (1998). Awareness of errors in naturalistic action after traumatic brain injury. *Journal of Head Trauma Rehabilitation, 13,* 16–28.

Hartman-Maeir, A., Soroker, N., & Katz, N. (2001). Anosognosia for hemiplegia in stroke rehabilitation. *Neurorehabilitation and Neural Repair, 15,* 213–222.

Hartman-Maeir, A., Soroker, N., Oman, S. D., & Katz, N. (2003). Awareness of disabilities after stroke. *Disability and Rehabilitation, 25,* 35–44.

Hartman-Maeir, A., Soroker, N., Ring, H., & Katz, N. (2002). Awareness of deficits after stroke. *Journal of Rehabilitation Medicine, 34,* 158–164.

Heilman, K. M. (1991). Anosognosia: Possible neuropsychological mechanisms. In G. P. Prigatano & D. L. Schacter (Eds.), *Awareness of deficit after brain injury* (pp. 53–62). New York: Oxford University Press.

Heilman, K. M., Barrett, A. M., & Adair, J. C. (1998). Possible mechanisms of anosognosia: A defect in self-awareness. *Philosophical Transactions of the Royal Society of London Biological Science, 353,* 1903–1909.

Hutton, S. B., Purl, B. K., Duncan, L.-J., Robbins, T. W., Barnes, T. R. E., & Joyce, E. M. (1998). Executive function in first-episode schizophrenia. *Psychological Medicine, 28,* 463–473.

Jarman, R. F., Vavrik, J., & Walton, P. D. (1995). Metacognition and frontal lobe processes: At the interface of cognitive psychology and neuropsychology. *Genetic, Social, and General Psychology Monographs, 121,* 155–210.

Katz, N., Fleming, J., Keren, N., Lightbody S., & Hartman-Maeir, A. (2002). Unawareness and/or denial of disability: Implications for occupational therapy intervention. *Canadian Journal of Occupational Therapy, 69,* 281–292.

Keshevan, M. S., Rabinowitz, J., DeSmedt, G., Harvey, P. D., & Schooler, N. (in press). Correlates of insight in first episode psychosis. *Schizophrenia Research.*

Klonoff, P. S., O'Brien, K. P., Prigatano, G. P., Chiapello, D. A., & Cunningham, M. (1989). Cognitive retraining after traumatic brain injury and its role in facilitating awareness. *Journal of Head Trauma Rehabilitation, 4,* 37–45.

Knight, C., Alderman, N., & Burgess, P. W. (2002). Development of a simplified version of the multiple errands test for use in hospital settings. *Neuropsychological Rehabilitation, 12,* 231–255.

Kortte, K. M. B., Wegener, S. T., & Chwalisz, K. (2003). Anosognosia and denial: Their relationship to coping and depression in acquired brain injury. *Rehabilitation Psychology, 48,* 131–136.

Labuda, J., & Lichtenberg, P. (1999). The role of cognition, depression, and awareness of deficit in predicting geriatric rehabilitation patients' IADL performance. *Clinical Neuropsychologist, 13,* 258–267.

Levine, B., Robertson, I. H., Clare, L., Carter, G., Hong, J., Wilson, B., et al. (2000). Rehabilitation of executive functioning: An experimental–clinical validation of goal management training. *Journal of International Neuropsychological Society, 6,* 299–312.

Levine, B., Stuss, D. T., Milberg, W. P., Alexander, M. P. Schwartz, M., & Macdonald, R. (1998). The effects of focal and diffuse brain damage on strategy application: Evidence from focal lesions, traumatic brain injury, and normal aging. *Journal of the International Neuropsychological Society, 4,* 247–264.

Levine, D. N. (1990). Unawareness of visual and sensorimotor defects: A hypothesis. *Brain and Cognition, 13,* 233–281.

Lewis, L. (1991). Role of psychological factors in disordered awareness. In G. P. Prigatano & D. L. Schacter (Eds.), *Awareness of deficits after brain injury: Clinical and theoretical issues* (pp. 223–239). New York: Oxford University Press.

Lezak, M. D. (1993). Newer contributions to the neuropsychological assessment of executive functions. *Journal of Head Trauma Rehabilitation, 8,* 24–31.

Lezak, M. D. (1995). *Neuropsychological assessment.* New York: Oxford University Press.

Luria, A. R. (1966). *Higher cortical functions in man.* London: Tavistock.

Lysaker, P. H., Lancaster, R. S., Davis, L. W., & Clements, C. A. (2003). Patterns of neurocognitive deficits and unawareness of illness in schizophrenia. *Journal of Nervous and Mental Disease, 191,* 38–44.

Malia, K. B., Bewick, K. C., Raymond, M. J., & Bennett, T. L. (1997). *Brainwave–R: Cognitive strategies and techniques for brain injury rehabilitation—Executive functions workbooks.* Austin, TX: PRO-ED.

Manly, T., Hawkins, K., Evans, J., Woldt, K., & Robertson, I. H. (2002). Rehabilitation of executive function: Facilitation of effective goal management on complex tasks using periodic auditory alerts. *Neuropsychologia, 40,* 271–281.

Marcel, A. J., Tegner, R., & Nimmo-Smith, I. (2004). Anosognosia for plegia: Specificity, extension, partiality, and disunity of bodily unawareness. *Cortex, 40,* 19–40.

Mateer, C. A. (1999). The rehabilitation of executive disorders. In D. T. Stuss, G. Winocur, & I. H. Robertson (Eds.), *Cognitive neurorehabilitation* (pp. 314–332). Cambridge, England: Cambridge University Press

McEvoy, J. P., Hartman, M., Gottlieb, D., Goswin, S., Apperson, L. J., & Wilson, W. (1996). Common sense, insight, and neuropsychological test performance in schizophrenia patients. *Schizophrenia Bulletin, 22,* 635–641.

Mesulam, M. M. (1985). *Principles of behavioral neurology.* Philadelphia: F. A. Davis.

Migliorelli, R., Teson, R., Sabe, L., Petracca, G., Petracchi, M., Leiguardia, R., et al. (1995). Anosognosia in Alzheimer's disease: A study of associated factors. *Journal of Neuroscience, 7,* 338–344.

Mintz, S. R., Dobson, K. S., & Romney, D. M. (2003). Insight in schizophrenia: A meta-analysis. *Schizophrenia Research, 61,* 75–78.

Nelson, O., & Narrens, L. (1994). Why investigate metacognition? In J. Metcalfe & A. P. Shimamura (Eds.), *Metacognition* (pp. 1–25). Cambridge, MA: MIT Press.

Norman, D. A., & Shallice, T. (1986). Attention to action: Willed and automatic control of behavior. In R. J. Davidson, G. E. Schwartz, & D. Shapiro (Eds.), *Consciousness and self regulation: Advances in research and theory* (pp. 1–18). New York: Plenum Press. (Original work published 1980)

Norris, G., & Tate, R. L. (2000). The Behavioural Assessment of the Dysexecutive Syndrome (BADS): Ecological, concurrent, and construct validity. *Neuropsychological Rehabilitation, 10,* 33–45.

Pachalska, M., Kurzbauer, H., Talar, J., & MacQueen, B. D. (2002). Active and passive executive function disorder subsequent to closed-head injury. *Medical Science Monitor, 8,* 1–9.

Pantelis, C., Barber, F. Z., Barnes, T. R. E., Nelson, H. E., Owen, A. D., & Robbins, T. W. (1999). Comparison of set-shifting ability in patients with chronic schizophrenia and frontal lobe damage. *Schizophrenia Research, 37,* 251–270.

Pantelis, C., Barnes, T. R. E., Nelson, H. E., Tanner, S., Weatherley, L., Owen A. M., et al. (1997). Frontal-striatal cognitive deficits in patients with chronic schizophrenia. *Brain, 120,* 1823–1843.

Pedrelli, P., McQuaid, J. R., Granholm, E., Patterson, T. L., McClure, F., Beck, A., et al. (in press). Measuring cognitive insight in middle-aged and older patients with psychotic disorders. *Schizophrenia Research.*

Phinney, A., Wallhagen, M., & Sands, L. (2002). Exploring the meaning of symptom awareness and unawareness in dementia. *Journal of Neuroscience Nursing, 34,* 79–90.

Pohjasvaara, T., Leskela, M., Vataja, R., Kalska, H., Ylikoski, R., Hietanen, M., et al. (2002). Post-stroke depression, executive dysfunction and functional outcomes. *European Journal of Neurology, 9,* 269–275.

Prigatano, G. P. (1986). *Neuropsychological rehabilitation after brain injury.* Baltimore: Johns Hopkins University Press.

Prigatano, G. P. (1991). Disturbances of self-awareness of deficit after traumatic brain injury. In G. P. Prigatano & D. L. Schacter (Eds.), *Awareness of deficit after brain injury* (pp. 111–126). New York: Oxford University Press.

Prigatano, G. P. (1996). Behavioural limitation TBI patients tend to underestimate: A replication and extension to patients with lateralized cerebral dysfunction. *Clinical Neuropsychologist, 12,* 56–67.

Prigatano, G. P. (1999). Disorders of self-awareness after brain injury. In G. P. Prigatano (Ed.), *Principles of neuropsychological rehabilitation* (pp. 265–293). New York: Oxford University Press.

Prigatano, G. P., Altman, I. M., & O'Brien, K. P. (1990). Behavioral limitations that traumatic-brain-injured patients tend to underestimate. *Clinical Neuropsychologist, 4,* 163–176.

Prigatano, G. P., Bruna, O., Mataro, M., Munoz, J. M., Fernandez, S., & Junque, C. (1998). Initial disturbances of consciousness and resultant impaired awareness in Spanish patients with traumatic brain injury. *Journal of Head Trauma Rehabilitation, 13,* 29–38.

Prigatano, G. P., & Klonoff, P. S. (1998). A clinician's rating scale for evaluating impaired self-awareness and denial of disability after brain injury. *Clinical Neuropsychologist, 12,* 56–67.

Prigatano, G. P., Ogano, M., & Amakusa, B. (1997). A cross-cultural study on impaired self-awareness in Japanese patients with brain dysfunction. *Neuropsychiatry, Neuropsychology, and Behavioural Neurology, 10,* 135–143.

Prigatano, G. P., & Schacter, D. L. (1991). *Awareness of deficit after brain injury.* New York: Oxford University Press.

Prigatano, G. P., & Weinstein, E. A. (1996). Edwin A. Weinstein's contribution to neuropsychological rehabilitation. *Neuropsychological Rehabilitation, 6,* 305–326.

Ramachandran, V. S. (1995). Anosognosia in parietal lobe syndrome. *Consciousness and Cognition, 4,* 22–51.

Ramachandran, V. S., & Rogers-Ramachandran, D. (1996). Denial of disabilities in anosognosia. *Nature, 382,* 501.

Rebman, M. J., & Hannon, R. (1995). Treatment of unawareness of memory deficits in adults with brain injury: Three case studies. *Rehabilitation Psychology, 40,* 279–287.

Royall, D. R., Cordes, J. A., & Polk, M. (1998). CLOX: An executive clock drawing task. *Journal of Neurology, Neurosurgery and Psychiatry, 64,* 588–594.

Royall, D. R., Lauterbach, E. C., Cummigs, J. L., Reeve, A., Rummans, T. A., Kaufer, D. I., et al. (2002). Executive control function: A review of its promise and challenges for clinical research. *Journal of Neuropsychiatry and Clinical Neuroscience, 14,* 377–405.

Royall, D. R., Mahurin, R. K., & Gray, K. (1992). Bedside assessment of executive impairment: The Executive Interview (EXIT). *Journal of the American Geriatric Society, 40,* 1221–1226.

Rubens, A. B., & Garrett, M. F. (1991). Anosognosia of linguistic deficits in patients with neurological deficits. In G. P. Prigatano & D. L. Schacter (Eds.), *Awareness of deficit after brain injury* (pp. 40–53). New York: Oxford University Press.

Schlund, M. W. (1999). Self-awareness: Effects of feedback and review on verbal self reports and remembering following brain injury. *Brain Injury, 13,* 375–380.

Sevy, S., Nathanson, K., Visweswaraiah, H., & Amador, X. (2004). The relationship between insight and symptoms in schizophrenia. *Comprehensive Psychiatry, 45*(1), 16–19.

Shallice, T., & Burgess, P. W. (1991). Deficits in strategy application following frontal lobe damage in man. *Brain, 114,* 727–741.

Sherer, M., Bergloff, P., Boake, C., High, W., & Levin, E. (1998). The Awareness Questionnaire: Factor structure and internal consistency. *Brain Injury, 1,* 63–68.

Sherer, M., Bergloff, P., Levin, E., High, W. M., Oden, K. E., & Nick, T. G. (1998). Impaired awareness and employment outcome after traumatic brain injury. *Journal of Head Trauma Rehabilitation, 13,* 52–61.

Sherer, M., Hart, T., Nick, T. G., Whyte, J., Thompson, R. J., & Yablone, S. A. (2003). Early impaired self awareness after traumatic brain injury. *Archives of Physical Medicine and Rehabilitation, 84,* 168–176.

Simon, A. E., Giacomini, V., Ferrero, F., & Mohr, S. (2003). Dysexecutive syndrome and social adjustment in schizophrenia. *Australian and New Zealand Journal of Psychiatry, 37,* 340–346.

Sohlberg, M. M. (2000). Assessing and managing unawareness of self. *Seminars in Speech and Language, 21,* 135–151.

Sohlberg, M. M., & Mateer, C. A. (2001a). *Cognitive rehabilitation: An integrative neuropsychological approach.* New York: Guilford Press.

Sohlberg, M. M., & Mateer, C. A. (2001b). Introduction to cognitive rehabilitation. In M. M. Sohlberg & C. A. Mateer (Eds.), *Cognitive rehabilitation: An integrative neuropsychological approach* (pp. 3–24). New York: Guilford Press.

Sohlberg, M. M., & Mateer, C. A. (2001c). Management of dysexecutive symptoms. In M. M. Sohlberg & C. A. Matter (Eds.), *Cognitive rehabilitation: An integrative neuropsychological approach* (pp. 230–268). New York: Guilford Press.

Sohlberg, M. M., Mateer, C. A, Penkman, L., Glang, A., & Todis, B. (1998). Awareness intervention: Who needs it? *Journal of Head Trauma Rehabilitation, 13,* 62–78.

Sohlberg, M. M., Mateer, C. A., & Stuss, D. T. (1993). Contemporary approaches to the management of executive control dysfunction. *Journal of Head Trauma Rehabilitation, 8,* 45–58.

Starkstein, S. E., Fedoroff, P., Price, T. R., Leiguardia, R., & Robinson, R. G. (1992). Anosognosia in patients with cerebrovascular lesions. *Stroke, 23,* 1446–1453.

Stratta, P., Arduini, L., Daneluzzo, E., Rinaldi, O., di Genova, A., & Rossi, A. (2003). Relationship of good and poor Wisconsin Card Sorting Test performance to illness duration in schizophrenia: A cross sectional analysis. *Psychiatry Research, 121,* 219–227.

Stuss, D. T. (1992). Biological and psychological development of executive functions. *Brain and Cognition, 20,* 8–23.

Stuss, D. T., & Alexander, M. P. (2000). Executive functions and the frontal lobes: A conceptual view. *Psychological Research, 63,* 289–298.

Stuss, D. T., & Levine, B. (2002). Adult clinical neuropsychology: Lessons from studies in frontal lobes. *Annual Review of Psychology, 53,* 401–433.

Swanberg, M. M., Tractenberg, R. E., Mohs, R., Thal, L. J., & Cummings, J. L. (2004). Executive dysfunction in Alzheimer's disease. *Archives of Neurology, 61,* 556–560.

Sylvester, C. Y. C., Wager, T. D., Lacey, S. C., Hernandez, L., Nichols, T. E., Smith, E. E., et al. (2003). Switching attention and resolving interference: fMRI measures of executive functions. *Neuropsychologia, 41,* 357–370.

Tham, K., Bernspang, B., & Fisher A. G. (1999). The development of the Awareness of Disabilities (AAD). *Scandinavian Journal of Occupational Therapy, 6,* 184–190.

Tham, K., Ginsburg, E., Fisher, A. G., & Tegner, R. (2001). Training to improve awareness of disabilities in clients with unilateral neglect. *American Journal of Occupational Therapy, 55,* 46–54.

Toglia, J. P. (1993). *Contextual Memory Test manual.* San Antonio, TX: Therapy SkillBuilders.

Toglia, J., & Kirk, U. (2000). Understanding awareness deficits following brain injury. *Neurorehabilitation, 15,* 57–70.

Vataja, R., Pohjasvaara, T., Mantyla, R., Ylikoski, R., Leppavuori, A., Leskela, M., et al. (2003). MRI correlates of executive dysfunction in patients with ischaemic stroke. *European Journal of Neurology, 10,* 625–631.

Wagner, M. T., & Cushman, L. A. (1994). Neuroanatomic and neuropsychological predictors of unawareness of cognitive deficit in vascular population. *Archives of Clinical Neuropsychology, 9,* 57–69.

Weinstein, E. A. (1991). Anosognosia and denial of illness. In G. P. Prigatano & D. L. Schacter (Eds.), *Awareness of deficit in brain injury: Clinical and theoretical issues* (pp. 240–257). New York: Oxford University Press.

Wild, K., & Cotrell, V. (2003). Identifying driving impairment in Alzheimer's disease: A comparison of self and observer reports versus driving evaluation. *Alzheimer Disease and Associated Disorders, 17,* 27–34.

Wilson, B. A., Alderman, N., Burgess, P. W., Emslie, H., & Evans, J. J. (1996). *Behavioral assessment of dysexecutive syndrome.* St. Edmunds, England: Thames Valley Test Company.

Wilson, B. A., Evans, J. J., Alderman, N., Burgess, P. W., & Emslie, H. (1997). Behavioral assessment of dysexecutive syndrome. In P. Rabbit (Ed.), *Methodology of frontal and executive functions* (pp. 239–250). London: Psychology Press.

Wilson, B. A., Evans, J. J., Emslie, H., Alderman, N., & Burgess, P. (1998). The development of an ecologically valid test for assessing patients with a dysexecutive syndrome. *Neuropsychological Rehabilitation, 8,* 213–228.

World Health Organization. (2001). *International classification of functioning, disability and health (ICF).* Geneva, Switzerland: Author.

Wykes, T., Reeder, C., Corner, J., Williams, C., & Everitt, B. (1999). The effects of neurocognitive remediation on executive processing in patients with schizophrenia. *Schizophrenia Bulletin, 25,* 291–307.

Ylvisaker, M., & DeBonis, D. (2000). Executive functions impairment in adolescence: TBI and ADHD. *Topics in Language Disorders, 20,* 29–57.

Ylvisaker, M., Jacobs, H. E., & Feeney, T. (2003). Positive supports for people who experience behavioral and cognitive disability after brain injury: A review. *Journal of Head Trauma Rehabilitation, 18,* 7–32.

Ylvisaker, M., Szekeres, S. F., & Feneey, T. J. (1998). Cognitive rehabilitation: Executive functions. In M. Ylvisaker (Ed.), *Towards brain injury rehabilitation: Children and adolescents* (rev. ed., pp. 221–269). Boston: Butterworth-Heinemann.

Youngjohn, J. R., & Altman, I. M. (1989). A performance-based group approach to the treatment of anosognosia and denial. *Rehabilitation Psychology, 3,* 217–222.

Zakzanis, K. K., & Heinrichs, W. (1999). Schizophrenia and the frontal brain: A quantitative review. *Journal of the International Neuropsychological Society, 5,* 556–566.

Zalla, T., Joyce, C., Szoke, A., Schurhoff, F., Pillon, B., Komano, O., et al. (2004). Executive dysfunctions as potential markers of familial vulnerability to bipolar disorder and schizophrenia. *Psychiatry Research, 121,* 207–217.

Zhou, J., Chittum, R., Johnson, K., Poppen, R., Guerico, J., & McMorrow, M. M. (1996). The utilization of a game format to increase the knowledge of residuals among people with acquired brain injury. *Journal of Head Trauma Rehabilitation, 11,* 51–61.

Part

Neurological Disabilities

2

Joan Pascale Toglia, PhD, OTR, FAOTA

A Dynamic Interactional Approach to Cognitive Rehabilitation

What one addresses in cognitive rehabilitation depends to a large extent on how one conceptualizes cognition and the scope of cognitive functioning. Traditional cognitive rehabilitation approaches have been guided by the assumption that cognition can be divided into distinct subskills (Trexler, 1987). In this chapter, I propose a dynamic interactional view of cognition as an alternative to traditional deficit and syndrome-specific approaches. In this dynamic approach, the clinician is urged to abandon classical taxonomies of dysfunction and instead to investigate dynamically the underlying conditions and processing strategies that influence performance. Assessment uses cues and task alterations to identify the person's potential for change. Treatment may focus on changing the person's strategies and self-awareness; modifying external factors such as the activity demands and environment; or simultaneously addressing the person, activity, and environment to facilitate performance.

This chapter draws heavily from cognitive and educational psychology literature that addresses how normal people process, learn, and generalize information. It integrates this material with occupational therapy practice and the rehabilitation of clients with cognitive dysfunction.

Cognitive dysfunction can be seen in people with developmental, neurological, or psychiatric dysfunction. The theoretical concepts presented in this chapter are broad and apply to all populations. However, the specific assessment and treatment techniques described later have been developed for adults with brain injury. Some of these techniques also have been used with adults who have schizophrenia (see Chapter 6) and school-age children or adolescents who have learning disabilities (see Chapter 10).

THEORETICAL FOUNDATIONS FOR A DYNAMIC INTERACTIONAL MODEL OF COGNITION

Cognition is defined as the person's capacity to acquire and use information to adapt to environmental demands (Lidz, 1987). This definition encompasses information-processing skills, learning, and generalization. The capacity to acquire information involves information-processing skills or the ability to take in, organize, assimilate, and integrate new information with previous experiences. Adaptation involves using information that has been previously acquired to plan and structure behavior for goal attainment. Thus, the ability to apply what has been learned to a variety of different situations is inherent within the concept of cognition (Lidz, 1987).

This description of cognition cuts across specific domains. Cognition is not divided into separate subskills such as attention, memory, organization, or reasoning.

Instead, cognitive abilities and deficiencies are analyzed according to underlying strategies, ability to monitor performance, and potential for learning.

Essential to the conceptualization of cognition is the idea that cognition is an ongoing product of the dynamic interaction among the person, activity, and environment (see Figure 2.1). Cognition is not static, stable, or fixed; it changes with our interaction with the external world (Feuerstein & Falik, 2004; Lidz, 1987). This implies that cognition is modifiable under certain conditions.

The dynamic nature of cognition is reflected in the way that information-processing resources are allocated and used. Normally, we can process only a limited amount of information at any one time. Although there is a fixed or structural limit in the capacity to process information (structural capacity), there are differences in the way that this fixed capacity can be used. The same activity can require different amounts of information-processing capacity depending on how one goes about performing it. The term *functional capacity* refers to the ability to use our limited information-processing capacity efficiently. The ability to monitor performance and select appropriate processing strategies maximizes use of functional information-processing capacity. The efficient allocation of limited processing resources is central to learning and cognition. Functional information-processing capacity is modifiable and varies with characteristics of the activity, the environment, and the person (Flavell, Miller, & Miller, 1993). For example, the cognitive-processing demands for a task involving cooking

an old recipe in a familiar kitchen are different than cooking the same recipe in an unfamiliar kitchen. The processing resources required for efficient performance change with the demands of the activity and environment. This implies that performance can be facilitated by changing the activity demands, the environment, the person's use of strategies and self-awareness, or all of the above.

Figure 2.1 illustrates the dynamic interactions among the person, activity, and environment. The person factors or internal variables are shaded and include (a) structural information-processing capacity; (b) personal context such as lifestyle, personality, and emotions; (c) self-awareness; and (d) processing strategies. Processing strategies and self-awareness are highlighted in bold and are the personal factors that represent core aspects of cognition. These aspects of cognition are modifiable and may be targeted during intervention as a means of maximizing information processing and enhancing occupational performance. External variables are depicted in the right-hand box and include the demands of the activity and the environment (social, physical, and cultural). Both external variables as well as other internal variables (personal context and structural capacity) influence the core aspects of cognition: self-awareness and efficient use of processing strategies. Strategy use and self-awareness have a reciprocal relationship with each other.

FIGURE 2.1. The dynamic interactional model of cognition.

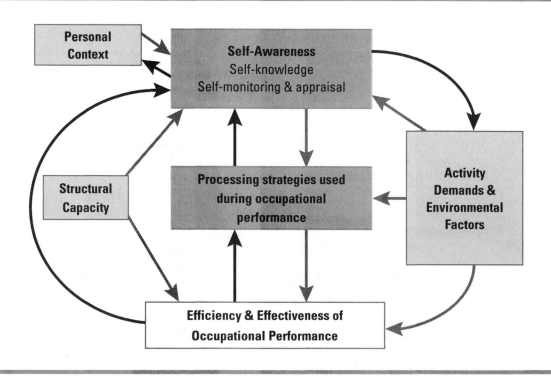

Self-awareness influences strategy use, but use of a different strategy also can increase awareness.

Independent occupational performance requires the ability to recognize one's limitations, self-monitor performance, and use efficient processing strategies. External cues and modifications of the activity or environment can directly support and enhance occupational performance (without changes in strategy use or self-awareness); however, another person is required for implementation and ongoing monitoring.

The dynamic interactional model (Figure 2.1) indicates that occupational performance can provide feedback that influences a person's self-perceptions and beliefs about his or her abilities and performance. Feedback also may be provided by another person or external source. In either case, performance difficulties may cause the person to choose different processing strategies, move to a different environment, or modify the demands of the activity. Thus, occupational performance and cognitive abilities may be modified as a result of experiences. Each component illustrated in the model and the dynamic interaction among them are described below. The overlap among the descriptions of each area reflects the close interaction among them.

COMPONENTS OF THE MODEL

Structural Capacity

Structural capacity refers to physical limits in the ability to process and interpret information. Structural capacity may be related to the severity and nature of the injury, length of time since the injury, person's age, and other health factors. Although there are inherent limitations in the ability to take in and process information (structural capacity), there are aspects of information processing that are modifiable and that can extend the range of abilities (functional capacity; Flavell et al., 1993). The full range of a person's processing capacity and potential for change can best be ascertained by examining the person's performance when information processing is guided, mediated, or structured by another person or by manipulating activity and environmental demands (Sternberg & Grigorenko, 2002). The distance between independent performance and performance with assistance or under optimal conditions has been described by Vygotsky (1978) as the zone of proximal development and has been used by researchers as a measure of cognitive modifiability (Wiedl, 1999) or cognitive plasticity (Baltes, Kühl, & Sowarka, 1992; Baltes, Kühl, Gutzmann, & Sowarka, 1995). I describe the zone of proximal development further later in the chapter.

Personal Context

The unique characteristics of a person, such as one's personality, coping style, beliefs, values, expectations, lifestyle, motivation, and emotions, can significantly influence the extent to which information is processed deeply and is monitored (Brown, 1988). For example, a person who believes that he will not get better no matter how hard he tries may not persist, put forth effort, or actively participate in treatment (Gage & Polatajko, 1994). Emotional states such as anxiety or depression decrease the ability to process information deeply and use effective strategies. For example, a person may be so depressed that she is unable to fully attend to the activity. She may lack the mental energy or motivation to initiate use of a compensatory strategy even though she is aware of her difficulties and is capable of using strategies effectively. In addition, the meaningfulness and relevancy of an activity can influence motivation, effort, and cognitive processing. If activities are perceived as irrelevant to one's life and recovery process, the person is not likely to be attentive or actively engaged in monitoring performance or using efficient processing strategies.

Premorbid personality characteristics such as a lifelong pattern of resistance to change or a tendency to be set in one's own ways of doings things also may influence the way in which new information is processed and feedback is used (Toglia, 2003a). A person who never liked to admit mistakes or ask for help may have difficulty accepting the changes that have occurred and may be more likely to use denial as a coping strategy. Denial can prevent the person from setting realistic goals, allocating effort, actively monitoring, and adjusting performance. It is important to keep in mind that one's view of one's cognitive abilities may be closely associated with self-identity and independence. For example, a person may describe himself or herself as someone who is detail oriented and well organized. Acknowledging and accepting difficulties in these areas can threaten one's sense of self. In addition, acknowledging that one cannot drive or return to work indicates a loss of independence. The ability to recognize errors may be harder in tasks that are highly valued and closer to one's sense of self-identity (Toglia & Kirk, 2000). Engagement in one's daily occupations contributes to shaping one's sense of self-identity and place within the world. Cognitive impairments can result in a loss of self-confidence and self-control as well as a loss of sense of self.

The ability to self-monitor performance and use efficient processing strategies requires acceptance of the changes that have occurred and a willingness to change or adjust methods used to perform an activity. At the same time, the results of activity experiences can gradually restructure over time one's self-expectations, sense of control, self-beliefs, and self-identity (Toglia & Kirk, 2000).

Self-Awareness

The concept of *self-awareness* is viewed as a multi-dimensional construct that includes two distinct but interrelated concepts: self-knowledge and on-line awareness. *Self-knowledge* includes understanding one's cognitive strengths and the limitations that exist outside the context of a particular task. *On-line awareness* refers to metacognitive skills such as the ability to accurately judge task demands; anticipate the likelihood of problems; and monitor, regulate, and evaluate performance within the context of an activity. Thus, on-line awareness changes within an activity, whereas self-knowledge is relatively stable and changes slowly with experiences (Cornoldi, 1998; Toglia & Kirk, 2000). Pre-existing knowledge and expectations about oneself influence how activity demands are perceived and shape expectations regarding outcome.

Understanding of one's abilities may be distorted due to poor coping mechanisms and inability to accept changes in performance or due to limitations in processing that prevent the person from perceiving errors in performance. Regardless of the origin, decreased understanding of one's cognitive abilities results in distorted judgments and expectations that can disrupt self-monitoring and self-regulatory processes and further impede effective use of strategies or ability to benefit from external cues and modifications. For example, if a person does not acknowledge having memory difficulties, he or she is unlikely to initiate use of compensatory strategies such as writing down a list of things to get at the store or taking notes while reading. If people perceive a task as easy, they are not likely to put forth effort and mobilize concentration or mental energy because they may not think it is needed. As a result, performance is not closely monitored or adjusted. At the opposite end of the continuum, a person may be acutely aware of difficulties in performance but may lack a clear understanding of why these difficulties are occurring. Performance may be paralyzed by diminished self-confidence and high anxiety. Self-perceptions of abilities affect the speed and intensity of performance as well as allocation of resources and strategy use. It also influences the activities one chooses to engage in (Toglia & Kirk, 2000).

A significant number of clients with brain injury are unaware of their limitations in occupational performance (Abreu et al., 2001; Hartman-Maeir, Soroker, Ring, & Katz, 2002). People who are unable to accurately judge the

difficulty of an activity in relationship to their own abilities tend to go beyond what they are capable of and show impairments in judgment and safety (Toglia & Kirk, 2000). For example, a person with severe unilateral neglect may try to drive a car when it is unsafe to do so because he or she does not recognize whether visual information is missing. Diminished awareness affects the ability to learn from one's mistakes and use feedback to modify behavior. Self-awareness is critical to judgment, safety, and independence across all areas of occupational performance. It has been linked to effective use of compensatory strategies (Dirette, 2002; Tham, Borell, & Gustavsson, 2000), motivation (Fleming, Strong, & Ashton, 1998), ability to set realistic goals (Fischer, Siegrfried, & Trexler, 2004), generalization of learning (Belmont, Butterfield, & Ferretti, 1982; Resing & Roth-Van der Werf, 2002), and rehabilitation outcome (Hartman-Maeir, Soroker, Oman, & Katz, 2003).

Differences in self-awareness may be observed in different contexts and across different activities (Abreu et al., 2001). Difficulty level, familiarity, and value of an activity can influence self-awareness (Tham et al., 2000). Self-monitoring skills are most likely to emerge in activities that are at the "just right level of challenge." Activities that are beyond the person's information-processing capabilities can lead to a failure to understand and integrate the experience (Toglia & Kirk, 2000). Engagement in familiar and meaningful occupations has been found to be more effective in facilitating the emergence of awareness because they provide a basis for comparison of performance (Dirette, 2002; Katz, Fleming, Keren, Lightbody, & Hartman-Maeir, 2002; Tham et al., 2000). Familiarity and previous experiences with activities provides a benchmark or standard that can be used to self-evaluate current performance. In the initial stages of treatment, however, activities that are familiar, relevant, and meaningful to one's life may need to be balanced with the degree of emotional value. For example, in some situations, it may be easier for a person to initially accept and recognize difficulties in familiar activities that are not closely associated with one's sense of self (Toglia & Kirk, 2000).

Self-efficacy is described as judgments and beliefs of one's performance capabilities with respect to a task. It includes the beliefs he or she has regarding his or her control over a situation (Bandura, 1997; Gage & Polatajko, 1994). Problems in self-awareness can lead to unanticipated consequences or unanticipated difficulties in occupational performance. This inevitably leads to a loss of a sense of control. The person who is unable to anticipate or recognize errors is taken by surprise with unexpected task outcomes (Toglia & Kirk, 2000). Similarly, people who are aware of their errors may experience intense anxiety because they are not sure why the errors are occurring. In both situations, there is diminished self-efficacy (Toglia & Kirk, 2000). A strong sense of self-efficacy is related to persistence and effort in an activity, commitment to goals, high self-esteem, psychological well-being, and motivation. The more an individual believes he or she has control over a situation, the better he or she will perform (Bandura, 1997; Gage & Polatajko, 1994). Thus, self-awareness is closely related to self-efficacy, persistence, motivation, and learning.

A discrepancy between occupational performance and one's expectations may lead to adjustment of response and selection of a different strategy. This is most likely to occur if a person recognizes or discovers errors in himself or herself and achieves a sense of control over performance. The outcome of performance can contribute to restructuring and shaping one's knowledge and beliefs about abilities under certain conditions (Toglia & Kirk, 2000).

Processing Strategies

Processing strategies can be described as small units of behavior that contribute to the effectiveness and efficiency of performance (Toglia, 2003a). They are the most observable aspects of a learner's performance and the aspects most accessible to intervention and modification. Processing strategies include behaviors that cut across specific cognitive domains. Table 2.1 includes examples of some of the processing strategies and behaviors that underlie task performance in cognitive skill areas. As the table shows, there is considerable overlap among the different areas. Attention to relevant or critical information underlies performance in attention, visual processing, memory, organization, and problem solving. The same underlying processing strategies and behaviors can influence performance in several areas.

The appropriate selection of processing strategies increases efficient use of information-processing resources. Processing strategies include organized approaches, methods, or tactics that operate to select and guide the efficient processing of information (Abreu & Toglia, 1987; Toglia, 1991). For example, if confronted with a large amount of information we may automatically prioritize information and decide where to start and what to do first, second, and so on. We may select the most important stimuli and ignore the unimportant stimuli. We may organize or cluster related information together or decide to shift our attention among various stimuli (Abreu & Toglia, 1987). All of these behaviors enhance our ability to take in and assimilate information. People with brain injury do not automatically use effective strategies. Similarly, students with learning disabilities have been described as "inefficient processors of information" because they do not automatically initiate use of efficient strategies (Swanson & Deshler, 2003). Table 2.2 lists examples of efficient and inefficient processing strategies. Inefficient processing strategies can impede information processing.

As described in the preceding section, strategy use requires the ability to anticipate difficulties and accurately judge activity demands in relationship to one's current abilities (Brown, Bransford, Ferrara, & Campione, 1983; Schneider, 1998). Similarly, the demands of the activity and environment influence the type of strategies that are most appropriate. If the complexity of the activity is above the processing capabilities of the person, efficient strategies cannot be used.

The type of processing strategies used by the person determines the depth at which information is processed. Deep processing strategies are characterized by active elaboration, organization, and attempts to relate new information to previous experiences or knowledge. The more one attends to an item and actively thinks about its meaning in relation to other concepts, the more deeply the information will be processed (Toglia, 1993b). Surface-level strategies include memorizing words without actively elaborating or reorganizing the material to obtain meaning (Nolen, 1988). Information that is processed at deep levels is more easily understood and retained than information processed at shallow levels (Anderson, 1985). Thus, the type of processing strategies used is a critical variable in learning and retention. Evidence suggests that by modifying processing strategies one can increase performance and that, unlike poor learners, good learners spontaneously apply deep processing strategies (Lidz, 1987).

Processing strategies can be external or internal in nature. External strategies involve interaction with external items, aids, or cues, whereas internal strategies involve mental repetition; practice or visualization; and use of self-cues, questions, or instructions. External and internal strategies can be further described by their range of application. Situational strategies are effective in specific tasks or environments, whereas nonsituational strategies are applicable in a wide range of tasks and environments (Toglia, 1991). One example of a situational strategy is rehearsal, or repeating information to oneself over and over. This strategy may be useful if the amount of information to be remembered is small, but it is not effective in situations in which the amount to be recalled is large. Nonsituational strategies are nonspecific in nature and may include pacing

TABLE 2.1. Underlying Elements of Cognitive Function

Structure	Processing Strategies and Behaviors
Attention	• Detects subtle changes in task conditions • Initiates exploration (search of the environment) • Searches for information in a planned, systematic manner • Is unhindered by internal or external distractions peripheral to the task • Paces and monitors speed of response • Identifies relevant information • Simultaneously attends to overall stimulus as well as to details • Keeps track of rules, facts, pieces of information • Easily disengages focus of attention when necessary • Follows changes in task, stimuli, or rules without error
Visual Processing	• Plans and systematically explores the visual display • Distinguishes critical features of the object or picture • Attends to the overall configuration • Shifts scanning approach with different stimuli arrangements • Localizes information in space • Pays equal attention to all parts of the visual field or stimulus figure • Paces and monitors speed of response to visual information • Simultaneously attends to the parts and whole
Memory	• Recognizes overall context • Recognizes most important details or information • Focuses, fixates on stimulus to be recalled • Sustains focus of attention on material to be remembered • Spontaneously shifts focus of attention to the stimuli to be remembered • Summarizes or identifies the main points or theme • Uses rehearsal (requires sustained repetitive activity) • Uses association (requires ability to recognize similarities and differences between stimuli and organize information into concept categories)
Organization	• Attention to critical details • Shifts from one activity, stimulus, or thought to another • Anticipates; thinks ahead: What next? What if? • Recognizes most critical, relevant aspects of objects or situation • Keeps track of all task variables, steps, or stimuli • Associates, groups, or chunks related information • Keeps the "whole picture" in mind while arranging the pieces • Monitors pace or speed during the task
Problem Solving	• Analyzes the conditions of the problem • Distinguishes critical facts, assumptions, and irrelevant information • Summarizes the main issues • Simultaneously keeps track of all the relevant information • Goes beyond "here and now" and anticipates events or consequences • Shifts to alternate strategies, plans when needed • Flexibility and reversibility in thinking • Simultaneously holds in mind all the qualities of a situation or experience • Monitors speed or pace as carrying out the task

the speed of response, visualizing oneself performing a task prior to actual performance, and verbalizing the task steps or rules during task performance.

Activity

The ability to use efficient processing strategies and monitor performance varies with the activity demands as well as the meaningfulness and familiarity of the activity

(Toglia, 1991, 1993a). The ability to link new situations with previous experiences and knowledge influences the monitoring, strategy selection, organization, and processing speed of new information (Bransford, Sherwood, Vye, & Rieser, 1986). If people are presented with information in a way that helps them activate appropriate knowledge, it can have a powerful effect on their abilities to process information (Bransford, 1979). Information that is recognized as familiar is easier to organize and is processed

TABLE 2.2. Inefficient and Efficient
Processing Strategies

Inefficient Strategies/ Behaviors Targeted for Change	Efficient Strategies/Behaviors Emphasized in Treatment
Omits details or steps	Highlights, circles, underlines relevant details
Overfocuses on pieces	Attends to the whole context prior to attending to details
Haphazard approach	Prioritizes, plans, groups materials together; arranges items in order of use prior to activity
Responds impulsively	Paces and modulates speed of action
Sidetracked with irrelevant information	Covers, reduces, or removes information

Note. From "The Multicontext Approach," by J. Toglia, 2003. In E. B. Crepeau, E. S. Cohn, & B. A. B. Schell (Eds.), *Willard & Spackman's Occupational Therapy* (10th ed., p. 266). Philadelphia: Lippincott Williams & Wilkins. Copyright © 2003 by Lippincott Williams & Wilkins. Reprinted with permission.

with less effort and stress on the capacity limitations of the system (Toglia, 1991, 1993b). This indicates that people with cognitive impairments may be more likely to show higher levels of performance within activities and environments that are natural, familiar, and predictable.

The self-monitoring skills and processing strategies needed to perform an activity also are partially determined by activity demands. Table 2.3 illustrates how the manipulation of specific features of an activity can place different demands on the underlying skills and strategies required to perform an activity component such as finding an item on a kitchen shelf. In assessment and treatment one or two parameters of the activity are systematically changed, whereas the others are held constant to determine its effect on performance. For example, in a visual search task, differences in the familiarity of the stimuli, number of stimuli, contrast, degree of detail, and so forth determine the skills and strategies required to perform the task. Difficulty

TABLE 2.3. Visual Search: Choosing an Item in a Kitchen Cabinet

Activity Parameters	Easy/ Less Attention and Effort	Difficult/ Greater Attention and Effort	Demands With Increased Complexity
Familiarity	Familiar kitchen and food items	Unfamiliar kitchen (e.g., cabinet includes unfamiliar brands, mixed types of items)	More difficult to pick up distinctive features
Directions	Structured (e.g., matching or point to specific items)	Unstructured (e.g., "Tell me what you see," "Find all the food items")	Requires initiation and organized visual search strategies, persistence
Distinctive features	Readily apparent (e.g., boxes, jars, cans are different sizes, with clear labels facing the front)	Obscure or partially hidden features (e.g., jars, bottles are rotated and at different angles)	Greater part–whole synthesis, visual attention. More difficult to pick up critical features and recognize items; increased likelihood of misperception
Degree of detail	Little to no detail Items differ widely in color, shape, type (cans, boxes, jars)	Fine detail; several different types of items that are the same color, type, or shape item	Greater demands on visual acuity, scanning, and attention
Contrast	High contrast (e.g., silver can with red label)	Low contrast (e.g., same shape and color cans or boxes that differ only in writing on label)	Harder to determine where one item ends and another begins; greater demands on visual acuity and selective attention
Background	Solid shelf liner-nonpatterned	Shelf is lined with distracting patterned design	Greater selective attention
Context	Within context (e.g., finding item in kitchen while making breakfast)	Outside of context (e.g., food item, in therapy area)	Greater visual attention to critical features less cues for recognition
Amount	Less than 8 items are presented at any one time	15–25 items are presented simultaneously	Greater demands on selective attention and strategies to keep track of visual stimuli
Arrangement	Organized into predictable format (e.g., horizontal rows) with items spread apart	Randomly scattered or overlapping so that some features of objects are partially obscured items close together	Greater demands on saccadic eye movements, part–whole synthesis, strategies to keep track of visual stimuli, ability to change search pattern

Note. Adapted from "Cognitive–Perceptual Retraining and Rehabilitation," J. P. Toglia, 2003. In E. B. Crepeau, E. S. Cohn, & B. A. B. Schell (Eds.), *Willard & Spackman's Occupational Therapy* (10th ed., p. 621). Philadelphia: Lippincott Williams & Wilkins. Copyright © 2003 by Lippincott Williams & Wilkins. Adapted with permission.

on a visual search task can occur for many reasons. The extent to which cognitive perceptual symptoms are observed depends on the activity demands. A person may be able to quickly locate one object out of 10 familiar objects lined up on a shelf but may be unable to accurately locate target symbols on a detailed map. Both require visual search skills, but the demands of the activities and the additional activity characteristics such as the body alignment, positioning, and active movement patterns also can influence the selection of different processing strategies (Abreu & Toglia, 1987). By analyzing the demands of an activity, one can understand the conditions that cause information processing to break down. This contrasts to the deficit specific approach, in which the deficit is defined by the task. Thus, if the client cannot do a categorization task or a figure ground task he or she is assumed to have a categorization or figure ground deficit. The activity parameters that influence performance are not analyzed.

In addition to influencing the ability to process information, characteristics of an activity also can influence the ability to transfer learning. Transfer of learning occurs easily if two activities share physical characteristics or look nearly the same. On the other hand, transfer of learning is most challenging in situations that require the same underlying skills but look physically different than the original learning situation (Glick & Holyoak, 1987; Resing & Roth-Van der Werf, 2002). This indicates that activities and environments that are gradually changed in superficial appearance may facilitate the ability to transfer learning to multiple situations.

Environmental Factors

Environmental factors such as the social, physical, and cultural aspects of an environment can influence a person's ability to process information.

The social environment has occupied a central place in some theories of cognitive development and includes the people with whom the person interacts (Vygotsky, 1978). Vygotsky (1978) and Feuerstein (1979) have argued that much of learning and higher cognitive skills are mediated through social interaction. For example, in child development an experienced adult guides the child through problem-solving activities and structures the child's learning environment by selecting, focusing, and organizing incoming stimuli. Social interactions can transform or mediate incoming information either to enhance or impede information processing (Jensen & Feuerstein, 1987). An adult may speak rapidly and present the child with

complex directions to a task. The child may become overwhelmed by the information and withdraw or refuse to participate. Another adult may present the same information in a slow, simplified, and structured manner, and the child may readily participate in the task. In one case, information processing is inhibited, whereas in the other case, it is enhanced.

Mediation can help the learner attend to information that is relevant, extract meanings, make connections, and deepen experiences. Feuerstein has provided guidelines for effective mediation and has described the types of interactions that facilitate change (Feuerstein & Falik, 2004). When another person successfully mediates or structures incoming information, the person may begin to internalize this external structuring and adopt regulatory activities on his or her own (Brown & Ferrara, 1985). Intervention may involve gradually reducing external guidance and support so that the person learns to cue himself or herself. This highlights the importance of including significant others within the rehabilitation program and guiding them in use of effective mediation techniques. Other people can support and enhance the processing of information in a way that facilitates learning and performance.

Vygotsky (1978) described the distance between the level of a child's unaided performance and the level that can be accomplished through guidance or collaboration with a more knowledgeable participant as the *zone of proximal development*. Solving tasks with the assistance of a more knowledgeable person creates the zone of proximal development by tapping processes that "will mature tomorrow but are in the embryonic state" (p. 86). The level of performance the child can reach unaided characterizes the cognitive skills that have already developed, whereas the zone of proximal development characterizes cognitive skills that are in the developmental stage (Brown & French, 1979). Vygotsky (1978) and Feuerstein's (1979) theories imply that what an individual can accomplish with mediation or guidance from a more capable peer indicates the person's learning potential. This concept has direct implications for assessment and treatment of people with brain injury. It has been suggested that the zone of proximal development be called the *zone of rehabilitation potential* and used as a guiding principle in rehabilitation (Cicerone & Tupper, 1986). This zone is hypothesized to reflect the client's region of potential restoration of function or the degree of cerebral plasticity (Baltes et al., 1992, 1995).

In addition to the way that others can support information processing through cues, guidance, and structuring of information, the social environment also includes emotional support from others. Close family and social supports can provide a source of motivation, minimize emotional consequences of an illness or injury, enhance the ability to cope, and positively influence long-term outcome (Bhogal, Teasell, Foley, & Speechley, 2003). It is important that close relatives understand the nature of cognitive symptoms and are taught strategies to help them. Differences in perspectives between the client and significant others may result from awareness limitation. This can result in misunderstandings and tensions in relationships that can reduce emotional support. It is important therefore to include significant others in the early stages of treatment.

The cultural environment involves the beliefs, values, and expectations accepted by the person's cultural group. Culture influences the expression of emotion, views about personal independence, perceived role of the family, expectations of intervention, and what a person believes about illness and its meaning (Sohlberg & Mateer, 2001). It also influences the level of support that one receives at home or within the community. The physical environment includes the materials and objects that surround an individual. Familiar physical and cultural environments provide contextual cues that facilitate the access of previous knowledge and skills and guide in the selection and processing of new information (Abreu & Toglia, 1987).

Features of the physical context, such as the degree of auditory and visual distractions and the organization and arrangement of objects, can influence occupational performance. For example, a client may be asked to make cereal and toast for breakfast. In one situation, the kitchen may be familiar, quiet, and neatly organized. The refrigerator and cabinets may have only a few items on each shelf and the counter may contain only a toaster oven. In another situation, the kitchen may be unfamiliar, cluttered, and disorganized. The refrigerator and cabinets may be visually overcrowded with a large assortment of items. The counter may contain several appliances and unfamiliar gadgets. In addition, auditory distractions such as a ringing telephone, sirens, and busy traffic from the street may be present. Although the activity and goal remain the same, the strategies needed to perform the task are very different. In the latter example, the physical environment places greater demands on attention, visual discrimination, ability to keep track of information, and organization. The abilities of the client need to be matched with the demands of both the activity and the environment.

Summary of the Dynamic Model of Cognition

In this model, processing strategies and self-awareness represent core aspects of cognitive function that interact dynamically with external factors such as the activity and environment (social, physical, cultural) as well as with other internal variables (structural capacity, personal context). In some situations, performance is influenced most by personal factors such as the person's personality, emotions, self-awareness, or strategy use. In other situations, performance can be enhanced or impeded by manipulating external aspects of the activity or environment. Cognition and performance changes with experiences and the interaction among the person, activity, and environment (Bransford et al., 1986; Feuerstein & Falik, 2004; Lidz, 1987). The results of performance can restructure one's perceptions regarding performance and abilities. To understand cognitive function and occupational performance, one needs to analyze the interaction among person, activity, and environment. If the activity and environmental demands change, the type of cognitive strategies needed for efficient performance changes as well. Optimal performance is observed when there is a match between all three variables. Assessment and treatment reflect this dynamic view of cognition.

REDEFINING COGNITIVE FUNCTION AND DYSFUNCTION

Cognitive function, as previously described, requires the ability to receive, elaborate, and monitor incoming information. It involves the ability to flexibly use and apply information across task boundaries (Lidz, 1987). Cognitive problems reflect a reduced capacity to acquire and use new information. *Cognitive dysfunction* can be summarized as representing core deficiencies in (a) the ability to select and use efficient processing strategies to organize and structure incoming information; (b) the ability to anticipate, monitor, and verify the accuracy of performance; (c) the ability to access previous knowledge when needed; and (d) flexible application of knowledge and skills to a variety of situations (Toglia, 1991). These impairments may be observed in localized areas such as in visual processing, or they may exist regardless of the modality involved. Deficient functions are not completely absent but represent areas of weakness and vulnerability (Groveman, Brown, & Miller, 1985). The extent to which these deficiencies are observed depends on the activity demands (e.g., number of stimuli, complexity, and familiarity), the environment, and the person's characteristics (emotional status, motivation, personality). For example, a client's tendency to overfocus on irrelevant details or recognize and anticipate errors may emerge only under certain activities and environmental conditions. The underlying processes and behaviors that are interfering with the client's performance in the majority of tasks are the components that are analyzed during assessment and targeted as priorities for treatment.

This approach emphasizes the global capacities of cognition. Inefficient use or limits in information-processing resources underlie many cognitive symptoms. Cognitive dysfunction is conceptualized in terms of deficiencies in processing strategies and self-monitoring skills rather than by deficits in specific cognitive skills (Toglia, 1993b). People with brain injury often display inflexible and inefficient strategy use. There is a failure to initiate and apply self-regulatory or monitoring behaviors such as anticipating, monitoring, checking, and revising solutions. Difficulties in a wide range of attention, memory, visual-processing, and problem-solving tasks may reflect the same underlying behavior or inefficient strategy. For example, a tendency to overfocus on irrelevant details may interfere with a memory task, a visual-processing task, and a problem-solving task. The common behaviors that interfere with performance on several different tasks are analyzed rather than impairments in specific cognitive skills. In addition, the activity parameters and the environmental characteristics that increase and decrease cognitive perceptual symptoms during occupational performance are specified when describing cognitive dysfunction.

Cognitive dysfunction can affect functioning in all spheres of life: social and interpersonal, work, leisure, and daily living. Occupational activities may be performed inefficiently. The client may be unable to decide what to attend to first, how to prioritize, or how to break the task into steps. Excessive time may be spent processing nonessential details, and the client may have difficulty keeping track of previous events or associating related information (Toglia & Golisz, 1990). In social situations, cognitive dysfunction may interfere with the person's ability to accurately take in and integrate all parts of a situation. The client may have decreased awareness of another person's verbal and nonverbal reactions and may have difficulty following conversations. His or her behavior may, therefore, be inappropriate to the context (Toglia & Golisz, 1990). In addition, difficulty in shifting one's attention or viewing information from different perspectives may interfere with the ability to compromise and understand another person's point of view. Diminished social skills result in

social isolation and depression that further inhibits cognitive functioning (Fine, 1993).

ASSESSMENT

In this approach, the ability to learn and generalize information is central to the concept of cognition. Assessment, therefore, emphasizes the processes of change and learning and uses a dynamic approach (Lidz & Elliot, 2000). In this model, self-awareness and processing strategies are described as core aspects of cognition that are modifiable and critical to understanding occupational performance. Therefore, assessment of people with cognitive impairments emphasizes both self-awareness and use of processing strategies. At the same time, the internal and external variables that modify or influence the expression of cognitive abilities and symptoms are addressed. This includes the context of the person such as personality characteristics and lifestyle and external influences such as the demands of the activity and environment. An observed problem in occupational performance is the result of imbalances among person, activity, and environmental variables.

Personal Context

An important step in assessment is gaining an understanding of the personal context of the client, including the client's premorbid personality characteristics, beliefs, valued occupations, and previous lifestyle. This information can be gathered through questionnaires and interviews of the client or a relative, samples of previous work, and asking the client or relative to complete a schedule that indicates a typical week of activities and routines before the injury or illness as well as presently. For example, How does the client describe his or her personality? Lifestyle? Typical routines? How has the injury or illness affected the client's life?

Different routines, occupations, and lifestyles require different levels of cognitive skills. Cognitive limitations are best understood within the context of a person's life. The same cognitive impairments may affect two people's daily lives very differently, depending on their previous lifestyle. For example, subtle deficits in problem solving and reasoning may be devastating for a lawyer but may minimally affect the life of an elderly person who lives in a suburban retirement community. In addition, cognitive abilities may be closely associated with one's sense of self and personality. If what one perceives as a cognitive strength suddenly becomes one's greatest liability, it may be difficult for the person to accept. Intervention involves helping a person adjust to the cognitive changes that have occurred. This requires understanding and acknowledging the person's previous cognitive style and strengths.

Occupational Performance

Assessment includes gaining an understanding of the daily occupations and environments that the person previously functioned in as well as assessing current functional abilities. In many situations, the person may not have had the opportunity to resume normal daily routines and occupations, so the person as well as his or her relatives may not be fully aware of functional capabilities and limitations. This is particularly true if the person is in an inpatient setting or has not yet returned to his or her normal living situation. Cognitive impairments can be hidden and not readily observed by others (Golisz & Toglia, 2003). Therefore, it is essential to observe the person's performance in a range of familiar and unfamiliar activities and environments. If the person does not exhibit any cognitive symptoms within basic ADL skills, it is important to assess higher-level IADL skills, social skills, and work-related skills under unstructured situations. Independence in the community requires the ability to deal with unfamiliar, novel, and unpredictable situations.

Cognitive impairments may easily be missed in a structured clinical situation or within the narrow range of activities typically included in ADL scales. Unanticipated obstacles and problems need to be incorporated into a range of situations. The activities should require that the person make decisions and choices, initiate, plan and solve problems, and generate alternative methods. Distractions such as a radio playing in the background and the telephone intermittently ringing may need to be included to simulate the person's typical environment. For example, a person with brain injury may be able to make lunch without any difficulty if he is presented with all the items he needs on the table within a quiet environment. The same person, however, may show a tendency to become unorganized, get easily sidetracked, and lose track of information if the phone is ringing and interrupting the activity simultaneously or if he is provided with different instructions and told, "You can make whatever you would like for lunch. The refrigerator is filled with food."

The dynamic interactional model indicates that assessment of occupational performance needs to carefully consider the conditions of the activity and environment. It is not as simple as observing the quantity of assistance that the person needs to make lunch or get dressed. The conditions under which the activity is performed need to be specified. Occupational performance in a person with cognitive impairments can vary considerably under different conditions. Similarly, the person's social interactions across a range of natural contexts including meal time, talking to others while in the waiting room, and interacting with relatives should be observed. If difficulties in functioning or relationships are observed or reported, further assessment is necessary to understand why the difficulties are occurring and to obtain information that can guide intervention.

Self-Awareness

The client's views of his or her current abilities and limitations need to be explored in an in-depth manner, as self-knowledge and perceptions influence strategy use, activity choices, and performance. It also directly influences choices regarding the best approach to intervention. For example, What areas of functioning is the client most concerned with? Does the client perceive any changes in functioning? In attention, memory, thinking? Or in the ability to relate to others? What things does the client want to be able to do with less effort or less assistance?

Because awareness or clear self-knowledge of abilities is frequently limited following brain injury, the client's perceptions of performance need to be compared with a significant other's or clinician's direct observations of performance. The most commonly used method of assessing self-awareness involves measuring the discrepancy between the client's ratings of abilities and that of a relative (Sherer, Boake, et al., 1998). Other methods of assessing awareness include direct clinician rating and judgment of the client's awareness in response to questions. Several rating scales have been designed to measure awareness. They include the Self-Awareness Deficit Interview (Fleming, Strong, & Ashton, 1996), the Awareness Questionnaire (Sherer, Bergloff, Boake, High, & Levin, 1998), and the Patient Competency Rating Form (Prigatano, 1986).

It should be kept in mind, however, that these tools examine knowledge and perceptions of abilities outside the context of an activity. Awareness varies under different conditions. For example, people with brain injury tend to show greater unawareness if questions are open ended, as compared to specifically worded questions (Sherer, Boake, et al., 1998). Furthermore, response to awareness questions varies according to the timing of questions or whether questions are asked before or after an activity experience. Finally, awareness varies across different activities and contexts and can emerge with the experience of engaging in an activity (Abreu et al., 2001; Tham et al., 2000). Changes in awareness that may occur with activity experiences, guidance, or feedback are important to observe, as this information has implications for intervention.

Dynamic Assessment of Cognitive Modifiability

This model views cognition from a dynamic rather than a static perspective. In other words, cognitive abilities are not viewed as fixed traits or as a stable hierarchical set of subskills. Cognition is viewed as modifiable and as a process of ongoing learning and change that takes place with experience. It is important to recognize that this view of cognition is incompatible with traditional psychometrics that is the foundation for standardized tests. Traditional psychometrics is based on the assumption that abilities are fixed. Standardized tests expect performance to be stable and consistent. Changes that occur within a test condition are viewed as error that reduces reliability (Feuerstein & Feuerstein, 2001; Sternberg & Grigorenko, 2002). Measurement of cognitive impairments such as cognitive screening instruments and neuropsychological tests are based on traditional psychometric models. The end product of performance is emphasized. The objective of static assessments is to identify and quantify cognitive impairments. This information may be helpful for diagnosis, monitoring progress, discharge planning, and client or caregiver education regarding expected behaviors; however, it is limited in providing guidance for intervention (Toglia, 1989a). Table 2.4 summarizes and contrasts the characteristics of static and dynamic assessment. The different assessment approaches reflect differences in the purposes of assessment as well as in the perspectives of cognition.

Dynamic assessment offers a framework for taking the dynamic perspective of cognition into consideration rather than assuming that abilities are stable. Dynamic assessment assumes that changes and learning take place with task experience. Assessment focuses on change and examines what, how, and why change occurs. It requires a different way of thinking about assessment and the abilities that are being measured (Sternberg & Grigorenko, 2002). Dynamic methods focus on examining changes in performance with cues, mediation, feedback, or task alterations (Lidz & Elliot, 2000). They are designed to provide an estimate of cognitive modifiability or learning potential. In essence, the goal of dynamic assessment is "to see whether and how the participant will change if an opportunity is provided" (Sternberg & Grigorenko, 2002, p. 30). In essence, dynamic assessment provides a small snapshot of the person's response to intervention. It examines whether

T A B L E 2 . 4 . Comparison of Static and Dynamic Assessment Methods

	Static	Dynamic
Key characteristics	Quantitative	Qualitative but goes beyond observing the process and seeks to modify performance
	Identification of impairments	
	Degree of severity	
	Comparison to norm	
	Establishes a baseline	Focuses on the process of change
	Focuses on identifying deficits	Focuses on the best or optimal performance
	Examines independent performance	Examines changes with guided assistance or task alterations
	Derived from psychometrics	Derived from cognitive psychology theories (Vygotsky, Feuerstein)
Questions answered	Is there a problem?	Can performance be facilitated or changed?
	What is the problem?	
	What is the severity of the problem?	What cues or task alterations increase or decrease symptoms?

performance can be influenced through guided cues, demonstration of strategies, or restructuring the activity. Dynamic assessment is naturally linked with intervention.

In dynamic assessment, it is assumed that examination of performance with guided assistance provides a more comprehensive picture of the range of performance capabilities than independent performance. Assessment focuses on discovering the person's best performance or maximum level of function rather than identifying the severity of dysfunction. It taps into weakened skills that lie beneath the surface but have the potential for function. Assessment within the zone of proximal development has been thought to discriminate differences in abilities not identified using conventional methods (Brown & Ferrara, 1985; Brown & French, 1979).

Dynamic assessment does not refer to a specific procedure or technique but is a generic term that describes a wide range of methods. For example, dynamic assessments differ in the nature of tasks used, standardization of procedures, type of assistance provided, extent of the examiner–examinee interaction, length of time, and the methods used to measure responsiveness to instruction or change (Grigorenko & Sternberg, 1998; Lidz & Elliot, 2000). Despite these methodological differences, there is a core emphasis on providing guided assistance to facilitate changes in performance. This information is directly related to choosing and planning interventions.

The majority of dynamic assessment research has been conducted with children who have developmental disabilities or learning disorders (Hessels-Schlatter, 2002; Lauchlan & Elliot, 2001). There have been preliminary investigations in adults who have schizophrenia (Wiedl, 1999; Wiedl, Schoettke, & Garcia, 2001), elderly people with Alzheimer's disease (Baltes et al., 1995; Fernandez-Ballesteros, Zamarron, Tarraga, Moya, & Iniguez, 2003), brain injury (Haywood & Miller, 2003; Kolakowsky, 1998), and stroke (Kline, 2000; Toglia, 2004). More recently, the literature within the field of dynamic assessment has expanded considerably in quantity and in the range of applications. The majority of studies have found that dynamic assessment can produce statistically significant improvements in performance as compared to control groups (Haywood & Tzuriel, 2002; Swanson & Lussier, 2001) and even greater improvements in comparison to people who have similar static baseline scores or are within the same diagnostic category. Evidence across different populations indicates that dynamic assessment measures information that is unique and different than that of static assessment (Elliott, 2003). The extent to which dynamic assessment taps a separate construct of "cognitive modifiability" is an area that requires further investigation. Preliminary studies have supported use of dynamic assessment in the prediction of rehabilitation potential for people with chronic schizophrenia (Wiedl, 1999; Wiedl

et al., 2001; Wiedl, Wienobst, & Schoettke, 2001). Investigation of dynamic assessment with adults, however, is only in the preliminary stages.

Dynamic assessment as used within the framework of the dynamic interactional model of cognition consists of three components: (a) investigating self-perceptions of abilities prior to the task, (b) facilitating change in performance, and (c) investigating self-perceptions of performance and strategy use after the task. These components of dynamic assessment are summarized in Figure 2.2 and described below.

Self-Perceptions Prior to Task

Prior to activity performance, the client is asked general questions about their perceptions of their abilities: for example, Do you think your ability to do this sort of activity has changed in any way? In addition, the client can be asked to specifically rate perceived difficulty of an activity or anticipate or predict his performance. Sample items from an awareness interview that has been tested with adults who have had a right cerebrovascular accident and unilateral neglect is illustrated in Figure 2.3.

Facilitating Changes in Performance

If the client has difficulty during a task, the clinician attempts to facilitate performance either by providing a series of cues or teaching strategies or by reducing the demands of the activity. A sample sequence of graded cues used in a cancellation task to facilitate attention to the left side is presented in Table 2.5. Performance also may be facilitated by gradually changing one component of the

FIGURE 2.2. Components of dynamic assessment.

1. **Self-Perceptions of Performance and Abilities Prior to Task**
   - General questioning
   - Prediction

2. **Facilitating Changes in Performance**
   - Examining carryover from one item to the next (transfer of learning)

   → Cues or Strategy Teaching

   → Changes in Task Parameters

3. **Self-Perceptions of Performance During and After Task**
   - General questioning
   - Estimation
   - Strategy investigation

FIGURE 2.3. Sample items from unilateral neglect awareness interview.

General and Specific Questions Asked Before and After an Activity Experience

Since Your Stroke, Do You Experience	Not at All 1	A Little 2	Somewhat 3	A Lot 4
Difficulty locating, finding or seeing everything around you?	☐	☐	☐	☐
Difficulty finding all the items on tables, shelves, closets, drawers, or counters?	☐	☐	☐	☐
A tendency to miss things on the left side?	☐	☐	☐	☐
A tendency to miss numbers, letters, or words on the left side?	☐	☐	☐	☐
To what extent are any difficulties in finding or seeing things on the left side interfering with your overall ability to function?	☐	☐	☐	☐

Specific Prediction of Reading

I am going to ask you to read this paragraph. Do you think you will have any difficulty?
☐ I will not have any difficulties. ☐ I think I may have some difficulties. ☐ I am sure that I will have difficulties.

What kind of difficulty do you think you will have?

Do you think you will miss any words?
☐ No. ☐ I could miss a few words—less than 25%. ☐ I could miss several—up to one-half.
☐ I could miss many words—more than one-half.

After Task: Estimation of Performance (General and Specific Questioning)

How did you do on this task?
☐ I did not have any difficulties. ☐ I think I may have had some difficulties. ☐ I am sure that I had difficulties.

Do you think you would have performed any differently on this task before your stroke/injury?
☐ Yes   ☐ No

What was your accuracy on this task?
☐ I did not miss any words or numbers. ☐ I may have missed a few words—less than 25%. ☐ I may have missed up to one-half.
☐ I may have missed many words or numbers—more than one-half.

Note. Adapted from "The Multicontext Approach to Cognitive Rehabilitation," by J. P. Toglia, June, 1996 [Supplement manual to workshop conducted at New York Hospital, New York].

TABLE 2.5. Sample Graded Cue Sequence

Rationale	Example of Cues
Check and verify answer	Are you sure you found all the letter *A*s?
General feedback	There are still some left. Can you find them?
Specific feedback	There are still some on the left side.
Provide alternative approach	Try, beginning here. Go slower, and use your finger to point to each letter.
Task modification	Change one task parameter (e.g., number of items on the page are reduced; bright red line is placed in the left margin).

Note. From "The Multicontext Approach to Awareness, Memory, and Executive Function Impairments," by J. P. Toglia, 2003 [Supplement manual to workshops conducted at various locations].

activity at a time (e.g., decreasing the number of items or simplifying the instructions) rather than providing verbal cues. If a person's initial attempt at a task is completely unsuccessful (no partially accurate responses) activity modifications may be more appropriate rather than cues. An alternative method consists of teaching a person a strategy, providing feedback on strategy use, and observing the ability to apply the strategy across different tasks. In either case, alternative forms of the same task should be provided to examine the ability to transfer the effects of learning.

Initially, I used a hierarchical sequence of cues or hints (Table 2.5) during dynamic assessment. Currently, my emphasis has begun to shift to teaching strategies during assessment. This requires use of assessment tasks that provide opportunity to repeatedly apply what has been learned across different tasks so that patterns of change and transfer of learning can be directly examined. Some have argued that the use of strategies has the advantage of clearly identifying what is being trained and provides a concrete way to observe the effects of training (Klauer, 2002). Studies that include strategy training and feedback with children have produced larger effect sizes than those focusing on coaching or progressive hints (Swanson & Lussier, 2001).

Self-Perceptions of Performance During and After the Task

Examination of the client's perception of his or her performance, including the ability to recognize errors, can occur during an activity, after an activity component, or after the entire activity. Questions can be open-ended such as, How satisfied are you with your ability to do this activity? Do you think your ability to do this type of activity has changed in any way? How? Did you run into any difficulty as you were doing this activity? Tell me why. Why do you think you may have originally missed some of the information? Questions also can be structured by asking the client to rate the difficulty of a task (not difficult, slightly difficult, difficult, very difficult) or asking the client to estimate his or her score or performance on a rating scale. Typically, a combination of structured and unstructured questions is recommended. It is important for the clinician to compare responses with the same types of questions before, during, and after performance to examine any changes in awareness that may occur with activity experience (see Figure 2.3).

Strategy investigation involves probing the person's responses without suggesting the answers. For example, the person may be asked to explain why he or she chose a particular answer or approached an activity in a particular way: Tell me how you went about solving this problem; Tell me how you know these items are the same; Tell me how you kept track of everything that you needed to do. I noticed that you began to use your finger in the midst of the task; why do you think you did that? In addition, techniques such as reflection or repeating the client's answer may be used (Toglia, 1989a).

Dynamic assessment methods can be applied to a wide range of specific tasks to provide an in-depth snapshot of learning and response to intervention (Embretson, 1987; Toglia, 1989b). For example, dynamic assessment methods have been used with sorting tasks, visual search tasks, copying designs, and memory tasks. The following are examples of different types of dynamic assessment that have been developed for the adult who has brain injury. Some of the assessments also have been piloted with clients with chronic schizophrenia. The assessments vary in the methods used to facilitate and examine change. Each

assessment was developed through videotape analysis of clients performing tasks with nonstandardized cues and questions. From the videotape analysis, guidelines and sequences of cues and questioning were developed.

Four examples—the Contextual Memory Test (CMT; Toglia, 1993a), the Toglia Category Test (TCA), deductive reasoning tests (Toglia, 1994), and the Dynamic Object Search Task—are presented in the following section. Most of the dynamic assessments described require use of language skills; however, the principles of dynamic assessment can easily be adapted for clients with aphasia by using tactile or visual cues. An example of the application of dynamic assessment principles to functional tasks and people who have aphasia and apraxia is described below.

EXAMPLES OF DYNAMIC INTERACTIONAL ASSESSMENT

Contextual Memory Test

The Contextual Memory Test (CMT; Toglia, 1993a) investigates awareness of memory capacity, recall performance, and strategy use. The test begins by asking the client general questions about his or her memory functioning and requiring the client to predict his or her score. The person is then asked to study a picture card containing 20 line drawings of items for 90 seconds. The pictures are either related to a restaurant theme or a morning theme. In part I, the person is not told that the items pictured on the card are related to a theme (see Figure 2.4). The person is asked to recall the items immediately after presentation and then again after 15–20 minutes. After immediate recall, the person is asked to estimate his or her performance, and the use of strategies is probed with standard questions. Figure 2.4 presents an illustration of the morning scene as well as sample questions that are used to probe awareness and strategy use.

If the person demonstrates poor recall and poor strategy use in part I, part II is administered. Part II involves repeating the recall section with an equivalent form of the test. The major difference between part I and II is that the instructions for the test in part II provide information on the theme or context of the pictures. The purpose is to determine whether recall performance can be influenced by giving the person a cue to help him or her attend to the overall theme or background context. Contextual information can enhance the ability to categorize items and remember. If recall performance is not facilitated with cues, then recognition memory may be tested by presenting 40 cards one at a time and asking the individual to choose the target stimulus items (Toglia, 1993a).

FIGURE 2.4. Sample items from the Contextual Memory Test.

Awareness and Strategy Questions	Morning Scene

Prior to the task:

Have you noticed any changes in your memory?

If you studied 20 objects, for a minute and a half, how many do you think you would be able to remember?

After the task:

How difficult was this task for you?

Estimate the number of objects that you remembered.

When you were studying the information, what did you do to help you remember?

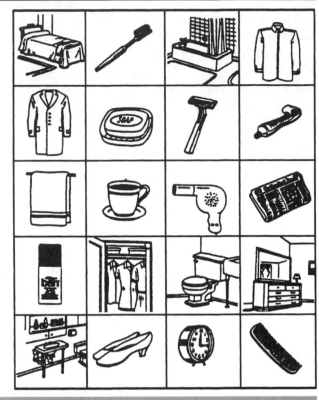

Note. From Toglia, J. P. (1993). *The Contextual Memory Test.* San Antonio, TX: Psychological Corporation. Copyright © 1993, Joan Toglia. Reprinted with permission.

The CMT has both static and dynamic qualities. Part I may be used alone to screen individuals for memory impairments. Part II provides a dynamic component to the assessment. One component of the activity (instructions) is changed to induce deeper processing and encoding of material. Assessment examines the effectiveness of a cue that emphasizes attention to the overall context. If contextual cues are effective, it implies that helping the person to initially attend to and process the overall context and environment of a situation, prior to attending to the specifics, may be helpful. Contextual information is normally processed automatically and provides a framework for organizing and remembering information; however, some people with brain injury may not automatically process contextual information. A person can have difficulty on the CMT for a variety of reasons. For example, poor recall can be related to difficulty in shifting visual attention to different items, tendency to overfocus on irrelevant details, poor attention span, decreased ability to recognize categories or create relationships and associations among items, and decreased ability to initiate active strategy use. The order of recall as well as the response to strategy investigation questions and cues provided in part II provide

insight into the underlying difficulties. Performance is analyzed by looking at the combination of results in the areas of awareness, recall, and strategy use. The test manual describes how different patterns of performance provide different implications for treatment (Toglia, 1993a).

Reliability and validity studies have been conducted on the CMT with people who have brain injury and are described in the test manual. Concurrent validity was established by examining the correlation between the recall scores of the CMT and the Rivermead Behavioral Memory Test (Wilson, Cockburn, & Baddley, 1985). Normative data have been collected on 375 adults in the New York area ranging in age from 18–86 years, with a mean age of 46. In addition, Josman and Hartman-Maier (2000) translated the test in Hebrew and collected normative data on 217 adults in Israel, ages 18–86. This study supported use of the CMT in clinical practice and provided recommendations regarding specific items that may be more difficult due to issues of cultural relevance.

The CMT has been studied in elderly people with and without Alzheimer's disease (Gil & Josman, 2001) as well as children with and without brain injury (Josman, Berney, & Jarus, 2000b). Results support the clinical usefulness and discriminant validity of the CMT in both of these populations. In addition Kizony and Katz (2002) found that visual contextual memory in people with stroke was moderately related to instrumental activities of daily living (IADL) performance. The immediate recall score of the CMT demonstrated one of the strongest correlations ($r = .59$) to Instrumental Activities of Daily Living as compared to other standardized cognitive measures.

Performance of 112 people with brain injury was compared with people without brain injury on awareness measures of the CMT. There were significant differences in both the direction and magnitude of predicted scores between people with and without brain injury. Individuals without brain injury tended to underestimate their scores by 1 or 2 items. People with brain injury tended to overestimate their actual scores by an average of 6 items. An interesting finding was that the actual predictions of those with brain injury were similar to the scores that individuals without brain injury predicted. Thus, it seems that people with brain injury tend to estimate their abilities on the basis of their premorbid capacities (Toglia, 1993a). A significant difference between predicted scores and actual recall performance also was noted between elderly people and those with Alzheimer's disease (Gil & Josman, 2001).

Responses to different aspects of awareness questions were examined. The results support the hypothesis that different aspects of awareness may be tapped by differences in the type and timing of the questions. For example, the correlation between general awareness questions and the ability to predict one's memory score was low, indicating little relationship between the two scores. The ability to generally acknowledge a memory problem does not seem to be related to the ability to predict memory capacity. Many clients readily admitted to and described memory problems but could not use this knowledge to accurately estimate the difficulty of a task or anticipate problems. In addition, there was little relationship between responses prior to the memory task and responses after the memory task, indicating that the questions asked before and after a task may measure different aspects of awareness. The results support the premise that awareness can be differentiated by systematic and objective assessment (Toglia, 1993a).

Responses to awareness questions provide important implications for treatment. For example, a person who has a tendency to considerably overestimate his or her score may have difficulty initiating memory compensatory techniques because he or she may be unable to anticipate when they might be needed. On the other hand, those who show good prediction scores may be good candidates for training in memory compensatory strategies (Toglia, 1993a).

Toglia Category Assessment

The Toglia Category Assessment (TCA) was designed to examine the ability to establish categories or switch conceptual sets (Toglia, 1994). Awareness is investigated by asking the client standard questions designed to investigate awareness before and after task performance. The test uses 18 plastic utensils that can be sorted according to size (small or large), color (red, yellow, and green), and utensil type (knife, fork, or spoon). The examiner asks the client to sort the 18 utensils into different groups so that the items in one group are different in one way from those of the other groups. Once the client correctly classifies the items according to one attribute (size, color, or type), he or she is then asked to sort the items again in a different way and then again in a third way. Strategy use is investigated by asking the client to explain how the groups are different after each classification. A sequence of cues is provided if the client has difficulty. The cues are semi-structured. They are organized into categories so that the examiner can choose the cue within a category that fits the client's needs (Toglia, 1994). Use of the cues helps to differentiate clients and their underlying problems. A person can have difficulty with the TCA for a variety of reasons, such as a tendency to become stuck or perseverative in one category or solution, to lose track of the sorting principle or categories, to use a concrete approach such as only grouping utensils according to use or function, or to take a disorganized approach to searching and sorting.

For example, one client with brain injury sorted the utensils into spoons, forks, and knives. When asked to sort the utensils a different way, the client shuffled the utensils around but ended up with the same three categories. Again the procedure was repeated, and the client did the same thing. However, when he was cued to attend to the individual attributes (size and color), he immediately sorted them in different ways. This indicated that the client's underlying problem was a tendency to become stuck in one response. Another client was able to sort the utensils into two separate groups (first color and then type of utensil) but could not think of a third way to sort them. Although he was provided with maximum cues, the client insisted there were only the two ways to sort the utensils and stated "size was not a good category." These two clients' responses to cues provide differential implications for treatment that are described in the test manual (Toglia, 1994).

The test results are interpreted by examining responses to awareness questions in combination with the person's responsiveness to cues. The extent that awareness can be facilitated during task performance and the person's ability to benefit from cues also are analyzed.

Josman (1999) established the reliability and validity of the TCA in a sample of 35 adults with brain injury and 35 adults with chronic schizophrenia. Josman (1993) also investigated the ability to estimate performance immediately following the tasks and found that there was a significant difference between the mean awareness scores of the brain-injured and psychiatric populations. These results suggest that awareness questions may be useful in differentiating among populations. She also found that people with brain injury who estimated that the task would be easy tended to have more difficulty than those who estimated that the test was hard. This is consistent with other studies that have found that a failure to recognize difficulty of a task associated with poorer task performance. Similarly, a study with children indicated that estimation of performance was significantly correlated with actual performance (Josman et al., 2000a).

The TCA also has been studied in the pediatric population. Josman and Jarus (2001) collected normative data on 235 typically developing children, ranging from age 5–11 years. In addition, the use of the TCA was explored with 30 children with severe brain injury and 30 children without neurological impairments, ages 8–14 years (Josman et al., 2000a). The results of these studies support the validity of the TCA with children.

Deductive Reasoning Test

The TCA utensils also may be used to dynamically assess deductive reasoning. In using the test for deductive reasoning, a question game is used to investigate the ability to formulate and test different hypotheses, keep track of previous responses, and modify hypotheses on the basis of feedback. In this task the examiner tells the client that he or she has to determine which utensil the examiner is thinking of, with the least amount of guessing and the fewest number of questions as possible. The client has to ask questions that can be answered as "yes" or "no." The examiner does not actually think of an item but answers "no" to all the questions (whenever possible) until there is only one possibility left. The answer is obtainable with 5 questions if 18 utensils of different colors (red, yellow, green), size (big, small), and type (fork, spoon, knife) are used. For example, if the following 5 questions are asked, the answer can be easily deduced: "Is it red? yellow? spoon? fork? small?" The answer must be a green, large knife. If the client does not solve the problem with 5 questions, another trial is given, with a maximum of up to 3 trials. The examiner gives a standard sequence of prompts when the client is unable to solve the problem with 4 questions.

Some people with brain injury tend to approach this task concretely, using single-item questions. For example, two clients asked about each utensil, one by one: "Is it this fork?" "Is it this spoon?" When cued to narrow down the questions, one client immediately generated an efficient set of questions. The other client required maximum cues and still could not generate a different set of questions. In both cases the client had the same initial baseline response, but again, there were significant differences in the ability to benefit from feedback and use cues to generate a more efficient strategy. These differences have different implications for treatment planning. In one case, the client requires only a general cue to think of an alternate approach to the task. In the other case, treatment needs to focus on helping the client to attend to and discriminate among the various attributes before attempting to solve a problem.

The interrater reliability and discriminant validity of the deductive reasoning test was established in a sample of 42 people with brain injury and 51 people without disabilities ranging in age from 18–84 years (Goverover & Hinojosa, 2004). In addition, Goverover and Hinojosa (2002) found that deductive reasoning and categorization scores of the TCA contributed to 71.4% of the variance in predicting IADL as measured by the Observed Tasks of Daily Living. The deductive reasoning scores were found to be a stronger predictor of IADL performance. However, the TCA appeared to capture a dimension of IADL that was different than that of the deductive reasoning test. This suggests that both scores contributed unique information that is important to performance on cognitively complex tasks of daily living (Goverover & Hinojosa, 2002).

Dynamic Object Search Test

The Dynamic Object Search Test uses a different method of dynamic assessment as compared to the TCA and the CMT. It places a greater emphasis on examining the ability to learn and apply a strategy within a series of search tasks. The Object Search Test was derived from the original Dynamic Visual Processing Test (Toglia & Finkelstein, 1991). It consists of 12 pages (or trials) of 24 line-drawn objects. Size of space and background distraction varies across four task conditions in the Object Search Task. In a preliminary study, the test was presented within a single session to 40 people who had a right cerebrovascular accident and unilateral neglect. Participants were randomly assigned to two groups: a control group ($n = 20$) and a dynamic assessment group ($n = 20$). The control group received the same object search test without guided assistance or dynamic methods. In the dynamic assessment group, participants were provided with strategies such as feeling the edge of the page and visualizing the size of space with eyes closed and covering part of the page if they had difficulty. Participants also were provided with feedback on performance and use of the strategy. On each of the 12 trials, a baseline score of independent performance was obtained as well as a score with cues. The baseline score on each trial, however, reflected the effects of previous learning or repeated cues in the dynamic assessment group. Thus, a learning curve or learning profile was plotted that indicated whether the person could internalize and apply targeted strategies and feedback across similar types of tasks. Figure 2.5 shows an example of a learning profile of 3 participants. All three participants had similar initial scores, but they differed in their response to instruction. For example, Case 1 demonstrated improvements with strategy instruction that were maintained across the object search trials, whereas Case 2 demonstrated an up-and-down pattern. Improvements were noted immediately after cues or instruction, but the effect was transient. When cues were provided, performance improved for the next trial but then reverted backward as assistance was withdrawn. This pattern was more apparent in Trials 7–12, when search conditions were more complex. Case 3 demonstrated initial improvements but then was unable to benefit from instruction when task conditions increased in complexity (Trials 7–12; Toglia, 2004).

Functional visual scanning tasks such as finding specific events on a calendar filled with events were presented after the dynamic assessment procedures to examine the ability to transfer strategies to a variety of tasks. Results indicated that clients demonstrated significant changes in

unilateral neglect across similar and somewhat similar tasks as compared to a control group that did not receive dynamic assessment procedures. In addition, significant differences between the two groups were observed in initiation of search on the left side and use of strategies. Awareness, as measured prior to dynamic assessment, did not predict whether or not a person would be responsive to cues and strategy instruction. This suggests that, although one may initially deny difficulties outside the context of a task, awareness might increase with feedback and training during actual task experiences. Far transfer to functional tasks was not observed if group means were examined, but individual differences in performance were observed that were masked if groups were compared (Toglia, 2004).

Different learning profiles were observed that can be described as follows: (a) no changes in performance, (b) changes in performance only when performance was supported by the examiner, (c) transitory changes in performance, (d) consistent increases in performance only when tasks remained similar, and (e) consistent increases in performance across tasks that varied. The differences observed in learning profiles have direct implications for intervention. Further research is needed to examine subgroups or clusters that reflect differences in learning.

This method of dynamic assessment is different than those previously described, as it focuses on the process of change as it is occurring within a task and directly examines the capacity to apply and reapply taught strategies. Learning within this task was not related to initial severity, and the task further differentiated people who had similar initial static scores. Repeated opportunity to provide feedback and strategy training, followed by observation of independent performance, yielded a performance profile that was useful in characterizing patterns of learning. In contrast, the highest score attainable with cues from the examiner was not helpful in differentiating among participants if attention to the left side was examined. The majority of participants exhibited near symmetrical performance when the examiner supported performance. The ability to apply a strategy independently, immediately after instruction and feedback, across tasks that varied in difficulty level and appearance appears to have potential as a valuable clinical tool. Presently, the Dynamic Object Search Test is undergoing further development (Toglia, 2004).

Application of Dynamic Assessment Concepts to Aphasia and Apraxia

Dynamic assessment concepts also may be applied to people with aphasia and apraxia. Table 2.6 illustrates four

FIGURE 2.5. Learning profile across 12 object search trials for 3 cases within the dynamic group. Lower numbers on the Laterality Index indicate greater inattention to the left.

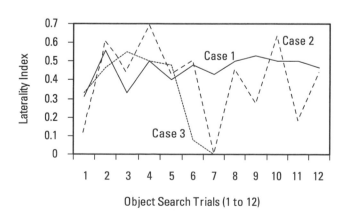

TABLE 2.6. Sample Dynamic Assessment of Clients With Aphasia and Apraxia

Task Direction	Objects on Table	Task Steps	Results	Number of Cues	Type of Cues
Peel the banana	banana, orange, apple	Selects banana	E	0	
		Orients banana			
		Peels all sides			
Butter the bread, and cut it in half	knife, spoon, fork, plate, butter, bread, cream cheese, sugar	Selects knife	E		
		Holds knife properly	■		
		Opens butter	C	2	P/G
		Puts butter on knife	●		
		Spreads butter on bread	■		
		Repeats spreading	●		
		Cuts bread	C	3	P/A/G
Pour the soda into he glass, and drink it with the straw	soda can, glass, straw, fork, can opener, coffee mug, bowl	Selects can	E		
		Opens can	■		
		Pours into glass	●		
		Opens straw	C	1	G
		Places straw in glass	●		
		Drinks	C	3	P/T/G
Fit the letter into the envelope, and put a stamp on it	Letter (8.5 × 11), envelope, stamp, letter opener, scissors, pen	Selects paper	E		
		Folds paper	C	2	G/P
		Selects envelope	E		
		Puts paper in envelope	C	3	P/T/G
		Takes stamp off packet	C	2	T/G
		Places stamp properly	E		
Make yourself a bowl of cereal	cereal, milk, bowl, spoon, fork, knife, can of soda, box of pan-cake mix, orange juice, can opener, scissors	Selects cereal	E		
		Opens cereal box	E		
		Pours into bowl	C	1	G
		Selects milk	C	2	A/T
		Opens milk	C*	1	G
		Pours milk	C	2	G
		Selects spoon	C	1	P
		Holds spoon properly	●		
		Eats cereal	C	1	G

Note. ● = Client performs step without cues; ■ = Client performs step in an awkward and clumsy manner without cues; C = Client performs step with cues; E = Examiner performs this step. Even with cues, client is unable to perform this step; * = Step occurred out of sequence.

Cues may include but are not limited to the following: V = Verbal cues: Repeating–rephrasing, simplifying directions, stating name of key object; SR = Stimuli reduction—Removing the unnecessary items; P = Visually focusing attention by pointing; A = Auditorily focusing attention by tapping; G = Visually gesturing action without object; G/O = Visually gesturing action with object; T = Tactile cues to initiate movement; TS = Task segmentation—Removing all items; Presenting one item at a time in the order in which it is used. If examiner places object in client's hand, then an E is used for item selection, because the examiner performed this step.

Adapted from *Treatment of Individuals With Limb Apraxia*, by J. Toglia, December 1993, presented at AOTA Neuroscience Institute: Treating Adults With Apraxia, Denver, CO.

sample items from a functional dynamic assessment. Each task is broken into substeps. The tasks range from those that are simple and include only three substeps (e.g., peel the banana) to those that are more complex (e.g., make a bowl of cereal). Each task is presented to the client with 3–4 unnecessary items. For example, in the cereal task, extra items such as a can opener, scissors, fork, and knife are placed on the table along with the cereal items. The ability to perform each substep is documented in the "result" section by using the codes on the bottom of the form. For example, if the individual requires cues, a "C" is placed next to the substep. If the individual is unable to perform the substep with cues, the examiner performs that particular substep for the client and records an

"E" next to that substep. The number of cues and type of cues required are recorded in the next two columns. Cues include visual gesturing or demonstration of the action by the examiner with or without the intended object, tapping or pointing to selected items, placing the correct item in the person's hand, and partial tactile guidance if necessary. Table 2.6 illustrates a client who was globally aphasic and apraxic following bilateral strokes. The test results indicate that performance was consistently facilitated by selecting the relevant items and initiating the task by placing the appropriate item in the client's hand. This information was used in training the caregiver to enhance the person's function. Rather than attempting to give the client verbal instructions, the caregiver was instructed to limit the number of items presented to the client at once. The caregiver was also trained to place the initial item in the client's hand and provide a visual gesture depicting the action of the item if needed.

Linking Assessment to Treatment

In the Dynamic Interactional Model, people are not classified as having deficits in separate cognitive areas. Little emphasis is placed on the absolute level of performance on specific tests. The clinician operates as a detective with each individual case and analyzes common underlying behaviors that interfere with performance on several different activities.

Dynamic assessment provides an in-depth look at self-perceptions of abilities and strategies as well as changes in self-perceptions and strategy use that may occur with mediation or alterations in activity parameters. The type of intervention approaches that may be most effective in facilitating performance depend to a large degree on the person's self-awareness and potential for learning or change. These aspects of performance are not directly assessed in a systematic way in traditional assessment approaches, but they play a critical role in guiding decision about treatment approaches.

For example, if dynamic assessment indicates that a person has poor self-awareness and shows little to no response to cues or guided assistance from another person, then it implies that performance may be best facilitated by changing the activity or environment or training specific functional skills without expectation for generalization, rather than trying to change the person's self-awareness and strategy use. On the other hand, if dynamic assessment provides evidence of potential for change in the person's self-awareness and use of strategies, an approach that targets changes in the person's cognitive processing, such as the multicontext approach, may be appropriate. In the multicontext approach, the behaviors or symptoms that impede performance on several different activities and are most responsive to cues are targeted for intervention. At the same time, the clinician also may choose to use other treatment approaches for other areas that show less responsiveness to change.

Different approaches to treatment, such as modifying the activity or environment, training specific tasks through repetitive practice, compensation, and remediation, inherently contain different assumptions regarding the person's awareness and ability to learn. However, they are not mutually exclusive. In clinical practice they often are used simultaneously, although sometimes a treatment emphasizes one approach more than another (Toglia, 2003a).

The clinician needs to carefully match the person's capabilities with assumptions and expectations regarding potential for change. In planning treatment, the clinician needs to ask the following questions: To what extent is change expected from the person? What is the person's potential for change or learning? Does the person recognize difficulties during or after an activity when feedback is provided? Is performance easily modified with cues? To what extent should treatment focus on changing the task and environment as opposed to changing the person's use of strategies? Dynamic assessment is designed to provide information that guides the clinician in addressing these questions.

Therapists should keep in mind that the client's overall rehabilitation outcome is based on several additional factors, including the nature and expected course of the illness or injury; degree of social, emotional, and economic supports; and length of time of expected treatment.

The Dynamic Interactional Model of Cognition provides a broad framework for using and simultaneously integrating different treatment approaches. Performance can be facilitated by changing the person's self-awareness and strategy use, by manipulating activity and environment demands, or by all of the above. This model provides the foundation for the multicontext approach, which is narrower in approach because it focuses on changing the person's strategies and self-awareness. The remaining part of this chapter focuses on the multicontext approach; however, it should be kept in mind that the multicontext approach describes one aspect of an intervention program.

MULTICONTEXT TREATMENT APPROACH

In the multicontext approach, the same strategy is practiced across activities and situations that gradually change. An emphasis on self-monitoring and self-evaluating performance is embedded throughout treatment. The multicontext approach targets areas that show some evidence of awareness and responsiveness to cues. It encompasses both compensatory and remedial methods (Toglia, 1991, 2003b).

Remedial treatment aims to improve or restore the areas impaired by the injury, whereas compensation focuses on areas of strength (Neistadt, 1990). Although remediation and compensation appear to target different areas of treatment, the line between them is questionable. For example, is a residual skill that has been weakened by brain injury an impairment or an area of strength? At times the skills that are considered to be impaired and the skills that are considered to be residual strengths may overlap or even be identical. Furthermore, in both remediation and compensation, the focus of change is the person. The person is required to learn a technique or strategy that needs to be applied across different situations. Neistadt (1994) reviewed neuroscience research on learning and concluded that, because both approaches involve learning, "neither approach can be said to take advantage of neural plasticity more than the other; both approaches can facilitate neural plasticity" (p. 428).

In addition to learning and generalization, awareness is required from the client in both remediation and compensation. A client who is unable to recognize his or her errors or predict when they are likely to occur will not initiate the use of compensatory strategies and will not actively participate in remedial interventions. The multicontext approach simultaneously integrates both compensatory and remedial strategies with awareness-training techniques. There is an emphasis on changing the person's use of strategies and self-awareness through guided assistance and manipulation of activity demands. In some situations, activities may need to be adapted or graded downward to meet the information-processing level of the client. In other words, processing strategies and self-monitoring skills are targeted for change within activities that may be adapted so that they are within the person's capabilities or processing range. The ability to use a strategy at one level of task difficulty does not indicate that the person can automatically use that strategy across all levels of complexity. The activity demands and conditions that facilitate or inhibit strategy use are analyzed and specified during treatment (Toglia, 1991, 2003b).

The components of the multicontext approach include consideration of personal context, awareness training, an emphasis on processing strategies, activity analysis, establishment of criteria for transfer, and practice in multiple environments. Each component is discussed below.

Personal Context

In the multicontext approach, treatment activities are not predetermined. The activities chosen depend on the client's personality characteristics, interests, goals, and occupational routines and activities. If the client previously enjoyed going to the theater, it is likely that activities involving theater schedules, listings, and price comparisons would be incorporated into treatment. On the other hand, spreadsheets, numbers, and calculations might be integrated into treatment activities for a person who worked as an accountant. Treatment activities for a client who is elderly and needs to take several medications may include organizing medications, loading pills into an organizer, reading and understanding instructions for medications, and responding to an alarm at specified times. If the client is concerned about his or her ability to organize and plan schedules, then treatment activities might include different types of calendars and schedules, recognizing conflicts in schedules, planning schedules, and transforming schedule information into a calendar or other format. Treatment activities include, whenever it is possible, a combination of simulated activities that have relevance or meaning to the person's lifestyle and activities practiced in the different contexts in which they occur.

Use of the multicontext approach within a clinic requires that treatment activities and materials that are relevant to everyday life be well organized and accessible. The Internet can be used to investigate information; plan a simulated trip; find recipes, restaurant menus, and movie or TV listings; compare prices or schedules (train, airplane, bus); look up directions to a specific location; or find information on the weather, business, news, sports, or upcoming concerts. Computer activities that can easily be structured or graded by the occupational therapist such as greeting card, calendar, or daily planner programs can also be useful. Computer programs that present drills of the same exercise graded in difficulty are avoided.

Clients lose interest if they do not understand the purpose or relevance of the activity. An initial step in treatment is using previous interviews and data gathered during assessment to create a written plan of action that includes goals, targeted strategies, and examples of treatment activities. A process of subgoaling may be used. For example, the client's goals can be broken into smaller subgoals and placed into a chart format to help the client see the connection among goals, strategies, and specific treatment activities (see Table 2.7). The client or significant other may be asked to provide input and make additional suggestions or revisions to the plan and the activities. If the client demonstrates limited awareness, he or she may not be able to actively participate in setting realistic goals or choosing appropriate activities. A close relative may be asked to participate in goal setting and identifying activities that fit the interests, needs, and lifestyle of the client.

Client-centered practice should be viewed on a continuum. In some situations, the clinician may take a greater role in structuring treatment and identifying goals in the

TABLE 2.7. Subgoaling Worksheet

Main Goals

1. Increase independence in daily activities (less verbal reminders and less reliance on family)
2. Increase participation in social and leisure activities
3. Enhance ability to resume volunteer job

Areas of Concern (Subgoals)	Strengths Within Skill Area	Subskills That Need to Be Strengthened and Sample Strategies	Simulated Tasks Agreed on by Client or Family Member
Spontaneously initiate household tasks without reminders	Can do all household tasks	Getting started without reminders and recognizing things that need to be done • Follow written lists or auditory reminder cues	Practice looking around at different environments (kitchen, clinic, home living room) and initiate making written lists of things that need to be done
Initiate social conversations and activities (letters, telephone calls)*	Gets along well with people	Ability to generate or initiate a variety of ideas or topics • Cue card of topics • Outlines with broad categories	Practice in tasks requiring generating ideas or different options for conversations, letters
Initiate previous interests Ability to plan and organize open-ended activities*	Wide range of previous interests (music, movies, poetry, juice, woodworking)	• Tendency to get "stuck" • Ability to shift attention and keep track of all parts • Use strategies such as checklists and metal practice	• Practice in unstructured activities requiring generating alter natives, planning, and organizing • Plan and organize a woodworking project, investigate and concerts, compare prices
Less reliance on others to keep track of things to do and recall events that have occurred**	Can follow routine lists, remembers parts of things	Ability to keep track of information: • Use of an organizer system (daily planner) • Initiate efficient use of strategies: key retrieval cues, mental rehearsal	• Practice initiating and using an organizer book for retrieval • Practice rehearsing and summarizing key points from conversations, readings, movies, events
Following instructions and lists to completion without verbal assistance or reminders	Can follow routine lists	Sometimes gets stuck on pieces, "gets thrown off" Misinterprets instruction due to failure to "shift" • Time-monitoring strategies • Underline key steps • Self-checking and comparison to original instructions	Practice in following tasks with multiple-step task instructions (follow a list requiring photocopying and collating forms according to rules, follow directions for an unfamiliar electronic device, follow directions on a map)

Note. *Identified as important areas of concern. **Identified as area of greatest concern.

initial stages of treatment. The emphasis may be to enhance self-awareness and understanding of difficulties so that the client can gradually take a more active role in setting realistic goals and identifying activities that he or she would like to be able to perform with less difficulty or effort. This may require structured practice in a variety of familiar activities that gradually differ in surface appearance using the awareness-training techniques described below.

Awareness Training

Methods designed to enhance the person's self-understanding of abilities and limitations are deeply embedded throughout every treatment session. The client can move from a cued to an uncued condition only if he or she has internalized the ability to self-monitor and regulate per-

formance. If the client does not understand the full extent of his or her impairments, he or she will be unable to accurately estimate the difficulty of activities and will not perceive the need to approach an activity in a more efficient way. The effectiveness and stability of independent strategy use requires understanding of one's limitations (Dirette, 2002; Tham, Ginsburg, Fisher, & Tegner, 2001; Toglia, 2003a; Toglia & Kirk, 2000). Strategy training and techniques to enhance awareness need to be simultaneously interwoven into treatment.

Awareness training involves rebuilding a sense of self. It uses structured occupational experiences and self-monitoring techniques to help someone gradually rediscover themselves and redefine their knowledge of their own strengths and weaknesses. This requires helping someone to let go of previous ways of doing things and to explore new methods and strategies. Awareness training promotes self-efficacy or perceived sense of control over occupational performance (Toglia & Kirk, 2000). Clients are taught how to anticipate and evaluate their own performance within meaningful occupational situations. There is an emphasis on helping someone to recognize the situations that will be the most challenging for him or her or helping a person recognize when he or she will need to ask for assistance or do something special. The ability to anticipate, recognize, and monitor errors prevents surprises in task outcome and allows clients to stay a step ahead of their cognitive symptoms.

During awareness training, the responsibility of cueing and structuring activities is gradually transferred from the therapist to the client. The therapist is challenged to creatively think of ways to assist the client in using internal strategies or cues in the environment to enhance performance. Every external cue that is effective in enhancing the client's performance should be carefully analyzed. The therapist has the responsibility of thinking of ways to help the client initiate the same cue by himself or herself. Initially, the clinician may be more actively involved in guiding and structuring activity experiences. As awareness emerges, the clinician gradually removes support and shifts more responsibility for monitoring and evaluation to the client. Establishment of a close and trusting therapeutic relationship is a critical component in treatment (Sohlberg & Mateer, 2001; Toglia & Kirk, 2000).

The practitioner needs to provide a nonthreatening atmosphere so that clients can experience and recognize errors themselves and at the same time gain a sense of control over performance. The message conveyed in treatment needs to be positive, with an emphasis on "staying a step ahead" by using strategies. This is in contrast to approaches that focus on pointing out errors as soon as they occur.

There is a wide variety of techniques that can be used to help clients experience and integrate knowledge about changes in functioning. Methods of goal setting and self-evaluation of goals on a rating scale are especially valuable in focusing treatment and promoting self-awareness. Client self-ratings of specific goals can be compared with ratings of a significant other or practitioner. A goal may be to diminish wide differences between the client's self-assessment of performance and that of others. Malec, Smigielski, and DePompolo (1991) found that goal attainment scales offer a concrete focus that can be effective in increasing realistic goal orientation and self-awareness in people with brain injury. A sample of a goal rating scale is presented in Figure 2.6.

FIGURE 2.6. Goal rating scale.

Reliance on Others

1. Relies on others for information the majority of time
2. Relies on others for information frequently (about ½ of the time)
3. Relies on others for information some of the time (about ¼–⅓)
4. Relies on others for information occasionally (less than ¼)
5. Does not rely on others for information

Structured logs or journals of daily activities and occupational situations can be used to help clients self-reflect and interpret occupational experiences. For example, the client might record information such as activity experiences (writing a letter, planning a meal, following a new recipe, ordering from an online catalog, and comparing prices with other online stores), performance results, what was learned from the experience, and what might be done differently next time. Structured self-observation helps clients gain a better understanding of their own strengths and weaknesses and empowers them to think of strategies that may be helpful in preventing future difficulties (Toglia, 2003a; Toglia & Kirk, 2000). Additional strategies used to address different aspects of awareness are presented in Table 2.8 and include self-prediction, role reversal, self-questioning, self-evaluation, structured error monitoring systems, and videotape feedback (Toglia, 2003a). In addition, strategy cue cards that clients can look at whenever they run into difficulty can be used. Strategy tips also can be recorded on a voice memo. In either case, an alarm signal can be used to cue the person to review his or her self-questions or strategy tips at set intervals during an activity. These techniques are particularly useful within activities that are concrete, meaningful, and familiar, and have specific or clear outcomes, as in these situations; it is easier for clients to discover errors themselves (Katz et al., 2002; Tham et al., 2000). Directly telling a person that he or she made an error or pointing out errors is least effective in influencing performance and tends to elicit defensive reactions (Toglia & Kirk, 2000). Structured self-monitoring techniques such as cueing the person at set time intervals to pause ("Stop for a minute and carefully monitor or check your work") can encourage clients to detect errors by themselves. Additional structure for self-evaluation may be needed, such as a specific checklist of things to look for or covering part of a page and exposing one piece of information at a time during the self-checking process so that the client can easily detect any errors.

Some clients may not be ready to self-evaluate or reflect on their performance. In these situations, immediate feed-

TABLE 2.8. Awareness Strategies and Training Techniques

Behavior	Awareness Strategy or Technique	Description
Client uses strategies when cued but does not initiate use of a strategy.	Anticipation	Client is asked to anticipate any of the following: (a) the types of obstacles that might be encountered prior to performing the task, (b) the possible outcomes or consequences, and (c) the need to choose a strategy.
Client overestimates his or her abilities.	Self-prediction	Client is asked to predict the general difficulty level of the task on a rating scale or predict specific aspects of performance such as accuracy score, time score. Predictions are compared with actual performance.
Client does not spontaneously check work.	Self-checking and self-evaluation	After every 5 or 10 minutes, client is asked to self-check his work and fill out a self-evaluation form.
Client does not self-monitor performance during a task.	Self-questioning	Client is taught to ask self key questions during a task. The questions may be written on cue cards. External aids such as an alarm or buzzer may be used to remind the individual to read the cue card in the initial stages. Examples of questions include the following ● Do I understand the problem? ● Am I getting sidetracked by irrelevant details? ● Do I need more information? ● Am I getting stuck?
Client is unable to monitor time during a task, requires excessive time to perform tasks, performs unnecessary steps, gets caught up in unnecessary details, and becomes sidetracked.	Time monitoring	Estimate time; set time limits prior to initiation of the task and compare or evaluate results. Prior to performing the task, visualize oneself performing the task with and without getting sidetracked.
Client has poor error-monitoring and detection skills.	Role reversal	The therapist performs a task and makes errors due to distractibility, impulsivity, etc. The client observes the therapist's performance and gives the therapist feedback (points out errors and states why they may have occurred).

back in the form of a checkmark or point system can be used within an activity to reinforce positive behaviors such as use of a strategy. For example, the frequency of behaviors such as initiating use of a targeted strategy, spontaneously checking work, or recognizing errors as they are occurring can be objectively recorded and charted. The client also can be asked to self-rate, track, or record aspects of performance during an activity (Sohlberg & Mateer, 2001). This can enhance motivation and assist the client in staying focused on the treatment goals. Emphasis is not on the task outcome but on reinforcing the use of targeted behaviors or strategies. Performance with and without use of the targeted strategy can be contrasted and compared. An alternative method involves tracking problem behaviors. For example, a client can be asked to keep a log of memory or attention lapses that occur during daily occupations. The log of problems and the context of the situations in which they occurred are reviewed so that clients can learn more about themselves and the conditions under which problems are most likely to emerge. Methods of preventing future lapses are discussed for each daily life situation.

Processing Strategy

Treatment provides multiple opportunities to practice targeted processing strategies in a wide range of situations that are within a similar level of difficulty. The emphasis is on helping the person to control cognitive perceptual symptoms (e.g., in distractibility, impulsivity, inability to shift attention, disorganization, inattention to one side of the environment, tendency to overfocus on parts of an item or task) through use of effective strategies. In treatment, the person learns to recognize the conditions under which symptoms are least likely and most likely to emerge. This assists the person in identifying situations in which a particular strategy is needed. Case Examples 2.1 and 2.2 illustrate a focus on strategy training. Case Example 2.2 describes how treatment emphasizes the use of strategies to control impulsivity under specified activity parameters.

In each case example, treatment began by specifying the activity parameters at which the client could function. The client was taught to apply use of targeted processing strategies across different situations that stayed within similar

Case Example 2.1. Strategy Training and Unilateral Inattention

Mr. Jones tended to miss items on the left side whenever 10 or more objects were close together, similar in shape, and randomly scattered. When familiar objects with obvious differences were arranged horizontally and spaced evenly, he had no difficulty.

Treatment helped Mr. Jones learn to identify the situations in which he was most likely to have success and those in which he was most vulnerable to error. For example, prior to each activity, Mr. Jones was asked to predict the difficulty level of the task and to anticipate whether or not he would need to use special strategies such as an anchor. Strategies that were practiced in functional situations in which 10 or more items were randomly scattered included rearranging items on a counter prior to scanning, tactile exploration of space (eyes closed) to get an internal image of the size of the space to be explored prior to visual search, and placing a particular object on the left side to help him know when he was at the left side. An emphasis was placed on accurately anticipating task difficulty and the need to use a particular strategy rather than emphasizing the results. In addition, the therapist recorded the frequency of strategies such as tactile exploration and anchoring. Because Mr. Jones had difficulty writing, he used a voice memo recorder to summarize his activity experience, performance results, what he learned (e.g., strategies that were helpful), and what he should remember to do next time.

Case Example 2.2. Strategy Training for Impulsivity and Selective Attention

Gary demonstrated difficulty monitoring and adjusting the speed of response when 5–10 items were presented simultaneously and slight attention to detail was required. He tended to make numerous errors because he chose items quickly without fully attending to them. For example, when asked to make cereal, he quickly reached for a carton of orange juice in the refrigerator and did not realize his error until he had poured the orange juice into his cereal. If one or two items were presented at a time, Gary did not make errors. If Gary was cued to slow down his responses, performance was significantly improved.

Treatment involved teaching Gary to monitor and pace his speed of response in a variety of activities. Prior to an activity, Gary was asked to predict the number of responses that would be performed with "good timing" (e.g., looking around at all the items prior to making a choice) and the number of responses that would be "too quick" (e.g., reaching haphazardly without attending to all the choices and making errors). The emphasis was on increasing accuracy of predictions rather than on performance outcome. Gary also was asked to mentally rehearse or visualize himself performing the task with good timing and timing that was too quick. During the activity, Gary was encouraged to use his finger to point to each item to assist him in slowing down his responses. A chart was kept that allowed Gary to record the number of responses that he felt demonstrated good timing. Gary was cued during the task to stop, double check his work, and ask himself key questions: Am I going too quickly? Am I remembering to look and point to everything before I pick it up? This same strategy and self-monitoring system was emphasized in other card tasks, games, computer activities, and functional activities such as choosing all the items needed to make a sandwich. The motor demands of the tasks varied from tabletop tasks to tasks that involved standing, reaching, and weight shifting. Although the context of the task and environment were varied, the same strategy and self-monitoring system remained consistent throughout treatment. When Gary demonstrated improved ability to pace his speed of response under the task conditions described above, the tasks were then graded in difficulty, and the number of items presented simultaneously was increased to 15–20.

levels of complexity. The processing strategies were aimed at inhibiting or controlling the appearance of cognitive perceptual symptoms such as impulsivity and the tendency to miss information. At the same time, awareness-training techniques were integrated within each treatment session.

The case example involving unilateral inattention described use of external strategies such as tactile exploration of space, rearranging items, and use of an anchor. Examples of internal strategies for unilateral inattention include remembering to begin the task at the left margin; remembering to move one's eyes to the left; or remembering to ask oneself the same question periodically, "Am I remembering to look to the left?" The case example involving impulsivity included use of both an internal strategy (visualization prior to actual performance) and external strategy (finger-pointing). Additional internal strategies that may be used to assist the individual in monitoring impulsivity include counting silently to 10 before providing a response or verbalizing the rules or stimuli silently to oneself before responding. Additional external strategies include using an external timer to assist the individual in slowing down his or her responses (e.g., "Take your time and wait until you hear the buzzer before you respond").

Other examples of external strategies include blocking out or reducing the amount of information; task reorganization; use of task checklists, timers, alarm reminders, organizers, tape recorders, notebooks, and highlighters to focus attention on relevant stimuli; and use of rulers or measuring devices to ensure proper spacing or arrangement of items. Additional examples of internal strategies include using elaboration and association techniques, mental rehearsal, setting priorities, and remembering to attend to details before responding. Table 2.9 summarizes additional examples of various processing strategies that may be emphasized in treatment (Toglia, 1991). In addition, the processing strategies and behaviors listed in Table 2.1 and 2.2 are further examples of areas that may be targeted for treatment.

During all treatment sessions, the therapist analyzes the behaviors and processing strategies that the client is or is not using. Improvements in the ability to initiate use of a processing strategy should be reflected in several different activities.

Activity Analysis, Establishment of Criteria for Transfer, and Practice in Multiple Tasks and Environments

Processing strategies are practiced in a variety of situations during treatment to demonstrate the range of the strategy's applicability and to assist the client in understanding the

TABLE 2.9. Sample Processing Strategies

Sample Problem Behaviors and Symptoms	Sample Strategy	Description
Poor planning, attention, self-control	Verbal mediation or self-instructional procedures	Client says self-cues, task goals, plans, or task instructions out loud or silently before or during execution of a task.
Distracted by irrelevant information, difficulty selecting the main point	Underline, circle, or highlight critical details or facts Summarize with key words	Client highlights, circles, or lists information most critical to the task or problem.
Tendency to become overwhelmed by the amount of information.	Stimuli reduction	Client removes, covers, or visually blocks out information.
Loses track of steps, performs tasks incompletely, performs unnecessary steps, has poor planning and organization	Mental rehearsal or visual imagery prior to task performance	Client imagines self-performing task in an accurate and smooth manner, vividly imagines achieving the desired outcome, or imagines performing task with possible obstacles, and imagines effective coping strategies.
Poor visual object recognition	Verbalization of object characteristics	Client is taught to silently verbalize the characteristics of an object prior to determining what the object is.
Difficulty recognizing and locating objects	Visual imagery prior to visual search	Client vividly imagines the target item or object before searching for it.
Difficulty finding items; haphazard, disorganized approach	Categorization or identification of organization structure before beginning a task	Client is taught to rearrange similar items into meaningful clusters or smaller groups (e.g., grocery list, items in a closet or shelf).
Haphazard approach, difficulty focusing on task; does not know where to begin; appears overwhelmed by the amount of information	Task segmentation	Client is taught to simplify a task by breaking it down into smaller, more manageable components and to deal with one step or component of the task at a time.
Difficulty locating and finding items, tendency to omit items or steps during a task	Rearrangement of items	Client is taught to rearrange items prior to starting a task so that they are organized according to the sequence of use, there are spaces between them and they are arranged in a linear rather then scattered arrangement.
Tendency to overfocus on the parts of a visual scene or stimulus	Look all over before responding	Client is taught to gain an impression of the whole before attending to the parts. Look all over; actively scan the entire visual display from different perspectives prior to attending to pieces.
Impulsive, tendency to miss details, disorganized visual scanning	Point or use finger to help focus on details	Client is taught to point to stimuli prior to responding, to focus attention on details, and to slow down responses. Finger-pointing also may assist in facilitating an organized pattern of visual scanning.

conditions in which it is useful (Brown, 1988; Brown et al., 1983). The therapist avoids exclusive use of specific activities or environments because, if the skills taught are embedded in one context, they may be accessible only in relation to that specific context. Several authors have emphasized the importance of using a variety of situations and examples to promote generalization (Glick & Holyoak, 1987; Resing & Roth-Van der Werf, 2002; Sohlberg & Raskin, 1996). In the multicontext approach, the same processing strategies are practiced in a wide variety of activities; however, the range and variety of tasks are not randomly chosen. Treatment progresses along a horizontal continuum that gradually places more demands on the ability to transfer and generalize use of the targeted strategies (Toglia, 2003b).

Transfer of learning is not all or none. It can be conceptualized on a horizontal continuum that reflects different degrees of transfer of learning (see Figure 2.7). The continuum represents activities or situations that remain at a similar level of complexity but gradually differ in physical or superficial similarity. During intervention, the client practices the same strategy in a series of activities that gradually differ in physical appearance. When two situations are physically different, transfer becomes more difficult because the similarities of the two situations may not be recognized (Glick & Holyoak, 1987; Resing & Roth-Van der Werf, 2002). It is harder to recognize that the targeted strategy may be of use. The beginning of the continuum includes activities that are very similar to each other and represent alternate versions of the same activity. These activities share surface or physical characteristics. Ability to apply use of a strategy across activities that are similar represents *near-transfer* learning. The middle of the continuum includes activities that are somewhat similar to the original activities and represent *intermediate-transfer* activities. These activities share some physical features with the original activity, but the similarities are less obvious. *Far-transfer* activities are physically different from the original activity and *very-far transfer* activities are very different and include transfer of what one has learned in intervention to everyday functioning. The transfer continuum provides a guide for the sequence and progression of treatment activities. The physical similarity of activities or environments is gradually reduced while the underlying strategies required remain constant (Toglia, 2003b).

Treatment involves analyzing an activity to identify which of its parameters will stay constant in treatment and which will change. The observable or physical features of an activity or environment are those that are changed while the underlying strategy required stays constant. The same strategy can be practiced in different activities and environments and with different types of people. Examples of parameters that are likely to increase the difficulty of an activity include the number of items in the task, the degree of detail, the number of task steps or rules, the number of possible choices, the discriminability of the task and environmental stimuli, the degree of distractions in the environment, and the unpredictability or unfamiliarity of the environmental context. The parameters that are not likely to increase the difficulty of an activity include the type of stimuli; the attributes of the stimuli such as color, size, and shape; the task category; and the familiarity of the environment.

In many cases the parameters that increase the difficulty of the activity depend on the client's problem areas. For example, if a client has visual scanning problems, then increasing the size of the space to be explored and randomly scattering the items will significantly increase difficulty. On the other hand, if the client has difficulty in problem solving tasks and in generating alternative hypotheses, then increasing the size of space in which the task is performed is not likely to increase difficulty level. The

F I G U R E 2 . 7 . The activity transfer continuum: Same strategy emphasized across different activities and situations.

Very Similar		Somewhat Similar	Different		Very Different
Making instant coffee with a different cup, pot, or premeasured packages.	Making tea or hot chocolate, instant iced tea, lemonade, frozen orange juice	Making instant soup, oatmeal, jello, pudding, frozen vegetables	Making toast with butter and jelly or a peanut butter and jelly sandwich	Loading and starting the dishwasher, setting a table for two	Making a bed; doing a small load of laundry

Near-Transfer		Intermediate-Transfer		Far-Transfer	

task is only graded in difficulty when there is evidence that the person can apply use of the targeted strategy and self-monitoring skill across the transfer continuum (from near-transfer to far-transfer tasks).

Case Example 2.3 illustrates application of the multi-context treatment approach for a client, Ann, who con-fuses objects of similar size and shape. Treatment is focused on training Ann to monitor and improve her ability to visually attend to detail. The targeted strategy is using finger-pointing during visual search to assist her in attending to subtle differences between everyday objects. In addition, the strategy of stimuli reduction or visually

---

Case Example 2.3. Application of the Multicontext Treatment Approach: Ann

Ann is a 66-year-old female who had a right cerebrovascular accident 3 months ago. She was at a rehabilitation center for 9 weeks and is now receiving home care occupational and physical therapy.

Daily Life Problem
Ann has difficulty attending to critical visual details and makes frequent misinterpretations if there are 10 or more objects. For example, she frequently confuses items that are similar in shape (e.g., chooses tube of hand cream instead of toothpaste during brushing teeth, chooses a bottle of shampoo instead of liquid detergent). Requires occasional minimum assistance in dressing. Has difficulty locating armhole, collar, and so forth when clothing has a busy design or pattern. Has difficulty finding needed items, particularly in cluttered closets, drawers, or shelves. Ann can no longer follow a pattern in sewing or

knitting. Ann is aware that she is having visual difficulties but attributes it to needing new eyeglasses. Her near acuity is 20/30 with her corrective lenses.

Previous Activity Interests
Housewife—Enjoyed cooking, entertaining, sewing, knitting; playing cards with friends; attending local senior citizens center.

Activity Conditions That Remain the Same
All activities involve choosing target stimuli out of 10–20 familiar objects that are similar in size and shape. Objects may be scattered or overlapping one another.

Same Strategy Emphasized in All Activities
Attention to critical visual details using finger-pointing; stimuli reduction (blocking or covering part of the visual display).

Self-Monitoring Techniques
A strategy cue card stating "Pay attention to details; use finger and cover" was placed on the table or counter as a visual reminder. At 5–10 minute intervals, Ann was asked to stop and rate herself on the following: Am I using my finger to help me? Am I paying careful attention to the details? Am I removing or covering other objects if they are distracting to me? At the end of the session, Ann was asked to write what she learned from the session and what she would do differently next time.

Goal Rating
Each time that Ann met the goal of spontaneously using her finger during visual search or covered or removed other distracting visual stimuli, a check mark was recorded on a goal rating sheet.

ACTIVITY TRANSFER CONTINUUM

Very Similar		Somewhat Similar		Different		Very Different
20 spoons scattered on the kitchen counter. Find all the teaspoons out of scattered tablespoons, soupspoons, measuring spoons, teaspoons. Place each type of spoon in a drawer with an organizer.	Find all the butter knives in a drawer full of steak knives, dinner knives, and butter knives. Find the utensils with a certain handle or pattern.	Cabinet full of various types of canned goods; while standing, remove all the canned soups or all the canned vegetables.	While standing, empty the dishwasher and place saucers in one cabinet, dessert plates in another cabinet, or sort dishes, bowls, and cups into different cabinets.	Find matching fabric squares with similar patterns or designs scattered across a table. Find specific items spread across the table (e.g., shell, tile, bead) within the context of a craft task.	Sort white socks according to the size and pattern. Standing at a closet, choose all the short-sleeve shirts.

covering some of the visual information and systematically attending to one part of the visual display is practiced. Treatment activities progress from attending to details in kitchen activities, to sewing and craft activities, and to dressing and laundry. The example illustrates how the physical similarity between treatment tasks is gradually reduced along a horizontal continuum.

Activity parameters that remain constant across a variety of situations are identified so that treatment matches the level of the person and remains at approximately the same level of difficulty. For example, all treatment activities include 15–20 familiar objects that are similar in size and shape. Once the ability to successfully initiate finger pointing and stimuli reduction strategies is observed in different contexts with everyday objects, treatment activities can be increased in difficulty by using less-familiar objects or by requiring Ann to locate specific details in crowded pictures, catalogs, food circulars, bills, schedules, calendars, charts, recipes, menus, maps, newspapers, and sewing and knitting catalogs.

Treatment activities are graded in difficulty only if the person demonstrates the ability to use the same strategy across a variety of situations that are increasingly different in physical appearance. Treatment is horizontal in nature and emphasizes sideways learning. This is different than treatment approaches that emphasize a vertical approach to learning and gradually increase the activity demands as success at lower levels is achieved.

It should be kept in mind that the client's ability to effectively use a strategy depends on the level of difficulty. As soon as activity demands are increased in difficulty level (e.g., number of objects or steps is increased), the person may once again have difficulty using the same strategy beyond the near-transfer level. Thus, the ability to transfer strategies to different situations may be confined within a specified level of task difficulty. The multicontext approach suggests that the process of transfer may be enhanced in some clients by gradually changing the appearance of the activity and environment while emphasizing the same underlying behavior or strategy. In this way, the client learns that it is not the activity or the environment that is important but the strategy or behaviors (Toglia, 1991). Attention is drawn to the core similarity of the activities and away from the superficial similarities and differences.

The transfer continuum represents a guideline for treatment planning. However, it does not need to be strictly adhered to for all clients. For example, in situations in which the strategy to be trained is general or nonsituational (e.g., check work, plan ahead) and the deficits are mild, the individual may be able to recognize the similarity between near- and far-transfer tasks. Treatment may consist of practicing the targeted strategy within a variety of far-transfer tasks. However, if the individual has difficulty recognizing the similarity between two situations, the multicontext approach suggests that gradually changing the surface features of the task and moving treatment along the transfer continuum may increase the probability that transfer will occur in some individuals.

Group Treatment

It is important to keep in mind that individual treatment needs to be combined with group treatment activities. The same self-monitoring or task strategies that are emphasized in individual sessions can be reinforced within a group treatment session. Group activities can include problem solving and role-playing. For example, differences of opinion or conflicts between two people can be role-played in front of the group. Group members can be asked to think about a response to the situation, view the problem from different perspectives, and offer different alternative solutions (Toglia & Golisz, 1990).

Grattan and Eslinger (1989) found a significant correlation between flexibility of thinking and empathy, and they have suggested that treatment of clients with frontal lobe damage include training in social skills and social sensitivity. In addition to role-playing, tasks can involve cooperative effort, planning, and organization. Examples include putting together a newsletter, interviewing various people within the facility, or planning and organizing a bake sale, holiday party, raffle, or group outing. Each group session can end by asking members to complete a self-evaluation rating form that includes questions such as, "Did I listen to other group members? Did I compromise? Was I open and receptive to other opinions? Did I remain calm, even when I did not agree? Did I communicate my thoughts effectively? Did I help the group stay focused on the goal?" The self-rating form can be discussed openly, and members can receive feedback on their behavior from other group members. Strategies emphasized in individual treatment sessions, such as monitoring the tendency to get stuck in one perspective or viewpoint, listing or prioritizing task steps prior to beginning an activity, estimating a time goal, and summarizing the main points of a conversation, all can be emphasized within the group context.

The multicontext approach also has been applied to group programs for elderly people with mild cognitive impairment and women with lupus who have self-identified cognitive symptoms that are interfering with daily life. In both populations, participants completed pre- and post-questionnaires on memory functioning and memory self-efficacy. A focus group also was held before and after the group sessions to explore perceived difficulties in cognitive functioning and the impact on daily life activities, before and after the group.

The groups focused on teaching participants internal and external strategies that could be applied to a variety of activities. The group programs also emphasized increasing self-understanding and self-monitoring of cognitive or memory symptoms. Three techniques were integrated throughout each group and included (a) keeping a daily log of cognitive or memory lapses, including recording the lapse, the context in which it occurred, and strategies that can be used to prevent it from occurring in the future; (b) using a strategy worksheet or discussing and documenting how strategies explored in the group session could be used in each person's everyday life, weekly homework included practicing the strategy in identified activities and recording and evaluating the results; and (c) goal rating or self-evaluating personal goals that participants had established for themselves at midpoint and at the end of the group. Each group session began with a discussion of the cognitive logs and a review of the previous session. An activity was presented that required attention, memory, or executive functioning. Participants discussed how they went about doing the activity as well as any difficulties that they may have encountered. Strategies were introduced and participants practiced using different strategies in activities and discussed the results. Each group ended with discussion of the strategy worksheet. Both groups showed changes in self-efficacy and perceived everyday memory functioning. Themes from focus group discussions indicated participants perceived changes in their daily functioning and self-confidence. In addition, the groups with lupus were assessed with additional objective measures that showed changes in satisfaction with ability to function in daily life as well as perceived changes in activity limitations and participation in social or community activities. Findings from both groups indicated that group programs for people with subtle cognitive deficits can have a profound effect on one's ability to function in daily life (Harrison et al., 2003; Toglia et al., 2004).

Outcome of Treatment

Regardless of the treatment approach used, the desired outcomes of treatment for people with cognitive impairments are the same and include decreasing activity limitations and enhancing participation in everyday activities.

Outcome is multidimensional and goes beyond quantitative measures of cognitive impairment or standardized measures of ADL. A combination of a range of qualitative and quantitative methods can provide important information on intervention outcomes, regardless of the treatment approach used. Examples of outcome indicators may include changes in activity patterns; how one productively uses time; reliance on others; perceived caregiver burden; the frequency and satisfaction with participation in social, community, or productive activities; self-awareness and ability to identify realistic goals; the ability to meet targeted goals; and quality of life. Examples of rating scales and questionnaires that can be used as outcome measures of cognitive rehabilitation include the Frenchay Activities Index (Turnbell et al., 2000), Stroke Impact Scale (Duncan et al., 1999), Functional Activities Questionnaire (Pfeffer, Kurosaki, Harrah, Chance, & Filos, 1982), Memory Functioning Questionnaire (Gilewski, Zelinski, & Schaie, 1990); Mayo–Portland Adaptability Inventory, Community Integration Questionnaire (Willer, Ottenbacher, & Coad, 1994), Reintegration to Normal Living (Wood-Dauphinee, Opzoomer, Williams, Marchand, & Spitzwer, 1988), or the Canadian Occupational Performance Measure (Law et al., 1998).

CASE PRESENTATION: RON

Ron, a 53-year-old man who presented with subtle cognitive impairments as a result of a head injury sustained in a car accident 10 months ago, is ambulatory and independent in basic ADL skills. Prior to his injury, Ron had recently retired from his job as a firefighter and spent the majority of his week volunteering in a hospital. His responsibilities as a volunteer included visiting patients and helping office staff. Ron describes himself as a social person. He enjoyed his role as a volunteer because he found it personally rewarding to help other people. After the injury, Ron tried to resume his former volunteer work but experienced difficulty in keeping track of information. He was embarrassed that he forgot previous conversations and names of people that he had just met. He also reported that he found himself repeating the same conversation with each person he met because he could not think of other things to say.

Ron's wife works full-time and reports that Ron relies on her for her memory. Although she writes everything on calendars and daily lists, Ron calls her at work about his appointments or things he needs to do and does not initiate looking at the lists that she leaves for him. She reports that he often loses track of time and underestimates the length of time that a task may require. As a result, he often does not complete his list of daily errands. He also becomes easily frustrated if faced with new or unexpected situations and depends on her for guidance. Recently, he is spending a good deal of time watching TV and no longer initiates previous hobbies or interests such as getting together with friends, writing poetry, reading, woodworking, gardening, organizing his music and movie collections, or participating in community activities such as organizing church events or activities for the local firefighters' organization. Prior to his injury, Ron and his wife socialized a great deal with family and friends. However, Ron has increasingly avoided social situations.

A neuropsychological assessment revealed mild impairments in the areas of attention, memory, and executive functions. The occupational therapy assessment began by examining the congruence between Ron and his wife's perception of his difficulties by using a structured checklist called the Daily Living Questionnaire (DLQ; see sample items, Table 2.9). Ron readily acknowledged difficulties in memory and keeping track of information. There was, however, a discrepancy between his and his wife's perception of the magnitude of difficulties in the areas of IADL, memory, and organization. In addition, Ron's wife completed the Functional Activities Questionnaire (FAQ; (Pfeffer et al., 1982) to provide supplemental information. The FAQ is an informant-based measure of functional abilities that provides performance ratings on 10 higher-level everyday activities. Ron's wife's responses on the DLQ and FAQ indicated that Ron had difficulties with several activities, including following and remembering schedules; completing daily errands; recalling information from

books, TV programs, events, or conversations; following directions for tasks and filling out paperwork; initiating household tasks; organizing bills; initiating and following conversations in social situations; shopping (forgets items even with written lists); and initiating and planning activities (social events, planning own schedule).

Dynamic Assessment

Awareness

Upon general questioning, Ron stated that he was not able to function as he used to. He expressed greatest concern about his ability to remember and provided specific examples of forgetting appointments, parts of conversations, things that he had read, and persons' names. Despite acknowledgment of memory difficulties, Ron tended to overestimate his abilities within the context of specific memory tasks. For example, on the CMT, he overestimated his initial performance (he stated that he would recall 15–16 but recalled 9), but immediately after the task he accurately estimated his recall score. On other tasks that required organization, following multiple-step directions, or monitoring time, Ron was unable to anticipate difficulties or independently recognize errors. Structured methods for self-evaluation were necessary to help Ron recognize and correct errors.

Processing Strategies and Task Conditions

Ron was able to perform tasks that required visually detecting and locating targeted pieces of information such as finding specific items in crowded closets or drawers or

T A B L E 2.9. Sample Items From Daily Living Questionnaire

Place a check if your ability to do this activity has changed.

Part I

☐ Getting ready in the morning	☐ Organizing and scheduling own daily activities and errands
☐ Composing a letter or report	☐ Planning social arrangements
☐ Remembering appointments	☐ Participating in social activities with others
☐ Organizing and managing finances	☐ Participating in recreational activities, leisure, hobbies
☐ Reading books	☐ Driving

Part II

☐ Solving problems	☐ Understanding new instructions
☐ Performing daily activities at a normal speed	☐ Keeping track of time
☐ Taking initiative to start a new activity	☐ Staying focused on the task to be accomplished
☐ Resuming an activity without difficulty after being interrupted	

Note. From *The Multicontext Approach to Awareness, Memory, and Executive-Function Impairments*, by J. P. Toglia, 2003 [Supplement manual to workshops conducted at various locations].

finding the due date on bills. In other words, when Ron knew what he was looking for, he had no difficulty attending to details and discriminating among items.

Performance on the memory task CMT involving recall of 20 items related to a theme was characterized by a haphazard pattern of recall. Ron did not recognize the overall theme and did not appear to use efficient association or grouping strategies. He recalled 9 out of 20 items. When asked how he went about recalling the items he stated, "I just looked at them over and over." When given a list of strategies and asked to identify the memory strategy that would be most effective, he selected the association or grouping strategies. When Ron was cued to attend to the overall theme, prior to a memory task, his performance improved to within normal limits. This indicated that, although Ron had knowledge regarding the usefulness of different strategies, he did not initiate using an efficient strategy. On the TCA, he sorted the utensils in two ways but became stuck in previous responses and required moderate cues to attend to additional aspects of the utensils (size) and recognize an alternative method. On the deductive-reasoning task, he tended to repeat the same questions without realizing it and required cues to use an efficient strategy.

Observation of Simulated Functional Activities

On a catalog-ordering task that involved following multiple steps, keeping track of rules, and staying within imposed time limits, Ron demonstrated difficulty in attending to all aspects of the directions and shifting his attention to different parts of the task, and he lost track of time. He became stuck on one aspect of the activity and required moderate cues to switch his attention to other parts of the task. He also did not refer back to a card on the table that contained written directions and a checklist of rules and steps he needed to follow. On an unstructured task requiring him to create a checklist of all the things he would need to do to plan and leave for a trip, he had difficulty generating and organizing his ideas. He required cues to think of broad categories and to organize ideas within the categories.

A clerical activity, requiring following instructions to photocopy and collate forms and place them in different files, was used to simulate some of the clerical demands within Ron's volunteer job. Ron listened to the directions but did not ask for repetition and did not initiate writing anything down. The occupational therapist then wrote down the instructions on a piece of paper and cued Ron to refer to it during the activity. Ron read over the instructions, put them in his pocket, but did not refer to them during the

remainder of the task. He collated the papers incorrectly and placed some of the papers in the wrong file. He did not recognize any errors in performance until he was asked to check his work against a checklist that matched the original instructions.

Responsiveness to Cues

Ron was most responsive to cues that encouraged him to use strategies prior to initiating a task. If encouraged to check his work, he easily recognized memory difficulties (tendency to repeat himself or lose track of information), but he had difficulty recognizing errors in other areas. For example, once Ron became stuck in one approach or part of a task, he had difficulty viewing the task in a different way and required specific cues to generate alterative options or to switch attention to other aspects of the task or back to the overall goal.

Treatment

Data gathered from questionnaires, interviews with Ron and his wife, and assessments were used to create a sample subgoal chart that was presented to Ron and his wife for review, comments, and revisions (see Table 2.7). They were asked to identify the greatest areas of concern. Ron and his wife felt that it would be most important to help Ron keep track of things that he needed to do on a daily basis so that he would rely less on his wife for his memory. Ron's wife was feeling overwhelmed by Ron's constant and repetitive questions and increasing reliance on her, and this was creating underlying tensions in their relationship.

Several goal attainment scales were developed. For example, one scale was used to measure changes in the degree of Ron's reliance on his wife for remembering information (Figure 2.6). At the start of treatment, Ron was relying on others for information the majority of the time. Ron, his wife, and the occupational therapist each rated performance on the goal scale weekly and compared discrepancies. The emphasis was on obtaining agreement in perceptions, especially between Ron and his wife. Other goal scales involved rating the frequency and efficiency of targeted strategies.

Initially, an external strategy of using a daily planner that was divided into different sections was introduced. The first two sections included a to-do list and a calendar. Initially the focus was on increasing Ron's ability to initiate looking at his planner. Ron was not enthusiastic about use of the planner, as he stated that he never had to use to-do lists or refer to a daily schedule in the past because he always remembered everything he needed to do "in his head." Treatment sessions incorporated lists of daily errands that Ron needed to carry out at certain times within a session or during his visits to the program. Sample errands included delivering messages to office staff at specified times, photocopying his assigned homework, looking up information in a phone book, making phone calls, or checking prices of items at various sources. Ron was asked to estimate the number of errands he thought he would remember to carry out and to think of a list of possible strategies that he could use to help him complete everything that he was assigned to do. With structure and assistance from the practitioner, the strategy list included repeating the list to himself, recording the errands in his planner and crossing them off as they were completed, and using a timer or alarm at preset intervals to remind him to check his planner. Halfway through the session, Ron was asked to stop and monitor how he was doing in keeping track of what he needed to do. He also was asked to decide whether he wanted to change or initiate use of a different strategy. At the end of the session, Ron was asked to evaluate his ability to carry out the errands on a structured self-evaluation form and compare it with his initial predictions. He also was asked to comment on whether he would do anything differently next time.

Gradually, Ron began to recognize that his previous methods of keeping track of information were no longer as effective as they once were. He began to recognize that a written list in a consistent place (planner), along with a timer or alarm for activities that needed to be done at specified times, increased his probability of success. Treatment sessions also included organizing and prioritizing a list of errands from Ron's wife, predicting percentage of completion of errands at home, estimating time for each activity, and anticipating need for strategies. The clinician frequently asked Ron questions about upcoming events or appointments and recorded the number of times he spontaneously said "I don't know" instead of referring to his calendar. This was visually charted and provided Ron with concrete feedback regarding the focus of treatment. Although Ron continued to express a desire to remember everything he needed to do in his head, he began to realize that the planner helped him "test and evaluate his memory" and served as a "backup system" for his memory. This is reflective of the struggle that many clients have in letting go of their previous cognitive style and accepting different methods for task performance.

Goal attainment ratings indicated that, after 3 weeks of treatment, Ron's wife began to notice a decrease in the number of repetitive questions and calls she received about his schedule. He was initiating looking at his calendar and to-do list more frequently and was consistently initi-

ating setting a timer with an alarm signal to remind him of important activities. The positive feedback and change in one goal rating level from Ron's wife was motivating for Ron. He continued to rely on his wife, however, to help him "fill in information," such as remembering conversations, where they went, and what had occurred.

Sections were added to Ron's planner, including an event section and a self-reflection section. The event section included daily recordings of conversations, readings, or events. Ron was encouraged to record daily conversations, events that occurred, or things that transpired during the day. Initially, Ron tended to make long entries that were disorganized, difficult to reread, and incomplete. An outline was used to cue him to record when and where the event or conversation occurred, who was involved, and what happened. An emphasis was placed on helping Ron use lists of "key retrieval words" to summarize events. This required the ability to focus on the main themes of conversations, readings, or events. Summarizing and choosing keywords requires repetition, rehearsal, and reorganization of information so that retention and deeper encoding of material is facilitated.

Dynamic assessment previously indicated that cues that helped Ron focus on the main theme facilitated retention of information. A wide range of activities was used to practice efficiency in identifying keywords or themes. For example, Ron practiced writing keywords for newspaper and magazine articles, poems, telephone calls, conversations, movies, events, and activities that he participated in. Once again, within each activity, Ron was asked to predict task difficulty and self-assess his performance afterward, including rating his satisfaction and efficiency of notetaking. The purpose of the task evaluations was to increase his ability to monitor and self-reflect on his performance. A section of Ron's planner was used for self-reflections. In this section, Ron was asked to write about what he learned from activity experiences and about what he might do differently next time. He also was encouraged to write about any thoughts or feelings.

At this point, Ron began to resume his former volunteer job on a limited basis, with encouragement from his wife and occupational therapist. He used a separate section in his planner to record information on each patient he met and a summary of their conversation. With assistance, he also included a list of possible topics for conversation and conversation starters at the end of the book. His success in using the planner within his volunteer job helped Ron gain self-confidence.

Gradually Ron realized that writing keywords or self-retrieval cues helped him remember. He began to internalize these strategies by repeating keywords, ideas, and main themes to himself during activities such as reading, conversations, or an event. He used his written notes as a way of self-testing his ability to remember. For example, with his book closed, he would try to remember a telephone conversation and then open his book and underline the aspects that he had recalled. He discovered that, if he focused on the key ideas and repeated them to himself, he was able to retain more information without writing it down. After 3½ months of outpatient treatment, two times per week, Ron and his wife felt that the goal of decreasing reliance on others for memory had been met.

At this point, treatment continued for another 6 weeks and progressed to unstructured activities that required planning, organizing, and generating different alternatives. Additional strategies were introduced such as writing down the key steps of the task prior to performing it or creating a checklist, underlining key steps in written directions, mentally rehearsing performing a task, and visualizing the task outcome. During this phase of treatment, an emphasis was on helping Ron to monitor his tendency to forget about the overall goal and lose track of information within unstructured activities. Similarly, Ron was encouraged to monitor his tendency to repeat himself or "get stuck." Ron was given a cue card of helpful hints that was initially placed on the table and that he later kept in his pocket to refer to whenever he ran into difficulty. The card included hints such as the following: "Find the broad categories first before thinking about the specifics. Watch for repetitions. Mentally practice or imagine yourself performing each step of the activity." Ron practiced these strategies in activities that required generating different alternatives and options. For example, he practiced generating ideas for things to do on a rainy day, things to make for dinner, different questions to ask before you buy a used car, and different ways to start a conversation with someone you have just met. He also practiced thinking of different ways of organizing activities, including his schedule or to-do list. Examples of unstructured activities presented across the activity transfer continuum is presented in Case Example 2.4.

Case Example 2.4. Application of the Multicontext Treatment Approach: Ron

Activity Conditions That Remain the Same
All activities are higher-level unstructured activities that require initiation of ideas, planning, and organization.

Processing Strategy Emphasized in All Activities
Mentally practice or imagine yourself performing each step of the activity and the task outcome. Brainstorm broad categories prior to specifics. Create a checklist that can be used to guide task performance.

Self-Monitoring Techniques in All Activities
Identify potential obstacles and strategies that might be helpful prior to the task; use a cue card with hints and self-questions. Recognize when "getting stuck" or "losing track," and look at cue card.

Goal Ratings
Ron self-rates initiation of strategy use and effectiveness of task performance on a goal scale that is compared with ratings by clinician.

ACTIVITY TRANSFER CONTINUUM

Very Similar		Somewhat Similar		Different		Very Different
You are assisting in planning a barbecue picnic for the local firefighters' organization. What will need to be done?	You are assisting in planning a coffee social after Sunday mass. What will need to be done?	You would like to make something out of wood to donate to a raffle that the local church is holding. What do you do?	You would like to plan a get-together with 5 of your old friends, including dinner at a restaurant and bowling. What do you need to do?	You are planning a schedule of things to see and do for an old friend coming to the area for the first time. What would you need to do?	You would like to plant a garden in a small section of your yard. What do you need to do?

Ron and his wife were asked to generate cognitively challenging activities that required planning and organizing within his daily life. Their list included organizing a vast collection of music CDs and movies, organizing woodworking supplies, rearranging and organizing a bookcase, organizing into a binder poems that Ron had written, writing a checklist of steps to record a program with a new DVD player, and planning and organizing a get-together at a restaurant for lunch with a group of friends. Ron admitted that he had been avoiding some of these activities because they were too overwhelming. Specific goals to try 1–2 of these activities per week were established. Prior to each activity, Ron completed a worksheet that asked him to choose strategies that might be helpful, identify any potential obstacles or difficulties, and estimate length of time required and level of task difficulty. He then carried out the activity, recorded results, self-evaluated performance, and identified things to do differently next time.

At discharge, changes in functioning were documented with the FAQ and the DLQ. Initially, the FAQ yielded a score of 15, indicating that Ron's wife perceived that he had moderate levels of difficulty, whereas at discharge, the FAQ score was 5, indicating greater independence. At discharge, Ron's wife indicated difficulties in daily living on only 4% of the activities on the DLQ, whereas initially she had reported changes in nearly 50% of the daily living tasks. Initially, Ron's wife reported greater difficulties than Ron did. By the end of treatment, both Ron and his wife were closer in their perceptions of disability in all areas. In some instances, Ron rated himself lower than his wife did. For example, initially, Ron felt his memory and organization skills were higher than his wife had rated, but at the end of treatment, his wife rated him higher than he rated himself. This pattern is illustrated in Figure 2.8 and reflects increases in awareness that occurred during treatment. By the end of treatment, Ron had become more independent in keeping track of information, structuring his day, and carrying out daily responsibilities. He felt more comfortable in social situations and learned to move onto a "new thought" when he felt himself stuck in a conversation. He resumed participation in previous hobbies and, most importantly, he returned to his volunteer job. At discharge he stated "I may never be 100%," but he indicated satisfaction with his level of performance and an understanding of how strategy use helped him to improve his functioning.

A follow-up telephone call made to Ron and his wife approximately 3 months after discharge indicated that the gains he made continued to be maintained. Both Ron and

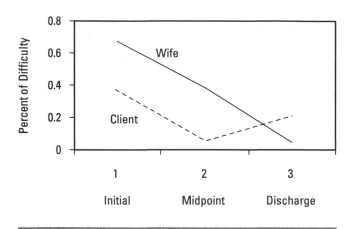

FIGURE 2.8. Changes in Daily Living Questionnaire.

his wife described improvements in his ability to organize, initiate, and carry out planned activities. They reported greater participation in social activities. For example, Ron independently planned a surprise party for a family member. He actively organized the event, including initiating phone calls, sending invitations, and decorating their home. Overall, Ron indicated an increase in his self-confidence.

Ron's case illustrates use of a combination of approaches and types of strategies. Methods that included modification of the environment (alarm, timer), compensation (writing down information), internal strategy training, and self-monitoring strategies were used simultaneously throughout treatment. The same strategies were practiced across a variety of situations, and self-monitoring and self-reflection were interwoven within treatment. Treatment began by addressing the area that the client was most concerned about and that had the greatest level of awareness and responsiveness to cues.

RESEARCH TO SUPPORT EVIDENCE-BASED PRACTICE

Several case reports have been used to describe the multicontext approach (Landa-Gonzalez, 2001; Toglia, 1989b, 1991). For example, Landa-Gonzalex described use of the multicontext approach with a 34-year-old man with traumatic brain injury. Intervention was carried out in the client's home and community and included practice in use of strategies such as a checklist and self-questioning across a wide range of functional activities. For example, he used a checklist to identify problems and safety hazards in a room, prepare a meal, and complete household cleaning chores. For each treatment activity, the client predicted his performance before the task and then self-evaluated his own performance after the task. Results after 6 months of intervention showed improvements in the client's awareness level, enhancement of his occupational function, increased satisfaction and quality of life, and decreased supervision. Application of the multicontext approach has also been described with a 66-year-old man with severe visual–perceptual impairments (Toglia, 1989b). Several strategies were practiced such as stimulus reduction, visual imagery, and pacing speed of responses across a variety of activities and environments. Self-monitoring strategies, including anticipating difficulties and checking outcomes, were integrated into all sessions. Treatment after 4 months resulted in improved functional performance as well as increases in self-confidence and ability to cope with his disability.

The multicontext treatment approach has not been compared with other treatment approaches; however, there are a growing number of studies and case reports that support the main components of the approach such as strategy training, awareness training, and practice in different contexts.

Strategy Training

Several studies and case reports in the literature document the effectiveness of strategy training such as use of verbal mediation (Cicerone & Giacino, 1992; Kray, Eber, & Lindenberger, 2004), self-instructional procedures (Stuss, 1991), mental rehearsal or visual imagery (Driskell, Cooper, & Moran, 1994; Niemeier, 1998), pacing, and task reduction methods. For example, verbal mediation and self-instructional strategies have been reported to be effective in improving concentration (Webster & Scott, 1983), planning and self-regulation skills (Cicerone & Wood, 1987), and unilateral neglect (Robertson, Tegner, Tham, Lo, & Smith, 1995). Self-instructional procedures involve saying self-cues, task goals, plans, or task instructions out loud before or during execution of a task. The technique also may include talking aloud each step of a task to focus attention on the task and inhibit distractions and stereotypic behaviors. The overt verbalization is gradually faded to a whisper, and eventually the client is asked to "talk silently to himself." Inner speech is thought to play an important role in regulation of action, planning, and executive functioning (Cicerone, 2002a).

Cicerone (2002b) described an intervention for attentional deficits for 4 adults with mild traumatic brain injury. The intervention included strategy training, use of verbal mediation, rehearsal and self-pacing, and imagined use of strategies in real-world situations. In addition, self-monitoring strategies, including anticipation of task demands and self-appraisal, were used. The treatment participants showed a reduction of self-reported attentional symptoms compared to a control group.

Freeman, Mittenberg, Dicowden, and Bat-Ami (1992) describe effective use of a combination of memory strategies and self-monitoring strategies to improve paragraph retention. The techniques used included use of visual imagery during reading, note-taking while reading, and use of a keyword list at the end of each paragraph. Individuals also were asked to restate the material or summarize information at the end of each page; pick out the main idea of the paragraph; and ask themselves questions such as, "Am I keeping track of everything? Am I following the story? Does it all make sense?" The effectiveness of training in a memory retrieval strategy using retrospection and self-questioning techniques has been described by Deelman, Berg, and Koning-Haanstra (1990). A 32-year-old client with head trauma was trained 9 months postinjury to use a systematic approach to retrieving information. First, she was taught to try to think back to the input situation and try to find a context by asking herself general questions such as, "Which activities are usual on that day?" Second, she was trained to search within the context by asking herself more specific questions such as, "Were other people involved in the activities?" Finally, she was trained to verify her answers.

Nelson and Lenhart (1996) described effective use of organizational and planning strategies such as categorizing items by location in the supermarket in a head trauma client who was 5 years postinjury. The use of strategies was possible only after the client became aware of her deficits.

Training in problem-solving strategies has been investigated in several studies (Levine et al., 2000; von Cramon, Matthes-von Cramon, & Mai, 1991). Typically, people with brain injury are taught to use task reduction methods to simplify a multistage problem by breaking it down into smaller subgoals or more manageable components. A systematic framework that includes an emphasis on problem definition, exploration of possible strategies, generation of alternate solutions, and self-checking is used to replace the impulsive, disorganized, and unsystematic approach that many people with brain injury exhibit when approaching problems. On the basis of their review of treatment studies, Cicerone and colleagues (2000) concluded that training in problem-solving strategies and the application of these strategies to everyday situations is recommended practice for postacute treatment of traumatic brain injury.

Niemeier, Cifu, and Kishore (2001) examined the effect of teaching a visual imagery strategy for 10 people with brain injury and unilateral neglect. Following training that included practicing the targeted strategy in a wide range of functional tasks, the treatment group demonstrated significantly better performance on functional tasks as compared to the control group.

The majority of studies that have incorporated strategy training have concluded or commented that successful strategy use depended on whether the person had awareness or became aware of their difficulties during the course of treatment. Similarly, a summary of research in educational psychology concludes that successful strategy intervention programs include an emphasis on self-monitoring skills, such as setting goals and planning, revising, and self-evaluating strategies (Pressley, 1995).

Practice Across Different Activities and Environments

In general, the studies that have shown greater success in cognitive rehabilitation are those that have used a broader range of treatment tasks, whereas those that have used only one or two graded training tasks have tended to produce task-specific effects (Antonucci et al., 1995; Levine et al., 2000; Neistadt, 1994; Niemeier, 1998; Niemeier et al., 2001; Sohlberg & Raskin, 1996). Lloyd and Cuvo (1994) reviewed 15 studies of adults with traumatic brain injury and found that those studies reporting more successful outcomes included training in a variety of examples. Likewise, in a review of 14 studies on remediation of attentional deficits, Mateer, Sohlberg, and Youngman (1990) found that those studies reporting positive outcomes used a wider variety of training tasks. In Neistadt's (1994) review of studies on perceptual retraining, she concluded that intermediate- and far-transfer "will only occur for clients with localized brain lesions and good cognitive skills who have been trained with a variety of treatment tasks" (p. 232). Raskin and Gordon (1992) describe three case studies of adults who had brain injury and cognitive deficits. Treatment included remedial and compensation training. Generalization was addressed in each treatment program by using a variety of treatment tasks, including those relevant to everyday life. They reported positive outcomes and argued that "no matter what approach one uses to treat cognitive deficits (remedial or compensation), generalization is only achieved when it is built into the training program" (p. 44).

Awareness Training

Awareness-training strategies such as anticipating possible difficulties, generating alternate strategies, self-prediction, structured error monitoring, self-evaluation, and videotape feedback have been described in case reports or studies with small numbers of participants (Cicerone, 2002a, 2002b; Cicerone & Giacino, 1992; Katz et al., 2002; Liu, Chan, Lee, Li, & Hui-Chan, 2002; Soderback, Bengtsson, Ginsberg, & Ekholm, 1992; Tham et al., 2001; von Cramon & Matthes-von Cramon, 1994). Cicerone and Giacino reported success in the use of self-prediction for two clients with head injuries and executive dysfunction. Clients were required to predict how many moves it would take them to complete the Tower of London puzzle. The authors observed that one client was able to spontaneously apply the strategy of prediction to his time management of daily activities. They suggested that the use of self-predictions may be effective in assisting clients to anticipate the effects of their own behavior.

Cicerone and Giacino (1992) also described a structured error-monitoring procedure. In this procedure, the client's performance was stopped immediately when an error was made and the client's attention was focused on the error. The client was required to keep a record of his own errors and systematically compare them with his rsponses on subsequent trials. The authors observed the ability of the client to apply the error-monitoring routine to a clerical task, although the client continued to require some prompts.

Videotape feedback has been used successfully in several studies to help clients become more aware of their difficulties (Liu et al., 2002; Soderback et al., 1992; Tham et al., 2001). In videotape feedback, a videotape is stopped at different points and the client is guided in identifying problems and generating possible strategies or solutions for the future. Liu and colleagues (2002) reported three case studies using videotape feedback and self-regulation methods within the context of meaningful daily tasks. They reported that clients demonstrated increased awareness of their problems as well as increased strategy use across a variety of daily tasks. Similarly, Tham and colleagues (2001) described an awareness training program for four clients with right-brain damage and unilateral neglect. The program included participation in meaningful activities, anticipation of difficulties, self-evaluation of performance, discussion of alternative strategies, and videotape feedback. The participants became more aware of their difficulties and demonstrated improved ADL performance.

SUMMARY AND IMPLICATIONS FOR FUTURE RESEARCH

In this chapter, I have presented a dynamic interactional model of cognition as a foundation for occupational therapy assessment and treatment of cognitive dysfunction. In the dynamic interactional model of cognition, treatment is reactive and individualized to the person's interests and responses. Learning and the ability to transfer information flexibly across task boundaries are seen as integral components of cognition. Therefore, learning potential and learning transfer is directly addressed in assessment. Dynamic assessment uses guided assistance and task alterations to determine the degree of cognitive modifiability. It examines the conditions that increase or decrease self-monitoring abilities and effective use of strategies. This information is used to guide treatment planning. The dynamic interactional model of cognition provides a framework for addressing cognitive impairments by changing the person (strategies and self-awareness), activity, or environment. It provides a broad framework for using different treatment approaches, including the multicontext approach. This is in contrast to traditional cognitive remedial treatment approaches that have been guided by a narrow conceptualization of cognition.

The multicontext treatment approach involves practicing the same processing strategy across a variety of selected activities and environments. Learning transfer occurs across a horizontal continuum that emphasizes "sideways learning." Treatment attempts to facilitate the transfer process by combining training in multiple situations with strategy training and awareness training. The ability to transfer skills learned in one situation to another situation is constantly observed and worked for within a specific level of task difficulty. The multicontext approach is used to address behaviors that show potential for change. The client is expected to learn to apply a targeted strategy within a variety of situations. Thus, change or generalization of learning is expected from the person. At the same time, however, activity and environmental demands may be changed so that strategies are practiced within the information-processing capabilities of the person. The multicontext approach simultaneously addresses changes in the activity, environment, and person. In cases in which the person does not demonstrate the potential to learn or apply information across situations, adaptation of the environment or functional skill training may be more appropriate treatment emphases.

Although case reports have supported the effectiveness of the components of the multicontext approach, such as strategy training, awareness training, and practice in multiple situations, the multicontext approach needs to be systematically tested and compared to other approaches developed for the adult with brain injury. Different people with brain injury may respond differently to various approaches. The level of severity, stage of recovery, available external supports, and type of cognitive dysfunction may influence the technique or approach that is most effective in enhancing function.

This approach needs to be explored further with other populations such as children with learning disabilities and adults with mental illness. The specific assessment and treatment techniques presented in this chapter rely heavily on verbal mediation. Clients with significant language impairment may not be capable of responding to verbal cues. In these cases, the same theoretical concepts described in this chapter can be applied, but the specific assessment and treatment techniques must be adapted. An example of an informal assessment that analyzes a client's response to nonverbal cues and changes in task parameters was presented but needs further development. Although awareness-training techniques and self-monitoring strategies described in this chapter would not be appropriate for these clients, awareness of cognitive capacity and the ability to recognize and correct errors could be promoted through tactile, kinesthetic, or visual feedback.

The concept of dynamic assessment deserves further attention within occupational therapy practice, as it assumes that learning and change can take place during activity experiences. This is more compatible with occupational therapists' view of human abilities as compared with the psychometric tradition that assumes that abilities remain relatively stable. For example, in standardized testing, changes in performance that occur within a task are considered noise, error, or unreliability, whereas in dynamic assessment, changes in performance are the focus of interest. Dynamic assessment therefore requires a paradigmatic shift. Traditional psychometric concepts of reliability and error do not fit with the dynamic assessment approach (Feuerstein & Feuerstein, 2001; Sternberg & Grigorenko, 2002).

The goals and concepts of dynamic assessment are appealing; however, it has been argued that empirical evidence is limited (Sternberg & Grigorenko, 2002). This is particularly true regarding use of dynamic assessment with adults who have brain injury. Sternberg and Grigorenko asserted that the field of dynamic assessment has experienced insufficient critical attention from the scientific community. They concluded a review of research on dynamic assessment by stating that they believe dynamic assessment will ultimately meet the challenges ahead and will prove to be a valuable resource to a wide range of disciplines.

There is still much to be learned about treatment of people with cognitive impairments. The effect of the nature of the environment and the activity on learning has been virtually unexplored in adults with brain injury. Comparing treatment that takes place in the same environment versus multiple environments needs further investigation. In addition, research is needed directly comparing treatment using a single graded tabletop or computer activity with treatment using different types of activities. Currently, a review of the literature indicates that studies that have found task-specific effects used a narrow range of treatment tasks, whereas studies that have documented more positive outcome have incorporated a wider variety of treatment activities; however, there have been no studies of direct comparison. The conditions that promote and facilitate learning transfer have been investigated in normal adults and children but, again, this area has not been adequately investigated with adults who have brain injury. Strategy use and strategy training also need further investigation. What strategies appear to be most effective or least effective? What strategies do clients perceive are most useful? Are there qualitative differences in the processing strategies used or not used among different clients? Which awareness-training techniques are most effective? Which types of patients benefit most from different approaches or strategies? Finally, treatment conducted in a predetermined hierarchical sequence needs to be contrasted with programs that are not conducted in a fixed sequence. In other words, the remedial approach to cognitive rehabilitation needs to be compared with the multicontext treatment approach.

This chapter provided a theoretical foundation as a guide for assessment, treatment, and future research. In it, I touched on many issues that need further exploration with the cognitively disabled population. In the absence of evidence that demonstrates that one cognitive rehabilitation approach is better than another, clinicians need to continue to keep a broad perspective, critically analyze the results of their treatment, and ask many questions.

REVIEW QUESTIONS

1. Discuss how cognition is conceptualized as a dynamic interaction among the person, activity, and environment. Explain how this conceptualization guides the evaluation and treatment process.

2. Describe the concept of processing strategies. Explain how processing strategies are influenced by the person's self-awareness, personal context, activity demands, and environment. Explain how they might be targeted during intervention as a means of enhancing occupational performance.

3. Explain the components of dynamic assessment as used within the framework of the dynamic interactional model of cognition. How is dynamic assessment different from static assessment? Give two examples of different dynamic assessment methods.

4. Describe the characteristics of the multicontext approach. How does this approach address transfer of learning?

5. Explain the concept of self-awareness and its relationship to the context of the person and self-efficacy. Describe different methods for evaluating self-awareness.

6. Explain how self-awareness (self-knowledge and on-line awareness) may be addressed in treatment as a means of increasing safety and independence in occupational performance. Provide examples of awareness treatment methods.

ACKNOWLEDGMENT

A special thank you is extended to D. Burstiner, OTR; M. Burke, OTR; and L. Smith, OTR, for their contributions with the second case presentation.

REFERENCES

Abreu, B. C., Seale, G. S., Scheibel, R. S., Huddleston, N., Zhang, L., & Ottenbacher, K. J. (2001). Levels of self-awareness after acute brain injury: How patients' and rehabilitation specialists' perceptions compare. *Archives of Physical Medicine and Rehabilitation, 82,* 49–56.

Abreu, B. C., & Toglia, J. P. (1987). Cognitive rehabilitation: A model for occupational therapy. *American Journal of Occupational Therapy, 41,* 439–448.

Anderson, J. (1985). *Cognitive psychology and its implications.* New York: W. H. Freeman.

Antonucci, G., Guariglia, C., Judica, A., Magnotti, L., Paolucci, S., Pizzamiglio, L., et al. (1995). Effectiveness of neglect rehabilitation in a randomized group study. *Journal of Clinical and Experimental Neuropsychology, 17,* 383–389.

Baltes, M. M., Kühl, K. P., Gutzmann, H., & Sowarka, D. (1995). Potential of cognitive plasticity as a diagnostic instrument: A cross-validation and extension. *Psychology and Aging, 10,* 167–172.

Baltes, M. M., Kühl, K. P., & Sowarka, D. (1992). Testing for limits of cognitive reserve capacity: A promising strategy for early diagnosis of dementia? *Journal of Gerontology, 17,* 165–167.

Bandura, A. (1997). *Self-efficacy: The exercise of control.* New York: W. H. Freeman.

Belmont, J. M., Butterfield, E. C., & Ferretti, R. P. (1982). To secure transfer of training: Instruct self-management skills. In D. K. Detterman & R. J. Sternberg (Eds.), *How and how much can intelligence be increased* (pp. 147–154). Norwood, NJ: Ablex.

Bhogal, S. K., Teasell, R. W., Foley, N. C., & Speechley, M. R. (2003). Community reintegration after stroke. *Topics in Stroke Rehabilitation, 10,* 107–109.

Bransford, J. (1979). *Human cognition: Learning, understanding, and remembering.* Belmont, CA: Wadsworth.

Bransford, J., Sherwood, R., Vye, N., & Rieser, J. (1986). Teaching thinking and problem solving: Research foundations. *American Psychologist, 41,* 1078–1089.

Brown, A. (1988). Motivation to learn and understand: On taking charge of one's own learning. *Cognition and Instruction, 5,* 311–321.

Brown, A., Bransford, J., Ferrara, R., & Campione, J. (1983). Learning, remembering and understanding. In J. Flavell & E. Markman (Eds.), *Handbook of child psychology* (Vol. 3, pp. 77–158). New York: John Wiley & Sons.

Brown, A. L., & Ferrara, R. A. (1985). Diagnosing zones of proximal development. In J. Wertsch (Ed.), *Culture, communication and cognition: Vygotskian perspectives* (pp. 272–305). Cambridge, England: Cambridge University Press.

Brown, A. L., & French, L. A. (1979). The zone of potential development: Implications for intelligence testing in the year 2000. *Intelligence, 3,* 255–277.

Cicerone, K. D. (2002a). The enigma of executive functioning. In P. J. Eslinger (Ed.), *Neuropsychological interventions: Clinical research and practice* (pp. 246–265). New York: Guilford Press.

Cicerone, K. D. (2002b). Remediation of "working attention" in mild traumatic brain injury. *Brain Injury, 16,* 185–195.

Cicerone, K. D., Dahlberg, C., Kalmar, K., Langenbahn, D. M., Malec, J. F., Bergquist, T. F., et al. (2000). Evidence-based cognitive rehabilitation: Recommendations for clinical practice. *Archives of Physical Medicine and Rehabilitation, 81,* 1596–1615.

Cicerone, K. D., & Giacino, J. T. (1992). Remediation of executive function deficits after traumatic brain injury. *Neuro-Rehabilitation, 2*(3), 12–22.

Cicerone, K. D., & Tupper, D. E. (1986). Cognitive assessment in the neuropsychological rehabilitation of head-injured adults. In B. P. Uzzell & Y. Gross (Eds.), *The clinical neuropsychology of intervention* (pp. 59–84). Boston: Martinus Nijhoff.

Cicerone, K. D., & Wood, J. C. (1987). Planning disorder after closed head injury: A case study. *Archives of Physical Medicine and Rehabilitation, 68,* 111–115.

Cornoldi, C. (1998). The impact of metacognitive reflection on cognitive control. In D. J. Hacker, J. Dunlosky, & A.

Graesser (Eds.), *Metacognition in educational theory and practice* (pp. 139–159). Mahwah, NJ: Lawrence Erlbaum.

Deelman, B. G., Berg, I. J., & Koning-Haanstra, M. (1990). Memory strategies for closed-head-injured patients. Do lessons in cognitive psychology help? In R. Wood & I. Fussy (Eds.), *Cognitive rehabilitation in perspective* (pp. 117–144). London: Taylor & Francis.

Dirette, D. K. (2002). The development of awareness and the use of compensatory strategies for cognitive deficits. *Brain Injury, 16,* 861–871.

Driskell, J. E., Cooper, C., & Moran, A. (1994). Does mental practice enhance performance? *Journal of Applied Psychology, 79,* 481–492.

Duncan, P. W., Wallace, D., MinLai, S., Johnson, D., Embrestson, S., & Jacobs-Laster, L. (1999). The Stroke Impact Scale, version 2.0: Evaluation of reliability, validity, and sensitivity to change. *Stroke, 30,* 2131–2140.

Elliott, J. (2003). Dynamic assessment in educational settings: Realizing potential. *Educational Review, 55,* 15–32.

Embretson, S. (1987). Toward development of a psychometric approach. In C. S. Lidz (Ed.), *Dynamic assessment* (pp. 141–170). New York: Guilford.

Fernandez-Ballesteros, R., Zamarron, M. D., Tarraga, L., Moya, R., & Iniguez, J. (2003). Cognitive plasticity in healthy, mild cognitive impairment (MCI) subjects and Alzheimer's disease patients: A research project in Spain. *European Psychologist, 8,* 148–159.

Feuerstein, R. (1979). *The dynamic assessment of retarded performers: The learning potential device, theory, instruments, and techniques.* Baltimore: University Park Press.

Feuerstein, R., & Falik, L. H. (2004). *Cognitive modifiability: A needed perspective on learning for the 21st century.* Retrieved April 2004 from http://www.icelp.org/asp/Dynamic_Cognitive_Assessment.shtm.

Feuerstein, R., & Feuerstein, R. S. (2001). Is dynamic assessment compatible with the psychometric model? In A. S. Kaufman & N. L. Kaufman (Ed.), *Specific learning disabilities and difficulties in children and adolescents* (pp. 218–246). Cambridge, England: Cambridge University Press.

Fine, S. (1993). Lesson 3: Interaction between psychosocial variables and cognitive function. In C. B. Royeen (Ed.), *AOTA Self-Study Series: Cognitive rehabilitation* (pp. 1–40). Rockville, MD: American Occupational Therapy Association.

Fischer, S., Gauggel, S., & Trexler, L. E. (2004). Awareness of activity limitations, goal setting, and rehabilitation outcome in patients with brain injuries. *Brain Injury, 18,* 547–562.

Flavell, J. H., Miller, P. H., & Miller, S. A. (1993). *Cognitive development* (3rd ed.). Englewood Cliffs, NJ: Prentice Hall.

Fleming, J. M., Strong, J., & Ashton, R. (1996). Self-awareness of deficits in adults with traumatic brain injury: How best to measure? *Brain Injury, 10*(1), 1–15.

Fleming, J. M., Strong, J., & Ashton, R. (1998). Cluster analysis of self-awareness levels in adults with traumatic brain injury and relationship to outcome. *Journal of Head Trauma Rehabilitation, 13,* 39–51.

Freeman, M. R., Mittenberg, W., Dicowden, M., & Bat-Ami, M. (1992). Executive and compensatory memory retraining in traumatic brain injury. *Brain Injury, 6*(1), 65–70.

Gage, M., & Polatajko, H. (1994). Enhancing occupational performance through an understanding of perceived self-efficacy. *American Journal of Occupational Therapy, 48,* 452–461.

Gil, N., & Josman, N. (2001). Memory and metamemory performance in Alzheimer's disease and healthy elderly: The Contextual Memory Test (CMT). *Aging Clinical Experimental Research, 13,* 309–315.

Gilewski, M. J., Zelinski, E. M., & Schaie, K. W. (1990). The memory functioning questionnaire for assessment of memory complaints in adulthood and old age. *Psychology and Aging, 5,* 482–490.

Glick, M. L., & Holyoak, K. J. (1987). Transfer of learning: Contemporary research and applications. In S. M. Cormier & J. D. Hagman (Eds.), *The cognitive basis of knowledge transfer* (pp. 9–42). London: Academic Press.

Golisz, K., & Toglia, J. P. (2003). Perception and cognition. In E. B. Crepeau, E. S. Cohn, & B. A. B. Schell (Eds.), *Willard and Spackman's occupational therapy* (10th ed., pp. 395–416). Philadelphia: Lippincott Williams & Wilkins.

Goverover, Y., & Hinojosa, J. (2002). Categorization and deductive reasoning: Predictors of instrumental activities of daily living performance in adults with brain injury. *American Journal of Occupational Therapy, 56,* 509–516.

Goverover, Y., & Hinojosa, J. (2004). Interrater reliability and discriminant validity of the deductive reasoning test. *American Journal of Occupational Therapy, 58,* 104–108.

Grattan, L. M., & Eslinger P. J. (1989). Higher cognition and social behavior: Changes in cognitive flexibility and empathy after cerebral lesions. *Neuropsychologia, 3,* 175–185.

Grigorenko, E. L., & Sternberg, R. J. (1998). Dynamic testing. *Psychological Bulletin, 124,* 75–111.

Groveman, A. M., Brown, E. W., & Miller, M. H. (1985). Moving toward common ground: Utilizing Feuerstein's model in cognitive rehabilitation. *Cognitive Rehabilitation, 3,* 28–30.

Harrison, M. J., Morris, K. A., Barsky, J., Toglia, J., Horton, R., & Robbins, L. (2003, October). *Development of a unique and novel psycho-educational program for active SLE patients with self-perceived cognitive dysfunction.* Paper presented at the 67th Annual Scientific Meeting of the American College of Rheumatology, Orlando, FL.

Hartman-Maeir, A., Soroker, N., Oman, S. D., & Katz, N. (2003). Awareness of disabilities in stroke rehabilitation: A clinical trial. *Disability and Rehabilitation, 25,* 35–44.

Hartman-Maeir, A., Soroker, N., Ring, H., & Katz, N. (2002). Awareness of deficits in stroke rehabilitation. *Journal of Rehabilitation Medicine, 34,* 158–164.

Haywood, H. C., & Miller, M. B. (2003). Dynamic assessment of adults with traumatic brain injuries. *Journal of Cognitive Education and Psychology Online, 3,* 137–158.

Haywood, H. C., & Tzuriel, D. (2002). Applications and challenges in dynamic assessment. *Peabody Journal of Education, 77,* 40–63.

Hessels-Schlatter, C. (2002). A dynamic test to assess learning capacity in people with severe impairments. *American Journal on Mental Retardation, 107,* 340–351.

Jensen, M. R., & Feuerstein, R. (1987). The learning potential assessment device: From philosophy to practice. In C. S. Lidz (Ed.), *Dynamic assessment: An interactional approach to evaluation learning potential* (pp. 379–402). New York: Guilford.

Josman, N. (1993). *Assessment of categorization skills in brain-injured and schizophrenic persons: Validation of the Toglia Category Assessment (TCA).* Unpublished doctoral dissertation, New York University, New York.

Josman, N. (1999). Reliability and validity of the Toglia Category Assessment Test. *Canadian Journal of Occupational Therapy, 66,* 33–41.

Josman, N., Berney, T., & Jarus, T. (2000a). Evaluating categorization skills in children following severe brain injury. *Occupational Therapy Journal of Research, 20,* 241–255.

Josman, N., Berney, T., & Jarus, T. (2000b). Performance of children with and without traumatic brain injury on the contextual memory test (CMT). *Physical and Occupational Therapy in Pediatrics, 19,* 39–51.

Josman, N., & Hartman-Maeir, A. (2000). Cross-cultural assessment of the Contextual Memory Test (CMT). *Occupational Therapy International, 7,* 246–258.

Josman, N., & Jarus, T. (2001). Construct-related validity of the Toglia Category Assessment and the Deductive Reasoning Test with children who are typically developing. *American Journal of Occupational Therapy, 55,* 524–530.

Katz, N., Fleming, J., Keren, N., Lightbody, S., & Hartman-Maeir, A. (2002). Unawareness and/or denial of disability: Implications for occupational therapy intervention. *Canadian Journal of Occupational Therapy, 69,* 281–292.

Kizony, R., & Katz, N. (2002). Relationships between cognitive abilities and the process scale and skills of the Assessment of Motor and Process Skills (AMPS) in patients with stroke. *OTJR: Occupation, Participation, and Health, 22,* 82–92.

Klauer, K. J. (2002). A new generation of cognitive training for children: A European perspective. In G. M. Van der Aalsvoort, W. C. M. Resing, & A. J. J. M. Ruijssenaars (Eds.), *Advances in cognition and educational practice: Learning potential assessment and cognitive training—Actual research and perspectives in theory building and methodology.* (Vol. 7, pp. 147–174). Amsterdam: Elsevier Science.

Kline, N. K. (2000). Validity of the Modified Dynamic Visual Processing Assessment. *Israel Journal of Occupational Therapy, 9,* 69–88.

Kolakowsky, S. A. (1998). Assessing learning potential in ptients with brain injury: Dynamic assessment. *Neurorehabilitation, 11,* 227–238.

Kray, J., Eber, E., & Lindenberger, U. (2004). Age differences in executive functioning across the lifespan: The role of verbalization in task preparation. *Acta Psychologica, 115,* 143–165.

Landa-Gonzalez, B. (2001). Multicontextual occupational therapy intervention: A case study of traumatic brain injury. *Occupational Therapy International, 8,* 49–62.

Lauchlan, F., & Elliot, J. (2001). The psychological assessment of learning potential. *British Journal of Educational Psychology, 71,* 647–665.

Law, M., Baptiste, S., McColl, S., Opzoomer, A., Polatajko, H., & Pollock, N. (1998). *The Canadian Occupational Performance Measure* (3rd ed.). Toronto: Canadian Association of Occupational Therapists.

Levine, B., Robertson, I. H., Clare, L., Carter, G., Hong, I., Wilson, B. A., et al. (2000). Rehabilitation of executive functioning: An experimental clinical validation of goal management training. *Journal of the International Neuropsychological Society, 6,* 299–312.

Lidz, C. S. (1987). Cognitive deficiencies revisited. In C. S. Lidz (Ed.), *Dynamic assessment: Evaluating learning potential* (pp. 444–478). New York: Guilford.

Lidz, C. S., & Elliot, J. G. (2000). Introduction to dynamic assessment. In C. S. Lidz & J. G. Elliot (Eds.), *Advances in cognition and educational practice: Vol. 6. Dynamic assessment: Prevailing models and applications* (pp. 3–16). Amsterdam: Elsevier Science.

Liu, K. P. Y., Chan, C. C. H., Lee, T. M. C., Li, L. S. W., & Hui-Chan, C. W. Y. (2002). Self-regulatory learning and generalization for people with brain injury. *Brain Injury, 16,* 817–824.

Lloyd, L. F, & Cuvo, A. J. (1994). Maintenance and generalization of behaviors after treatment of persons with traumatic brain injury. *Brain Injury, 8,* 529–540.

Malec, J. F., Smigielski, J. S., & DePompolo, R. W. (1991). Goal attainment scaling and outcome measurement in postacute brain injury rehabilitation. *Archives of Physical Medicine and Rehabilitation, 72,* 138–143.

Mateer, C., Sohlberg, M., & Youngman, P. (1990). The management of acquired attention and memory deficits. In R. Wood & I. Fussey (Eds.), *Cognitive rehabilitation in perspective* (pp. 68–95). London: Taylor & Francis.

Neistadt, M. E. (1990). A critical analysis of occupational therapy approaches for perceptual deficits in adults with brain injury. *American Journal of Occupational Therapy, 44,* 229–304.

Neistadt, M. E. (1994). Perceptual retraining for adults with diffuse brain injury. *American Journal of Occupational Therapy, 48,* 225–233.

Nelson, D. L., & Lenhart, D. A. (1996). Resumption of outpatient occupational therapy for a young woman five years after traumatic brain injury. *American Journal of Occupational Therapy, 50,* 223–228.

Niemeier, J. P. (1998). The Lighthouse Strategy: Use of a visual imagery technique to treat visual inattention in stroke patients. *Brain Injury, 12,* 399–406.

Niemeier, J. P., Cifu, D. X., & Kishore, R. (2001). The Lighthouse Strategy: Improving the functional status of patients with unilateral neglect after stroke and brain injury using a visual imagery intervention. *Topics in Stroke Rehabilitation, 8*(2), 10–18.

Nolen, S. B. (1988). Reasons for studying: Motivational orientations and study strategies. *Cognition and Instruction, 5,* 269–287.

Pfeffer, R. I., Kurosaki, T. T., Harrah, C. H., Chance, J. M., & Filos, S. (1982). Measurement of functional activities in older adults in the community. *Journal of Gerontology, 37,* 323–329.

Pressley, M. (1995). More about the development of self-regulation: Complex, long-term, and thoroughly social. *Educational Psychologist, 30,* 207–212.

Prigatano, G. (1986). *Neuropsychological rehabilitation after brain injury.* Baltimore: Johns Hopkins University Press.

Raskin, S. A., & Gordon, W. A. (1992). The impact of different approaches to cognitive remediation on generalization. *NeuroRehabilitation, 2,* 38–45.

Resing, W. C. M., & Roth-Van der Werf, T. J. M. (2002). Learning potential assessment and cognitive training in inductive reasoning: Emergent relationship? In G. M. Van der Aalsvoort, W. C. M. Resing, & A. J. J. M. Ruijssenaars (Eds.), *Advances in cognition and educational practice: Vol. 7. Learning potential assessment and cognitive training: Actual research and perspectives in theory building and methodology* (pp. 175–208). Amsterdam: Elsevier Science.

Robertson, H. I., Tegner, R., Tham, K., Lo, A., & Smith, N. I. (1995). Sustained attention training for unilateral neglect: Theoretical and rehabilitation implications. *Journal of Clinical and Experimental Neuropsychology, 17,* 416–430.

Schneider, W. (1998). The development of procedural metamemory in childhood and adolescence. In G. Mazzoni & T. O. Nelson (Eds.), *Metacognition and cognitive neuropsychology: Monitoring and control processes* (pp. 1–21). Mahwah, NJ: Lawrence Erlbaum.

Sherer, M., Bergloff, P., Boake, C., High, W., & Levin, E. (1998). The awareness questionnaire: Factor structure and internal consistency. *Brain Injury, 12*(1), 63–68.

Sherer, M., Boake, C., Levin, E., Silver, B. V., Ringholz, G., & High, W. M., Jr. (1998). Characteristics of impaired awareness after traumatic brain injury. *Journal of the International Neuropsychological Society, 4,* 380–387.

Soderback, I., Bengtsson, I., Ginsberg, E., & Ekholm, J. (1992). Video feedback in occupational therapy: Its effect in patients with neglect syndrome. *Archives of Physical Medicine and Rehabilitation, 73,* 1140–1146.

Sohlberg, M. M., & Mateer, C. A. (2001). *Cognitive rehabilitation: An integrative neuropsychological approach.* New York: Guilford.

Sohlberg, M. M., & Raskin, S. A. (1996). Principles of generalization applied to attention and memory interventions. *Journal of Head Trauma Rehabilitation, 11*(2), 65–78.

Sternberg, R. J., & Grigorenko, E. L. (2002). *Dynamic testing: The nature and measurement of learning potential.* Cambridge, England: Cambridge University Press.

Stuss, D. T. (1991). Disturbances of self-awareness after frontal system damage. In G. P. Prigatano & D. L. Schacter (Eds.), *Awareness of deficit after brain injury* (pp. 63–83). New York: Oxford University Press.

Swanson, H. L., & Deshler, D. (2003). Instructing adolescents with learning disabilities: Converting a meta-analysis to practice. *Journal of Learning Disabilities, 36,* 124–135.

Swanson, H. L., & Lussier, C. M. (2001). A selective synthesis of the experimental literature on dynamic assessment. *Review of Educational Research, 71,* 321–363.

Tham, K., Borell, L., & Gustavsson, A. (2000). The discovery of disability: A phenomenological study of unilateral neglect. *American Journal of Occupational Therapy, 54,* 398–405.

Tham, K., Ginsburg, E., Fisher, A., & Tegner, R. (2001). Training to improve awareness of disabilities in clients with unilateral neglect. *American Journal of Occupational Therapy, 55,* 46–54.

Toglia, J. (2004). *Dynamic assessment and unilateral neglect.* Unpublished doctoral dissertation, Teachers College, Columbia University, New York.

Toglia, J., & Kirk, U. (2000). Understanding awareness deficits following brain injury. *NeuroRehabilitation, 15,* 57–70.

Toglia, J., Morris, K. A., Harrison, M. J., Barsky, J., Horton, R., & Robbins, L. (2004, May). *A group program for persons with systemic lupus erythematosus and subtle cognitive difficulties.* Paper presented at the American Occupational Therapy Association Conference, Minneapolis, MN.

Toglia, J. P. (1989a). Approaches to cognitive assessment of the brain-injured adult: Traditional methods and dynamic investigation. *Occupational Therapy Practice, 1,* 36–57.

Toglia, J. P. (1989b). Visual perception of objects: A model for assessment and intervention. *American Journal of Occupational Therapy, 44,* 587–595.

Toglia, J. P. (1991). Generalization of treatment: A multicontextual approach to cognitive–perceptual impairment in the brain-injured adult. *American Journal of Occupational Therapy, 45,* 505–516.

Toglia, J. P. (1993a). *Contextual Memory Test.* San Antonio, TX: Psychological Corporation.

Toglia, J. P. (1993b). Lesson 4: Attention and memory. In C. B. Royeen (Ed.), *AOTA Self-Study Series: Cognitive rehabilitation* (pp. 4–72). Rockville, MD: American Occupational Therapy Association.

Toglia, J. P. (1994). *Dynamic assessment of categorization skills: The Toglia Category Assessment.* Pequannock, NJ: Maddak.

Toglia, J. P. (2003a). Cognitive-perceptual retraining and rehabilitation. In E. B. Crepeau, E. S. Cohn, & B. A. B. Schell (Eds.), *Willard and Spackman's occupational therapy* (10th ed., pp. 607–629). Philadelphia: Lippincott Williams & Wilkins.

Toglia, J. P. (2003b). The multicontext approach. In E. B. Crepeau, E. S. Cohn, & B. A. B. Schell (Eds.), *Willard and Spackman's occupational therapy* (10th ed., pp. 264–267). Philadelphia: Lippincott Williams & Wilkins.

Toglia, J. P., & Finkelstein, N. (1991). *Test protocol: The Dynamic Visual Processing Assessment.* New York: New York Hospital Cornell Medical Center.

Toglia, J. P., & Golisz, K. (1990). *Cognitive rehabilitation: Group games and activities.* Tucson, AZ: Therapy SkillBuilders.

Trexler, L. (1987). Neuropsychological rehabilitation in the United States. In M. Meier, A. Benton, & L. Diller (Eds.), *Neuropsychological rehabilitation* (pp. 437–460). New York: Guilford.

Turnbell, J. C., Kersten, P., Habib, M., McLellan, L., Mullee, M. A., & George, S. (2000). Validation of the Frenchay Activities Index in a general population aged 16 years and older. *Archives of Physical Medicine and Rehabilitation, 81,* 1034–1038.

von Cramon, D. Y., & Matthes-von Cramon, G. (1994). Back to work with a chronic dysexecutive syndrome? (A case report). *Neuropsychological Rehabilitation, 4,* 399–417.

von Cramon, D. Y., Matthes-von Cramon, G., & Mai, N. (1991). Problem solving deficits in brain-injured patients: A therapeutic approach. *Neuropsychological Rehabilitation, 1*(1), 45–64.

Vygotsky, L. S. (1978). *Mind in society: The development of higher psychological processes.* Cambridge, MA: Harvard University Press.

Webster, J. S., & Scott, R. R. (1983). The effects of self-instructional training on attentional deficits following head injury. *Journal of Clinical Neuropsychology, 5*(2), 69–74.

Wiedl, K. H. (1999). Cognitive modifiability as a measure of readiness for rehabilitation. *Psychiatric Services, 50,* 1411–1419.

Wiedl, K. H., Schoettke, H., & Garcia, D. C. (2001). Dynamic assessment of cognitive rehabilitation potential in schizophrenic persons and in elderly persons with and without dementia. *European Journal of Psychological Assessment, 17,* 112–119.

Wiedl, K. H., Wienobst, J., & Schoettke, H. (2001). Estimating rehabilitation potential in schizophrenic subjects. In H. D. Brenner, W. Boker, & R. Genner (Eds.), *The treatment of schizophrenia: Status and emerging trends* (pp. 88–120). Seattle: Hogrefe & Huber.

Willer, B., Ottenbacher, K. J., & Coad, M. L. (1994). The Community Integration Questionnaire: A comparative examination. *American Journal of Physical Medicine and Rehabilitation, 73,* 103–111.

Wilson, B., Cockburn, J., & Baddley, A. (1985). *The Rivermead Behavioral Memory Test.* Reading, England: Thames Valley Test Company.

Wood-Dauphinee, S. L., Opzoomer, A., Williams, J. I., Marchand, B., & Spitzwer, W. O. (1988). Assessment of global function: The Reintegration to Normal Living Index. *Archives of Physical Medicine and Rehabilitation, 69,* 583–590.

Beatriz C. Abreu, PhD, OTR, FAOTA
Suzanne M. Peloquin, PhD, OTR, FAOTA

The Quadraphonic Approach

A Holistic Rehabilitation Model for Brain Injury

LEARNING OBJECTIVES

By the end of this chapter, readers will

1. Describe the assessment and intervention features within the quadraphonic approach

2. Distinguish between macro client characteristics and micro theories (voices)

3. Describe at least three levels of intervention and recovery for cognitive rehabilitation after traumatic brain injury

4. Describe confluence and narrative as the two complementary constructs foundational to the macro approach.

In this chapter we propose a holistic system for the rehabilitation, health, and well-being of adults with cognitive disabilities after brain injury. The quadraphonic approach combines an analysis of performance skills with a synthesis of meaningful human occupations from the perspectives of both the medical and social models. The approach emerged from more than 38 years of Abreu's clinical practice in cognitive rehabilitation among a broad spectrum of clients ranging from those in coma to those planning community re-entries.

Abreu introduced the quadraphonic approach in 1990 from a medical model perspective, also called a *micro perspective* in this chapter (Krinsky, 1990). At that time, the approach was influenced by the construct of frame of reference, or guidelines to practice, taught in Anne Cronin Mosey's graduate courses at New York University. Two years later, Abreu relocated to Los Angeles and expanded what had been a cognitive frame of reference into a more holistic interpretation of practice. Occupational scientists at the University of Southern California influenced the shaping of a more holistic approach through the introduction of a social model (Wood, Abreu, Duval, & Gerber, 1994). And finally, collaborations with Suzanne Peloquin around her work on the art of practice and the construct of confluence have refined the approach into a more humanistic model of practice.

The quadraphonic approach proposes a fluid movement back and forth between micro and macro perspectives, a dual consideration that attends to performance skills and whole-person engagement in occupation. This chap-ter summarizes the quadraphonic approach in six sections:

1. Theoretical background,
2. Main concepts of the model,
3. Evaluation process and instruments,
4. Treatment principles,
5. Case example, and
6. Research needs and support for the model.

THEORETICAL BACKGROUND FOR THE MICRO PERSPECTIVE

The micro perspective of the quadraphonic approach uses four complementary functional theories, the four voices suggested by the term *quadraphonic*. The four theories that both explain and predict behaviors are information processing, teaching–learning, neurodevelopmental, and biomechanical (see Figure 3.1). Together, these four theories facilitate a collaborative design of therapeutic interventions to improve a client's adaptive strategies.

Information-Processing Theory

Information-processing theory explains how an individual's mind functions—that is, how individuals perceive and react to the environment. This theory postulates that there are three successive processing stages within the nervous system: (a) detection of the stimulus, (b) discrimination and analysis of the stimulus, and (c) selection and determination of the response based on hypotheses derived from the relationship between sensory stimuli and past experience (Abreu, 1992; Klatzy, 1980; Light, 1990). Information processing includes

FIGURE 3.1. Quadraphonic approach evaluation model.

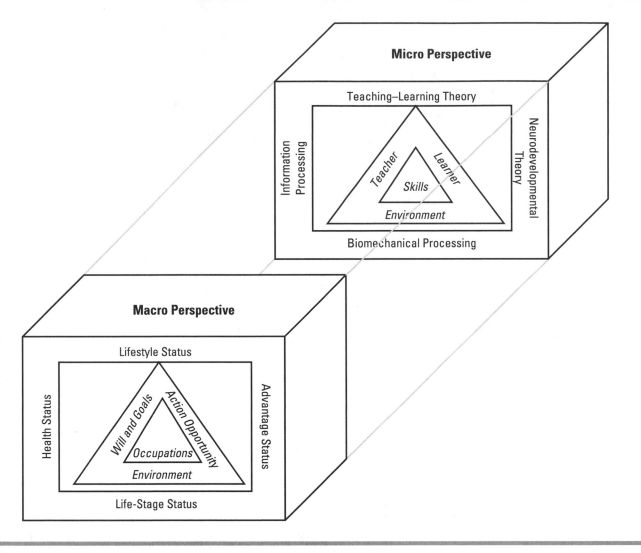

Note. From *The Quadraphonic Approach: Course Handouts,* by B. Abreu, 1997. Galveston, TX: Therapeutic Service Systems. Copyright © 1997 by Therapeutic Service Systems. Reprinted with permission.

stimulus and conceptually driven responses also called *bottom-up* and *top-down* responses (Engel, Fries, & Singer, 2001).

The detection stage of information processing entails the discovery, registration, and recognition of sensory cues. The discrimination and analysis stage includes the interpretation and organization of raw sensory information into a code. This code, or new communication system, is used by the individual's nervous system to determine a response. Discrimination and analysis also depend on the integrity of the sensory receptors (e.g., tactile, vestibular, ocular). The clarity of the stimulus as well as its intensity, pattern, complexity, and significance for the individual affect the discrimination and analysis of stimuli (Abreu,

1981). The response selection and determination stage involves comparing the stimulus with experiences in long-term memory and relating the stimulus in question to the overall purpose and goal of the response. In this stage, the response is planned, structured, and activated. The complexity and the duration of the activity will affect the response. The three successive stages of information processing occur at various levels within the central nervous system and at rates faster than a millisecond. The stages are fully interactive and interdependent in nature.

A response can be data driven, conceptually driven, or both (Norman, 1969, 1979). A data driven response is dependent on a client's analysis of incoming data. If a client is given, as a test, an unfamiliar drawing to reproduce, he or she may focus on all the details to understand what to do. That response can be said to be data driven. A conceptually driven response is more dependent on the environmental context of the stimulus event and is shaped by the individual's memories, personality, and culture (Norman, 1969, 1979). If a client is given a drawing of an object that resembles a childhood toy or game, he or she may say, "I'm not doing this test, it's for kids." That response is more conceptually driven.

Brain trauma or disease compromises information-processing skills. The dysfunction can occur at any stage of processing: stimulus detection, stimulus discrimination and analysis, or response selection and determination. Although information-processing theory can be used to explain some behaviors seen after brain injury and to identify the information-processing stages, the theory does not explain how an individual evaluates or uses cues gathered from the environment. Therefore, a theory that addresses the individual's process of capturing information from the environment is needed to complement information processing.

Teaching–Learning Theory

Explanations for the manner in which a client might use cues to facilitate information processing can be drawn from teaching–learning theory. This theory explains how individuals use cues to alter their capacity and methods of response to increase cognitive awareness and enhance control. There are several teaching–learning theories. Two theories that relate to the capturing of information from the environment are self-generated or natural learning and externally generated or mediated learning (Schwartz, 1991).

Self-generated or natural learning refers to the inherent ability of an individual to learn skills, tasks, or behaviors without external mediation (Schwartz, 1991). Examples are the ability to learn how to sit, walk, and manipulate objects spontaneously using natural strategies for gathering cues from the environment without the aid of an external resource such as a therapist. By comparison, externally generated or mediated learning requires input from an outside source such as a therapist, computer, or self-instructional packet. Although cognitive and functional rehabilitation relies heavily on externally generated learning, therapists must remember that some of their clients also are capable of self-generated learning (Zimmerman, 1995). According to Schwartz, therapists and clients who use external mediators predetermine (a) the structure of the learning environment; (b) the nature of the learning material; (c) the type of learning activity, role, and task; (d) the type of feedback; and (e) the manner of evaluation of the learning experience.

Two types of strategies, behavioral and cognitive, can be used for either self-generated or externally generated learning in cognitive–functional rehabilitation (Jacobs, 1993; Schwartz 1985). A comparison of the behavioral- and cognitive-learning strategies is provided in Table 3.1.

Metacognitive theory is a part of teaching–learning theory that has particular relevance for clients who function at higher levels and have competence in communication. Metacognitive theory explains the conscious thinking and feeling that accompany and pertain to problem solving (Berry, 1983; Bewick, Raymond, Malia, & Bennett, 1995; Brown & Palincsar, 1989; Paris & Winograd, 1990; Winnie, 1995). An individual who uses metacognitive strategies will engage in a conscious prediction, monitoring, and planning that considers the capacities of the self, the demands of the task, and the parameters of the strategy (Brown, 1988; Flavell, 1979, 1985). Metacognitive strategies can be either self-generated or externally

TABLE 3.1. Behavioral- and Cognitive-Learning Strategies

Behavioral-Learning Strategies	Cognitive-Learning Strategies
Are based on behavior modification	Are based on information processing from cognitive psychology
Analyze observable behavior	Analyze behavior that cannot be directly observed
Identify functional relationships	Describe how information is processed, structured, and modified
Prescribe cause–effect and reward–punishment guidelines to gain better control of specified behavior in treatment	Prescribe person-specific tasks, situations, and strategies to increase information-processing capabilities
Assume that consequences influence behavior	Assume that conscious awareness and prediction of outcomes influence behavior
Do not include ideation, imagery, or meaning	Include ideation, imagery, and meaning
Use positive and negative behaviors as reinforcement	Use self-esteem and a sense of mastery as reinforcement

Note. From *The Quadraphonic Approach: Evaluation and Treatment of the Brain-Injured Patient,* by B. C. Abreu, 1990, New York: Therapeutic Systems. Copyright © 1990 by Therapeutic Service Systems. Reprinted with permission.

generated. Metacognitive training uses language to influence the degree of interaction that the client has with the environment (Abreu, 1992). Language gives meaning to objects and allows individuals to know what objects are and what objects can do or allow an individual to do (Gibson, 1979; Luria, 1973). Language is used as an interactive means of influencing new and more effective learning strategies that increase independence and life satisfaction after the challenge of brain injury. Language cues are words, phrases, or signals used as a part of the learning strategy. An example of a client's use of metacognitive theory might be when he or she uses self-talk in analyzing a problem before engaging in its solution ("If I slow down, I am more apt to succeed").

The theoretical foundations provided by information processing and teaching–learning explain cognition from "the eyebrows up," as if this function resided only in the brain. The rest of the body, including head, neck, trunk, and limb functioning, is addressed by the biomechanical and neuromuscular systems that function intimately with the cognitive–perceptual system. The artificial separation of the brain from the rest of the body does not acknowledge the mind–body relationship. Our bodies are vehicles for the biomechanical expressions of a nervous system that shapes postural control. The control and posture gained through the ability to preposition, position, and maintain body alignments are critical for functional activity. Treatments that address movement also need to consider their influences on cognition. The next two theories are used to provide an explanation of movement as it relates to brain injury.

Neurodevelopmental Theory

Neurodevelopmental theory is concerned with the quality of movement as it relates to the client with developmental or acquired brain injury. Historically, this theory has explained techniques on the basis of a hardwired, hierarchical view of the nervous system and has encouraged a genetic-reflex constraint model to explain the individual's inherent capacities to develop normal movement patterns on the basis of genetic endowment and a fixed hierarchical reflex control mechanism. The current view is that the nervous system is more flexible and adaptive. This newer environmental (physical–social–cultural) constraint model does not deny the hardwired and hierarchical nature of some structures within the nervous system, but it also explains and supports the nervous system's variability. This variability is shown when different movements in different circumstances activate a variety of nervous system

structures and communication strategies (Reed, 1989a, 1989b). The communication functions within the nervous system rely on redundancy wherein a variety of multimodal sensory receptors generate the same information, guaranteeing an effective interaction with the environment (Nashner, 1982). For example, if a client with a brain injury moves around in a given environment, he or she derives overlapping visual, vestibular, and proprioceptive information relative to position in space. Success in his or her mobility is possible given this multimodal input, even if one or more receptors is impaired.

The environment includes the aggregate of all relevant characteristics derived from people, objects, circumstances, and conditions that surround the individual (Gentile, 2000). Characteristics that influence actions are called *environmental regulators* because they direct and organize (regulate) an individual's movements for action. Gentile described three types of critical environmental regulators that relate to perceptual motor skills: *stationary, moving,* and *intervariable*.

Stationary regulators do not move. They include supportive surfaces for clients in both standing and seated positions as well as stationary objects that surround the client in the environment. To be included as regulators, such objects must influence the client's actions; an example of a stationary regulator is a piece of furniture around which a client must walk. A stationary environment allows for self-paced actions (Gentile, 2000).

Moving regulators are people, support surfaces, and objects that move within the individual's environment. One example of a moving regulator is an escalator. The speed of movement of such a regulator can vary and affect the ability of the individual to achieve goals. In a slow-moving environment, an individual is better able to self-pace. In a fast-moving environment, the individual must predict and anticipate what to do and thus demonstrate more diversification of response. In this context, the moving environment also requires external timing and faster reaction time responses (Gentile, 2000).

Intervariable regulators are people, support surfaces, and objects that move at variable speeds and in changing directions: They fluctuate from one encounter to the next. An example of an intervariable regulator is a bouncing ball. If dealing with intervariable regulators, the individual must perform as many response variations as there are changes in the environmental regulator. The individual must maintain vigilance to detect changes.

Developmental or acquired brain injury can reduce an individual's capacity to detect and discriminate stimuli as well as to respond to relevant environmental regulators

(Abreu, 1992, 1994a, 1995; Lee, 1989). Brain injury can affect environmental interactions and may hinder the formulation of postural control strategies during the experience of external and internal perturbations or disturbances of balance (Abreu, 1995; Nashner, 1982; Newton, 1995). A client may, for example, be hampered in formulating a postural control response because of a preoccupying thought (internal perturbation), the sound of a siren (auditory external perturbation), or being jostled in a crowd (physical external perturbation). Most of the regulators discussed to this point are purely physical. Social and cultural regulators also are critical, and these are discussed later in this chapter.

Biomechanical Theory

The ability of an individual to adapt to the demands of environmental regulators depends on the integrity of the central and peripheral nervous system that is expressed through the musculoskeletal system of the body. The body is the biomechanical effector of centrally and peripherally determined motor plans. Biomechanical theory is useful in explaining and analyzing a client's movement; it enables the therapist to better understand the integration of the nervous and musculoskeletal systems with perceptual–motor skills. The individual's musculoskeletal system expresses the generation, scaling, and coordination of movement but also can be a movement regulator or constraint. The integrity and function of bones, tendons, ligaments, and muscles may facilitate or frustrate movement strategies.

Biomechanics relates to the laws and principles of human movement and assists in understanding the client with brain injury. Mechanical kinesiology is the study and analysis of movement from two perspectives that are important in cognitive and functional rehabilitation: Kinematics and kinetics. *Kinematics* describes the mechanical components of the body without consideration of the balanced and unbalanced forces that cause motion. Examples of kinematics are the therapist's naming a motion such as flexion and counting and measuring the movements. This process is similar to that which occurs in goniometry. *Kinetics,* on the other hand, describes the causal analysis of motion with consideration of the interacting forces that cause motion. Kinetics is divided into static and dynamic analysis. An example of kinetics is the therapist's determination that the client cannot flex because extensor tone is high and flexors are weak.

Brain injury can affect head and trunk movements and lead to a biomechanical disarrangement sometimes associated with the disappearance of symmetrical motor behaviors. Body displacement, velocity, and angular joint movements may be adversely affected after brain injury, thereby causing deterioration of the quality and quantity of the client's movement dynamics. Therefore, evaluation of client performance using kinetics to analyze the mechanical components and kinematics to analyze the interactive forces can provide guidelines for practice.

THEORETICAL BACKGROUND OF THE MACRO PERSPECTIVE

Peloquin's (2002a) articulation of confluence provides guidelines that assist practitioners to refocus cognitive rehabilitation in the grounded, integrated, and individualized manner that Yerxa (1992) suggested. *Confluence* is the flowing together of two or more streams of thought; for the occupational therapy profession, it is the integration of the art and science of practice, the synthetic blend of competence and caring in practice (Peloquin, 2002a). *Confluent education* is the deliberate and purposeful evocation by responsible agents of knowledge, skills, attitudes, and feelings that flow together to produce wholeness in the person (Brown, 1971). Peloquin (1996) suggested that integration of the affective and cognitive elements in individual and group learning is advantageous in helping students to cultivate desirable knowledge, attitudes, and behavior. We propose that the confluent model for education also is appropriate for a holistic clinical practice. If cognitive rehabilitation must include a reductionistic focus on performance skills such as memory, that focus does not preclude a confluent approach to the treatment of memory problems, wherein affective considerations are integrated into cognitive rehabilitation strategies. If asked to use memory, for example, a client might be asked to remember highly pleasant childhood or teen memories rather than more factual elements that are devoid of affect.

A *holistic practice* recognizes that individuals are meaningfully interconnected within a societal context and are capable of maintaining and restoring equilibrium in a global health environment (McColl, 1994; McColl, Gerein, & Valentine, 1997; Miller, 1992). Adherence to these beliefs can energize occupational therapists to refocus cognitive rehabilitation along functional lines by changing the manner in which they relate to their clients (Peloquin, 1993a, 1993b). Changes can occur through an expanded focus on the client–therapist relationship to include explicit reciprocity, the sharing of treatment control, establishment of authentic interactions, acceptance of a client's responsibility for choice and, ultimately, the acceptance of both the client and the therapist as thinking–feeling individuals (Peloquin, 1989, 1990, 1993a, 1993b, 1995, 1996). Given this expanded focus, a therapist will include in rehabilitation those issues that relate to the affective domain: emotion, motivation, satisfaction, intuition, imagination, creativity, interpersonal capacities, values, norms, spirituality, ethics, and culture. A holistic practice will deliberately use methods, actions, and interactions that develop the affective domain. The environmental design of such a practice is nurturing and supports the interconnection of cognition, function, and affect in both teachers and learners.

In confluent practice, the teaching–learning partners engage in the cognitive–functional rehabilitation process with the goal of health and optimal adaptation through which clients adjust behaviors, attitudes, and values to make them more congruent with new external and internal demands following disease or trauma (Abreu, 1992, 1994a). Empowered by this holistic refocusing of cognitive–functional rehabilitation, let us proceed to consider a client–learner-centered model of therapy in a holistic and confluent practice.

We propose that cognition and learning should be viewed within an occupations framework that supports the inclusion of a macro (or functional) analysis and synthesis of a client's occupational story (Abreu, 1994a; Wood et al., 1994). The macro perspective is based on the use of narrative and functional analysis to explain and predict individual behavior on the basis of four status characteristics that define behavior. The four characteristics are lifestyle status, life-stage status, health status, and disadvantage status. *Lifestyle status* describes and predicts the individual's manner of expressing, producing, and performing day-to-day occupations. Examples of parameters within lifestyle status include the client's personal characteristics and use of economic resources. *Life-stage status* describes the individual's physical, emotional, and spiritual periods of growth and development— turning points and life-markers. Examples of life-stage status include childhood, adolescence, and adulthood as well as marriage, divorce, accomplishments, failures, and death. *Health status* describes the presence of premorbid conditions such as arthritis or back pain as well as any changes in behaviors, values, or attitude after the illness or injury. *Disadvantage status* describes the degree of functional restriction that results from impairment, including personal as well as social disadvantage. One example of a parameter within disadvantage status is a client's inability to go to the movies, shop, or cook because of physical, cognitive, or psychosocial impairments.

Another example is a client's inability to be a financial provider, spouse, parent, or caretaker as a result of disability. Figure 3.1 has a depiction of the four characteristics in the macro perspective.

Storytelling and narrative modes of analysis have been used by Mattingly and Fleming (1993) as a way to help therapists reflect on their practice. These researchers used an interpretative strategy of asking participating therapists to view segments of videotapes of occupational therapy practice and to analyze the segments and categorize the results as if they were chapters in a story. One outcome of these studies was that participating therapists became more conscious of their assumptions that oppose what actually mattered to the client. Narrative reflections also increased the therapists' awareness that practice is only partially shaped by a therapist's original evaluation and treatment plan. The occupational therapy process unfolds with interferences, surprises, improvisations, and dynamic interactions among a variety of team players, two of whom are the occupational therapist and the client.

One of the goals of the quadraphonic approach is to increase the awareness of both the therapist and the client with regard to the affective domain of the therapeutic experience. Narrative thinking can guide a therapist toward a focus on the affective experience of adaptation after disease, injury, or trauma for more effective cognitive and functional rehabilitation. The humanistic orientation provided by the use of narrative enhances the capacity of the occupational therapist to consider the client's experience of brain injury and the manner in which personal restrictions and social disadvantages affect a life. Examples of narrative strategies in occupational therapy are the interview, occupational storytelling, and occupational storymaking (Clark, 1993; Clark, Ennevor, & Richardson, 1996; Mattingly & Fleming, 1993). Bateson (1989) described how narratives or personal stories provide a framework for reflecting about the unique shape, relationships, and commitments of individual lives (Krefting & Krefting, 1991). Nachmanovitch (1990) emphasized the power of improvisation in life and the arts. That same power can be tapped in cognitive rehabilitation.

The use of narrative in the macro framework for occupation yields a client-centered therapeutic orientation in which the therapist functions as a professional consultant who advises on the management of various aspects of the client's life (Bridge & Twible, 1997; Herzberg, 1990; Patterson & Marks, 1992). This macro framework can also respond to recent changes in the health care delivery system such as demedicalization and consumerism, both of which place the patient in a more central role in rehabilitation (Bridge & Twible, 1997; Holyoke & Elkan, 1995; Pollock, 1993). The interview is a tool used to elicit information. Storytelling considers a client's short- and long-term memories, whereas storymaking involves the creation or playing out of rehabilitation outcomes—what the client and rehabilitation team would like to accomplish or see happen. Progression toward planned cognitive and functional outcomes is not linear but full of tricks, reversals, and surprises. The predicted outcomes are uncertain and not predetermined by critical pathways. Because the main character in the rehabilitation process is the client who has experienced the brain injury, the narrative, enfranchised alongside the medical diagnosis, is an important factor in developing a holistic treatment plan.

The quadraphonic approach uses narrative to embrace a real-life occupations framework from both the macro and the micro perspectives and to maximize the performance and satisfaction of clients in a holistic and confluent manner. Wood and colleagues (1994) defined the macro framework for cognitive rehabilitation as a clinical orientation that relies on daily living, leisure, recreation, work, and other ordinary occupations as primary therapeutic modalities. Effective adaptation and optimal health are identified as outcomes. The macro perspective also has been referred to as "adaptive," "functional," and "top-down" (Abreu, 1994a; Siev, Freishtat, & Zoltan, 1986; Trombly, 1993).

In contrast, the micro perspective of occupational functioning focuses on the foundational subskills or performance skills, including attention, memory, categorization, and problem solving. These subskills can be further broken into visual and auditory memory or categories such as short-term and long-term memory. The micro perspective also has been called "restorative" and "bottom-up" (Abreu, 1994a; Trombly, 1993; Wood et al., 1994). We propose that practitioners reject the underlying assumptions that support a treatment dichotomy within which therapists must choose between macro and micro, or between functional or restorative perspectives. The dual system of rehabilitation proposed herein facilitates a free-flowing movement between macro and micro perspectives to embrace both remediation and compensation techniques.

MAIN CONCEPTS OF THE MODEL FROM THE MICRO PERSPECTIVE

From the micro perspective, the quadraphonic approach constitutes a frame of reference that integrates four theoretical foundations to guide the evaluation and treatment of cognitive–perceptual and postural control dysfunction. When considering such impairments, the therapist must be aware that these do not occur in isolation but are influenced by factors such as the client's mood and motivational dynamics (Diller, 1993). The format used for the development of this particular micro frame of reference (Abreu, 1992, 1994a) includes three components: a theoretical base, a functional–dysfunction continuum, and applications to practice that describe examples of evaluation and treatment.

The three assumptions for this frame of reference are as follows:

1. Continuous analysis of the components of occupational performance (bottom-up approach) combined with analysis of total performance or occupations (top-down approach) is critical for rehabilitation, and cognitive impairment has an effect on perceptual–motor function.
2. The integration of the cognitive–perceptual and postural control systems is required in cognitive rehabilitation because their separation excludes the role of cognition in movement.
3. Applied phenomenology (Fleming, 1991) is necessary to understand the meaning that clients attribute to their illnesses and other life experiences. The narrative process is critical to individualize treatment so that it will be optimally useful to clients who need to improve adaptive strategies after brain injury or trauma (Clark, 1993).

EVALUATION PROCESS: THE MICRO PERSPECTIVE

Evaluation from the micro perspective provides a biomedical orientation in which the occupational therapist functions as a professional who offers specialized services for the management of cognitive and functional rehabilitation (Bridge & Twible, 1997; McColl et al., 1997; McColl, Law, & Stewart, 1993; World Health Organization, 1980). The micro perspective is an affirmation of the need for the detection, identification, and measurement of impairments that cause disability; it is important because the therapist may need to assume responsibility for the client until the medical situation stabilizes and the client's cognitive and functional capacities improve (Bridge & Twible, 1997; McColl et al., 1997).

Three Interactive Forces for the Micro Perspective

Guided by the theoretical foundations just described, the therapist and client develop strategies for evaluation and intervention from the micro perspective while also analyzing the effect of three interactive forces and their affective elements: the client–learner, the environment, and the therapist–teacher. Table 3.2 outlines these forces.

TABLE 3.2. Three Interactive Forces for Micro Evaluation

The Client–Learner	The Environment	The Therapist–Teacher
1. Story of the client's adaptation and losses	1. Physical	1. Procedural
2. The client's stages of awareness impairment, disability, and restrictions	2. Social	2. Interactive
3. The client's stages of motor learning or relearning	3. Cultural	3. Conditional
4. The stage of recovery and acceptance		

Note. From *The Quadraphonic Approach: Evaluation and Treatment of the Brain-Injured Patient,* by B. C. Abreu, 1990, New York: Therapeutic Systems. Copyright © 1990 by Therapeutic Service Systems. Reprinted with permission.

The Client–Learner

Four significant factors contribute to the client–learner's agency as the first interactive force. These factors offer a comprehensive view of the client and include the client's story of adaptation and losses, awareness, motor-learning capacity, stage of recovery, and acceptance.

The *story* of the client is the narrative of the incidents, events, and changes leading up to the current time. Told by the client and significant others, documented by the therapist, and used as a basis for evaluation and treatment, this narrative can reveal the strategies for adaptation used by the client both before and after the injury. Adaptation is the process by which clients adjust their behaviors, attitudes, and values to make themselves more congruent with the new external and internal demands subsequent to disease or trauma. The client's ability to deal with loss is a significant strategy to consider in treatment of brain injury.

The client's *awareness* of disability also contributes to his or her agency as an interactive force (Fischer, Trexler, & Gauggel, 2004; Hoofien, Gilboa, Vakil, & Barak, 2004). Unawareness is common after brain injury and plays a critical role in rehabilitation (Bogod, Mateer, & MacDonald, 2003; Sherer et al., 2003). In 1989, Crosson and colleagues identified three types of awareness that occur among clients with brain injury: intellectual, emergent, and anticipatory. *Intellectual awareness* is defined as some level of understanding on the part of the client that a particular function is impaired. *Emergent awareness* is the client's recognition of a problem as it happens. *Anticipatory awareness* is the client's ability to predict that a problem will occur on the basis of a solid awareness of the impairment. Although Crosson and colleagues proposed a hierarchy among the levels of awareness, we found no evidence supporting such a hierarchy (Abreu et al., 2001). The multidimensional nature of awareness requires a more comprehensive model of awareness after brain injury (Hartman-Maeir, Soroker, Oman, & Katz,

2003; Simmond & Fleming, 2003; Toglia & Kirk, 2000). A client's disposition at re-entry depends on awareness and many other factors, including recovery of function, social support systems, and insurance coverage.

The third important factor that shapes the manner in which the client acts as an interactive force is the client's motor learning capacity. *Motor learning* is the acquisition of skilled movements as a result of practice. In cognitive rehabilitation, the requisite motor skills are considered new skills because they have been lost because of disease or trauma. Motor learning occurs in a social context because the client's performance is facilitated by the therapist's guided participation or scaffolding interventions. This apprenticeship relative to motor learning also is time dependent because some learning can persist whereas other learning is transitory (Newell, 2003). Motor learning can occur years after the brain injury, even in the chronic stages of recovery (Hammond et al., 2004; Incoccia, Formisano, Muscato, Reali, & Zoccolotti, 2004). We propose that the interpretation of a client's performance at evaluation be flexible, recognize interdependence among many factors, and reflect knowledge of a dynamic interface between awareness and motor learning. Furthermore, the client's response to any test, activity, task, or role depends on personal ability, developmental history, emotional condition, and perception of meaning (Nelson, 1987).

The final factor related to the client's role as an interactive force is his or her ability to accept and cope with each stage of recovery. *Acceptance* depends to a great extent on an individual's motivation, hope, and commitment to reshape lifestyle and personal identity (Corbin & Strauss, 1988).

The Environment

The second major interactive force at the micro level is the environment. There are three types of environments: physical, social, and cultural. In cognitive and functional rehabilitation, the *physical environment* has historically received the most emphasis (Abreu, 1981, 1992; Abreu & Toglia, 1987). The physical environment includes the characteristics, both relevant and irrelevant, that are associated with the activities, conditions, circumstances, objects, and people surrounding the client (Gentile, 2000). These characteristics include the quantity, size, spatial orientation, speed, and duration of the stimuli, as well as whether these are stationary or moving. All of these characteristics or task parameters interact to regulate a client's movement and posture; this interaction was discussed at length in the section on neurodevelopmental and biomechanical theory.

The *social environment* includes the client's voluntary relationships or social networks, the family structure, and community resources (Mosey, 1986). Additionally, the social environment includes the client's perspective about personal roles, rights, duties, and privileges (Mosey, 1986). These aspects of the environment are critical in guiding the client's discharge plans and in formulating adaptive strategies for community reentry. These adaptations are greatly affected by the actions of the client, family, and friends with regard to the rehabilitation process (Corbin & Strauss, 1988). An adaptation can occur within both the personal context (the client's function) and the social context (the client's support systems; Pierce & Frank, 1992).

The *cultural environment* is a complex subject that includes the traditions, values, norms, language, and symbolic meanings that are shared as cultural agreements between the client and any group (Mosey, 1986). These agreements describe how things should be done in ethical and aesthetic terms. Cultural environment regulates the types of activities, tasks, and roles in which a client will participate, as well as the individuals with whom he or she will engage.

The Therapist–Facilitator

The third force to consider at the micro level is the therapist–facilitator, who must use clinical reasoning and the principles of therapeutic relationships to make clinical judgments. Clinical pathways, flowcharts, mathematical models, or judgmental formulations may represent this type of reasoning, which is based on a series of analytical steps. Clinical reasoning helps the therapist formulate an educated evaluation, create an effective treatment plan, and re-evaluate the plan as required.

Fleming (1991) described three types of reasoning that influence clinical judgments: procedural, interactive, and conditional. *Procedural reasoning* can be described as the way in which therapists think about the diagnosis and impairment and the manner in which they initially interact with a client. *Interactive reasoning* is the way therapists think about and interact with clients to determine their current needs and values. *Conditional reasoning* occurs when the therapist engages in the acts of thinking about, interpreting, and interacting while considering brain injury in a broader social and temporal context that goes beyond disability to the client's view of the future (Fleming, 1991).

The therapist must be aware that all clinical decision-making processes are based on imperfect measurements that are subject to some degree of ambiguity, contain some possibility of error, and need to be continually re-evaluated.

Guidelines for Evaluation From the Micro Perspective

Evaluation from the micro perspective is characterized by five guidelines that parallel those used with the macro perspective:

1. An examination of the client's cognitive (mind) and postural control (body strategies);
2. A precise determination and definition of those processes that will be assessed (e.g., attention, memory, problem solving, motor planning) and a selection of the evaluative strategies that correspond with these definitions;
3. A consideration of the client's choices and degree of control within the evaluation process;
4. A scoring and documentation of results that include commentary about the client's personal awareness and responsivity as well as his or her interaction with the therapist, task, and environment; and
5. A consideration of the psychometric character of the evaluation and whether it yields both qualitative and quantitative data about the client's performance.

These factors guide the therapist when selecting which assessments or activities to use for evaluation. For example, the client named Edgar reports a moderate memory deficit and indicates that his primary aim is to return home to his wife Daisy and to continue working as a chemical engineer. By stating this impairment, Edgar determines the therapist's starting point. From this point, the therapist will move more deeply into an evaluation, attending to the five guidelines as they relate to Edgar's use of memory strategies.

The micro evaluation uses a cuing system to aid in the development of treatment plans for adults with brain injury (Abreu, 1992; Abreu & Toglia, 1987). Throughout the evaluation, the therapist uses questions and probes in an attempt to clarify whether the client understands instructions and to investigate more deeply the performance and responses given during the task or test. This investigation is conducted to specify the factors contributing to the client's use of inefficient strategies and to identify the contextual modifications that may improve his or her performance. Tables 3.3 and 3.4 show examples of evaluations that might have been used with Edgar.

MAIN CONCEPTS OF THE MODEL FROM THE MACRO PERSPECTIVE

We believe that the view of health taken from a medical perspective, which targets health problems, should be integrated with a view of health taken from a social perspective that facilitates wellness. That integration occurs within the quadraphonic approach. From the macro perspective, the quadraphonic approach relies on a definition

TABLE 3.3. Micro Evaluation Samples: Coma and Minimal Responsive

The Four Theories Are the Statements That Describe and Predict the Micro Perspective Evaluation Guidelines.

Information-Processing Evaluation	Teaching–Learning Evaluation	Neurodevelopmental Evaluation	Biomechanical Evaluation
1. Coma–Near Coma Scale	1. Stimulus–response transfer or carryover	1. Modified tasks based on neurodevelopmental analysis	1. Modified tasks based on kinematic and kinetic analysis
2. Coma Recovery Scale	2. Personalized target stimulation such as	2. Observational findings such as	2. Observational findings such as
3. Sensory Stimulation Assessment Measure	a. Gustatory memories	a. Balance and postural control	a. Active range of motion
4. Western Neurosensory Stimulation	b. Tactile memories	b. Musculoskeletal tone	b. Passive range of motion
	c. Auditory memories	c. Symmetry	c. Muscle power
5. Quadraphonic Evaluation System: Personalized form tracking a 24-hour spectrum	d. Visual memories	d. Movement disassociations	d. Joint-play movements
		e. Reaction and movement time	e. Endurance
		f. Mobility and stability	f. Coordination
*Determine arousal patterns and changes in response in arousal and attention as a result of interventions			

The Three Forces Are the Regulators of the Evaluation Micro Perspective. It Predicts the Evaluation Interaction Process.

The Client–Learner	The Therapist–Teacher	The Training–Compensatory Environment
Losses • Could you tell me how Edgar handled previous losses? • How are you handling the loss of Edgar as you know him?	1. Are you primarily controlling the evaluation–treatment session? 2. Are your judgments focused or driven primarily by the protocols, procedures, test and measurement methods, or Edgar's diagnosis?	1. Are the physical traits of the environment stable, unchangeable, and as familiar as possible to provide a close fit to the minimal processing Edgar has at this stage?
Awareness Edgar most likely will not have a general sense that there is a problem (intellectual awareness), be able to recognize a problem exists (emergent awareness), nor be able to predict problems in the future (anticipatory awareness).	3. Are your judgments focused or driven primarily by Edgar's needs and values (what Edgar feels is good, meaningful, and important)?	2. Are Edgar's cultural and personal system traits represented and included during the intervention process? 3. Are Edgar's social personal support systems represented and included during the intervention process?
Motor Learning Edgar's motor relearning actions and sequences at this stage are full of error and variable performance. The actions are reflexive, conscious, or both.	4. Are your judgments focused or driven primarily by Edgar's social support system and the timing of his disadvantage?	
Stage of Acceptance • Could you tell me how Edgar may accept or cope with illness as he recovers?		

TABLE 3.4. Micro Evaluation Samples: Acute and Community Re-entry

---

The Four Theories Are the Statements That Describe and Predict the Micro Perspective Evaluation Guidelines.

Information-Processing Evaluation and Teaching–Learning Evaluation	Neurodevelopmental Evaluation	Biomechanical Evaluation
1. Attentional battery: modified tests, eye fixations, visual scanning, modified Stroop, and modified trail-making	1. Modified task based on neurodevelopmental analysis	1. Modified tasks based on kinematic and kinetic analysis
2. Visual–perception battery: visual acuity, visual analysis, visual spatial, visual motor	2. Observational findings such as	2. Observational findings such as
3. Recognition and recall battery: storytelling, visual action picture, 20 associated photos, 20 associated words, repeating story, belonging item	a. Balance and postural control b. Musculoskeletal tone c. Symmetry d. Movement disassociations	a. Active range of motion b. Passive range of motion c. Muscle power d. Joint-play movements
4. Problem-solving battery: list to make shopping easier, categorize in groups, functional hypothetical, discovery photograph rules	e. Reaction and movement time f. Mobility and stability	e. Endurance f. Coordination
5. Motor-planning battery: gesture imitations, metronome movement patterns, object manipulation, blocks construction		
6. Postural-control battery: asymmetry assessment, theoretical base of support assessment, self-perturbation, external perturbations, T form		

The Three Forces Are the Regulators of the Evaluation Micro Perspective. It Predicts the Evaluation Interaction Process.

The Client–Learner	The Therapist–Teacher	The Training–Compensatory Environment
Losses • Could you tell me how you handled previous losses? • Let's talk about how you are different now from before the injury/accident/illness. **Awareness** Before you test: • Have you ever taken these types of tests before? • Do you remember what the results of tests like these were? • Why are you taking these tests? • How well do you think you will do on this test/task/activity? **During** • How are you doing with this test/task/activity? • Can you tell me what just happened? (error–problem recognition) **After Test** • How well did you do? • Did you perform better or worse than you expected? • How may this problem affect your plans to go back to life/work/school independently? (Specify areas.) **Motor Learning** • Are your motor actions and sequences conscious, full of errors, and variable performance, requiring constant feedback? • Are motor actions and sequences associative with less errors and requiring less feedback? • Are motor actions automatic, with no errors, and independent? **Stage of Acceptance** • Describe your life as if it were a book. • Describe how well you have accepted changes and illnesses in the past. Let's talk about how it feels to be at this stage of your recovery.	1. Are you primarily controlling the evaluation–treatment session? 2. Are your judgments focused or driven primarily by the protocols, procedures, test and measurement methods, or Edgar's diagnosis? 3. Are your judgments focused or driven primarily by Edgar's needs and values (what Edgar feels is good, meaningful, and important)? 4. Are your judgments focused or driven primarily by Edgar's social support system and the timing of his disadvantage?	1. Are the physical traits of the environment an additional task demand, which tends to inhibit initial acquisition of task competency but ultimately to facilitate transfer? 2. Are Edgar's cultural and personal systems' traits represented and included during the intervention process? 3. Are Edgar's social and personal support systems represented and included during the intervention process?

Note. From *The Quadraphonic Approach: Evaluation and Treatment of the Brain-Injured Patient,* by B. C. Abreu, 1990, New York: Therapeutic Systems. Copyright © 1990 by Therapeutic Service Systems. Reprinted with permission.

of health adapted from a holistic health model. We see health as a state of *wellness* that emerges from three interactive forces and their affective elements (Porn, 1993). These interactive forces are the client's (a) will and goals, (b) capacity for actions, and (c) opportunities for action. These interactive forces shape health and adaptation both before and after illness or trauma. Within this section, we focus on adaptation that is related to health, also known as *health adaptation*.

In spite of an illness or disability that may be interpreted by many as a lack of health, health adaptation and wellness can occur. Individuals with brain injury continue to have a repertoire of adaptive behaviors that can enhance health and the rehabilitation process. This repertoire reflects personal styles, values, and an individualized sense of meaningfulness. Therapists need to connect personally with their clients, tap this repertoire, and share power in the processes of rehabilitation, health adaptation, and prevention. Such a sharing of power requires deliberate and collaborative efforts that begin with the first interview and continue through discharge planning.

The first interactive force within the macro perspective on evaluation is the client's will. Will shapes an individual's personal determination to set goals and to act as an agent in life planning after brain injury. Discernment of a client's will depends on the client's communication skills and capacity as a narrator, combined with the therapist's ability to elicit the client's story. The client's expression of will and goals can occur through verbal as well as nonverbal means, such as the use of photos, if communication problems exist. Only if the client's will is known, through whatever creative means the therapist may use to discern it, can real collaboration occur.

An intimate relationship exists between the first interactive force, the client's will, and the second force, the client's capacity for action. Highly important in unleashing this second force is the therapist's ability to probe for values and to prompt volition during exchanges within which the client senses that that which is personally meaningful is also what the therapist values. Mutual attention can then turn to facilitating the capacities of the client in the actions of recovery and rehabilitation and in the development of wellness behaviors.

Serving as the third interactive force in health adaptation are the client's opportunities for desired action. Such opportunities include the type, frequency, and intensity of situations and events offered that engage the client in activities of daily living, productive activities, education, play, and leisure activities congruent with his or her physical, social, and cultural environments. Critical to mar-

shalling this interactive force is the therapist's creativity in facilitating opportunities of all kinds that align with a client's sense of purpose, meaning, and satisfaction.

The idea of health advocated through the quadraphonic approach is that health after illness or disability occurs through a confluence of self-direction and personal adaptation (Hellstrom, 1993; Rudnick, 2002). Within the quadraphonic approach, the therapist's role is seen as that of coach and partner in any client's reclamation of health. Even with what seem to be best efforts, the results of rehabilitation can be highly variable, however. We know that people free from illness or disability can lack health and wellness. Because we also know that health and wellness can occur in people with chronic disability and deadly disease, we strive toward that end (Taljedal, 1997).

The rehabilitation process offers opportunities for therapists and clients alike to expand their understanding of health and its reclamation through continued reflections and observations. The evaluations described in the next section offer occasions for the kinds of reflection and observation that may enhance such understanding and thus facilitate healthy outcomes after brain injury.

EVALUATION PROCESS: THE MACRO PERSPECTIVE

From the macro perspective, therapists may use a wide range of functional assessment tools. We do not suggest a rigid protocol in proposing the assessments that follow. Rather, we offer possibilities for therapists to consider, hoping that other creative ways of eliciting required data may also emerge. We begin with standardized functional outcome scales, the specific tools used in evaluation to compare the results of individual assessments with national standards. The determination of which scale to use in the evaluation process is a matter of clinical judgment. In addition to using these scales, the therapist may want to survey clients and their families regarding their perceptions of outcomes and their satisfaction with achievement (Ottenbacher & Christiansen, 1997). Two such surveys are the Craig Handicap Assessment and Reporting Technique (Segal & Schall, 1995) and the Community Integration Questionnaire (Willer, Ottenbacher, & Coad, 1994). The importance of maintaining a focus on functional outcomes is underscored by the development of classifications known as functional reading groups (Stineman et al., 1994).

Cognitive and functional evaluations from the macro perspective examine the individual's subjective sense of satisfaction and adaptation after a breach in health (Abreu, 1994a; Trombly, 1993). For this element of the evaluation, the therapist will rely on narrative communications from the client and from family members as well as functional assessments of the client's real-life occupations. Occupations have been described as the meaningful ordinary and familiar things that people do every day for personal or cultural reasons (Clark, 1993; Zemke & Clark, 1996). These activities undergo constant change according to the individual's lifestyle, life stage, health, and disadvantage status. Chunks of meaningful activities are orchestrated in a nonlinear progression from day to day (Clark, 1993).

Through interview questions that prompt personal sharing, the therapist seeks to better understand the client's personal story and orchestration of occupations; the client might be asked to bring personal documents, photographs, or meaningful objects that can enhance communications (Clark, 1993). Because brain injury can cause expressive and receptive disorders of communication, flexible methods of eliciting information are quite important. The use of narrative for the macro evaluation helps the therapist to discover the way in which the client makes sense of his or her life experiences (Polkinghorne, 1988; Riessman, 1993).

In the quadraphonic approach, Abreu provides a system of six assessment strips for the cognitive and functional classification of each client (see Figure 3.2). Four of the strips are based on a macro perspective and two strips on the micro. The strips are used to classify each client along one of seven functional performance levels listed in Table 3.5. On the basis of this classification of functional performance, the therapist works with the client to design functional treatment guidelines that enable advancement to the next functional level. The six treatment guidelines leading from coma to community re-entry are discussed later in this chapter.

The Interview, Storytelling, and Storymaking

The interview is one of the assessment tools used to elicit the client's narrative. The interview is conducted in a face-to-face meeting during which the therapist engages with the client and documents the information that is reported. The interview process can be expanded by including the client's family members as well as significant others and also may include a written survey that does not involve a face-to-face meeting. The interview should be a dynamic and interactive process during which the therapist documents direct observation of the client's social responses together with the client's descriptions of personal behaviors. The interview should be an effort to guide and engage the client in meaningful communication about everyday experiences (Holstein & Gubrium, 1995). This process assists in the discovery of an individual's patterns of interaction and self-organization within society (Psathas, 1995). The individual's cognitive and functional skills can be better understood with reference to the social milieu within which the individual is embedded (Vygotsky, 1978).

Facilitated storytelling can shed light on the personal and social disadvantages that can emerge from the individual's societal embeddedness (Josselson & Lieblich, 1995). To study a whole person, one cannot rely exclusively on logical numerical methods and objective descriptions. The interview constitutes a search for and discovery of the individual's perceptions of the real-life setting, the significance to the client of the everyday, and the manner in which the client establishes an "under-life" (those behaviors that may not be typical of the individual but that characterize functioning in the treatment facility or in the institutions that provide rehabilitation services).

Stories that emerge during an active interview can be prompted either by something that is said or done by the client or by the therapist's pursuit of clarity on a comment that is not topically coherent. The active interview is an improvisational production. It is structured and focused, yet allows for spontaneity and responsivity within parameters provided by the interviewer (Holstein & Gubrium, 1995). Considerations that affect the framework of the interview include (a) the client's competency as narrator given his or her state of impairment, disability, and disadvantage; (b) the client's capacity to demonstrate and communicate what is meaningful and what societal interactions are like; (c) the opportunity to evaluate the client's satisfaction with personal roles (e.g., mother, brother, client) as well as satisfaction with the occupational therapy services being provided; (d) the facilitation of ordinary exchanges that rely on mutual attentiveness, monitoring, and responsiveness (e.g., being sensitive to turn-taking in the conversation); (e) the climate of mutual disclosure; (f) the emphasis on sentiment and emotion that are the core of human experience, accepting that the interview is biased and multidirectional; and (g) the use of improvisation during the interview process.

Storytelling also may be influenced by the client's reduced ability to acquire, store, and recall information about personally experienced events (episodic memory) or general world knowledge (semantic memory). An example of episodic memory is a client's recollection of what he or she ate for breakfast or how he or she participated in the high school graduation ceremony. By comparison, an

FIGURE 3.2. Occupational therapy department evaluation/discharge form.

Client: ____________ DOA: ____________ DOI: ____________ Initial Date: ____________ Discharge Date: ____________ Discharge Environment: ____________

SCALE: **7** = Independent 100% **6** = Modified Independence 90% **5** = Supervised Assistance 80% **4** = Minimal Assistance 75% **3** = Moderate Assistance 50% **2** = Maximum Assistance 25% **1** = Dependent < 25%

CODE: **IL** = Initial Level **DL** = Discharge Level **DP** = Deferred Per Pathway

Client Goal(s): ____________

Family Goal(s): ____________

☐ **1. Personal Management**

Scale	IL	DL	Scale	IL	DL	Scale	IL	DL	Scale	IL	DL	Scale	IL	DL	Scale	IL	DL	Scale	IL	DL
7			7			7			7			7			7			7		
6			6			6			6			6			6			6		
5			5			5			5			5			5			5		
4			4			4			4			4			4			4		
3			3			3			3			3			3			3		
2			2			2			2			2			2			2		
1			1			1			1			1			1			1		
Basic ADL 1 Hair, Oral, Dress, Face			**Basic ADL 2 Bath, Toilet, Shave**			**Housekeeping**			**Laundry**			**Safety**			**Awareness**			**Satisfaction**		

Outcome Goals: ____________

Discharge Outcomes: ____________

☐ **2. Meal Planning & Meal Preparation**

Scale	IL	DL	Scale	IL	DL	Scale	IL	DL	Scale	IL	DL	Scale	IL	DL	Scale	IL	DL	Scale	IL	DL
7			7			7			7			7			7			7		
6			6			6			6			6			6			6		
5			5			5			5			5			5			5		
4			4			4			4			4			4			4		
3			3			3			3			3			3			3		
2			2			2			2			2			2			2		
1			1			1			1			1			1			1		
Meal Planning			**Cold Prep**			**Microwave Prep**			**Stove Prep**			**Clean-Up**			**Awareness**			**Safety**		

Outcome Goals: ____________

Discharge Outcomes: ____________

☐ **3. Mobility**

Scale	IL	DL	Scale	IL	DL	Scale	IL	DL	Scale	IL	DL	Scale	IL	DL	Scale	IL	DL	Scale	IL	DL
7			7			7			7			7			7			7		
6			6			6			6			6			6			6		
5			5			5			5			5			5			5		
4			4			4			4			4			4			4		
3			3			3			3			3			3			3		
2			2			2			2			2			2			2		
1			1			1			1			1			1			1		
Mobility Planning			**TLC Grounds Mobility**			**TLC Block Mobility**			**Postural Stability**			**Postural Mobility**			**Awareness**			**Safety**		

Outcome Goals: ____________

Discharge Outcomes: ____________

T A B L E 3 . 5 . Seven Functional Performance Levels in the Quadraphonic Approach

Goals	Environmental Condition
Totally Dependent To increase the performance level and satisfy to 25%. Increase awareness of relevant environmental characteristics and inhibit irrelevant characteristics.	At this level, clients require a therapeutic environment with minimal processing demands. The instructions are simple, with one-step commands. Continuous cuing is required. Objects should be familiar and nonrotated. The duration of engagement in the activity should be brief and the speed of presentation slow. Treatment emphasizes a multisensory approach, using a variety of limited stimuli and movement patterns. The focus should be on functional outcome. The therapist must determine when breakdown occurs. Cues are generated primarily by the therapist and are task- and goal-specific. Performance may not increase with cuing. A feedback program is used to provide information on performance and results. Emphasis on micro and match functional context.
Maximum Dependence To increase the performance level to 50%. Increase error detection in performance guided by external cues.	Exposure to predictable and unpredictable conditions. At this stage, the environmental regulations require a higher processing demand. The instructions are short and simple, with two-step commands. Continuous cuing may be required. Objects remain familiar and nonrotated. The duration and speed of the presentation is increased. Treatment emphasizes cortical and subcortical strategies. Cues are generated primarily by the therapist and are task-, goal-, and strategy-specific. A feedback program is used to provide information on performance and results. Once client is able to perform task or activity more than 50% of the time (not chance), a variation of mix–match and adopt environments can follow.
Moderate Dependence To increase performance level and satisfaction to 75%. Facilitate the client's error detection and error correction performance, guided through external cues and self-monitoring.	Combine a variety of environments, postural supports, and body positions. Continue to increase processing demands. The instructions are short and simple, with two-step commands. Unfamiliar objects are used and rotated. The duration and speed of the activity are again increased. The duration of activities is 45 minutes. Treatment emphasizes cortical and subcortical strategies. Cues are encouraged to be self-generated and are task-, goal-, and strategy-specific. Performance may increase with cues. A feedback program is used to provide information on performance and results.
Minimal Assistance To increase performance level and satisfaction to above 75%. Promote client's ability to set up and restructure the environment.	**Mixmatch and adapt:** Combine a variety of environments, postural supports, and body positions; high processing demands. The instructions are given with three-step or more commands. Objects are similar, unfamiliar, abstract, rotated, and nonrotated. The duration is greater than 1 hour. Treatment emphasizes the client's control and decision making. Performance may not be dependent on cues. A feedback frequency program is used to change, diminish, or delete external feedback.
Supervised Assistance To increase client's performance and satisfaction to above 80%. Promote the client's function and control in structured and unstructured environments.	**Mixmatch and adapt:** Combine a variety of environments, postural supports, and body positions; high processing demands. The instructions are given with three-step or more commands. Objects are similar, unfamiliar, abstract, rotated, and nonrotated. The duration is greater than 1 hour. Treatment emphasizes the client's control and decision making. Performance may not be dependent on cues. A feedback frequency program is used to change, diminish, or delete external feedback.
Independent With Modification To increase the client's performance level to above 90%, so that the client is able to perform with minimal modification; promote client's selection and control in a variety of environments.	**Mixmatch and adapt:** Combine and match a variety of environments, postural supports, and body positions; high processing demands. The instructions are with three-step or more commands. Objects are familiar, unfamiliar, abstract, rotated, and nonrotated. The duration of the activity is for 1.5 hours or more. Cues should be self-generated. A feedback frequency program is used to change, diminish, or delete external feedback.
Independent Client is independent without modification. Client does not need occupational therapy services.	**Mixmatch and adapt:** No modifications are required in physical, social, or cultural context.

Note. From *The Quadraphonic Approach: Management of Cognitive and Postural Dysfunction,* by B. Abreu, 1990, New York: Therapeutic Service Systems. Copyright © 1990 by Therapeutic Service Systems. Reprinted with permission.

example of semantic memory is the client's recollection of what Americans eat for breakfast or what type of celebrations adolescents have when they complete high school.

Individuals who have experienced brain injury show a diversity of symptoms that reflect different aspects of cognition. Impairment is reported in almost every aspect of cognitive functioning following brain injury: general cognitive ability (Duchek & Abreu, 1997; Lezak, 1983), attention (Toglia, 1993; Van Zomeren & Brouwer, 1994), memory (Toglia, 1993; Wilson, 1987), visual–spatial perception and integration (Gianutsos & Matheson, 1987; Warren, 1993a, 1993b), and language (Hartley, 1995). All of these impairments contribute to a decrease in the capacity to communicate. The characteristics of the client's social communication also may vary depending on the location and extent of the lesion. For example, if the posterior region of the right hemisphere or the frontal lobe is affected, the therapist may have difficulty obtaining information that requires visual–spatial processing such as making or reading facial expressions, visual scanning, respecting personal space, and interpreting complex visual information (Braun, Baribeau, Ethier, Daigneault, & Proulx, 1989).

Such impairments may affect the client's storytelling abilities, diminishing the ability to relate personal history and reconstructions. Examples may include reduced mastery of vocabulary, diminished capacity to name words and speak fluently, reduced comprehension of lengthy and complex visual and auditory information, inability to follow instructions with three or more steps, and decreased ability to make the social connections necessary for politeness and courteous conversation (Coelho, Liles, & Duffy, 1991; Hartley, 1995; Hartley & Jensen, 1992; Rehak et al., 1992).

The client's comprehension or fluidity in communicating may fluctuate because of lapses in alertness and attention, decreased empathy, and reduced initiation or motivation. The net effect of the client's difficulties may be the production of a broken story. The story will warrant a therapist's increased sensitivity and trust in the client's capacity to communicate what is meaningful. The client's impairments are not static; they are context- and goal-dependent, and they may vary depending on where and when the therapist chooses to conduct a portion of the interview. In a restaurant favored by the client, for example, the client's affect, tone, and fluidity may change.

The goal of the interview and its associated storytelling is to create a partnership that helps clients to share their messages about morals and beliefs and the meaning that they find in their lives and social worlds. These messages are sometimes more important than the specific events or details uncovered in the interview. The therapist may discover, through communicative improvisations, information about a client's norms and values that may not be apparent in his or her institutional under-life. See Table 3.6 for a list of sample questions that can be included in the interview done from the macro perspective. The result of the narrative process is a summary of the client's story that can be used as a basis for the evaluation.

Guidelines for Evaluation From the Macro Perspective

After the narrative information has been collected, the evaluation process continues with the classification of the client's performance through the use of the six cognitive and functional evaluation strips mentioned earlier. The six strips are personal management, independent meal planning and preparation, mobility planning and mobility, money management, upper-extremities subskills, and cognitive–perceptual subskills (see Figure 3.2). The first four of the evaluation strips view occupation from the macro perspective. Each time a strip is used in the macro perspective, the therapist may consider the following actions as guidelines: (a) an examination of the characteristics that affect the client's behavior, including lifestyle, life-stage, health, and disability status; (b) a precise operational definition of the assessment area; (c) a consideration of the client's choices and degree of control within the evaluation process; (d) documentation of the results that include commentary about the client's personal awareness and responsivity as well as his or her interaction with therapist, task, and environment; and (e) a consideration of the psychometric character of the evaluation and whether it yields both qualitative and quantitative performance data.

The use of the four evaluation strips that assess the macro perspective will depend on the individual circumstances of each client. The therapist will seek to understand the big picture of a client's lifestyle by eliciting a detailed discussion of individual circumstances in an interview that is structured around open-ended questions. To focus the evaluation, the therapist may ask a client questions about personal status, such as "How much help would you like to contribute to managing the household?" or "What are some of the more frustrating aspects of your present situation?" Given a response that suggests the client wants to continue helping with shopping and food preparation but is having problems being efficient in the grocery store, the therapist might offer to assess these areas.

TABLE 3.6. Sample Questions for the Client Interview

Content (What to Ask: The Wording)	Process (How to Ask: The Way to Ask)	Context (Where to Ask: The Place to Ask)
1. Describe your life as if it were a book. Describe this stage of your life as a chapter.	1. Attend to the content.	1. Change the locations of the interview to evoke the story.
2. How do you feel about being admitted to this institution?	2. Attend to the flow of the topic.	2. Restaurants.
3. Let's talk about how it feels to be diagnosed with a brain injury.	3. Encourage elaboration.	3. Churches, synagogues, religious institutions.
4. Let's talk about how it feels to have a cognitive impairment.	4. Provide self-disclosing incidents.	4. Schools.
5. What happened to your life when you decided to be admitted to this institution?	5. Provide clarification of the collaborative role.	5. Theaters, movies.
6. Overall, what has been your experience after your incident (tumor, accident, stroke, illness)?	6. Discuss events at length.	6. Outdoor areas.
7. Teach about dressing with one hand.	7. Cultivate the art of hearing.	7. Other personally meaningful locations.
8. Could you tell me what happened to your family after your brain injury?	8. Recognize the gestalt of the story.	
9. What was your role in your family?	9. Analyze and narrow the themes of the story (verbal, nonverbal).	
10. Could you tell me how different your role as a (father, sister, wife, worker) is now?	10. Interview until saturation: Nothing new comes out.	
11. After the rehabilitation program ends, what happens next?		

For example, consider the client named Edgar who was mentioned above. Recall that he was diagnosed with a brain injury and shows a moderate memory deficit. He also has been admitted into a community re-entry facility from a rehabilitation hospital. In the initial interview, Edgar indicates that his primary goals are to return home to his wife Daisy, to contribute to the management of the household, and to return to work as a chemical engineer. By stating these goals, Edgar determines the point at which the therapist starts the assessment. To focus the assessment, the therapist may ask Edgar questions, such as "What skills do you need to return home? How much help were you giving Daisy at home? What are the skills required as a chemical engineer? What do you do for fun?" The answers to these questions will lead to the follow-up assessment related to the cognitive and functional macro evaluation strips.

During the evaluation, the therapist and Edgar decide to use grocery shopping as one of the skills to be tested. The shopping task is divided into four components, each valued at a score of 25%: plan a shopping list, plan a budget, plan how to get to the store, and go to the store and shop. During the evaluation, the therapist assesses the four com-

ponents and records the score. If the client is unable to perform any function, the therapist uses a tutoring approach that includes questions, cues, prompts, and repetition to determine if the client can improve his or her performance. For example, the therapist may use a hierarchical cue procedure that would include awareness cues ("Look carefully"), general directives ("Look in the frozen food section"), or specific directives ("Look for ice cream"). This cuing process will reveal whether a client can benefit from cues and therefore benefit from further rehabilitation. Some clients will be able to benefit from remediation, and others will require compensatory techniques.

In the case of Edgar, the therapist will test his planning skills and accompany him to the store to assess and document his performance. The therapist and Edgar will establish the targeted performance level and supplement the assessment with narrative information. Prior to shopping, Edgar might be asked how well he anticipates doing; after completing the task, he might be asked how well he thought he did. During the shopping test, the therapist will observe Edgar's response to other shoppers and his effectiveness with the cashier. The therapist will also note the strategies Edgar uses to remember, the responses he gives, and the results of any suggestions or modifications given to him. This information will contribute to the qualitative aspects of the evaluation. Throughout the evaluation process, Edgar will be a collaborator and thus continually learn about his performance. When the therapist completes the macro evaluation of those functions identified as important by Edgar and Daisy, focus can then shift to the micro perspective.

TREATMENT PRINCIPLES: HOLISTIC AND CONFLUENT TREATMENT IN EDGAR'S CASE

On completion of the macro and micro evaluation, the therapist is ready to work with the client to develop a holistic and confluent treatment plan. As previously stated, holistic treatment is based on a global health notion that clients are capable of maintaining and restoring equilibrium in their lives (McColl, 1994). Holistic treatment will use confluent methods, actions, and interactions that develop the affective domain. The holistic and confluent approach is particularly important if one aims to preserve the personalization of the rehabilitation process in a managed care environment (Abreu & Price-Lackey, 1994; Peloquin, 1996).

In the current managed care environment, critical pathways can be used to organize treatment plans in a holistic fashion, avoiding duplication of services and maximizing interdisciplinary cooperation. These pathways can become the blueprint created by a health care team (including client and family) on the basis of the diagnosis and desired functional outcomes (Abreu, Seale, Podlesak, & Hartley, 1996). The efficiency and effectiveness of any critical pathway are measured by functional outcomes that match the client's goals and satisfaction with the services rendered (Abreu et al., 1996).

The case study of Edgar will be used to demonstrate select methods of a treatment approach that is holistic and confluent. The reader is reminded that, in the quadraphonic approach, there is always a free-flowing movement between the macro and micro perspectives. Abreu designed six treatment environments to match seven cognitive and functional levels (the seventh level, that of independence, warrants no therapeutic intervention). The six treatment environments are total dependence, maximum dependence, moderate dependence, minimal assistance, supervised assistance, and independence with no modification. In the story of Edgar's recovery, total dependence, moderate dependence, and supervised assistance is highlighted in three practice settings: a coma unit, a rehabilitation unit, and a community re-entry setting.

Treatment Guidelines for Functional Levels

During treatment, therapists tutor, coach, and encourage the client and his or her social support systems (family and friends) to develop strategies for dealing with the impairments, disabilities, and disadvantages resulting from brain injury. If a client is evaluated with a functional performance level below 50%, the therapist may use traditional as well as more affective approaches to encourage the client with both verbal and nonverbal exchanges that communicate support (Peloquin, 1995).

On the other hand, for those clients who have shown functional performance ranging from 50% to 90% independence, the most beneficial therapeutic environment is variable and with increasing task demands. These additional task demands create contextual interference that facilitates successful performance (Druckman & Bjork, 1991, 1994; Schmidt & Bjork, 1992). For a more detailed delineation of the suggested therapeutic environment for each level of client function, see Figure 3.2.

Phases of Treatment

In addition to the functional performance guidelines, we propose three phases for every treatment level: preparatory, performance, and postperformance (see Figure 3.3).

Preparatory Phase

The preparatory phase addresses four types of treatment techniques that precede the demand for performance: emotional and mental, attentional recruitment, organizational and reorganizational, and practice schedules and feedback plan. By using emotional and mental techniques in the preparatory phase, the therapist is better able to engage the client as a partner in the treatment process. This engagement is accomplished through the use of the macro assessment tools that are used to establish a connection with the client's story and personal goals. Through specific explanations of the purpose of treatment and through body language that communicates interest and empathy, the therapist invites the client into a critical collaborative relationship. The preparatory phase also may include relaxation techniques. Quiet and stable environments are recommended, and the use of meditation and subliminal self-help techniques may help some clients.

Attentional recruitment techniques include a wide range of strategies for increasing the client's readiness and capacity to gather and retain information. These techniques also facilitate the client's letting go of irrelevant in-

FIGURE 3.3. Quadraphonic approach treatment model.

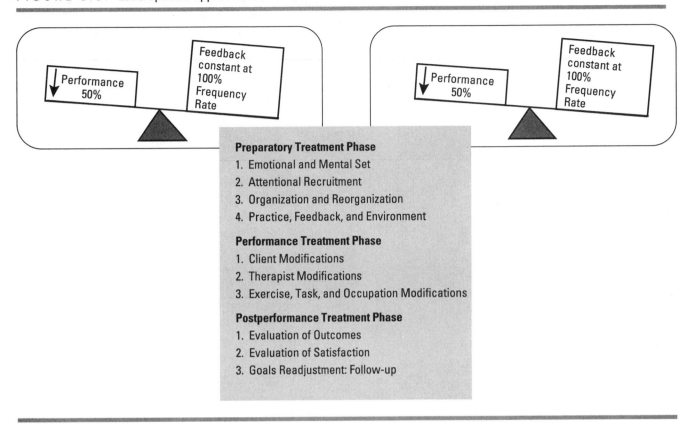

Preparatory Treatment Phase

1. Emotional and Mental Set
2. Attentional Recruitment
3. Organization and Reorganization
4. Practice, Feedback, and Environment

Performance Treatment Phase

1. Client Modifications
2. Therapist Modifications
3. Exercise, Task, and Occupation Modifications

Postperformance Treatment Phase

1. Evaluation of Outcomes
2. Evaluation of Satisfaction
3. Goals Readjustment: Follow-up

Note. From *The Quadraphonic Approach: Course Handouts*, by B. C. Abreu, 1997, Galveston, TX: Therapeutic Service Systems. Copyright © 1997 by Therapeutic Service Systems. Reprinted with permission.

formation so it will not interfere with his or her functional performance. As a technique for awareness and self-monitoring, the therapist can invite the client to describe aloud what to do and how to do it. For visual acuity and perception training, Abreu recommended increasing luminance and the use of large print. In addition, the therapist can increase background contrast, increase light, and decrease shadows (Lampert & Lapolice, 1995; Warren, 1995). A multimodal approach to instructions (visual, auditory, kinesthetic, verbal, nonverbal) is recommended.

Neurodevelopmental and biomechanical techniques are also used as attentional motor recruitment techniques to provide the client with sufficient trunk control or trunk support to ensure postural readiness. Poor bodily alignment because of muscle tone and musculoskeletal changes can rob the client of the appropriate postural support required to attend to incoming information. The client may not be able to simultaneously focus on controlling posture (sitting or standing) while gathering visual and auditory information. Therefore, the clinician either provides faci-

litation or inhibition motor techniques for postural control and support or uses external support devices to compensate for the impaired postural control.

In addition, the therapist can use traditional information-processing techniques and cognitive rehabilitation techniques that help the client notice the critical traits of activity, task, or role: verbal repetitions, cues to initiate, simplifications through concrete instructions, and changes in the pace or duration of instructions and stimuli presented.

The third sets of treatment techniques in the preparation phase are organizational and reorganizational techniques. These include a wide variety of strategies for planning and arranging information and procedures in an orderly fashion so that the client will gain more understanding and develop more skills from any training session. Organization is the act of thinking about what one is either doing or going to do. Organizational strategies help us to consciously monitor and control the way in which we plan and execute instructions so as to produce a unified action with coherent relations among steps. This conscious

self-awareness and self-monitoring about how to organize learning before it happens and while it happens is
also called *metacognition* or *reflection*.

Organizational strategies help clients to monitor and control behavior through reflection about the factual knowledge
given about the skill or task, its components, its controls,
and its functions. Factual knowledge is called declarative
knowledge and is known as *declarative memory* when retained or stored in memory. Organizational strategies can
also be used to help clients monitor and control behavior
through reflection on procedural knowledge or the rules
given regarding how to perform a task. When rule-based
or procedural knowledge is retained or stored, it is called
procedural memory. Finally, organizational strategies
help with a client's introspection about his or her ability
to handle a task that is actually being attempted.

Psychologists and educators, particularly Chi and
colleagues (Chi & Bassok, 1989; Chi, de Leeuw, Chiu, &
LaVancher, 1994; Chi & Glaser, 1985; Chi, Glaser, & Rees,
1982), have supported the idea that self-regulation of cognitive skills in the classroom can help individuals solve
mathematics and physics problems and play chess
(Dreyfus & Dreyfus, 1986; Gagné & Smith, 1962; Kluwe,
1987; Paris & Winograd, 1990; Schoenfield, 1987; Silver,
1987; Swanson, 1990). Other studies, with special populations, support the use of self-regulation to assist in speech
and language (Blackmer & Mitton, 1991; Dabbs, Evans,
Hooper, & Purvis, 1980; Koegel, Koegel, & Ingham, 1986;
Schloss & Wood, 1990; Shriberg & Kwiatkowski; 1990;
Whitney & Goldstein, 1989). The use of self-regulation
in cognitive rehabilitation after acquired brain injury is
growing, and further studies are needed to establish validation and efficacy (Abreu, 1992; Abreu & Toglia, 1987;
Bewick et al., 1995; Toglia, 1991; Webster & Scott, 1983;
Ylvisaker & Szekeres, 1989).

The value of reflective problem solving using metacognitive and affective techniques has been advocated by several occupational therapists for use in both the clinic and
the classroom (Abreu, 1992, 1994a; Abreu & Toglia, 1987;
Neistadt, 1992; Parham, 1987; Peloquin, 1996; Schon,
1987; Toglia, 1991, 1993). Introspective analysis that allows individuals to understand the reasons for their failures
is a process of learning to learn (Stuss, 1992).

Good learners comprehend the problem, represent the
principles of the problem in formal terms, plan a solution,
execute the plan, and interpret and evaluate the solution
(Posner, 1988). Metacognitive techniques include developing a plan of action; maintaining and monitoring
the plan; and evaluating the plan before, during, and after
the action (Brown, 1978, 1987; Flavell, 1985, 1987). The

metacognitive approach uses questions, cues, and prompts
to bring awareness to the client's rules of behavior, task
performance, and use of strategies. The client is encouraged to engage in self-explanation and self-monitoring
through talk-aloud or think-aloud methods. However, if a
client is unable to self-explain and monitor, the therapist
can cue with questions and prompts. The four basic questions that a client can ask about any task are

1. What should I do before I start this training session?
2. What should I do during this training session?
3. What should I do after this training session?
4. Do I need to do anything else to perform better during
   training?

The educational literature suggests that good students
use more self-talk about actions that exemplify the solutions. They also use more self-monitoring for evaluating
their accuracy than do other students (Chi & Bassok,
1989; Chi et al., 1994; VanLehn, Jones, & Chi, 1991,
1992). Similar procedures have been described in the occupational therapy rehabilitation literature for clients with
head injury (Abreu, 1992; Abreu & Toglia, 1987; Toglia,
1993; Webster & Scott, 1983).

The fourth set of techniques used in the preparatory
phase includes the practice schedule and feedback plan.
A practice schedule defines the type and quantity of the
repeated performances needed by the client for learning
to occur. The therapist proposes the best practice schedule for a client depending on the level of recovery and the
physical and cognitive tolerance for training. No evidence
in the literature supports one particular schedule over
another. Therefore, therapists must use clinical judgment
to decide which type of evidence and which order of practice training to use. The training can be an intense practice process or more distributed (spread out). Training can
be designed to include partial or complete tasks and can
use forward or backward chaining. In clinical retrospect,
Abreu has not perceived a proportional relationship between the number of practice performances and the mastery or retention of a skill. Practice does not guarantee
performance with brain injury. During the preparatory
phase, the client–learner helps the therapist to establish a
timeline for the achievement of outcome goals.

A feedback plan defines the type and quantity of the responses that will be given to modify, correct, or strengthen
a behavior displayed by the client during the practice session. In the quadraphonic approach, Abreu advocated the
use of consistent feedback with clients who perform at a
level of independence from 0 to 49%. On the other hand,
for clients who are performing at a level of independence

above 50%, the use of random feedback is highly recommended (Abreu, 1994a).

Certain motor learning and action system theorists have stated that using variability in practice improves the retention and transfer of motor skills (Druckman & Bjork, 1991, 1994; Reed, 1982; Schmidt, 1988; Schmidt & Bjork, 1992). Abreu (1990) has noted that not all clients benefit from random and less frequent feedback and that clients with low cognitive levels and those in early recovery stages perform better with the use of constant and amplified feedback. But as soon as the clients show understanding of the goal and some stability in their responses that is not attributable to chance (i.e., above 50% accuracy), Abreu implements a lower frequency feedback schedule.

Performance Phase

The performance phase is the stage in treatment during which the client–learner executes an action or creates something for purposes of learning or relearning and for satisfaction. For Abreu, the performance phase of treatment includes an improvisation by the therapist to spontaneously create a caring and effective bond with the client. In this phase, the client, who has recently become a novice in ordinary occupations in which he or she was previously an expert, must regain expertise. The literature on tutoring individuals to progress from novice to expert levels has given guidelines for the performance phase of treatment.

Information on identifying effective strategies that move learners toward expertise has been the subject of investigation in cognitive psychology and artificial intelligence (Chi et al., 1982). Research in artificial intelligence attempts to simulate human capacities in a mechanized environment via expert systems. The characteristics of an expert, whether human or machine, can be considered as broad guidelines for engaging the client in ordinary occupations. In general, experts excel in their own domain; perceive larger meaningful patterns and conceptual frames and have vast organizational strategies, process information and problem-solve faster, have superior short-term and long-term memory, use more associations with more principles, spend a great deal of time analyzing a problem qualitatively, and have strong self-monitoring skills (Chi & Glaser, 1985).

Experts must explicitly know how to use effective strategies in conjunction with their content knowledge for mastery of any skill or knowledge (Glaser & Chi, 1988; Posner, 1988). The use of strategies can enhance problem solving through the discovery of better ways to express, recognize, and use diverse and particular forms of knowledge.

In collaboration with an interdisciplinary rehabilitation team, we created a list of contextual modifiers that can enhance client success during the performance phase. Contextual modifications are cues that can originate from three primary sources as well as the interplay among them that occurs during task performance: the therapist, the task or environment, and the client. Although these contextual modifications interact closely, it is important to articulate and distinguish between them for purposes of evaluation, treatment, and research.

The contextual modifiers listed in Figure 3.4 are recommended for use as treatment tools and for documenting the qualitative aspects of the client's performance. The first column describes the contextual dimension or type of modifier. Some of these modifiers are not totally exclusive or discreet; they may be nested or embedded in others. Because the modifiers are qualitative tools, their goal is to identify, describe, and analyze the patterns of a client's changes in performance. These tools are classified as soft, but they enhance the therapist's awareness of interactional considerations essential for treatment and aid in the identification of the kind of strategy that improves performance. Therapists must remember that improved performance does not always correlate with client satisfaction.

The second column lists the standard approach or the first strategy in treatment: After giving standard instructions, the therapist observes the client's behavior without modification. The process is one of "wait and see what happens." The therapist then repeats the instructions and modifies the environment. This step is represented with various recommendations for modifications or contextual modifiers listed in the third column. Notice that these items specify either training or compensatory techniques. For example, consider error detection and correction technique as it relates to the case of Edgar.

Edgar was unable to detect or correct errors in money management when balancing his checking account. With verbal and visual cueing, Edgar was able to increase his functional performance level and balance the account accurately. Even so, Daisy was taught to supervise Edgar because, after eight 1-hr therapy sessions, there was no generalization of performance. Edgar was successful only with cueing to initiate, increased illumination, and concrete explanations. Use of pictorial representation did not help him. Edgar was aware that he was cue-dependent and needed external monitoring. He was able to perform all cash transactions using self-generated cues such as "count your change twice" before putting it in his pocket. The contextual modifiers listed in the third column include both self-specific and task-specific strategies.

FIGURE 3.4. Contextual modifiers for client performance.

Contextual modifications are cues that can originate from three primary sources—the therapist, the task or environment, and the client—and from an interplay among them that occurs during task performance. Although clinically these modifications interact closely, it is important to articulate and distinguish them for purposes of evaluation, treatment, and research.

Contextual Dimension	Standard Approach	Contextual Modification (Therapist/Client/Task)	Outcome Successful (Given)	Unsuccessful
1. Activity Phase The phase during an activity when the client's functioning breaks down and the therapist offers feedback	☐ Standard No modification throughout any phase of the test, task, or activity	*Give feedback:* ☐ Before preparatory stage ☐ At initiation stage ☐ At middle stage ☐ At end stage ☐ After completion	*Given feedback:* ☐ At preparatory stage ☐ At initiation stage ☐ At middle stage ☐ At end stage ☐ After completion	☐ ☐ ☐ ☐ ☐
2. Postural Readiness The bodily positions that facilitate the client's execution of a task	☐ Standard position assumed by client	*Cue the client to position:* ☐ Eyes ☐ Head/Neck ☐ Limbs ☐ Hand ☐ Hips ☐ None ☐ Other _____	*Given cueing to position:* ☐ Eyes ☐ Head/Neck ☐ Limbs ☐ Hand ☐ Hips ☐ None ☐ Other _____	☐ ☐ ☐ ☐ ☐ ☐
3. Error Detection/ Correction Information provided the client relative to the presence of error	☐ Standard Client initiates response to error in the absence of observable cueing	☐ Cue for error detection ☐ Cue for error correction ☐ Client self-cues for error detection ☐ Client self-cues for error correction ☐ Other _____	☐ Therapist cueing for error detection ☐ Therapist cueing for error correction ☐ Client self-cueing for error detection ☐ Client self-cueing for error correction ☐ Other _____	☐ ☐ ☐ ☐
4. Social Milieu Manipulation made to the client's social environment	☐ Standard No modification of social milieu (client's family, friends, social, and institutional support system)	☐ Seat the client near a friend ☐ Ask the client to help another ☐ Ask client helper to work with the client ☐ Ask a question to elicit interaction ☐ Other _____	☐ Seating near a friend ☐ A request to help another ☐ A client + L83 helper ☐ A question to elicit interaction ☐ Other _____	☐ ☐ ☐ ☐
5. Safety The information that the client requires to perform safely + C11	☐ Standard No modification of set-up, equipment, and safety demands	☐ Explain safety measures ☐ Explain preventive measures ☐ Explain dangerous consequences ☐ Explain emergency procedures ☐ Repeat preventive measures ☐ Other _____	☐ Explanation of safety measures ☐ Explanation of preventive measures ☐ Explanation of dangerous consequences ☐ Explanation of emergency procedures ☐ Repetition of preventive measures ☐ Other _____	☐ ☐ ☐ ☐ ☐
6. Awareness of a Problem Awareness of impairment, dysfunction, restriction, or personal or social	☐ Standard No modification of awareness capacities and limitation	☐ Give general cues that a problem exists ☐ Give specific cues when error happens or problem exists ☐ Give specific cues after error happens or problem occurs ☐ Give gentle confrontation about the undetected problem ☐ Give away the answer or solution ☐ Other _____	☐ General cues that a problem exists ☐ Specific cues when error happened or problem existed ☐ Specific cues after error happened or problem occurred ☐ Gentle confrontation about undetected problem ☐ An answer or solution ☐ Other _____	☐ ☐ ☐ ☐ ☐

(continued)

FIGURE 3.4. Contextual modifiers for client performance *(Continued)*.

Contextual Dimension	Standard Approach	Contextual Modification (Therapist/Client/Task)	Outcome Successful (Given)	Unsuccessful
7. Feedback Type The structuring of corrective verbal information that the client is given in which to respond to an instruction	☐ Standard No modification of feedback	☐ Give knowledge of performance feedback: Corrective information about a component of part of task, test, or movement	☐ Knowledge of performance feedback	☐
		☐ Give knowledge of results feedback: Corrective information about the total or whole task, test, or movement goal	☐ Knowledge of results feedback	☐
		☐ Give positive feedback: Corrective information in form of approvals, assurances, reinforcers	☐ Positive feedback	☐
		☐ Give negative feedback: Corrective information in form of disapprovals or negative reinforcers	☐ Negative feedback	☐
		☐ Give private feedback: Corrective information in a confidential or private environment	☐ Private feedback	☐
		☐ Give public feedback: Corrective information provided in a group view or community environment	☐ Public feedback	☐
8. Medications Substances used to affect client's cognitive function	☐ Standard No medications	☐ _____ ☐ _____ ☐ _____ ☐ _____	Medication _____ Medication _____ Medication _____ Medication _____	☐ ☐ ☐ ☐
9. Expectations for Accuracy/ Correctness The therapist's anticipation or expectation relative to the client's success or failure	☐ Standard expectations	☐ Therapist anticipates task failure ☐ Therapist anticipates task success ☐ No anticipation ☐ Other _____	☐ But therapist's expectation was a failure ☐ And therapist's expectation was a success ☐ In the absence of any particular expectation ☐ Other _____	☐ ☐ ☐
10. Organizational Strategy Organizational methods, guidelines provided	☐ Standard organization offered	☐ Provide guidelines about where to start or end ☐ Provide guidelines about where to look ☐ Provide guidelines about what to say ☐ Provide rules and guidelines for behavior ☐ Reorganize information ☐ Client self-initiates strategy ☐ Other _____	☐ Guidelines about where to start or end ☐ Guidelines about where to look ☐ Guidelines about what to say ☐ Rules and guidelines for behavior ☐ Reorganized information ☐ Self-initiated strategy ☐ Other _____	☐ ☐ ☐ ☐ ☐ ☐
11. Therapy Set Information given the client about the goal or performance of the task or therapy	☐ Standard request to perform	☐ Explain goal, purpose of task ☐ Explain goal, purpose of therapy ☐ Explain role of the therapist ☐ Other _____	☐ Explanation of the goal, purpose of task ☐ Explanation of the goal, purpose of therapy ☐ Explanation of the role of the therapist ☐ Other _____	☐ ☐ ☐

(continued)

FIGURE 3.4. Contextual modifiers for client performance *(Continued)*.

Contextual Dimension	Standard Approach	Contextual Modification (Therapist/Client/Task)	Outcome Successful (Given)	Unsuccessful
12. Personal History References to the client's needs, values, interests, or preferences	☐ Standard request to perform	☐ Connect task with client's interests, preferences ☐ Connect task with client's hobbies ☐ Refer to client's needs, goals ☐ Refer to client's values ☐ Use personally relevant task ☐ Use personally concrete task ☐ Other _____	☐ Connection made with client's interests, preferences ☐ Connection made with client's hobbies ☐ Reference to client's needs, goals ☐ Reference to client's values ☐ Use of personally relevant task ☐ Use of personally concrete task ☐ Other _____	☐ ☐ ☐ ☐ ☐ ☐
13. Voice Tone Changes The modification of verbal tone that the client is given	☐ Standard No modification in voice	☐ Use a therapy voice: formal therapeutic language ☐ Use a directive voice: interpersonal control, commanding ☐ Use a sympathetic voice: calm, confident, yet gentle ☐ Use a modulated voice: modified to increase understanding (e.g., slower, louder, shorter statements) ☐ Other _____	☐ Formal tone ☐ Commanding tone ☐ Calm and gentle tone ☐ Modulated tone to increase understanding ☐ Other _____	☐ ☐ ☐ ☐
14. Therapist's Use of Self The conscious use of personal strength and interpersonal capacities	☐ Standard No deliberate use of personal interventions	☐ Give expressive touch ☐ Use gentle humor ☐ Move closer to client ☐ Actively listen to a client's concern ☐ Use of encouraging words or gestures ☐ Give power of choice	☐ Expressive touch ☐ Gentle humor ☐ Proximity of the therapist ☐ Active listening ☐ Encouragement ☐ Choices	☐ ☐ ☐ ☐ ☐ ☐
15. Sensory Modality The visual, verbal tactile, or movement cues provided	☐ Standard No modification of sensory input	☐ Give verbal repetition ☐ Give verbal cues (includes questions/probes) ☐ Give visual cue/nonverbal feedback ☐ Give tactile/kinesthetic cue ☐ Give pictorial representation ☐ Give written cues ☐ Increase illumination, contrast, brightness ☐ Other _____	☐ Verbal repetition ☐ Verbal cues ☐ Visual cue/nonverbal feedback ☐ Tactile/kinesthetic cue ☐ Pictorial representation ☐ Written cues ☐ Increased illumination, contrast, brightness ☐ Other _____	☐ ☐ ☐ ☐ ☐ ☐ ☐
16. Amount of Information The number of instructive steps, choices, or pieces of information presented	☐ Standard No modification to amount of information	☐ Cue to initiate ☐ Give one step at a time ☐ Reduce the number of steps ☐ Shorten the task ☐ Other _____	☐ Cueing to initiate ☐ One step at a time ☐ Reduced number of steps ☐ Shortening of the task ☐ Other _____	☐ ☐ ☐ ☐

(continued)

FIGURE 3.4. Contextual modifiers for client performance *(Continued)*.

Contextual Dimension	Standard Approach	Contextual Modification (Therapist/Client/Task)	Outcome Successful (Given)	Unsuccessful
17. Complexity The level of difficulty of the pieces of information given	☐ Standard No modification of level of difficulty	☐ Simplify by using concrete explanations ☐ Simplify by demonstrating ☐ Simplify by using familiar tasks ☐ Simplify by using self-related items ☐ Simplify by increasing the spacing between items or objects (nonscattered) ☐ Simplify by decreasing spatial traits or position of objects ☐ Other _____	☐ Concrete explanations ☐ Demonstrations ☐ Familiar tasks only ☐ Self-related items ☐ Increased spacing between items or objects (nonscattered) ☐ Decreased spatial traits or position of objects ☐ Other _____	☐ ☐ ☐ ☐ ☐ ☐
18. Pace The speed and consistency with which information is presented	☐ Standard No modification of pace	☐ Give slow presentation ☐ Give fast presentation ☐ Give predictable, stable presentation ☐ Give random, unpredictable presentation ☐ Other _____	☐ Slow presentation ☐ Fast presentation ☐ Predictable, stable presentation ☐ Random, unpredictable presentation ☐ Other _____	☐ ☐ ☐ ☐
19. Duration The interval of time that the client is given in which to respond to an instructions	☐ Standard No modification of duration time	☐ Give 15 seconds ☐ Give 30 seconds ☐ Give 1 minute ☐ Other _____	☐ 15 seconds ☐ 30 seconds ☐ 1 minute ☐ Other _____	☐ ☐ ☐

Note. A Formula
Client's performance was successful in _____ when given _____.
  (Indicate the task or module)   (Indicate the contextual modifiers that helped)
Use of _____ did not help. Client's level of awareness of his or her
  (Indicate other modifiers used that were not successful)
problems / _____.
  (State client level of awareness)

Note. A Sample
Client's performance was successful in money management when given cueing to initiate, increased illumination, and concrete explanations. Use of pictorial representations did not help. Client is aware of his limitations.

The fourth column, outcome, is a guide used to indicate performance. The outcome results can be further developed to frame a narrative that describes the task and the successful and unsuccessful modifications.

The contextual modifier tools are used to gather data that can be stored and analyzed through a variety of methods. Computer software, such as the Nonnumerical Unstructured Data *Indexing, Searching, and Theorizing (NUD*IST) can be used to analyze the qualitative data provided by the use of contextual modifiers (Weitzman & Miles, 1995). The results can show which learning patterns and compensation techniques are best used for cognitive rehabilitation.

Postperformance Phase

The postperformance phase is reflective and consists of an intense review of the training session after performance. The review includes an evaluation of the training strategies used, the actions used to reinforce client confidence, and the client's and therapist's reactions to personal performance, including mutual satisfaction or dissatisfaction, self-confidence, and goal readjustment. Examples of post-performance reflective questions are, "What kind of reminders or help did you give Edgar? Was the type and amount of help provided to Edgar successful and satisfying for him and you?"

Many of the contextual modifiers used are based on cognitive apprenticeship as well as information-processing and teaching–learning techniques. These teaching–learning techniques focus on the qualitative analysis of both verbal and nonverbal instructions. One example, scaffolding, is used to refer to the guided learning techniques generated by the therapist–teacher to provide support in the form of cues, reminders, and other help necessary for the apprentice to perform an approximation of the training goal or task.

The therapist–teacher acts as a guide, shaping the learning and relearning efforts of the client with brain injury until the adjustable and temporary support is no longer needed. Many times, however, this support cannot be removed either because clients cannot generalize their training from clinic to environment or because they have not been able to achieve performance levels that are safe and do not require supervision. Self-efficacy judgments are decisions based on what people believe they can do in varied circumstances. A client's self-efficacy beliefs can change through occupational therapy interventions that offer direct mastery experiences and opportunities to make inferences from social comparisons, influences, and physiological states (Bandura, 1977). The postperformance phase of reflection includes inquiry into the effects of social learning during occupational therapy.

CASE EXAMPLE: EDGAR

Following is a brief discussion of three stages of Edgar's recovery with samples of treatment plans. For didactic purposes, the case of Edgar is based on a composite of many cases I encountered over the years. Remember that the quadraphonic approach advocates that the therapist should act as a collaborator in treatment, freely moving between the macro and micro perspectives.

Stage 1: The Coma—Low Arousal

Had it not been for recent medical advances, Edgar, like many other clients with head injury, might have died from secondary complications such as metabolic imbalance or urinary tract and respiratory infections (Bartkowski & Lovely, 1986; O'Dell & Riggs, 1996). In addition, medical technology now allows clients like Edgar to both survive and prosper. Medical practitioners involved with the

rehabilitation of brain injury are faced with therapeutic and ethical challenges for those involved in their care (O'Dell, Jasin, Lyons, Stivers, & Meszaros, 1996; O'Dell & Riggs, 1996; Rosenberg & Ashwal, 1996).

Edgar is a 25-year old traffic accident survivor who was in a coma for 1 week. He was recorded as Glasgow scale 7, and his multimodal–evoked potential data were considered good predictors of his recovery and mortality (Bartkowski & Lovely, 1986; O'Dell & Riggs, 1996). During coma, Edgar lacked meaningful interaction with people and the environment; however, he showed sleep and wake rhythms (Shaw, 1986). His decerebrate motor reactions began to fade after 7 days, and prehension, chewing, sucking, and postural adjustment reflexes began to emerge. He moved from coma to resumption of vegetative functions in 1 month and entered a persistent vegetative state (PVS). In this new state, he was able to control his respiration, blood pressure, digestive, and excretory functions (Rappaport, 1986). During PVS, the therapist and the other team members instructed Edgar's family and social support system to evaluate and track the length of arousal time, the presence of volitional versus coincidental movement, and the nature of the multimodal stimuli required to elicit appropriate responses. The family's participation in the treatment process provided them with some opportunity for control and responsibility and for the expression of their love.

During PVS stage, the occupational therapist used both macro and micro perspectives for rehabilitation. Tactile stimulation, so essential for eliciting arousal responses, became a form of expressive touch and part of the attempt to communicate with and encourage Edgar during this stage of his recovery. The therapist's communication with Edgar, in both words and nonverbal interactions, reflected respect for and sensitivity to the image of Edgar that was constructed through interviews with Daisy. Family and friends also contributed stimulation through narratives, pictures, and visits to the intensive care unit.

Time use is a constraint that can enhance occupational therapy practice at the coma level and throughout recovery (Christiansen, 1996; Kielhofner, 1977, 1985; Neville, 1980; White, 1996). The therapist and the members of the coma rehabilitation team each made an attempt to simulate and facilitate the functioning of Edgar's internal time clock with cues related to external time. While treating Edgar in the coma phase, the therapist would greet him with a resounding "Good morning, Edgar," and a team member added the specific time of day such as "it's 7:00 a.m." or "it's 8:00 a.m." In addition, when greeting those other individuals who were sometimes also present, the therapist used the same approach.

Other external cues designed to help Edgar regulate his internal clock were putting the television or radio on with Edgar's favorite programs, reading the newspaper, and turning on the news or weather channels (White, 1996). Each action aimed to influence Edgar's time clocks so that he could regain a sense of sleep–awake time or a rest–activity cycle (Christiansen, 1996). The internal time clocks such as the sleep–awake cycle, hormonal activity, and variations in blood pressure and body temperature as well as the external time clocks such as daylight, noise, and social rituals resemble the increase or decrease in social activity and interaction associated with the start and end of daily occupations (Christiansen, 1996).

The occupational therapist working with the allied health team and the family monitored, collected, analyzed, and reported the rate of Edgar's recovery to predict outcomes during this minimally responsive stage. The *minimally responsive state* should be differentiated from coma. The minimally responsive patient demonstrates some evidence of consciousness, whereas the patient in coma does not. At this stage, it is extremely important to monitor such changes precisely (Abreu, 1992; Giacino, Kezmarsky, DeLuca, & Cicerone, 1991). A monitoring form was used to track daily changes in Edgar's responsiveness (see Figure 3.5). This form was kept at Edgar's bedside in a binder. All team members were instructed in how to use the monitoring system, and each team member was given a different-colored pencil with which to check and record observable responses. The occupational therapist summarized the findings daily and noted them in the medical record. The 24-hr monitoring chart proved effective and useful in revealing Edgar's individual pattern of arousal. Edgar showed progress in corneal reflexes, papillary reactivity, oculomotor responses, and spontaneous eye opening (Giacino, Kezmarsky, et al., 1991). He also improved in the duration of time of his arousal, the presence of volitional versus coincidental movement, and a lessened degree of intensity of the multimodal stimuli required to elicit his responses.

A second tracking system based on the coma intervention program treatment procedures used at the JFK Johnson Rehabilitation Institute designed by Giacino and colleagues (Giacino, 1996; Giacino, Kezmarsky, et al., 1991; Giacino, Sharlow-Galella, et al., 1991) was also used with Edgar. This progress-tracking chart can be used to record progress on a monthly basis. The baseline response relates to 2 commands chosen from a list of 10 (close eyes, move arm, move leg, move fingers, open mouth, look away from me,

look at me, look up, look down, touch my hand) observed over four consecutive trials (estimated at 15, 30, 45, and 60 s) and then translated into percentages.

In the process, every time a team member interacted with Edgar, he or she oriented him to his or her name, the time of day, the reason for the visit, and the protocol being used. Closing remarks also were provided at the end of the visit, with statements indicating when the team member would see Edgar again. The team members changed the instructions given to distinguish whether Edgar's corresponding movements were voluntary or incidental. For example "Edgar, move your right arm" was alternated with "Edgar, stop moving your right arm." All stimuli, whether tactile, visual, or auditory, were followed by ample processing time. Stimuli were also manipulated to allow for Edgar's maximally efficient manual exploration, visual location, and fixation.

The team was encouraged to systematically record Edgar's response 15 s after stimulation. They asked Edgar to use two different movements in communicating (e.g., one for "yes" and another for "no") rather than relying on the execution of a single movement. Arousal was measured by the wakefulness revealed by eye opening; attention was determined by the number of times Edgar responded each time a stimulus was presented. The stimulus was personalized by using symbolic items such as Daisy's perfume or an audiotaped message from his family and friends.

Stage 2: Rehabilitation

After emerging from coma, Edgar was ready for more dynamic interventions. Edgar's capacity for independent living, work, and leisure occupations was predictably limited by the sequelae of brain injury: impairments in attention, memory, capacity to learn, and postural control (Abreu, 1981, 1995; Arce, Katz, & Sugarman, 2004; Hoofien, Gilboa, Vakil, & Barak, 2004). These sequelae are treated clinically in two manners: retraining and compensation. Although the effectiveness of either technique has yet to be fully supported in the literature, both techniques are used in the clinic. Retraining programs involve the use of exercises, repetitive practice, or drills (Sohlberg & Mateer, 2001). Compensatory programs involve the use of externally and internally based rule behaviors such as mnemonic devices, memory notebooks, and electronic watches (Harrell, Parente, Bellingrath, & Lisicia, 1992). Another example of compensation is the use of systematic training that specifies the establishment of routines and the development of procedural strategies

F I G U R E 3.5. Quadraphonic approach evaluation system behavioral hourly chart.

Patient: _____   Handedness: _____

Date: _____   Lesion Site: _____

Age: _____   Education: _____

Dx: _____   Native Language: _____

Onset: _____   Therapist: _____

Period of Observation: From: _____ (a.m./p.m)   To: _____ (a.m./p.m.)

Observation Location: _____

Characteristics of **Behavior**

Indicate whether each behavior was Present (P) or Absent (A).

	1a	2	3	4	5	6	7	8	9	10	11	12n	1	2	3	4	5	6	7	8	9	10	11	12m
1.																								
2.																								
3.																								
4.																								
5.																								
6.																								
7.																								
8.																								
9.																								
10.																								
11.																								
12.																								
13.																								
14.																								
15.																								
16.																								
17.																								
18.																								
19.																								
20.																								

PUPIL GAUGE (mm)

2 3 4 5 6 7 8 9

Test for Pupillary Constriction: (a) Darken the room to enlarge the pupils; (b) shine the light from a small penlight directly into the pupil of the eye; (c) note whether the pupil constricts briskly or sluggishly; (d) repeat the procedure for the the other eye; (e) shine the light into both eyes simultaneously so that the same amount of light reaches both; turn the light on and off; (f) note whether the two pupils dilate and constrict together and simultaneously, to the same degree. The chart above is a guide for determining pupil size.

or rule-based actions (Bewick et al., 1995; Sohlberg & Mateer, 2001).

Edgar benefited from the use of these mechanistic organizational strategies. For example, an enlarged laminated instruction card placed near the equipment Edgar used served as a compensatory memory strategy. Enlarged simplified instructions were used in a very systematic manner. Edgar initially read the instructions aloud and, when questioned, answered why he was reading them aloud. Later, he was able to read instructions silently. Many times Edgar did not remember doing specific actions, but he continued to perform accurately, in a safe and timely manner, while depending on cues.

Given his moderate memory loss, Edgar also used a compensatory memory notebook divided into sections that provided a rich repository of information to help reconstruct his life after brain injury. The notebook was divided into sections different from those more traditionally used in cognitive rehabilitation (Sohlberg & Mateer, 2001). The sections reflected a more holistic and confluent approach to rehabilitation. They included the following:

1. *"My story"*: This section included photographs, pictures, and names with brief descriptions of family members, friends, pets, coworkers, favorite occupations, hobbies, and happy moments before the injury.
2. *"My time use"*: This section contained Edgar's schedule of therapies, meals, and to-do lists of more personal projects with their times and dates (a page that allowed reflection about time use was filled in weekly).
3. *"My temporary support system"*: This section included photographs and names with brief descriptions of therapists, doctors, nurses, dietitians, and aides who worked with Edgar daily. The brief descriptions identified each person by role, function, and participation in Edgar's rehabilitation program. A page that allowed reflections about Edgar's satisfaction with services was filled in weekly.
4. *"My private thoughts"*: This section contained feelings, reactions, and responses that Edgar felt during his interventions. This section was shared with others only at Edgar's initiation, thus providing Edgar with a sense of privacy and control over self-disclosure.

For postural control issues, Edgar engaged in a motor work-up program in occupational therapy. Edgar engaged in relaxation and breathing exercises for 10 min before starting the motor work-up module. The therapist performed these exercises with Edgar in a quiet room assigned for individual therapy. The therapist also engaged Edgar in neurodevelopmental and biomechanical maneuvers for the improvement of his more affected hemiparetic side, upper and lower extremities, and neck and trunk. The therapist started with the scapular and shoulder muscle and joint complex as well as wrist and hand muscle and joint complex to free these limitations and to establish a better balance between flexor and extensor muscles, adductors and abductors, and supinators and pronators. Weight-shifting and weight-bearing exercises for scapula, elbow, hand, hip, knee, and feet were also performed. The therapist used landmarks on Edgar's body prominences such as the inferior angle of the scapula and the superior anterior posterior iliac crest to visualize whether Edgar's body asymmetry improved after the manual maneuver. To monitor weight distribution bilaterally, the therapist used videotaping with reflectors and sensors taped on the joint, as well as T-foam (dense foam that registers bodily indentations), before and after the session. Realigning Edgar's body using key points of control resulted in an increase in Edgar's symmetry, a disassociation of movements (or an ability to move each individual body segment in isolation), improved joint mobility, and increased awareness.

After the motor work-up, Edgar chose tasks and occupations that he enjoyed so as to provide him with an opportunity to increase his endurance and coordination and control his posture. These activities were monitored with the goal of increasing his coordination in timed tasks from 10- to 7-s response rates in 1 week (a subskill goal). Another goal was for Edgar to engage in some of his favorite activities, carpentry and antiquing, within a 3-week period for a 2-hr standing session. Edgar's long-term goal for postural control was to be able to dance with Daisy within 8 weeks.

Some of Edgar's postural control issues were related to his mild attentional problems. While standing, Edgar was unable to attend to all aspects of the environment without missing information. Postural control demands were interfering with his attentional capacity, and his strategy was to respond too quickly or slowly. He was taught to self-monitor and self-talk through the activity so that he could concentrate and maintain his focus while working on his tolerance for standing. Organizations and metacognitive strategies reflecting on person, task, and strategy were facilitated. Edgar was able to accomplish his goal and danced with Daisy at a friend's wedding.

Edgar had a general awareness about his strength and limitations. He was able to recognize and appraise the difficulties he was having as he did a task and when cued, but he was unable to foresee potential limitations secondary to his disability in the future.

Stage 3: Community Re-entry

After receiving rehabilitation services in a hospital and after achieving medical stability, Edgar was discharged even though he had not reached his optimal potential. At this time, he was admitted to a transitional living community. Many clients achieve maximum benefit from training and compensatory strategies at such community re-entry centers, which bridge hospitals, nursing homes, and long-term centers with the community. The interventions that Edgar received in the acute hospital were limited by time constraints as well as by the nature of the rehabilitation techniques that could be efficiently administered. Documentation indicated that Edgar had reached independence in basic personal management and that, although he improved in the use of self-mediated learning strategies, he was still unable to return home. Daisy was working full-time as a teacher, and she felt that Edgar would not be safe at home alone.

Edgar previously worked as a high-salaried chemical engineer who supervised seven other engineers in a water purification plant. At the community re-entry level, the focus is primarily on functional outcomes and, in Edgar's case, the goal was transition to the highest degree of independence using community-based services as well as community resources for medical needs. Daisy complained about Edgar's memory and reported problems involving Edgar getting lost. Edgar dismissed the memory issue, claiming it was not that bad and saying, "I was forgetful before." Daisy also was concerned with changes in Edgar's social behaviors. Previously gregarious, Edgar now preferred to be only with her and discouraged visitors.

By the third month at the transitional center, Edgar and Daisy had both received extensive training in memory and compensatory strategies from the entire rehabilitation team. The memory book that he brought from the hospital was reduced in size, and Daisy and Edgar were taught how to keep personal memory books that included a section called "my private thoughts." This section was set up differently from the one that Edgar had used in the hospital. The pages were divided in half. On one half, Edgar and Daisy were instructed to track positive and negative feelings experienced during the day. Once a week, they were to each analyze their logs, clustering the themes that emerged from their notes. They were both taught this process to increase their affective communication and increase their awareness of patterns of behavior that invited encouragement or compliments from their partner.

As noted earlier, Edgar could not attend to all aspects of a task or situation without missing information. Therefore,

the kitchen at home was rearranged and reorganized with labels and pictures that made it easier for Edgar to recognize where utensils and food were located instead of having to use his memory. For easier detection and recognition, many of the foods were kept in see-through containers or plastic bags rather than opaque containers.

Edgar showed moderate impairment in free recall of visual and auditory information during short-term and long-term memory tasks. His performance improved if the task involved recognition and retrieval of auditory and visual information. In naturalistic environments, Edgar performed more poorly. He got lost moving from building to building or office to office in the center. He did not seem to recognize the impact that this impairment would have on his goal of returning to work. He stated, "I'll do better in my office. I have worked there for years." He showed low anticipatory awareness of his disability. Abreu has seen a high degree of inaccuracy when individuals give personal accounts of their abilities to remember everyday items (Abreu, Seale, Scheibel, Huddleston, Zhang, & Ottenbacher, 2001). Some clinicians question the reliability of self-report techniques because they correlate only minimally with performance on memory tests (Bennett-Levy, Polkey, & Powell, 1980; Sunderland, Harris, & Gleave, 1984).

Edgar was unable to categorize information based on many characteristics. He was unable to understand jokes; he showed decreased empathy and reflection. His ability either to reason deductively from general abstractions to specific rules or to inductively go beyond the obvious or specific evidence also was impaired (Johnson-Laird, 1995; Pellegrino, 1985).

Edgar brought some of his personal projects to occupational therapy treatment sessions and, with moderate assistance, completed several of these. He identified the type of work project that he was managing before the accident: purifying the water for a small city in Texas. Prior to the start of training, the internal case manager contacted Edgar's employer to verify Edgar's previous workload and responsibilities. At the transitional center, the internal case manager monitors communication with employer, family, and external case managers (third-party payers). Edgar's employer confirmed the high degree of responsibility required of his position, and the case manager passed this information to the occupational therapist and the rest of the team. Following two individual simulated work sessions, a situational assessment in Edgar's workplace was performed. The results confirmed Edgar's dependency on external cues, mediation, and supervision. Edgar was unable to perform the work tasks that he had done before the injury.

In addition to individual therapy sessions, Edgar engaged in group interventions. One of the interventions was the "relax and have fun" group. The group was given this name by former clients because they found that it helped them relax and have fun during evenings and weekends when therapy schedules addressed leisure and recreational activities. As its central focus, the group planned two or three community outings each week. Edgar's participation and behaviors were evaluated and documented according to the skills required to plan and enact the "relax and have fun" activities. Edgar took great pleasure in planning and participating in fishing and sailing outings.

Clients at transitional centers are given opportunities to participate in community rituals, including an induction ceremony and a graduation ceremony. Edgar participated in both. The clients performed the induction ceremony with staff guidance as needed so as to identify and support the individual goals of each new client. Such a ritual fosters solidarity among the clients and the rehabilitation team. The graduation ceremony celebrates the achievement of the clients when they are ready for community re-entry.

Graduation was a very powerful and emotional treatment tool for Edgar, Daisy, and the rehabilitation community as a whole. This ritualized social encounter gave increased meaning and legitimacy to the completion of his rehabilitation experience (Crepeau, 1995). The graduation ceremony also represented Edgar's reclamation of membership in the community at large rather than a sustained membership in a group of clients living an "under-life" in an institution of care. Edgar regained his status as husband, lover, and friend and found employment with his company in a different capacity.

RESEARCH NEEDS AND SUPPORT FOR THE MODEL

Abreu and others have engaged in several inquiries into constructs associated with the quadraphonic approach. This section constitutes an overview of related quantitative, qualitative, and other inquiries as well as a review of relevant studies within the broader occupational therapy literature. We have organized these inquiries according to their relationship to the micro or the macro perspective.

One point seems important to make at the outset of this review. Testing a frame of reference or a model such as the quadraphonic approach is a complex and extensive process. To facilitate that process, we have conducted our own research, but we also draw support from work conducted by others within the Transitional Learning Center and found in the broader literature.

Our testing of the model has occurred within the institutional context of the Transitional Learning Center. One organizing framework within our center has been the implementation of critical pathways. The heterogeneity of a brain-injured population and the variations in neurobehavioral consequences of brain injury among our clients have mandated a systematic coordination of all direct-care services and research at our center through the establishment of differing goals and treatment tracks for our clients. At our facility, critical pathways delineate the services to be rendered from admission to discharge toward optimal goal achievement in one of four treatment programs or tracks: Return to Work, Return to School, Functional Independence, and Neurorehabilitation (Abreu et al., 1996). Within this system of case management, our department's use of the quadraphonic approach has become well known. We recommend that individuals work with others in their settings to establish frameworks that enhance interdisciplinary understanding.

In our facility, we also conduct research related to instruments that enable our understanding of the outcomes of interventions across disciplines. We use the Community Integration Questionnaire (CIQ; Willer, Ottenbacher, & Coad, 1994), the Craig Handicap Assessment and Reporting Technique (Whiteneck, Charlifue, Gerhart, Overholser, & Richardson, 1992), and the Disability Rating Scale (Hall, Cope, & Rappaport, 1985). Our occupational therapy team contributes to research into such outcome measures. For example, Reistetter and colleagues (Reistetter, Spencer, Trujillon, & Abreu, in press) recently completed a systematic review of the literature on the community integration (CI) of people with traumatic brain injury to answer four questions:

1. How does one best measure CI?
2. Can one predict CI following rehabilitation?
3. Do social and activity participation have an effect on CI?
4. Does CI have an effect on quality of life and life satisfaction?

The evidence found in the rehabilitation literature indicated that the most prominent tool used to measure CI was the CIQ. In addition, results of the review indicated that there was mixed evidence supporting the ability to predict CI. Prominent variables for predicting community integration after brain injury were severity of the injury and the individual's age, gender, education, prior work, living environment, cognition, emotional status, and degree of disability. Other results found in the review were that social relationships influence CI and that CI in turn affects quality of life and life satisfaction. Although we cannot measure direct links between the quadraphonic approach and community integration per se, some of these results support our use of constructs that ground both macro and micro perspectives.

Other studies from outside of the Transitional Learning Center address constructs found within the macro perspective that emphasize affective and interpersonal considerations. A qualitative study by Allison and Strong (1994) supported the use of complex and personalized verbal strategies for effective rehabilitation. The researchers discovered four major categories of strategies used by therapists in their interactions with clients: therapy voice, modified information, directive voice, and sympathetic voice. Such strategies resemble the kinds of therapeutic adjustments suggested within the contextual modifiers listed in Table 3.5.

To discover practitioner traits and qualities considered important by clients, Darragh, Sample, and Krieger (2001) interviewed an opportunistic sample of 51 individuals with brain injury. Individuals with head injury perceived services rendered by occupational therapists helpful if they were seen as relevant, meaningful, practical, and innovative in replacing lost skills and if framed with periodic feedback. These same individuals perceived providers as helpful if they were clear, honest, respectful, not overly optimistic or pessimistic, supportive, listening, and understanding. The authors suggested that, if attention is not paid to the interpersonal relationship, the rehabilitation services offered may seem incomplete and ineffective. Their suggestion aligns with Peloquin's (1993b) inquiry into patient's perceptions of the nature and negative effects of depersonalized practitioner behaviors in practice. Contextual modifiers used within the quadraphonic approach include affective and interpersonal considerations found important in these inquiries.

Schwartzberg (1994) also researched the experience of clients with brain injury, specifically high-functioning individuals who participated in self-help groups. She discovered perceptions of 10 helping factors that included telling others about one's own pain, actively listening to familiar pain in others, the recognition of the existence of a problem, grieving and laughing about daily situations, receiving validation from similar experiences, being so accepted that one had a respite from hiding one's disability, and giving and receiving practical suggestions. The net effect of the overall experience was a legitimization of head injury—that is, the acceptance of the injury as real. Emphasis in the macro perspective on making every effort to truly hear and empower the client draws support from this study. Also supported by this inquiry is encouragement

in the quadraphonic approach of mutual client support through group interventions and contextual modifiers.

Some researchers have explored the experiences of therapists who treat individuals with brain injury. Because such research relates to the humanistic dynamic within the macro perspective, Abreu (1990) studied the interaction of one occupational therapist with two clients, one post-stroke and one post–head injury. The study was conducted in a cognitive rehabilitation setting in the Northeast for a period of 3 months. Four major themes emerged:

1. There were communication differences depending on the diagnosis, with the observed therapist (a woman with 3 years of experience) interacting more dynamically with a young male client than with an older female client who had had a stroke.
2. The therapist perceived both clients as having little cognitive and physical control or personal power.
3. The cognitive rehabilitation specialty is draining.
4. The physical therapist's role in cognitive rehabilitation seems much more easily described and understood than that of the occupational therapist.

Another study by Crepeau (1994) inspired a research project within this center. Crepeau had explored the interactions within an interdisciplinary team meeting and discussed the various images of the team meeting, including those commonly described in the literature and those less explicitly discussed. One of her conclusions was that a tightly organized team meeting does not allow for the collective discussion of the meaning of illness to the patient and the patient's family, a consideration important within the macro perspective of the quadraphonic approach.

Prompted by this study, Abreu and colleagues (Abreu, Zhang, Seale, Primeau, & Jones, 2002) conducted a qualitative descriptive case study that included participant's observations of 51 interdisciplinary rehabilitation team meetings that involved clients with brain injury. Research participants discovered two patterns of interactions: the meetings were too lengthy, and the clients were subservient to the rehabilitation professionals, present almost as ghosts. Perhaps unaware of or insensitive to this subservience, team members noted in meeting reports that a transformation of the client had occurred, yielding a more functional and healthy individual. The results of this study suggest that the mere physical presence of the client in interdisciplinary rehabilitation meetings does not necessarily lead to collective discussions of meaning or to collaboration.

The macro perspective relies heavily on the use of narrative among those with head injury. Clark's (1993) work lent support to that approach. She used narrative analysis in her exploration of direct clinical practice with an individual post-stroke. Her successful practice with this client consisted of a facilitation of the reconstruction of childhood occupations, storytelling, and storymaking. Each of these occurs within the quadraphonic approach.

Another inquiry related to humanistic aspects of the macro perspective was more reflective than research-oriented and emerged from our thinking about cognitive biases and about the negative stereotyping that is often felt by individuals with head injury (Abreu & Peloquin, 2004). Development of the capacity to cognitively categorize is a normal process, but stereotyping and negative biases that are prejudicial and detrimental also can develop on the basis of life experiences as well as a person's style of information processing (Abreu & Peloquin, 2004). Additionally, personal optimism or negativism can be viewed as a specific style of information processing that may result in a generalized expectation for positive or negative outcomes (Schweizer, Beck-Seyffer, & Schneider, 1999). In practice among individuals with head injury, a positive cognitive bias toward individual differences seems essential to a practitioner's cultural competence and his or her perception of diversity as strength. Further research assessing the role that any negativism or bias against difference may play in a therapist's facilitation of client's lifestyles seems needed.

Addressing yet another vital construct within the macro perspective's use of story and narrative, Krefting (1989) noted the client's tendency to cope with loss of capacity and self-identity through concealment strategies such as that of describing the self as a silent versus talkative type rather than openly declaring difficulties participating in conversation. Additionally, Krefting reframed a client's lack of awareness of disability more broadly as being a "blind spot," arguing that the concept of a blind spot was less reductionistic than was labeling the phenomenon a lack of awareness.

Turning to a client's functioning in the diverse areas of occupation that are important within the macro perspective, our team has studied the potential of virtual environments in occupational therapy evaluation (Christiansen et al., 1998). The prototype of a computer-generated virtual kitchen environment was tested among 30 people with traumatic brain injury. Adequate initial reliability was found: The intracorrelational coefficient value for total task performance based on all steps involved in the meal task was .73. When three items with low variance were removed, the intracorrelational coefficient improved to .81. Little evidence of vestibular optical side effects was noted in the people tested.

Using our computer-generated virtual kitchen in 2001, our research team investigated select cognitive functions of 30 people with brain injury and 30 without (Zhang et al., 2001). The results of this study had implications for the micro perspective of the quadraphonic approach with its focus on performance skills. People with brain injuries consistently demonstrated a significant decrease in the ability to process information ($p = 0.04$–0.01), identify logical sequencing ($p = 0.04$–0.01), and complete the overall assessment ($p < 0.01$), as compared with people without brain injury. The time needed to process tasks, which we interpreted as the speed of cognitive responding, was also significantly different between the two groups ($p < 0.01$). The findings of this study suggested that this virtual reality environment is a replicable supplemental tool for the assessment of select cognitive functions.

Using the same environment later in 2003, our research team performed a prospective correlational study examining 3-week test–retest results for equivalence reliability between computer-simulated and natural environments in 54 people with traumatic brain injury (Zhang et al., 2003). The results of the study showed adequate reliability (intraclass correlation .76 at $p < .01$) and validity of the virtual kitchen environment as a method of assessment. A multiple regression analysis revealed that the virtual environment test was a good predictor of results on the real-life kitchen assessment. As a result of these studies, we use our virtual kitchen evaluation alongside the regular kitchen evaluation to assess meal preparation of a peanut butter sandwich and soup, a typical meal for Americans of modest means.

We have conducted additional studies that relate to the micro perspective of the quadraphonic approach. One postulate proposed within the micro perspective, and already noted within our discussion of the virtual kitchen, is that the surrounding environment can enhance the cognitive system, which in turn can enhance motor performance among clients with brain injury. Such influence is due in part to the demands for cognitive processing that the environment imposes on the arousal and attention systems.

In 1995, Abreu published the results of her doctoral dissertation that examined the effects of environmental predictability on postural control in 50 people with post-stroke hemiplegia and 50 who had not had stroke. The effect of predictability of condition on posture was significant but not as predicted. There was greater postural stability under unpredictable conditions when clients reached to the right side as measured in both anterior–posterior and medial–lateral planes and also when they reached to the left. The findings refute the assumption that a hierarchical, predictable environmental model of moving from predictable to unpredictable environments is necessary for the evaluation and treatment of postural control. Instead, the findings suggest that rehabilitation strategies should use predictable and unpredictable environmental conditions concurrently and not necessarily sequentially.

In 2002, our research team duplicated this 1995 study among 10 clients with traumatic brain injury and 10 people without. These study findings again refuted the hierarchical model of moving from predictable to unpredictable environments for postural control and its treatment (Zhang, Abreu, Gonzales, Huddleston, & Ottenbacher, 2002). The relationship between information-processing demands and postural skills appears more complex than a simple linear association. The results of this study suggested a similar clinical application to that of Abreu's 1995 study: Rehabilitation strategies should use predictable and unpredictable conditions concurrently, not necessarily sequentially.

More recently, we have completed a new study examining the effects of environmental factors on postural stability. In the first study, we investigated the effects of and associations among postural stability, reaching time, cognition, and walking ability as measured by the Minimal Data Set for Nursing Home Residents. We used the Minimal Data Set version 2.0 on 38 nursing home volunteer residents older than age 67 years (Abreu et al., in press). The findings support the assumption that postural stability and response time result from an interaction among individual factors as well as environmental factors such as predictability. Unpredictable or variable environments may enhance postural stability and shorten response time in older adults. These findings suggest that further studies are needed to understand the characteristics of environments that enhance postural control for older nursing home residents (Abreu et al., in press).

Another construct within the micro perspective of the quadraphonic approach is that of awareness. Krefting's (1989) comments about a blind spot, mentioned earlier, also relate to this construct. Abreu and colleagues (2001) examined self-awareness of performance on selected daily living tasks completed by 55 people with acquired brain injury. Ten people without brain injury provided comparison data. Three self-awareness criteria were examined during dressing, meal planning, and money management: intellectual, emergent, and anticipatory awareness. Statistically significant differences ($p < .05$) were found for all levels of self-awareness across all daily living tasks tested. No evidence was found for supporting a hierarchy among intellectual, emergent, and anticipatory awareness.

We began this section by acknowledging the complexity involved in the process of researching a model. Although these studies seem supportive of select constructs within the quadraphonic approach, a significant amount of work needs to supplement what has been done thus far.

CONCLUSION

The aim of the quadraphonic approach and its complementary macro and micro perspectives is to offer a holistic system for the rehabilitation, health, and well-being of people with cognitive disabilities after brain injury. Inherent within the approach is the realization of the profession's art alongside its science and the actualization of both competent and caring actions. This confluence of aim and function is an enactment of the profession's integrative ethos (Peloquin, 2002b). Ora Ruggles, early reconstruction aide and later occupational therapist in many settings, elegantly captured that ethos in a visionary statement: "It is not enough to give a patient something to do with his hands. You must reach for the heart as well as the hands. It's the heart that really does the healing" (Carlova & Ruggles, 1946, p. 69). That same vision continues to inspire the quadraphonic approach today.

REVIEW QUESTIONS

1. What differences are there within the quadraphonic approach between the macro and micro perspectives?
2. Discuss the four theories and client characteristics.
3. Explain why people with traumatic brain injury benefit from a multifaceted approach.
4. Exemplify the use of confluence and narrative using the case of Edgar.

ACKNOWLEDGMENT

Dr. Abreu was supported in part by grants from the Moody Foundation and the Department of Health and Human Services (DHHS) No. 3R01AG17638-01A1S1. We thank Renee Pearcy for her research assistance. This chapter is based on *The Quadraphonic Approach* workshops, formatted here in condensed form.

REFERENCES

Abreu, B. C. (1981). Interdisciplinary approach to adult visual perceptual function–dysfunction continuum. In B. C. Abreu (Ed.), *Physical disabilities manual* (pp. 151–181). New York: Raven Press.

Abreu, B. C. (1990). *The quadraphonic approach: Management of cognitive and postural dysfunction.* New York: Therapeutic Service Systems.

Abreu, B. C. (1992). The quadraphonic approach: Management of cognitive–perceptual and postural control dysfunction. *Occupational Therapy Practice, 3*(4), 12–29.

Abreu, B. C. (1994a). Perceptual motor skills. In C. B. Royeen (Ed.), *AOTA Self-Study Series: Cognitive rehabilitation* (pp. 1–48). Rockville, MD: American Occupational Therapy Association.

Abreu, B. C. (1994b). *The quadraphonic approach: Evaluation and treatment of the brain-injured patient.* New York: Therapeutic Service Systems.

Abreu, B. C. (1995). The effect of environmental regulations on postural control after stroke. *American Journal of Occupational Therapy, 49,* 517–525.

Abreu, B. C. (1997). *The quadraphonic approach: Course handouts.* Galveston, TX: Therapeutic Service Systems.

Abreu, B. C., Heyn, P., Reistetter, T. A., Zhang, L., Milton, S., Masel, B., et al. (2003). The effects of the predictability of an arm reaching target on seated postural stability, reaching time, and selected Minimum Data Set for nursing home residents. *Physical and Occupational Therapy in Geriatrics 22*(2), 1–13.

Abreu, B. C., & Peloquin, S. M. (2004). Embracing diversity in our profession. *American Journal of Occupational Therapy, 58,* 353–359.

Abreu, B. C., & Price-Lackey, P. (1994). Documentation and additional considerations. In C. B. Royeen (Ed.), *Cognitive rehabilitation* (pp. 1–44). Rockville, MD: American Occupational Therapy Association.

Abreu, B. C., Seale, G. S., Podlesak, J., & Hartley, L. (1996). Development of critical paths for postacute brain injury rehabilitation: Lessons learned. *American Journal of Occupational Therapy, 50,* 417–427.

Abreu, B. C., Seale, G., Scheibel, R. S., Huddleston, N., Zhang, L., & Ottenbacher, K. J. (2001). Levels of self-awareness after acute brain injury: How patients' and rehabilitation specialists' perceptions compare. *Archives of Physical Medicine and Rehabilitation, 82*(1), 49–56.

Abreu, B. C., & Toglia, J. P. (1987). Cognitive rehabilitation: A model for occupational therapy. *American Journal of Occupational Therapy, 41,* 439–448.

Abreu, B. C., Zhang, L., Seale, G., Primeau, L., & Jones, J. (2002). Interdisciplinary meetings: Investigating the collaboration between persons with brain injury and treatment teams. *Brain Injury, 16,* 691–704.

Allison, H., & Strong, J. (1994). Verbal strategies used by occupational therapists in direct client encounters. *Occupational Therapy Journal of Research, 14,* 112–129.

Arce, F. I., Katz, N., & Sugarman, H. (2004). The scaling of postural adjustments during bimanual load-lifting in traumatic brain-injured adults. *Human Movement Science, 22,* 749–768.

Bandura, A. (1977). Self-efficacy: Toward a unifying theory of behavioral change. *Psychological Review, 84,* 191–215.

Bartkowski, H. M., & Lovely, M. P. (1986). Prognosis in coma and the persistent vegetative state. *Journal of Head Trauma Rehabilitation, 1*(1), 1–5.

Bateson, M. C. (1989). *Composing a life.* New York: Penguin.

Bennett-Levy, J., Polkey, C. E., & Powell, G. E. (1980). Self-report of memory skills after temporal lobectomy: The effect of clinical variables. *Cortex, 15,* 543–557.

Berry, D. C. (1983). Metacognitive experience and transfer of logical reasoning. *Quarterly Journal of Experimental Psychology, 35A,* 39–49.

Bewick, K. C., Raymond, M. J., Malia, K. B., & Bennett, T. L. (1995). Metacognition as the ultimate executive: Techniques and tasks to facilitate executive functions. *NeuroRehabilitation, 5,* 367–375.

Blackmer, E. R., & Mitton, J. L. (1991). Theories of monitoring and the timing of repairs in spontaneous speech. *Cognition, 39,* 173–194.

Bogod, N. M., Mateer, C. A., & MacDonald, S. W. S. (2003). Self-awareness after traumatic brain injury: A comparison of measures and their relationship to executive functions. *Journal of the International Neuropsychological Society, 9,* 450–458.

Braun, C. M., Baribeau, J. M., Ethier, M., Daigneault, S., & Proulx, R. (1989). Processing of pragmatic and facial affective information by patients with closed-head injuries. *Brain Injury, 3*(1), 5–17.

Bridge, C., & Twible, R. (1997). Clinical reasoning. In C. Christiansen & C. Baum (Eds.), *Occupational therapy: Enabling function and well-being* (pp. 158–179). Thorofare, NJ: Slack.

Brown, A. (1988). Motivation to learn and understand: On taking charge of one's own learning. *Cognition and Instruction, 5,* 311–321.

Brown, A. L. (1978). Knowing when, where, and how to remember: A problem of metacognition. In L. B. Resnick (Ed.), *Knowing, learning, and instruction: Essays in honor of Robert Glaser* (pp. 77–165). Hillsdale, NJ: Lawrence Erlbaum.

Brown, A. L. (1987). Metacognition, executive control, self-regulation, and other more mysterious mechanisms. In F. E. Weinert & R. H. Kluwe (Eds.), *Metacognition, motivation, and understanding* (pp. 65–116). Hillsdale, NJ: Lawrence Erlbaum.

Brown, A. L., & Palincsar, A. S. (1989). Guided, cooperative learning and individual knowledge acquisition. In L. B. Resnick (Ed.), *Knowing, learning, and instruction: Essays in honor of Robert Glaser* (pp. 393–451). Hillsdale, NJ: Lawrence Erlbaum.

Brown, G. I. (1971). *Human teaching for human learning: An introduction to confluent education.* New York: Viking.

Carlova, J., & Ruggles, O. (1946). *The healing heart.* New York: J. Messner.

Chi, M. T. H., & Bassok, M. (1989). Learning from examples via self-explanations. In L. B. Resnick (Ed.), *Knowing, learning, and instruction: Essays in honor of Robert Glaser* (pp. 251–282). Hillsdale, NJ: Lawrence Erlbaum.

Chi, M. T. H., de Leeuw, N., Chiu, M. H., & LaVancher, C. (1994). Eliciting self-explanations improves understanding. *Cognitive Science, 18,* 434–477.

Chi, M. T. H., & Glaser, R. (1985). Problem-solving ability. In R. J. Sternberg (Ed.), *Human abilities: An information-processing approach* (pp. 227–257). New York: W. H. Freeman.

Chi, M. T. H., Glaser, R., & Rees, E. (1982). Expertise in problem solving. In R. J. Sternberg (Ed.), *Advances in psychology of human intelligence* (Vol. 1, pp. 7–76). Hillsdale, NJ: Lawrence Erlbaum.

Christiansen, C. (1996). Three perspectives on balance in occupation. In R. Zemke & F. Clark (Eds.), *Occupational science: The evolving discipline* (pp. 431–451). Philadelphia: F. A. Davis.

Christiansen, C., Abreu, B., Ottenbacher, K., Huffman, K., Masel, B., & Culpepper, R. (1998). Task performance in virtual environments used for cognitive rehabilitation after traumatic brain injury. *Archives of Physical Medicine and Rehabilitation, 79,* 888–892.

Clark, F. (1993). Occupation embedded in a real life: Interweaving occupational science and occupational therapy—1993 Eleanor Clarke Slagle Lecture. *American Journal of Occupational Therapy, 47,* 1067–1078.

Clark, F., Ennevor, B. L., & Richardson, P. L. (1996). A grounded theory of techniques for occupational storytelling and occupational storymaking. In R. Zemke & F. Clark (Eds.), *Occupational science: The evolving discipline* (pp. 373–397). Philadelphia: F. A. Davis.

Coelho, C. A., Liles, B. Z., & Duffy, R. J. (1991). Discourse analyses with closed-head-injured adults: Evidence for differing patterns of deficits. *Archives of Physical Medicine and Rehabilitation, 72,* 465–468.

Corbin, J. M., & Strauss, A. (1988). *Unending work and care: Managing chronic illness at home.* San Francisco: Jossey-Bass.

Crepeau, E. B. (1994). Three images of interdisciplinary team meetings. *American Journal of Occupational Therapy, 48,* 717–772.

Crepeau, E. B. (1995). Lesson 6: Rituals. In C. B. Royeen (Ed.), *AOTA Self-Study Series: The practice of the future: Putting occupation back into therapy* (pp. 1–29). Bethesda, MD: American Occupational Therapy Association.

Crosson, B., Barco, P. P., Velozo, C. A., Bolesta, M. M., Cooper, P. V., Werts, D., et al. (1989). Awareness and compensation in post-acute head injury rehabilitation. *Journal of Head Trauma Rehabilitation, 4*(3), 46–54.

Dabbs, J. M., Evans, M. S., Hooper, C. H., & Purvis, J. A. (1980). Self-monitors in conversation: What do they monitor? *Journal of Personality and Social Psychology, 39,* 278–284.

Darragh, A. R., Sample, P., & Krieger, S. R. (2001). "Tears in my eyes 'cause somebody finally understood": Client perceptions of practitioners following brain injury. *American Journal of Occupational Therapy, 55,* 191–199.

Diller, L. (1993). Introduction to cognitive rehabilitation. In C. B. Royeen (Ed.), *AOTA Self-Study Series: Cognitive rehabilitation.* Bethesda, MD: American Occupational Therapy Association.

Dreyfus, H., & Dreyfus, S. (Eds.). (1986). *Mind over machine.* New York: Free Press.

Druckman, D., & Bjork, R. A. (Eds.). (1991). *In the mind's eye: Enhancing human performance.* Washington, DC: National Academy Press.

Druckman, D., & Bjork, R. A. (Eds.). (1994). *Learning, remembering, believing: Enhancing human performance.* Washington, DC: National Academy Press.

Duchek, J. M., & Abreu, B. C. (1997). Meeting the challenges of cognitive disabilities. In C. Christiansen & C. Baum (Eds.), *Occupational therapy: Enabling function and well-being* (pp. 288–311). Thorofare, NJ: Slack.

Engel, A. K., Fries, P., & Singer, W. (2001). Dynamic predictions: Oscillations and synchrony in top-down processing. *Nature Reviews Neuroscience, 2,* 704–716.

Fischer, S. Trexler, L. E., & Gauggel, S. (2004). Awareness of activity limitations and prediction of performance in patients with brain injuries and orthopedic disorders. *Journal of the International Neuropsychological Society, 10*(2), 190–199.

Flavell, J. H. (1979). Metacognition and cognitive monitoring: A new area of cognitive–developmental inquiry. *American Psychologist, 34,* 906–911.

Flavell, J. H. (1985). *Cognitive development.* Englewood Cliffs, NJ: Prentice Hall.

Flavell, J. H. (1987). Speculations about the nature and development of metacognition. In F. E. Weinert & R. H. Kluwe (Eds.), *Metacognition, motivation, and understanding* (pp. 21–29). Hillsdale, NJ: Lawrence Erlbaum.

Fleming, M. H. (1991). The therapist with the three-track mind. *American Journal of Occupational Therapy, 45,* 1007–1014.

Gagné, R. M., & Smith, E. C., Jr. (1962). A study of the effects of verbalization on problem solving. *Journal of Experimental Psychology, 63*(1), 12–18.

Gentile, A. M. (2000). Skill acquisition: Action, movement, and neuromotor processes. In J. Carr & R. Shepherd (Eds.), *Movement science: Foundations for physical therapy in rehabilitation* (2nd ed., pp. 111–186). Gaithersburg, MD: Aspen.

Giacino, J. T. (1996). Sensory stimulation: Theoretical perspectives and the evidence for effectiveness. *NeuroRehabilitation, 6,* 69–78.

Giacino, J. T., Kezmarsky, M. A., DeLuca, J., & Cicerone, K. D. (1991). Monitoring rate of recovery to predict outcome in minimally responsive patients. *Archives of Physical Medicine and Rehabilitation, 72,* 897–901.

Giacino, J. T., Sharlow-Galella, M., Kexmarsky, M. A., McKenna, K., Nelson, P., King, M., et al. (1991). *JFK coma recovery scale and coma intervention program treatment procedures.* Edison, NJ: JFK Medical Center.

Gianutsos, R., & Matheson, P. (1987). The rehabilitation of visual–perceptual disorders attributable to brain injury. In M. J. Meier, A. L. Benton, & L. Diller (Eds.), *Neuropsychological rehabilitation* (pp. 202–241). New York: Guilford.

Gibson, J. J. (1979). *The ecological approach to visual perception.* Boston: Houghton-Mifflin.

Glaser, R., & Chi, M. T. H. (1988). Overview. In M. T. H. Chi, R. Glaser, & M. J. Farr (Eds.), *The nature of expertise* (pp. xv–xxviii). Hillsdale, NJ: Lawrence Erlbaum.

Hall, K., Cope, N., & Rappaport, M. (1985). Glasgow Outcome Scale and Disability Rating Scale: Comparative usefulness in following recovery in traumatic head injury. *Archives of Physical Medicine and Rehabilitation, 66,* 35–37.

Hammond, F. M., Grattan, K. D., Sasser, H. C., Corrigan, J. D., Rosenthal, M., Bushnik, T., et al. (2004). Five years after traumatic brain injury: A study of individual outcomes and predictors of change in function. *NeuroRehabilitation, 19*(4), 25–35.

Harrell, M., Parente, F., Bellingrath, E., & Lisicia, K. (1992). *Cognitive rehabilitation of memory: A practical guide.* Gaithersburg, MD: Aspen.

Hartley, L. L. (1995). *Cognitive–communicative abilities following brain injury: A functional approach.* San Diego, CA: Singular.

Hartley, L. L., & Jensen, P. J. (1992). Three discourse profiles of closed-head-injury speakers: Theoretical and clinical implications. *Brain Injury, 6,* 271–282.

Hartman-Maeir, A., Soroker, N., Oman, S. D., & Katz, N. (2003). Awareness of disabilities in stroke rehabilitation: A clinical trial. *Disability and Rehabilitation, 25*(1), 35–44.

Hellstrom, O. (1993). The importance of a holistic concept of health for health-care-examples from the clinic. *Theoretical Medicine, 14,* 325–342.

Herzberg, S. R. (1990). Client or patient: Which term is more appropriate for use in occupational therapy? *American Journal of Occupational Therapy, 44,* 561–565.

Holstein, J. A., & Gubrium, J. F. (1995). *The active interview* (Vol. 37). Thousand Oaks, CA: Sage.

Holyoke, P., & Elkan, L. (1995). *Rehabilitation services inventory and quality.* Toronto, Ontario: Institute for Work and Health.

Hoofien, D., Gilboa, A., Vakil, E., & Barak, O. (2004). Unawareness of cognitive deficits and daily functions among persons with traumatic brain injuries. *Journal of Clinical and Experimental Neuropsychology, 26,* 278–290.

Incoccia, C., Formisano, R., Muscato, P., Reali, G., & Zoccolotti, P. (2004). Reaction and movement times in individuals with chronic traumatic brain injury with good motor skills. *Cortex, 40,* 111–115.

Jacobs, H. E. (1993). *Behavior analysis guidelines and brain injury rehabilitation: People, principles, and programs.* Gaithersburg, MD: Aspen.

Johnson-Laird, P. N. (1995). Deductive reasoning ability. In R. J. Sternberg (Ed.), *Human abilities: An information-processing approach* (pp. 173–194). New York: W. H. Freeman.

Josselson, R., & Lieblich, A. (Eds.). (1995). *Interpreting experience: The narrative study of lives* (Vol. 3). Thousand Oaks, CA: Sage.

Kielhofner, G. (1977). Temporal adaptation: A conceptual framework for occupational therapy. *American Journal of Occupational Therapy, 31,* 235–242.

Kielhofner, G. (1985). *A model of human occupation.* Baltimore: Williams & Wilkins.

Klatzy, K. (1980). *Human memory: Structure and processes.* San Francisco: Freeman, Cooper.

Kluwe, R. H. (1987). Executive decisions and regulation of problem-solving behavior. In F. E. Weinert & R. H. Kluwe (Eds.), *Metacognition, motivation, and understanding* (pp. 31–64). Hillsdale, NJ: Lawrence Erlbaum.

Koegel, L. K., Koegel, R. L., & Ingham, J. C. (1986). Programming rapid generalization of correct articulation through self-monitoring procedures. *Journal of Speech and Hearing Disorders, 51,* 24–32.

Krefting, L. (1989). Reintegration into the community after head injury: The results of an ethnographic study. *Occupational Therapy Journal of Research, 9*(2), 67–83.

Krefting, L., & Krefting, D. (1991). Leisure activities after a stroke: An ethnographic approach. *American Journal of Occupational Therapy, 45,* 429–436.

Krinsky, R. (1990). The visionary world of Beatriz Abreu. *Advance, 6*(11), 7, 13.

Lampert, J., & Lapolice, D. J. (1995). Functional considerations in evaluation and treatment of the client with low vision. *American Journal of Occupational Therapy, 49,* 885–890.

Lee, W. A. (1989). A control systems framework for understanding normal and abnormal posture. *American Journal of Occupational Therapy, 42,* 291–301.

Lezak, M. D. (1983). *Neuropsychological assessment.* New York: Oxford University Press.

Light, K. E. (1990). Information processing for motor performance in aging adults. *Physical Therapy, 10,* 820–826.

Luria, A. R. (1973). *The working brain.* New York: Basic Books.

Mattingly, C., & Fleming, M. H. (1993). *Clinical reasoning: Forms of inquiry in a therapeutic practice.* Philadelphia: F. A. Davis.

McColl, M. A. (1994). Holistic occupational therapy: Historical meaning and contemporary implications. *Canadian Journal of Occupational Therapy, 61*(2), 72–77.

McColl, M. A., Gerein, N., & Valentine, F. (1997). Occupational therapy: Meeting the challenges of disability. In C. Christiansen & C. Baum (Eds.), *Occupational therapy: Enabling function and well-being* (pp. 508–528). Thorofare, NJ: Slack.

McColl, M. A., Law, M., & Stewart, D. (1993). *Theoretical basis of occupational therapy: An annotated bibliography.* Thorofare, NJ: Slack.

Miller, R. (1992). Introducing holistic education: The historical and pedagogical context of the 1990 Chicago statement. *Teacher Education Quarterly, 19*(1), 5–13.

Mosey, A. C. (1986). *Psychosocial components of occupational therapy.* New York: Raven Press.

Nachmanovitch, S. (1990). *Free play: The power of improvisation in life and the arts.* Los Angeles: Jeremy P. Tarcher.

Nashner, L. M. (1982). Adaption of human movement to altered environments. *Trends in Neuroscience, 5,* 358–366.

Neistadt, M. E. (1992). The classroom as a clinic: Applications for a method of teaching clinical reasoning. *American Journal of Occupational Therapy, 46,* 814–817.

Nelson, D. L. (1987). Occupation: Form and performance. *American Journal of Occupational Therapy, 42,* 633–641.

Neville, A. (1980). Temporal adaptation: Applications with short-term psychiatric patients. *American Journal of Occupational Therapy, 34,* 328–331.

Newell, K. M. (2003). Schema theory (1975): Retrospectives and prospectives. *Research Quarterly for Exercise and Sport, 74,* 383–388.

Newton, R. A. (1995). Balance abilities in individuals with moderate and severe traumatic brain injury. *Brain Injury, 9,* 445–451.

Norman, D. A. (1969). *Memory and attention: An introduction to human information processing.* New York: Wiley.

Norman, D. A. (1979). Perception, memory, and mental processes. In L. Nilsson (Ed.), *Perspectives on memory research* (pp. 121–144). Hillsdale, NJ: Lawrence Erlbaum.

O'Dell, M. W., Jasin, P., Lyons, N., Stivers, M., & Meszaros, F. (1996). Standardized assessment instruments for minimally-responsive, brain-injured patients. *NeuroRehabilitation, 6,* 45–55.

O'Dell, M. W., & Riggs, R. V. (1996). Management of the minimally responsive patient. In L. J. Horn & N. D. Zasler (Eds.), *Medical rehabilitation of traumatic brain injury* (pp. 103–132). Philadelphia: Hanley & Belfus.

Ottenbacher, K. J., & Christiansen, C. (1997). Occupational performance assessment. In C. Christiansen & C. Baum (Eds.), *Occupational therapy: Enabling function and well-being* (pp. 104–135). Thorofare, NJ: Slack.

Parham, L. D. (1987). Toward professionalism: The reflective therapist. *American Journal of Occupational Therapy, 41,* 555–561.

Paris, S. G., & Winograd, P. (1990). How metacognition can promote academic learning and instruction. In B. F. Jones & L. Idol (Eds.), *Dimensions of thinking and cognitive instruction* (pp. 15–52). Hillsdale, NJ: Lawrence Erlbaum.

Patterson, J. B., & Marks, C. (1992). The client as customer: Achieving service quality and customer satisfaction in rehabilitation. *Journal of Rehabilitation, 58*(4), 16–20.

Pellegrino, J. W. (1985). Inductive reasoning ability. In R. J. Sternberg (Ed.), *Human abilities: An information-processing approach* (pp. 195–225). New York: W. H. Freeman.

Peloquin, S. M. (1989). Helping through touch: The embodiment of caring. *Journal of Religion and Health, 28*(4), 299–322.

Peloquin, S. M. (1990). The patient–therapist relationship in occupational therapy: Understanding visions and images. *American Journal of Occupational Therapy, 44,* 13–21.

Peloquin, S. M. (1993a). Beliefs that shape care: Reflections from narratives. *American Journal of Occupational Therapy, 47,* 935–942.

Peloquin, S. M. (1993b). The depersonalization of patients: A profile gleaned from narratives. *American Journal of Occupational Therapy, 47,* 830–837.

Peloquin, S. M. (1995). The fullness of empathy: Reflections and illustrations. *American Journal of Occupational Therapy, 49,* 24–31.

Peloquin, S. M. (1996). Using the arts to enhance confluent learning. *American Journal of Occupational Therapy, 50,* 148–151.

Peloquin, S. M. (2002a). Confluence: Moving forward with affective strength. *American Journal of Occupational Therapy, 56,* 69–77.

Peloquin, S. M. (2002b). Reclaiming the vision of *Reaching for Heart as Well as Hands. American Journal of Occupational Therapy, 56,* 517–526.

Pierce, D., & Frank, G. (1992). A mother's work: Two levels of feminist analysis of family-centered care. *American Journal of Occupational Therapy, 46,* 972–980.

Polkinghorne, D. E. (1988). *Narrative knowing and the human sciences.* Albany: State University of New York Press.

Pollock, N. (1993). Client-centered assessment. *American Journal of Occupational Therapy, 47,* 298–301.

Porn, I. (1993). Health and adaptedness. *Theoretical Medicine, 14,* 295–303.

Posner, M. I. (1988). Introduction: What is it to be an expert? In M. T. H. Chi, R. Glaser, & M. J. Farr (Eds.), *The nature of expertise* (pp. xxix–xxvi). Hillsdale, NJ: Lawrence Erlbaum.

Psathas, G. (1995). *Conversation analysis: The study of talk-in-interaction* (Vol. 35). Thousands Oaks, CA: Sage.

Rappaport, M. (1986). Brain evoked potentials in coma and the vegetative state. *Journal of Head Trauma Rehabilitation, 1*(1), 15–29.

Reed, E. S. (1982). An outline of a theory of action systems. *Journal of Motor Behavior, 14,* 98–134.

Reed, E. S. (1989a). Changing theories of postural development. In M. H. Wollacott & A. Shumway-Cook (Eds.), *Development of posture and gait across the life span* (pp. 3–24). Columbia: University of South Carolina Press.

Reed, E. S. (1989b). Neural regulation of adaptive behavior. *Ecological Psychology, 1,* 97–118.

Rehak, A., Kaplan, J. A., Weylman, S. T., Kelly, B., Brownell, H. H., & Gardner, H. (1992). Story processing in right-hemisphere brain-damaged patients. *Brain and Language, 42,* 320–336.

Reistetter, T. A., Spencer, J. C., Trujillo, L., & Abreu, B. C. (in press). Examining the Community Integration Measure (CIM): A replication study with life satisfaction. *Neuro-Rehabilitation.*

Riessman, C. K. (1993). *Narrative analysis* (Vol. 30). Newbury Park, CA: Sage.

Rosenberg, J., & Ashwal, S. (1996). Recent advances in the development of practice parameters: The vegetative state. *NeuroRehabilitation, 6,* 79–87.

Rudnick, A. (2002). The notion of health: A conceptual analysis. *Israel Medical Association Journal, 42*(4), 83–85.

Schloss, P. J., & Wood, C. E. (1990). Effect of self-monitoring on maintenance and generalization of conversational skills of persons with mental retardation. *Mental Retardation, 28,* 105–113.

Schmidt, R. A. (1988). *Motor control and learning: A behavioral emphasis* (2nd ed.). Champaign, IL: Human Kinetics.

Schmidt, R. A., & Bjork, R. A. (1992). New conceptualizations of practice: Common principles in three paradigms suggest new concept for training. *Psychological Science, 3,* 207–217.

Schoenfield, A. H. (1987). What's all the fuss about metacognition? In A. H. Schoenfield (Ed.), *Cognitive science and mathematics education* (pp. 189–215). Hillsdale, NJ: Lawrence Erlbaum.

Schon, D. A. (1987). *Educating the reflective practitioner.* San Francisco: Jossey-Bass.

Shriberg, L. D., & Kwiatkowski, J. (1990). Self-monitoring and generalization in preschool speech-delayed children. *Language, Speech, and Hearing Services in Schools, 21,* 157–170.

Schwartz, R. A. (1985). *Therapy as learning.* Dubuque, IA: Kendall.

Schwartz, R. K. (1991). Education and training strategies: Therapy is learning. In C. Christiansen & C. Baum (Eds.), *Occupational therapy: Overcoming human performance deficits.* Thorofare, NJ: Slack.

Schwartzberg, S. L. (1994). Helping factors in a peer-developed support group for persons with head injury: Part I: Participant observer perspective. *American Journal of Occupational Therapy, 48,* 297–304.

Schweizer, K., Beck-Seyffer, A., & Schneider, R. (1999). Cognitive bias of optimism and its influence on psychological well-being. *Psychological Reports, 84,* 627–636.

Segal, M. E., & Schall, R. R. (1995). Assessing handicap of stroke survivors: A validation study of the Craig Handicap Assessment and Reporting Technique. *American Journal of Physical Medicine and Rehabilitation, 74,* 276–286.

Shaw, R. (1986). Persistent vegetative state: Principles and techniques for seating and positioning. *Journal of Head Trauma Rehabilitation, 1*(1), 31–37.

Sherer, M., Hart, T., Nick, T. G., Whyte, J., Thompson, R. N., & Yablon, S. A. (2003). Early impaired self-awareness after traumatic brain injury. *Archives of Physical Medicine and Rehabilitation, 84,* 168–176.

Siev, E., Freishtat, B., & Zoltan, B. (1986). *Perceptual and cognitive dysfunction in the adult stroke patient* (rev. ed.). Thorofare, NJ: Slack.

Silver, E. A. (1987). Foundations of cognitive theory and research for mathematics problem-solving instruction. In A. H. Schoenfield (Ed.), *Cognitive science and mathematics education* (pp. 33–60). Hillsdale, NJ: Lawrence Erlbaum.

Simmond, M., & Fleming, J. (2003). Reliability of the self-awareness of deficits interview for adults with traumatic brain injury. *Brain Injury, 17,* 325–337.

Sohlberg, M. M., & Mateer, C. A. (2001). *Cognitive rehabilitation: An integrative neuropsychological approach.* New York: Guilford.

Stineman, M. G., Hamilton, B. B., Granger, C. V., Goin, J. E., Escarce, J. J., & Williams, S. V. (1994). Four methods for characterizing disability in the formation of function related groups. *Archives of Physical Medicine and Rehabilitation, 75,* 1277–1283.

Stuss, D. T. (1992). Biological and psychological development of executive functions. *Brain and Cognition, 20,* 8–23.

Sunderland, A., Harris, J. E., & Gleave, J. (1984). Memory failures in everyday life following severe head injury. *Journal of Clinical Neuropsychology, 6,* 127–142.

Swanson, H. L. (1990). Influence of metacognitive knowledge and aptitude on problem solving. *Journal of Educational Psychology, 82,* 306–314.

Taljedal, I. B. (1997). Weak and strong holism. *Scandinavian Journal of Social Medicine, 25*(2), 67–69.

Toglia, J. P. (1991). Generalization of treatment: A multi-context approach to cognitive–perceptual impairments in adults with brain injury. *American Journal of Occupational Therapy, 45,* 505–516.

Toglia, J. (1993). Attention and memory. In C. B. Royeen (Ed.), *AOTA Self-Study Series: Cognitive rehabilitation.* Bethesda, MD: American Occupational Therapy Association.

Toglia, J., & Kirk, U. (2000). Understanding awareness of deficits following brain injury. *NeuroRehabilitation, 15*(1), 57–70.

Trombly, C. A. (1993). The Issue Is: Anticipating the future: Assessment of occupational function. *American Journal of Occupational Therapy, 47,* 253–257.

VanLehn, K., Jones, R. M., & Chi, M. T. H. (1991). Modeling the self-explanation effects with Cascade 3. In K. Hammond & D. Gentner (Eds.), *Proceedings of the Thirteenth Annual Conference of the Cognitive Science Society* (pp. 137–142). Hillsdale, NJ: Lawrence Erlbaum.

VanLehn, K., Jones, R. M., & Chi, M. T. H. (1992). A model of the self-explanation effects. *Journal of the Learning Sciences, 2*(1), 1–59.

Van Zomeren, A. H., & Brouwer, W. H. (1994). *Clinical neuropsychology of attention.* Oxford, England: Oxford University Press.

Vygotsky, L. S. (1978). *Mind in society: The development of higher psychological processes.* Cambridge, MA: Harvard University Press.

Warren, M. (1993a). A hierarchical model for evaluation and treatment of visual–perceptual dysfunction in adult acquired brain injury, Part 1. *American Journal of Occupational Therapy, 47,* 42–54.

Warren, M. (1993b). A hierarchical model for evaluation and treatment of visual–perceptual dysfunction in adult acquired brain injury, Part 2. *American Journal of Occupational Therapy, 47,* 55–65.

Warren, M. (1995). Providing low vision rehabilitation services with occupational therapy and ophthalmology: A program description. *American Journal of Occupational Therapy, 49,* 877–883.

Webster, J. S., & Scott, R. R. (1983). The effects of self-instructional training on attentional deficits following head injury. *Clinical Neuropsychology, 5*(2), 69–74.

Weitzman, E. A., & Miles, M. B. (1995). *Computer programs for qualitative data analysis.* Thousand Oaks, CA: Sage.

White, J. A. (1996). Temporal adaptation in the intensive care unit. In R. Zemke & F. Clark (Eds.), *Occupational science: The evolving discipline* (pp. 363–361). Philadelphia: F. A. Davis.

Whiteneck, G. G., Charlifue, S. W., Gerhart, K. A., Overholser, J. D., & Richardson, G. N. (1992). Quantifying handicap: A new measure of long-term rehabilitation outcomes. *Archives of Physical Medicine and Rehabilitation, 73,* 519–526.

Whitney, J. L., & Goldstein, H. (1989). Using self-monitoring to reduce disfluencies in speakers with mild aphasia. *Journal of Speech and Hearing Disorders, 54,* 576–589.

Willer, B., Ottenbacher, K. J., & Coad, M. L. (1994). The Community Integration Questionnaire. A comparative examination. *American Journal of Physical Medicine and Rehabilitation, 73,* 103–111.

Wilson, B. A. (1987). *Rehabilitation of memory.* New York: Guilford.

Winnie, P. H. (1995). Inherent details in self-regulated learning. *Educational Psychologist, 30,* 173–187.

Wood, W., Abreu, B., Duval, M., & Gerber, D. (1994). Occupational performance and the function approach. In C. B. Royeen (Ed.), *AOTA Self-Study Series: Cognitive rehabilitation* (pp. 1–44). Rockville, MD: American Occupational Therapy Association.

World Health Organization. (1980). *International classification of impairments, disabilities, and handicaps.* Geneva, Switzerland: Author.

Yerxa, E. J. (1992). Foreword. In N. Katz (Ed.), *Cognitive rehabilitation: Models for intervention in occupational therapy* (pp. vii–ix). Stoneham, MA: Butterworth-Heineman.

Ylvisaker, M., & Szekeres, S. F. (1989). Metacognitive and executive impairments in head-injured children and adults. *Topics in Language Disorders, 9,* 34–49.

Zemke, R., & Clark, F. (1996). Preface. In R. Zemke & F. Clark (Eds.), *Occupational science: The evolving discipline.* Philadelphia: F. A. Davis.

Zhang, L., Abreu, B. C., Gonzales, V., Huddleston, N., & Ottenbacher, K. J. (2002). The effect of predictable and unpredictable motor tasks on postural control after traumatic brain injury. *NeuroRehabilitation, 17,* 225–230.

Zhang, L., Abreu, B. C., Masel, B., Scheibel, R. S., Christiansen, C., Huddleston, N., et al. (2001). Virtual reality in the assessment of selected cognitive function after brain injury. *American Journal of Physical Medicine and Rehabilitation, 80,* 597–604.

Zhang, L., Abreu, B. C., Seale, G. S., Masel, B., Christiansen, C., & Ottenbacher, K. J. (2003). A virtual reality environment for evaluation of a daily living skill in brain injury rehabilitation: Reliability and validity. *Archives of Physical Medicine and Rehabilitation, 84,* 1118–1124.

Zimmerman, B. J. (1995). Self-regulation involves more than metacognition: A social cognitive perspective. *Educational Psychologist, 30,* 217–221.

4

Sarah Averbuch, MA, OTR
Noomi Katz, PhD, OTR

Cognitive Rehabilitation

A Retraining Model for Clients With Neurological Disabilities

LEARNING OBJECTIVES

By the end of this chapter,
readers will
1. Understand the theoretical base
and the rationale behind the model
2. Be familiar with the instruments
used for assessment and their
psychometric properties and
learn their use
3. Understand the treatment, goals,
process, and methods and be able to
apply them
4. Be able to acknowledge the need
for evidence-based practice, be familiar with the research that exists,
and become part of the effort to
provide more evidence.

The purpose of this chapter is to describe an occupational therapy cognitive-retraining model for the rehabilitation of clients with neurological disabilities. The model was developed by occupational therapists at Loewenstein Rehabilitation Hospital and derives originally from clinical experience with clients following traumatic brain injury (TBI). The model is used to treat adults and adolescent clients with neurological and neuropsychological dysfunctions such as those that occur after stroke or TBI, as well as adolescents with learning difficulties or underachieving school students. Clients are treated throughout the rehabilitation process, from the acute phase until they reach a plateau, then as they progress to outpatient rehabilitation at the day center and continuing on into the community until they resume their place as productive members of society. Treatment methods focus on cognitive training by enhancing remaining skills and by teaching remediative cognitive strategies, learning strategies, or procedural strategies, depending on the client's abilities and stage of illness or disability.

This chapter discusses the theoretical basis for cognitive retraining, including the neuropsychological, cognitive, and neurobiological rationale, and an intervention that includes assessment tools with research findings, treatment goals, and methods. We supply case studies and group examples to illustrate the intervention and conclude the chapter with a discussion on evidence-based practice that includes descriptions of research studies in progress.

THEORETICAL BASE

Neuropsychological Rationale

The cortex is described as a network of fibers. Each brain region is involved in various functions and interacts with other regions in completing a specific task (Mesulam, 2000). Thus, every normal act is a result of a dynamic balance among all brain structures. According to Luria (1973), "Mental functions . . . cannot be localized in narrow zones of the cortex . . . but must be organized in systems of concretely working zones, each of which performs its role in a complex functional system" (p. 31). Luria also stated that the global function is constant, although the relationships among its components are variable and influenced by specific circumstances under which the function is performed. Thus, the ways or the actions through which the specific task is achieved vary according to circumstances. The system, the network of fibers of the higher mental processes in the human cortex, constantly changes during the development of the child and is influenced by the environment (learning and training process). The structures of higher mental processes change, and with them, so do their relationships with each other (i.e., their "intellectual organization"; Vygotsky, 1962). Thus, normal function is a result of a dynamic balance among all brain structures.

Modern observation shows that the structural foundations of cognitive and behavioral domains are partially overlapping with large-scale networks that are organized around reciprocally interconnected cortical centers. The components of these networks can be divided into critical versus participating areas. Lesions that impair performance in a specific cognitive domain, like speech disturbances, help to identify the critical components, whereas performing general tasks involving the impaired domain reveals the components that participate in its coordination (Mesulam, 2000, p. 2).

Brain injury causes a disturbance in the delicate balance between brain structures, which is not always the result of a localized lesion of one of the brain areas only. A lesion in each zone or area may lead to disintegration of the entire functional system (Luria, 1973, 1980; Mesulam, 2000). In other words, the functional system as a whole can be disturbed by a lesion affecting a very large number of areas, and it can be disturbed differently by lesions in different locations. Brain damage also can cause symptoms associated with undamaged areas of the brain due to disinhibition of an intact area caused by damage elsewhere. Therefore, treatment aims to regain a balance between the brain structures and to create compensatory strategies for improving function. There are several ways to perform cognitive functions, thus calling for training that creates alternative strategies and achieves the reorganization of impaired intellectual abilities.

In summary,

the multiplicity of functions fulfilled by cortical regions, the variety of ways in which complex cognitive functions can be performed, and the different contingencies of learning tasks on an intact brain offer a substrate for the functional reorganization of impaired intellectual abilities. (Rahmani, Geva, Rochberg, Trope, & Bore, 1987, p. 45)

New evidence suggests that cortical circuits might be modifiable following brain injury. This property of modifiability of neurons is often referred to as *plasticity*. Plastic changes might support recovery and some type of functional changes. Recovery could result from the reorganization of remaining circuits as a result of change in the organization of regions directly and indirectly disrupted by the injury (Kolb & Gibb, 1999).

Cognitive Rationale

Cognitive theories concern the information processing of the normal intellect. The information an individual has to deal with comes from three sources: (a) his or her environment; (b) his or her memory, where the information is compared to previous experiences; and (c) the feedback

he or she receives after the action (Bourne, Dominski, & Loftus, 1979). Information passes through several stages, during which it is received, registered, and encoded. This processed information is then organized as a schema. Neisser (1976) defined *schema* as

that portion of the entire perceptual cycle which is internal to the perceiver, modifiable by experience, and somehow specific to what is being perceived. The schema accepts information as it becomes available at sensory surfaces and is changed by that information; it directs movements and exploratory activities that make more information available by which it is further modified. (p. 54)

It enables us to handle a large body of information by allowing us to compare new stimuli with previous experiences and then modify and change the schema. This is similar to Piaget's process of assimilation and accommodation (cited in Ginsburg & Opper, 1979).

The normal individual actively seeks and assimilates information in relation to his or her ability to understand and then remember it. This search is guided by schemata representing the layout of our memories and knowledge. Perception, thinking, and memory are constantly interacting. Comprehension and memory depend on what and how we perceive. Perception is influenced by the ability to

- Appreciate the relevance of the information,
- Distinguish among hierarchical constellations of attributes characteristic of different information, and
- Distinguish among hierarchical constellations of attributes that are characteristic of different information that is perceived.

These abilities further rely strongly on previous experiences and accumulated knowledge.

For example, visual identification is strongly affected by the ability to analyze the information according to its hierarchical attributes and previous experiences. Identification is much clearer when we deal with incomplete or partial information as presented in embedded figures. Identification is made according to characteristic features, the prototype of the groups to which the specific item belongs (Rahmani, 1982; Rahmani et al., 1987). As noted in studies by Rosch (1978; Rosch & Mervis, 1975), the formation and learning of components is based on forming preferential levels of abstraction, selecting prototypes, creating object categories, and determining the degree of category membership. In a similar way, the learning process and memory are strongly affected by the perception process.

The various mechanisms of the cognitive functions of perception, thinking operations, and memory provide the procedures for the cognitive retraining of impaired intellectual processes in clients with brain damage.

Neurobiological Rationale

As a result of advances in the neural sciences, in particular with respect to the analysis of how different aspects of mental functions are represented in the brain, our understanding of the relationship between the brain and behavior has expanded and so, too, has our understanding of the learning processes on which treatment interventions are based.

Kandel (1998; Kandel & Pittenger, 1999) emphasized the importance of interdisciplinary collaboration among theorists in the fields of cognitive psychology, psychiatry, psychoanalysis, and modern biology. The contribution of the first three disciplines is derived from the perspective of mental functions and their behavioral expression, whereas biology provides us with the understanding of the human brain. Such a collaboration can enable meaningful advances in the understanding of higher human mental processes, as well as help build a better and a stronger rationale on which to base treatment. Kandel (1998) suggested a framework for understanding the relationship between the mind and the brain that is based on five principles that represent the current thinking of biologists:

- *Principle 1:* "Mind is the range of functions carried out by the brain" (p. 460). That is, the action of the brain underlies all human behaviors, including complex cognitive functions.
- *Principle 2:* "Genes and their protein products are important determinants of the pattern of the interconnections between neurons in the brain and the details of their functioning" (p. 460). Therefore, genes and combinations of genes have a significant role in determining human behavior.
- *Principle 3:* "Just as combinations of genes contribute to behavior . . . so can behavior and social factors exert actions on the brain by feeding back upon it to modify the expression of genes and the function of nerve cells. *Learning* . . . produces alteration in gene expression" (p. 460).
- *Principle 4:* "Alterations in gene expression induced by learning give rise to changes in patterns of neuronal connections" (p. 460). These changes caused by learning are expressed in individual behavior.
- *Principle 5:* " Learning by producing changes in gene expression . . . alter the strength of synaptic connections and structural changes . . . alter the anatomical pattern of interconnections between nerve cells of the brain" (p. 460). In other words, learning causes structural and anatomical changes in the brain.

These statements empower the learning process as one of the main factors for cognitive–behavioral changes. To the question of how genes contribute to behavior, Kandel emphasized the process; behavior is generated by neural circuits that involve many cells, each of which express specific genes that direct production of specific proteins that underlie the development and function of neural circuits (Kandel, 1995).

Several studies presented by Merzenich, Recanzone, Jenkins, Allard, and Nudo (1988) provide evidence of how experience and practice changes the topographic organization of the somatosensory cortex. We can make deductions about the different ways learning takes place in humans from models of memory. For example, memory is divided into explicit and implicit learning: memory for what things are and memory for how to do things. Explicit memory encodes conscious information, whereas implicit memory encodes information about motor and perceptual strategies (Kandel & Pittenger, 1999). Our clinical experience shows that patients can learn without awareness: Individuals with severe explicit memory problems are still able to memorize complicated tasks through implicit learning without being aware that they can perform the given tasks. This emphasizes the fact that the process of implicit memory underlies the neural basis for a set of unconscious mental processes, which are different from implicit learning.

This framework for cognitive learning, as described briefly here, provides us with a stronger, evidence-based treatment rationale. "The capability of learning is so highly developed in humans that humankind changes much more by cultural evolution then by biological evolution" (Kandel, 1998, p. 461). In other words, humans have the capability of changing through learning and for adapting to multiple situations. The individual changes that occur in humans give them the capacity to change their environment socially, culturally, and physically. According to this theory, these changes are much more dynamic and significant, through the passage of generations, than are biological changes.

INTERVENTION

Assessment

The first phase of the intervention process is the assessment phase. It is important to assess the client's cognitive abilities and disabilities, level of awareness, and executive-functioning abilities. In performing a detailed anamnestic interview, we first collect data about the client's previous performance in occupational areas, including academic and work history, and everyday life activities, as well as his or her preferences and plans for the future. This information helps us understand the client's and his or her family's goals and what is being referred to when they state that they would like the client to be able "to do what he was able to do before" or "to return to how she was before."

Another important part of the assessment process is to identify the client's preferred learning patterns. If these patterns are no longer as effective as before due to the injury experienced, it is possible to deduce their preferred learning patterns through an examination of the client's previous patterns of performance. The integration of all this information allows us to tailor an individual and efficient treatment plan.

Cognitive rehabilitation theory assumes that most typical healthy adults achieve a basic cognitive task performance. We, therefore, start by assessing the client's current level of cognitive performance. This assessment serves as a baseline for measuring progress and, together with premorbid information, sensory motor evaluation, and functional status evaluation in daily activities, forms the basis for treatment planning and intervention (Katz, Hefner, & Ruben, 1990).

Assessment of cognition within this model is an essential and central component for further intervention planning. It includes an array of the following cognitive batteries listed in Table 4.1. The Loewenstein Occupational Therapy Cognitive Assessment (LOTCA) is used first as a baseline for every adolescent and adult client, and the LOTCA–Geriatric (LOTCA–G) is used for elderly clients. The Rivermead Behavioral Memory Test (RBMT), Test of Everyday Attention (TEA), Behavioral Inattention Test (BIT), Behavioral Assessment of Dysexecutive Syndrome (BADS), Multiple Errands Test Simplified (MET–SV), and Self-Awareness of Deficits Interview (SADI) are used if a more in-depth assessment of specific cognitive skills such as memory, attention, unilateral spatial neglect, and higher cognitive functions such as awareness or executive function are warranted. Although the Cognistat (Northern California Neurobehavioral Group, 1995) is used as a screening assessment in the acute stage in neurosurgical departments as part of the decision to refer patients to rehabilitation, the MET–SV is the only instrument that assesses higher-level cognitive skills of executive functions in a complex daily activity.

Loewenstein Occupational Therapy Cognitive Assessment

At the Loewenstein Rehabilitation Hospital in Israel, the staff developed the LOTCA to assess basic cognitive abil-

TABLE 4.1. Cognitive Assessment Instruments

Battery	Cognitive Skills Tested	Reference
Loewenstein Occupational Therapy Cognitive Assessment (LOTCA)	Orientation, visual, and spatial–perception, praxis, visuomotor organization, thinking operation, logical	Itzkovich, Elazar, Averbuch, & Katz, 2000
LOTCA–Geriatric	The same as above and, in addition, memory	Katz, Elazar, & Itzkovich, 1995; Elazar, Itzkovich, & Katz, 1996
Rivermead Behavioral Memory Test	Memory	Wilson, Cockburn, & Baddeley, 1985
Test of Everyday Attention	Attention (selective, sustained, switching, and divided)	Robertson, Ward, Ridgeway, & Nimmo-Smith, 1994
Behavioral Inattention Test	Unilateral spatial neglect	Wilson, Cockburn, & Halligan, 1987a, 1987b
Behavioral Assessment of Dysexecutive Syndrome	Executive functions	Wilson, Alderman, Burgess, Emslie, & Evans, 1996
Neurobehavioral Cognitive Status Examination	Level of consciousness, Orientation and Attention; Language, Constructions, Memory, Calculations, Reasoning.	Northern California Neurobehavioral Group (1995)
Multiple Errands Test Simplified	Executive functions in daily activity	Alderman, Burgess, Knight, & Henman, 2003
Self-Awareness of Deficits Interview	Awareness of deficits, awareness of disabilities, and ability to set realistic goals	Fleming, Strong, & Ashton, 1996, 1998; Fleming & Strong, 1999

ities of clients following brain injury (Katz, Itzkovich, Averbuch, & Elazar, 1989; Najenson, Rahmani, Elazar, & Averbuch, 1984). Basic cognitive abilities are those "intellectual functions thought to be prerequisite for managing everyday encounters with the environment" (Najenson et al., 1984, p. 315).

The staff derived foundations for the LOTCA battery from clinical experience as well as from Luria's (neuropsychological) and Piaget's (developmental) theories and evaluation procedures (Golden, 1984; Inhelder & Piaget, 1964). As a starting point for occupational therapy intervention and a screening test for further neuropsychological assessment, the battery provides an initial profile of cognitive abilities. It consists of 25 subtests and 6 areas of division: orientation, visual perception, spatial perception, praxis organization, visuomotor organization, and thinking operations. A 4- or 5-point scale is used for each subtest, from which the evaluator may obtain a general profile of functioning as well as profile of functioning in a specified area. Although the entire battery takes 30–50 minutes to administer, the evaluator can divide the testing into shorter sessions if necessary. The instructions include procedures for evaluating clients with expressive-language deficits.

In addition, evaluators used the LOTCA as a measure of the client's status over time (i.e., clinical change). In cases in which deficits were present at initial assessment, the evaluator used the LOTCA as a follow-up in reference to the client's progress. In general, to avoid simple memory carryover, it is best to repeat the assessment after an interval of at least 2 months. However, because clients practice many similar tasks during treatment, it is important to consider learning as a possible explanation for higher scores. The learning, if generalized, is precisely the purpose of treatment. Therefore, in contrast to the view of classic measurement theory, we should not regard it as a threat to validity (Katz et al., 1990).

Reliability and Validity

Initially, the researchers established the battery's measurement properties in different ways. They determined interrater reliability coefficients of .82 to .97 for the various subtests and, on using patient groups and a normal control group, found an alpha coefficient of .85 and above in reference to the internal consistency of perception, visuomotor organization, and thinking operations (Katz et al., 1989). Next, the researchers determined validity in differentiating between known groups. The Wilcoxon two-sample test showed that, between the control groups and

the client groups of TBI and cerebrovascular accidents (CVA), all subtests differentiated at the $p < .0001$ level of significance. Through the use of exploratory factor analysis, they examined initial construct validity, which showed a three-factor solution and a total amount of variance explained above 60% (i.e., substantial). This result supported the assumed structure of the LOTCA (Katz et al., 1989) and led to further investigation. To test the area of visuomotor organization in reference to criterion validity within the TBI group, the examiners used the Block Design subtest of the Wechsler Adult Intelligence Scale (Wechsler, 1981). They found a Pearson correlation coefficient of $r = .68$ between the score on the Block Design and the mean score of the visuomotor organization subtests of the LOTCA and a $r = .77$ when the testing did not measure time on the Block Design. The results were almost identical for a group of adult clients with chronic schizophrenia ($r = .69$ and $r = .78$; Katz & Hiemann, 1990).

To determine the validity of the LOTCA in reference to American participants, the researchers compared both Americans and Israeli healthy adults, as well as those among the two countries who experienced a stroke (Annes, Katz, & Cermak, 1996; Cermak et al., 1995). Comparison of means and standard deviations of each LOTCA subtest revealed strong similarities between the American and Israeli healthy adult samples. The similarities in ability to perform accurately between the two groups support the use of the LOTCA battery in the United States.

Comparison of clients who experienced a recent stroke showed that, on the majority of LOTCA subtests, there were no significant differences between American and Israeli participants. Thus, the LOTCA is an appropriate tool to assess Americans who have had a stroke. The American healthy sample data serve as standards of performance. In addition, in accordance with its design, the study compared the performance of clients post-right and post-left CVA (Cermak et al., 1995). Few differences existed between the two groups in both countries. Only one subtest, the pegboard construction, revealed significant differences among both American and Israeli participants. Therefore, the conclusions indicated that, for the most part, the LOTCA subtests are not specific to right or left cerebral hemisphere and show more integrative cognitive abilities.

However, through the use of one-way analysis of variance (ANOVA), comparison of clients following TBI ($n = 25$) and right CVA, both with neglect ($n = 19$) and without neglect ($n = 21$), showed significant F tests for three of the cognitive areas on the LOTCA (i.e., all except orientation). Sheffe post hoc tests showed that the source of difference was the neglect group, which performs lower in all areas. A Wilcoxon analysis, which compared all LOTCA subtests, showed the same results. In other words, clients post-TBI performed significantly higher than clients post-right CVA with neglect, while the nonneglect right CVA group was not significantly different from the TBI (Katz, Hartman-Maeir, Ring, & Soroker, 1999).

Annes and colleagues (1996) compared the performance on the LOTCA between older (40–70 years) and younger American adults (17–25 years) in two ways: accuracy on all subtests and length of time to perform the Visuomotor Organization subtests. Similarity in accuracy of performance between older and younger adults was significant on almost all subtests and supported the consideration of the group as one. However, although nearly all normal adults achieved maximum performance on the LOTCA subtests, younger adults required significantly less time to complete all the Visuomotor Organization subtests. On the basis of these results, it appears that time, at least for the Visuomotor Organization subtests, can be used as a more sensitive measure for screening among healthy adults or those with mild cognitive deficits.

Additionally, Katz, Champagne, and Cermak (1997) found similar results regarding the puzzle subtest. Groups of younger and older American adults were tested on three versions of the puzzle construction subtest. On all versions, the younger adults performed faster than the older adults. Older adults performed faster in the simplified version from the LOTCA–G than in the original LOTCA subtest in both conditions, either on top of the design (as required in the test) or in front of it.

The relationships of cognitive performance and daily functioning in clients following right CVA, with and without neglect, was studied by Katz and colleagues (1999). The study comprised 40 clients with right CVA and first stroke as its sample. On the basis of the BIT conventional subtests cutoff point (Wilson, Cockburn, & Halligan, 1987a), they assigned clients into neglect ($n = 19$) and nonneglect ($n = 21$) groups. Within both groups, the mean age of the participants was approximately 58 years. In both groups, the number of men outweighed the number of women. The functional measures included the Functional Independence Measure (FIM; Granger, Cotter, Hamilton, & Fiedler, 1993), activities of daily living (ADL) checklist (Hartman-Maeir & Katz, 1995), and the Rabideau Kitchen Evaluation–Revised, which includes drink and sandwich preparation (Neistadt, 1992).

Participants were assessed in three periods: at admission to the rehabilitation program, at the time of discharge, and at a 6 months' follow-up session. Results of Spearman correlation analysis of the four LOTCA areas with the functional measures at these three assessment periods were as follows: *At admission,* in the neglect group, perception correlated with ADL checklist ($r = .47$), visuomotor organization and thinking operations correlated with the FIM total and motor ($r \approx .50$). In the nonneglect group, all areas correlated with the FIM cognitive ($r = .50$ to $r = .67$); perception and thinking correlated with ADL checklist ($r \approx .45$). *At discharge,* in the neglect group, moderate to high correlations (ranging from $r = .48$ to $r = .80$) revealed a significant relationship between the LOTCA (except Orientation), and all performance measures. The highest correlations were between visuomotor and thinking and drink and sandwich preparation ($r \approx .80$). In general, within the non-neglect group, significant correlations were moderate (ranging from $r = .36$ to $r = .62$). The highest correlation appeared between the visuomotor organization area and the FIM total ($r = .62$). *At follow-up,* participants took part in only three LOTCA visuomotor subtests: colored block design, puzzle, and drawing a clock. In the neglect group, moderate to high correlations (ranging from $r = .40$ to $r = .77$) appeared with the functional measures (except for clock with FIM total and cognitive, which was $r \approx .30$). The puzzle subtest correlated the highest with all functional measures ($r = .70$). When comparing the two groups, the number of significant correlations within the non-neglect group was smaller and lower than in the neglect group. The highest correlation appeared between the puzzle and sandwich preparation ($r = .70$; Katz et al., 1999).

To explore the predictive validity of the LOTCA to daily function, from the time of admission to follow-up, the researchers computed a multiple regression analysis. In reference to the entire sample of right CVA participants ($n = 40$), the BIT conventional score explained about 60% of the variance of all functional measures at follow-up. Depending on the measure (FIM, drink, or sandwich), the LOTCA area scores of perception, visuomotor, or thinking operations explained only an approximate additional 5% of the variance. A separate analysis for the groups revealed that, in the non-neglect group, perception explained 57% and the visuomotor an additional 13% of the FIM total; perception explained 62% of the sandwich preparation; thinking explained 44% and perception an additional 12% of the drink preparation. Thus, these results identify neglect to be the major variable predicting daily functioning in clients post right CVA with neglect. However, for those clients who do not suffer from neglect, cognitive deficits have a major contribution to the level of daily functioning (Katz, Hartman-Maeir, Ring, & Soroker, 2000).

Children's Performance

The testing of 240 normal primary school children determined age-level standards among 40 participants in each age group, between ages 6 and 12 years. To determine age norms of the various subtests, as well as to verify the hierarchical order in which the various cognitive competencies included in the battery are acquired, the study assessed the performance of children on the LOTCA. The results showed a clear, developmental sequence in performance along the LOTCA subtests. Performance levels increased steadily with age, while the performance speed of visuomotor tasks decreased concomitant with the increase toward maximal performance (Averbuch & Katz, 1991; Itzkovich, Elazar, Averbuch, & Katz, 2000).

In addition, two cultural groups in Israel were assessed: typical Ethiopian children and Bedouin children in the same age groups. Results indicated significant differences between the two groups (Averbuch & Katz, 1991; Katz, Kizony, & Parush, 2002). These findings support the validity of the test and its sensitivity to cultural and environmentally based influences on children's cognitive developmental performance (Parush, Sharoni, Hahn-Markowitz, & Katz, 2000; Rosenblum, Katz, Hahn-Markowitz, & Parush, 2000).

Dynamic Occupational Therapy Cognitive Assessment for Children

Because we wanted to develop a means of assessing children's potential for learning through mediation in addition to measuring their static baseline cognitive abilities, the original LOTCA battery underwent a series of modifications to adapt it for use with children. Over the last few years the new Dynamic Occupational Therapy Cognitive Assessment for Children was adapted for the assessment of children ages 6 to 12 years as a dynamic evaluation based on the cueing system used by Toglia (1994, with her permission; Katz, Parush, & Traub Bar-Ilan, 2004). An extensive data collection was conducted under the guidance of Katz and Parush, which included the assessment of healthy children, children with learning disabilities, children following TBI, and children with attention-deficit/hyperactivity disorder

LOTCA–Geriatric Version

The LOTCA battery was used clinically with elderly patients, but data on elderly people older than age 70 years with the LOTCA has not been collected systematically. Clinical experience alerted us to the difficulties in admin-

istering the battery to elderly patients. Some items are too small to see or manipulate, and the battery as a whole is too long. Therefore, an adapted geriatric version of the LOTCA was developed and researched (Katz, Elazar, & Itzkovich, 1995, 1996). The geriatric version, LOTCA–G, was changed on the basis of the literature and clinical observations according to the following criteria: the enlargement of items to reduce vision and motor coordination difficulties; the reduction of details in some items for lower task complexity; the shortening of subtests, and thus the whole battery, to reduce general length of time; and the addition of three memory subtests.

The final LOTCA–G is comprised of 20 subtests (Elazar, Itzkovich, & Katz, 1996). Katz and colleagues (1995) determined construct validity for the LOTCA–G comparing 33 elderly post-stroke and 43 healthy independent elderly participants. Participants' mean age of 77 was similar for both groups, with a range of 70–91 years. Men represented a third of both groups. All subtests, except Praxis and Colored Block Design, differed significantly between the groups, with healthy elderly performing better. On all perception subtests, both groups performed well. In order of severity, the most noted decline in the stroke group was in visuomotor organization, thinking operations, and orientation.

Mean length of time to perform the whole assessment for both groups on the LOTCA was about 55 minutes, with a range of 30–90 minutes, showing a large variance. However, no significant difference was found between healthy elderly people and clients post-CVA, suggesting normal slowness at older age when complex performance is required. LOTCA–G performance length of time shows that there is a difference of 45 minutes (clients) compared to 31 minutes (healthy), with a larger range (20–60 compared to 20–45). Within the stroke group, the LOTCA took more time (57 vs. 45 minutes) but not statistically significantly more; however, within the healthy group, the difference in time is very significant (51 vs. 31 minutes). A two-way ANOVA shows overall significant statistical differences ($F = 11.26, p < .0001$); Scheffe's post hoc test showed that the differences are (a) in the healthy group between both versions LOTCA and LOTCA–G, and (b) between both groups, healthy and clients post-CVA, for the LOTCA–G.

More recently, Bar-Haim Erez and Katz (in press) studied the validity of the LOTCA–G in the assessment of individuals with dementia as compared with healthy elderly participants. Participants included 30 with dementia and 43 healthy elderly individuals. Results demonstrated significant differences between the groups on all

LOTCA–G areas scores. Most subtests differentiated also between individuals with mild dementia (score 20–23) on the Mini Mental Status Examination (MMSE; Folstein & Folstein, 1975) and moderate dementia (MMSE score 16–19), suggesting that the test is sensitive to levels of dementia. Significant moderate correlations were found between LOTCA–G area scores and the MMSE score. In conclusion, the LOTCA–G was recommended to use for elderly people with dementia to obtain a detailed cognitive profile beyond the MMSE cutoff score, thus enabling intervention planning.

Rivermead Behavioral Memory Test

Memory deficits are evaluated with the RBMT, which is a battery designed to assess memory abilities in everyday tasks. The RBMT is used to assess "skills necessary for adequate functioning in normal life and can also be used to help therapists identify areas for treatment" (Wilson, Cockburn, & Baddeley, 1985, p. 4).

The RBMT consists of 11 subtests that assess verbal and visual recognition and recall, learning and recall of instructions, and recall of a new spatial route (a given path in the room). Subtests include remembering a name, belonging, appointment, pictures, story (immediate and delayed), faces, route (immediate and delayed), message, orientation, and date. All subtests use simple and everyday items. For example, one of the instructions is to remember to ask when the next appointment is, when the clock rings, or to ask for a personal belonging at the end of the assessment that had been given to the therapist at the beginning of the session.

The test has four alternate versions so that it is possible to repeat the assessment a few times. Each subtest has a screening pass–fail score (maximum 12) and a standardized profile 3-point score: normal, marginal, and deficit (maximum 24).

The test was found valid in differentiating healthy people from clients following TBI and stroke (Goldberg & Katz, 1994; Van Balen, Westzaan, & Mulder, 1996; Wilson, Cockburn, & Baddeley, 1986). It also was found to be significantly more correlated with functional outcomes than other formal memory tests (Wilson et al., 1986). Norms for elderly people older than age 70 were determined by Cockburn and Smith (1989) for an English sample and by Van Balen et al. (1996) for a Dutch sample. The Hebrew translation of the RBMT is used in Israel by occupational therapists, apparently without many culture-related difficulties. Initial results from clients following stroke ($n = 20$) and a healthy control group ($n = 20$)

showed similar means for the RBMT screen and profile scores but within the stroke group mainly for right-CVA participants (Goldberg & Katz, 1994).

An extended version was created by De Wall, Wilson, and Baddeley (1994) to increase the difficulty of the test. The authors combined two parallel versions into one test, which extended the test to include double the amount of material in each subtest. Participants consisted of 26 healthy middle-age people and 22 healthy elderly people. Findings suggest that the test was more sensitive, detecting small age differences, but further work is needed to ascertain its ecological validity.

Behavioral Inattention Test

The BIT (Halligan, Cockburn & Wilson, 1991; Wilson, Cockburn, & Halligan, 1987a, 1987b) consists of 6 conventional subtests and 9 behavioral subtests designed to identify a wide variety of visual neglect behaviors. The conventional subtests are line crossing, letter cancellation, star cancellation, figure and shape copying, line bisection, and representational drawing. The scoring range varies within the conventional subtests totaling a maximum of 146 points.

The behavioral subtests evaluate aspects of daily life: scanning 3 pictures (plate of food, bathroom sink, and a room); telephone dialing; menu reading; article reading; telling time; coin sorting; address and sentence copying; map navigation; and card sorting. All subtests' score a maximum of 9 points totaling a maximum of 81. Scores can provide a functional profile of neglect and a meaningful guide for treatment.

The Hebrew translation of the BIT follows closely the original BIT with some minor adaptations of cultural items in menu reading; coin sorting; and address, sentence, and article wording. Normative data, as well as reliability and validity data, were obtained from 50 participants without brain damage and 80 CVA patients: 54 with right brain damage and 26 with left brain damage. Scores of the control participants were used to establish cutoff points for individual subtests and total scores. Interrater, parallel form, and test–retest reliability were all high ($r = .99, .91, .99, p < .001$, respectively). Validity was established in two ways: first, by examining the relationship between the conventional and behavioral test scores ($r = .92, p < .001$), a measure of concurrent validity, and second, by examining the relationship between the behavioral scores and therapists' observations of the patients' ADL ($r = .67, p < .001$; Halligan et al., 1991; Wilson et al., 1987a). Shiel and Wilson (1992) found a strong association between neglect, as assessed by the BIT, and ADL, as assessed by the Rivermead ADL assessment and Frenchay Activities Index. Their study contributes to enhancing the ecological validity of the BIT.

Hartman-Maeir and Katz (1995) studied 40 Israeli participants with right CVA, from both day center and hospital settings. Participants were evaluated on three measures: the BIT, performance tasks, and a checklist of ADLs. Results showed that 7 of the 9 BIT behavioral subtests differentiated significantly between participants with visual neglect and those without neglect; 6 of the 9 subtests correlated significantly with parallel performance tasks or ADL checklist items. These findings support the validity of the BIT in predicting daily function and suggest that the test is valid for use in Israel. Furthermore, as described above (Katz et al., 1999), the BIT conventional score explained about 60% of the variance of all functional measures at follow-up within an additional group of 40 right CVA clients.

Test of Everyday Attention

The TEA (Robertson, Ward, Ridgeway, & Nimmo-Smith, 1994, 1996) includes the visual selective, sustained attention, transfer of attention, divided memory, and working memory (auditory–verbal) components of attentions. The test includes 8 subtests and has 3 comparable versions. The subtests are Map Search (visual selective), Elevator Counting (sustained), Elevator Counting With Distraction (auditory selective and working memory), Visual Elevator (Transfer), Elevator Counting With Reversal (working memory auditory–verbal), Telephone Search (visual selective), Telephone Search While Counting (dual task decrement), and Lottery (sustained attention).

The test has norms for healthy individuals in four age groups (18–80 years old), and standard scores also are provided. The test has good reliability and validity. It was tested on patients following brain injury and on patients with Alzheimer's disease.

In the first study performed in Israel (Dvir et. al., 2003), the TEA was tested on 30 patients ages 20–50, following brain injury at the day treatment program at Loewenstein Rehabilitation Hospital, and results were compared with those of 30 matched healthy control patients. For 3 subtests that are based on reading in English, a Hebrew version was prepared (Map Search, Telephone Search, and Telephone Search With Counting). Participants were tested on both English and Hebrew versions, but no significant differences were found. The Lottery subtest was not included. Results indicated significant differences be-

tween the healthy and TBI groups on all subtests supporting the test's construct validity and its usage in Israel.

Behavioral Assessment of the Dysexecutive Syndrome

The BADS (Wilson, Alderman, Burgess, Emslie, & Evans, 1996) consists of 6 subtests: Rule Shift Cards, Action Program, Key Search, Zoo Map, Temporal Judgment, and Modified Six Elements. The profile scores of each subtest ranges from 0–4, and the total profile score ranges from 0–24. Interrater reliability was found to be $r = .88$ to 1.00; Test–retest reliability for a sample of 29, 6–12 months later, percentage of agreement was 27–90, was lowest for Zoo Map and highest for Action Program. Construct validity was established as significant differences were found between the control groups and TBI and schizophrenia groups; however, only differences on total profile were found between patients, TBI were higher than patients with schizophrenia (Evans, Chua, McKenna, & Wilson, 1997; Wilson, Evans, Alderman, Burgess, & Emslie, 1997; Wilson, Evans, Emslie, Alderman, & Burgess, 1998). Clark and O'Carroll (1998) examined the relationship between executive functions and memory with rehabilitation status of patients with schizophrenia. They used only the Modified Six Elements from the BADS, the RBMT, and 3 cognitive scales. The measures were correlated with chronicity, education, and ages but did not correlate significantly with the REHAB measure. These results raise some question about the measures used.

Norris and Tate (2000) studied the BADS in Australia and found a total profile score for 37 healthy control participants that was very similar to the UK data. The test also was found to differentiate significantly between TBI patients and control patients, especially with respect to the subtests Action, Zoo Map, Six Elements, and Total Profile ($p < .005, .007, .002, .004$, respectively).

A stratified convenience sample of 93 healthy participants in Israel were tested and results compared to the UK data in the manual (Dvir et al., 2003); ages 18–65 divided into three age groups (18–35, 36–50, 51–65) and three educational groups (<12, 12, >12 years); and 35 men and 58 women. Total profile was slightly higher for the UK data ($t = 1.71, p < .05$), as well as Action Plan and Temporal Judgment ($t = 2.27, 3.21$; both $p < .05$).

Multiple Errands Test Simplified

The MET–SV (Alderman, Burgess, Knight, & Henman, 2003) is conducted in a shopping mall. It is comprised of different tasks requiring multitasking with specific rules within a time frame. It is scored on inefficiencies, rule breaks, interpretation failure, task failures, total errors, and strategies used, and a 10-point scale is used to rate how well the individual performed the task.

The MET was used to examine clients following brain injury and was found to be reliable and valid. Results demonstrated high interrater reliability (.81–1.00) and internal consistency (.77). Construct validity was established by demonstrating significant difference between participants with brain injury and control participants. It is currently being studied with young clients following brain injury from the day treatment program at Loewenstein Rehabilitation Center. It is of paramount importance for us to have a higher-level functional test that can provide a better understanding of executive functions in everyday complex tasks. Thus, the MET provides us with the ability to evaluate higher-level functioning individuals who have performed well in standard tests such as the BADS and in specific daily tasks but demonstrates difficulties in performing novel, complex multitasks with time constraints.

The MET also has a hospital version (Knight, Alderman, & Burgess, 2002) that follows similar rules, but it is performed within a large hospital and thus can be used if patients are still hospitalized.

Self-Awareness of Deficits Interview

The SADI (Fleming & Strong, 1999; Fleming, Strong, & Ashton, 1996, 1998) is a structured interview that includes three parts related to awareness of deficits, awareness of disabilities, and ability to set realistic goals. Each of the three awareness areas is scored on a 4-point scale (0–3) and a total awareness score (range of 0–9). Interrater shows a high interclass correlation coefficient, $r = .82$; construct validity was found among groups of TBI patients and healthy controls using cluster analysis; and significant prediction of outcomes 12 months post-TBI.

The measures provides comprehensive information on a person's awareness of his or her deficits and their consequences, as well as his or her ability to set realistic goals, which makes for a good starting point for intervention. Its use was demonstrated in three case examples of clients following TBI, stroke, and diagnosis of schizophrenia (Katz, Fleming, Keren, Griffen, & Hartman-Maeir, 2002).

Neurobehavioral Cognitive Status Examination

The Cognistat (Northern California Neurobehavioral Group, 1995) is a screening test to determine the cognitive status of the client. In Israel, the test is used by occupational therapists in general hospitals as a screening of cognitive deficits and as a baseline in neurosurgical departments (Weiss, 1994). The Cognistat also is used in assessing elderly clients, as the test provides more information for intervention planning than the MMSE.

The Cognistat was developed in 1983 by the Northern California Group. The test assesses 5 major cognitive areas: Language, Constructions, Memory, Calculations, and Reasoning. Level of Consciousness, Orientation, and Attention are evaluated first and only then are the other areas assessed. All areas are tested in a screen and metric paradigm. The client is first presented with the screen task, which is the most difficult item. If the client performs well at the screen task, the cognitive skill involved is assumed normal, and no further testing is done in that area. If the client fails the screen task, the metric tasks are administered. The metric part consists of a series of test items of increasing difficulty. Performance on the metric determines whether and to what degree the cognitive skill is impaired. Scores are presented on a profile arranged into 4 performance levels: average, mild, moderate, and severe (Northern California Neurobehavioral Group, 1995).

Studies in a variety of client populations in which brain dysfunction is suspected show that the Cognistat is sensitive in detecting cognitive impairments, differentiating between groups, as well as measuring changes over time (Lezak, 1995; Logue, Tupler, D'Amico, & Schmitt, 1993; Mysiw, Beegan, & Gatens, 1989; Osmon, Smet, Winegarden, & Gandhavadi, 1992; Schwamm, Van Dyke, Kierman, Merrin, & Mueller, 1987).

A Hebrew translation was prepared and used with the author's permission by Katz, Elazar, and Itzkovich (1996) compared performance of 24 healthy independent elderly people with 15 clients post-CVA, all older than age 70. Results showed that healthy elderly people scored higher than patients post-CVA on all subtests. Significant correlations were found among compatible subtests of LOTCA and Cognistat and low correlations among cognitive skills from different domains, supporting validity of both tests. In an additional study, performance of 47 healthy independent elderly people, 47 neurosurgical patients, and 42 people with dementia were compared (Katz, Hartman-Maeir, Weiss, & Armon, 1997). Statistically significant differences were found among the three groups on raw scores of all individual subtests and on the 4 performance levels. Construction subtest scores were low for all groups and seemed to detect the aging process in addition to disease-related dysfunction. The mean scores and standard deviations of all groups for most subtests were similar or a little lower to those reported in the test manual, which supports the use of the test in Israel.

Kizony and colleagues (1998) established standards for Israeli adults and elderly people and compared their results with the data in the manual. Ninety-one participants in three age groups (20–39, 40–69, 70 and older) were tested; all performed the screening and metric parts. One-way ANOVA indicated significant differences between the three groups except for calculations and judgment, and post hoc Scheffe demonstrated that the elderly people achieved significantly lower scores than the other 2 groups. In general, the profile was found to be similar to the American data in the manual, with the exception of differences in 3 of the 11 subtests (Construction, Memory, and Similarities). It is suggested that the data in the manual can be used, but the Israeli standards should be considered as well.

Treatment Goals and Process

The overall purpose of cognitive retraining is to broaden the client's capacity to process information and to be able to transfer and generalize these capacities toward the performance of purposeful activities (Rahmani et al., 1987). Specifically, training is expected to support the client's ability to systematically search for relevant information, as well as to enhance the ability to register, retain, and retrieve this information through strategies that can be generalized into task performance.

The main goal of cognitive training is to enable the client to become independent in all aspects of daily life. By independence, we are referring not only to the capability of performing different given tasks well but also to be able to choose and manipulate the environment to suit one's needs and abilities, such that the individual can adapt and be productive within a given environment. In other words, clients are taught that, before they attempt to act, they must first learn to evaluate a given task or situation with respect to its complexity and the variety of ways they can act on it, to become aware of their abilities with respect to the performance of the task, and to use internal and external feedback, so that they can act in the most appropriate manner. In this context, the ability to choose refers to our ability to evaluate our strengths and weaknesses and to be aware of the ways through which we can improve our performance to achieve success and protect ourselves from failure. Under normal circumstances, we usually choose to act according to what we know we can do.

The rationale behind cognitive retraining is that, through learning and experience, we can improve our ability to evaluate and become aware of our abilities and thus avoid entering into situations that may be beyond our capabilities. That is, the goal of cognitive retraining is to improve the client's metacognitive abilities. Following *International Classification of Functioning, Disability, and Health* terminology (World Health Organization, 2001), *cognition* is a body function that enables us to live independently and according to our abilities. It is composed of basic cognitive skills and higher-level cognitive functions of awareness of our cognitive abilities and executive functioning and is developed through learning and experience.

Thus far, what we have described represents the primary treatment goals that we strive to achieve in our clients. The specific goals of cognitive intervention include techniques to enhance and strengthen first those cognitive abilities that remain intact or are at least stronger than others. As mentioned previously, when brain damage occurs, not all cognitive functions are equally affected. Thus, by strengthening those areas of cognitive ability that remain intact, we create a basis for new and improved cognitive strategies.

The creation of alternative cognitive strategies represents another goal of intervention. Alternative strategies refer to different patterns, or ways of receiving and accumulating information. Training the client to use these alternative strategies can enable him or her to systematically perceive, process, and act according to all available relevant information. In using alternative strategies, clients acquire the ability to decide what information is most relevant given the specific circumstance and to act accordingly so as to solve problems in new and different ways. Achieving such goals can lead to the creation of new functional patterns that can result in the acquisition of a different behavioral cognitive structure, which in turn can improve the client's functional performance.

Treatment Methods

The treatment process is composed of several phases as described above, beginning with assessment. The second phase is treatment through various methods, the choice of which depend on the client's status: (a) enhancing remaining abilities, (b) remedial cognitive-training strategies, (c) learning strategies, and (d) procedural strategies. The next section outlines these methods and provides case and group treatment examples.

Enhancing Remaining Abilities

The second phase of the intervention process involves the enhancement of the client's abilities to perform various tasks, which then forms a basis for developing new strategies. Once the client's ability to perform specific tasks has improved, it is important to make the client aware of his or her improved capabilities. Given the fact that, at the beginning stages of treatment, most clients find themselves in a very complicated and frustrating situation, the ability to experience and be aware of success can be instrumental in increasing their motivation and in enhancing the client–therapist bond.

As was mentioned previously, it is important to determine the goals of the client and the client's family prior to the specific determination of a detailed cognitive treatment plan. However, in certain circumstances it also is important to consult with the medical staff before prioritizing treatment goals to learn which daily living tasks they consider to be more urgent or crucial for the client to be able to perform. Usually, these refer to basic activities of daily living (BADL). In such cases, the client should first be trained to perform these specific tasks before the cognitive-training protocol is initiated.

BADL training should proceed according to the client's abilities in the here and now. It can be done through remedial or procedural training, according to the therapist's judgment as to which is preferable given the specific circumstances of the client and the treatment environment. People generally tend to automatically generate personalized routines for performing BADL. Often a client is under great pressure to be able to regain the ability to eat, dress, and bathe independently before hospital discharge and to generalize those skills on his or her return home. The therapist can help the client create new routines in the performance of those tasks based on his or her current abilities and in the context of his or her immediate environment. If environmental adaptations are needed to support task performance, then the client will be dependent on these human or physical adaptations to perform this task However, as the client responds to therapy and his or her cognitive functioning improves, these adaptations may no longer be required, resulting in independent performance.

Remedial Cognitive Training Strategies

The next phase of the intervention process involves the enhancement of the client's existing cognitive abilities through the development of improved cognitive strategies. First, it is vital that we determine which of the client's disabilities stem from the primary injury incurred and which of them represent secondary sequel of the injury. It is crucial that we treat the primary disabilities first because they represent the basis of the problem. Once we deal with the primary disabilities, many of the secondary problems will diminish as treatment progresses.

Cognitive training is structured according to different levels, each of which is characterized by the amount and complexity of information to be processed. Within each level the client is trained through strategies that are specifically suitable to him or her and to the particular training level. These new strategies are adapted according to the client's abilities and general performance rather than according to specific cognitive areas, and they are devised to enhance the client's ability to perceive, process, evaluate, and perform various tasks. Furthermore, these strategies form the basis for a functional scheme through which the client can develop the skill to handle increasingly more and more complex tasks as prerequisite training for the complex tasks he or she needs or wants to perform in daily life.

At each level, the client first needs to internalize the cognitive strategies so that he or she can manipulate them through the use of various modalities. Once the client has accomplished this, the therapist then teaches him or her to adapt these strategies to suit his or her real-life activities.

Specifically, the client first receives training in specific strategies to improve impaired cognitive functioning that are based on his or her intact cognitive skills. This training generally occurs in the occupational therapy department and involves the use of specially designed tools and manipulatives, much like it occurs in a laboratory environment. Once clients learn to use the strategies well enough so that they can use them with a variety of materials, they are instructed on ways to transfer this knowledge to real-life situations, first through performance of ADLs in the hospital environment and then later in the home. As a result of this treatment process, the client should be able to integrate the various newly learned strategies into schematic patterns and, finally, into a new functional behavioral pattern.

One of the most common problems that results from brain injury relates to impaired attentional abilities. In general, clients with TBI have difficulty focusing attention, maintaining concentration on given tasks or situations, and dividing their attention among various stimuli. Attention underlies our ability to function throughout the spectrum of life's activities. To develop an appropriate strategy for treating attentional problems, it is important to use the modality most suitable for the specific client, be it visual, auditory, thinking, memory, or executive-function components.

In general, training commences at a level in which the client is able to cope with the amount of information needed and the complexity of the task, yet still regard it as challenging. The client is trained to use specific strategies to perform skills relating to different areas of cognitive function, such as visual perception, visuomotor organization, or thinking operations. For example, within the area of visual perception, performance can be enhanced through learning a strategy for systematic and efficient scanning. To accomplish this, we begin with paper-and-pencil exercises in which the client is asked to scan letters, numbers, or figures from one side of the page to the other or, alternatively, from the top of the page to the bottom. Next, we add pictures with gradually increasing amounts of information and ask the patient to describe what she or he sees and then, if it contains information that is either incomplete or not completely clear, to create a hypothesis about what is in the picture. Later we use the same strategy to have the client attempt to find a number, word, or figure in his or her room, within the hospital, in the phone book, and so forth.

This strategy also will form the basis for searching for information when working on improving thinking operation strategies, like flexibility or planning, and for searching for information in academic texts or in complicated situations, which underlies thinking operations. The next step in this process is to add strategies to help the client identify the main ideas, exceptions, and hierarchical order of the gathered data and to organize this information. Finally, the client is trained in strategies to be used for operations such as classification, planning, using feedback, optional thinking, and the ability to evaluate outcomes. Intervention that includes the whole spectrum of these strategies will not be appropriate for all clients, but these are some of the strategies that are important to enhancing the thinking operations and executive functions that underlie the ability to function in areas such as academic performance.

By training the client to improve his or her attentional abilities through the use of activities related to different cognitive areas, we also enrich the client's experience. In addition, the use of a variety of didactic tools that relate to different cognitive skill areas allows the therapist to provide the client with "neutral materials." Neutral materials are especially important when training clients at the level of developing new strategies, as this allows them to focus on the new strategy without having to confront familiar material that, because they may have performed differently at the same task in the past, can trigger comparisons between past and present performance. Furthermore, neutral tasks are changeable and contain no specific or personal significance, thus reducing the potential for distraction or frustration.

Once clients demonstrate that they have internalized the new strategies, we begin training them to perform familiar tasks and lead them to make the transfer to other tasks. To clarify, we refer to the example of attention training. Training begins by addressing the client's ability to focus attention on a variety of tasks that require the use of different types of cognitive abilities, gradually increasing the difficulty and speed requirements of performance. Once the client demonstrates that he or she can use the strategy well, we begin to introduce tasks that he or she had performed previously.

In the next phase of treatment we introduce complex tasks that require the client to integrate different strategies for gradually increasing durations of time. During this phase, the client begins the process of transferring newly acquired strategies to the performance of daily, work, or academic life skills. The time to initiate this phase varies from client to client. Usually, it is begun after the completion of the acute rehabilitation phase, once the client has progressed and is in a phase of "Plato." Plato is an expression that refers to a client's cognitive abilities; it does not imply that he or she will not progress further over time, given appropriate treatment. If the client has made meaningful progress, is aware of his or her abilities and has learned to implement compensatory strategies, he or she will generally be able to deal with new and unfamiliar situations.

Although the process is not always smooth or easy and may require extended periods of time, nevertheless, at this stage the client should be able to use his or her newly acquired strategies to develop new behavioral patterns. The more clients practice the use of these strategies in a variety of situations, the more their awareness increases and their ability to use these behavioral patterns to cope with unfamiliar situations improves. The end result of the treatment is the integration of the different learned strategies into schematic patterns and finally into a new functional behavioral system.

Group Therapy for Improving Attention Abilities

At the Loewenstein Rehabilitation Hospital, we conduct a therapeutic group treatment for clients who have experienced TBI designed to improve their attention abilities in everyday life activities. The group focuses on improving a basic cognitive component: attention, which is essential for the performance of any activity in any occupational area, whether it be IADL, work, education, or leisure. The training methods implemented are derived from a variety of day-to-day living activities, including listening to news

Case Example 4.1. Remedial Strategies Training for Spatial Neglect

M. is a 56-year-old man, married with three children, a professor in economics, and a senior academic university staff member. During one of the research meetings abroad he experienced a CVA with right temporal intracerebral hemorrhage. M. underwent surgical craniotomy for evacuation of the hematoma. Subsequently, he suffered from mild left hemiparesis, cognitive disturbances, and suspected left hemineglect. A month after the accident, he returned to Israel and was hospitalized at Loewenstein Rehabilitation Hospital.

ASSESSMENT

Motor function: Slight left-sided weakness, hands both functional, able to walk short distances.
ADL: Required complete assistance for dressing and grooming.
Cognitive functioning: Evaluated through the LOTCA.

- *Orientation:* Able to report personal details; orientation of place and time partially intact.
- *Visual perception:* Basically intact, although had difficulty with unclear information such as embedded figures.
- *Spatial perception:* Had great difficulties discriminating directions on his body and within outside space.
- *Praxis:* Good performance on all subtests (imitation, ideamotor, ideational praxis).
- *Visual–motor organization:* Failed all subtests, appeared to have difficulty scanning within the left space.
- *Thinking operations:* Performed well on all subtests, but performance was better with auditory administration of the items.
- *Attention and concentration difficulties:* Apparent.

Because the clinical picture clearly indicated left hemineglect, the BIT was administered to evaluate its severity. The result of the BIT was 40 out of 146, demonstrating severe spatial neglect.

TREATMENT

Our treatment protocol for neglect is composed of 6 stages and includes 3 changeable parameters: the physical environment, the complexity of the task, and the amount of therapist intervention. The treatment is based on a combination of two theoretical models: Kinsbourn's model, which emphasizes the type of stimuli and encourages head movements, moving the stimulus gradually from right to left in the spatial field, and Posner's attention approach, which emphasizes the intended transfer of attention and structured cues to shift attention within the spatial field.

Stage 1: The treatment was conducted in a specially modified room with minimal visual or auditory distractions, during the morning hours when arousal level was higher. We began with a short basic scanning task, which included one type of stimulus (figures), scanning one row, with clear figures, large intervals, and only few items appearing on the page. The paper was placed in the patients' right field of vision; scanning was to be performed from left to right. An obvious cue was used to mark the left border of the task. M. was asked to move his gaze systematically to the left, and he was given uniform, consistent instructions to help him learn to scan the entire spectrum of targeted stimuli.

Stage 2: The physical conditions remained the same as in Stage 1. The task was gradually moved from the right side to the middle of the field and for increasing periods of time. In addition, the stimulus content was increased, changing in density and variety, with more rows added to the task. The same instructions were given, the patient was encouraged to repeat them to himself, and immediate feedback was provided.

Stage 3: The task was moved gradually from the middle to the left field. The task difficulty was increased by increasing the amount and variety of stimuli (e.g., numbers, letters, figures) in an unorganized format on the page. The patient was asked to mark the cues appearing at the border of the left field. Once again, the patient was asked to repeat to himself the instructions for moving his gaze, which have him systematically scan the rows from left to right.

Stage 4: The physical conditions of the task environment were changed by moving the patient to a more open space with more distractions. The task difficulty was increased by increasing the number and complexity of stimuli and by adding more distracters. In addition, the treatment time was increased, and the cues on the left borders were gradually removed. The patient was asked to self-instruct using self-talk or his inner voice, and he was encouraged to check his work and verbalize his mistakes.

Stage 5: At this stage of treatment, the patient was able to systematically scan and had learned the strategies needed to overcome his neglect. The treatment progressed to the use of more complex tasks in which the learned strategies supported performance, such as organizing and performing tasks of constructional praxis, finding his way around his room and the hospital, reading a route on a map, writing free text without the use of cues on the left side of the page, and reading and summarizing text. At this point another BIT test was administered, and M. achieved 130 out of 146, indicating no impact of neglect on this test. He used the learned strategies well and performed within a reasonable response time.

Stage 6: Treatment was modified from lab treatment to real-life situations such as scanning a big unfamiliar room or place, planning a street route and crossing only on the pedestrian crossing, becoming oriented within a house and a shopping mall, watching TV, and working on a computer (with relevant materials and not just exercises).

At this stage, M. was an outpatient in our day treatment center. He was fully aware of his neglect and had learned the strategies well. He was able to read the newspaper in

(continued)

Case Example 4.1. Remedial Strategies Training for Spatial Neglect *(Continued)*

a reasonable amount of time and enjoy it. At home, he was able to prepare light meals (despite his wife's complaints that he leaves the kitchen messy and disorganized, which he improved on with time). He gradually returned to his work at the university. At first he had an assistant type for him and prepare his papers; however, after 2 months he began doing these tasks himself, and by the beginning of the second semester he returned to his teaching duties.

M. reported that he is doing well, although he is aware that he sometimes dozes on the table or lectern. After 1½ years he had returned to full duty, resuming his research and even traveling abroad accompanied by his wife. The one thing he was still not able to do was drive. M. had to rely on taxis or his wife to drive him where he needed to go. What prevented him from driving at this stage was that he was unable to respond quickly

enough to unexpected stimuli on his left field. Otherwise, however, he conducted his life in a manner similar to how it was before he had the stroke. It was obvious that M. had assimilated the learned strategies he had been taught very well and that his neglect was not interfering with his everyday life.

reports, listening to music, handling messages recorded on an answering machine, and so forth.

Group treatment is offered in addition to daily individual therapy sessions, in which clients are taught strategies for coping with their attention deficits. The purpose of the group is to assimilate the strategies that they were taught and to facilitate their ability to functionally and independently implement them in activities that are part of their daily routine in the home environment, to which they return to shortly after the hospitalization period is over.

Rationale

Park and Ingles (2001) performed a meta-analysis (integrating the results of 30 research studies) examining the effectiveness of attention rehabilitation on participants with TBI. They found that acquired deficits of attention are treatable and that the importance of treating attention is widely recognized by rehabilitation professionals. Attention retraining typically requires participants to complete a series of repetitive exercises in which they respond to visual and auditory stimuli (e.g., they may be asked to press a buzzer when they hear the number 3). The results of the meta-analysis indicated that direct retraining of attention produced only small, statistically nonsignificant improvements in performance, whereas the few studies that examined the outcomes of treatment to remediate performance of skills requiring attention showed statistically significant improvements and a larger effect with respect to the transfer of performance to daily living. They found that the most rewarding programs will likely be those that focus on training skills that

also are of great functional importance to the individual participants.

Goals of the Group Treatment

The first focus of the treatment is improving functional attention, with simultaneous training in various specific components of attention. These include focused attention, sustained attention (concentration), alternating attention, and divided attention and the activation of these attentional abilities through both visual and auditory channels. In addition, treatment incorporates the use of attention distracters, such as external distractions (noise, temperature, scents) and internal distractions (thoughts, fatigue, pain, need for a cigarette).

The second goal is to increase clients' awareness of their attention deficits. According to Toglia and Kirk (2000), awareness of a disability is defined as the individual's ability to recognize his or her deficits or illness and its ramifications on safe and independent functioning. Awareness is necessary to sustain active effort, motivation, and the persistence required for rehabilitation. Awareness has been found to be related to attainment of rehabilitation goals and to employment outcomes.

As part of the process of achieving these goals, clients are provided with theoretical knowledge about attention, its components, and their impact on human function, with examples from daily life. Clients are encouraged to express what they perceive their attention problems to be and how these problems may affect their lives. Typically, participants present difficulties in reading, watching television, social functions (such as following a conversation), and computer use.

Case Example 4.2.   Remedial Strategies Training for Thinking Operations

I. is a 29-year-old woman with a BA in social work. She is single and living alone independently. She has right-handed motor dominance.

On February 14, 2003, she was involved in a car accident in which she was severely injured and accepted in the emergency room with Glasgow Coma Scale–3 (the scale ranges from 1—no response to 15—full consciousness; a rating of 3 indicates the patient opens his or her eyes to pain and speech). She was diagnosed as having TBI with multiple trauma and left hemiparesis. She was admitted for a full rehabilitation program at Loewenstein Rehabilitation Hospital on March 3, 2004.

ASSESSMENT

Motor function: She was independently mobile, with slight left-sided weakness, but both hands were functional.

Cognitive functions: The results of the LOTCA assessment indicated that she had no difficulty in orientation, visual and spatial perception, or praxis and visual motor organization. Her main problem was in thinking operations, primarily with respect to shifting and rationale sequencing. She demonstrated severe attention deficits and was easily distracted. She was highly motivated, and although she was not aware of her cognitive deficits and their possible functional consequences, she was fully engaged in treatment.

Our initial focus was to improve her thinking operations, with special emphasis on the mental ability to shift between tasks.

TREATMENT

The treatment protocol began with strategies of classification: scanning data, hierarchical ordering, and grouping according to different criteria. At first she was given tasks with simple, uncomplicated, concrete materials, such as everyday objects; then gradually we increased the task de-

mands with respect to the amount of information involved and its complexity. I. was attentive and a good learner. We added strategies for monitoring her work, deriving conclusions and using feedback. However, during the treatment other difficulties arouse. She had the tendency to work fast, be impulsive, and not review her work well enough. Difficulties of attention and being easily distracted were detected. Those problems became more meaningful as the complexity of the tasks increased.

We administered the RBMT for evaluating her memory process. She scored 23 out of 24, indicating that her memory was intact. She did not have memory problems in her daily life, although sometimes she did not remember things like meetings or messages, but that was more the result of her attention and distractibility deficits.

We taught her strategies for monitoring her work, such as checking it at every stage of the task, asking questions (at first aloud, and with time using her inner voice) about how she would implement her plan for performance of the task, and so forth. In this way, we hoped to contain her impulsivity and for her to become engaged and focused on the task and to be less distracted. Aside from her cognitive problems, she demonstrated behavioral problems as well. She became dependent on the staff for approval at every step of her work, and she regressed and became childish.

In parallel with the cognitive treatment, we began to work by carefully reflecting on how to modify her behavior. Instead of responding with immediate approval for a task she had performed, we trained her to judge her work for herself and then to describe what she had done well and what she could have done differently and why. Once she made progress using neutral materials, we applied the same strategies of evaluation, monitoring, and using internal and external feedback for when she performed real-life tasks and for monitoring her behavior.

At this point, 3 months from the initiation of treatment, we administered the BADS to evaluate her executive functions. She scored 17 out of 24, indicating that her performance was about average. Despite these results, her ability to monitor her performance and behavior were limited. She showed no problems in initiation or planning, but she found it difficult to implement her plan step by step, use feedback, and generate alternatives. These difficulties were especially apparent when she was confronted with novel materials and situations, at which time we observed her take one step back by responding impulsively and not planning her actions. Her attention problems were most significant when the task or situation were less structured. We worked on those deficits by having her apply insight and come up with alternative solutions. I. was able to implement the strategies learned to different situations at a similar level of task demands. Every time she confronted a novel or complex situation, she needed us to intervene by reintroducing the strategies she needed to use and monitoring her work. On April 1, 2004, she was advanced to our day treatment center, attending a daily treatment program created for her and learning to apply her skills to tasks outside the hospital. She continues to receive treatment twice a week in her community and began attending a course on religious studies.

She has resumed her independent daily living despite living alone and far from her family. She has no problem at housework, including financial tasks such as paying bills, banking, and dealing with bureaucracy. Recently she returned to work as a social worker in her community, with close supervision of a fellow professional. She still has episodic recurrences of impulsive behavior and attentional slips, but these have become less frequent as she progresses in treatment and continues to succeed in her everyday life.

Group Format

The group treatment consists of approximately eight structured meetings, but the number of meetings is adjusted according to the progression of the group and the cognitive level of the participants. It is a closed group, composed of six inpatients with TBI, ages 18 and older. Members are all clients approaching discharge from the hospital. The participants return to their homes on weekends and holidays.

Principles of the Group Treatment

From neutral exercises to functional training: The first few sessions are based on remedial auditory attention exercises, which are almost without functional significance. In this way, the participants come to understand and actualize the theoretical knowledge they acquired on attention and its components by the performance of activities that have no personal meaning and are, therefore, easier to comprehend. Gradually, the participants are exposed to activities with more functional significance, taken from daily life. For example, in one session clients practice various telephone tasks, such as listening to messages and announcements on answering machines and computerized voice mail and writing down specific pieces of information, such as the opening hours of a bank or a museum.

From concrete to abstract: Each session focuses on a certain category of activities, in which training begins with simple, concrete tasks and then progresses to more abstract tasks. For example, the third session usually focuses on songs. First, the clients are asked to perform tasks that require them to keep track of quantitative information, such as the amount of times they hear a certain pair of words. As the session progresses, the clients are asked to perform activities that require both auditory attention and higher thought processes, such as forming conclusions, culminating in a group analysis of the meaning of a song.

Increase in the level of difficulty: Both within each session and from one session to the next, the activities become more difficult with respect to the length of time and the load of information that must be processed.

Adaptation of the exercises and activities to the cognitive level of the patients: The groups are designed to be homogeneous with respect to the characteristics of group members, so that participants within each group are on similar levels of cognitive ability. In this way the activity requirements can be altered uniformly to suit the group participants. However, activities are sometimes changed or added according to participants' expressed needs or wishes.

Basic Structure of the Individual Group Sessions

The basic structure of the individual group sessions involves the following tasks and activities (listed by session number):

1. A short video is shown, followed by a group discussion on the task requirements of watching a video and a theoretical explanation of the components of attention.
2. Patients perform remedial auditory attention exercises, tasks based on repetitive recorded and written instructions.
3. Participants are asked to retrieve information from recorded songs.
4. Participants answer questions that are based on short recorded texts, verbally and in writing.
5. Participants perform a variety of telephone tasks such as finding a number in a phone book, recall of a phone message, and so forth.
6. Participants listen to radio and watch television advertisements, from which they are asked to retrieve relevant information.
7. Participants listen to radio and television newscasts and then answer related questions and list the news highlights.

Results and Summary

The improvement of attention abilities has great importance in the rehabilitation of clients with TBI. According to Parente and Herrmann (1996), training attention through functional activities that arouse the client's interest has a greater chance of being transferred and implemented into daily life. Thus, the rehabilitation of attention through real-life activities gives a clearer indication of the effectiveness of the therapy and the quality of transference to daily living. During group sessions, the participants process their experiences from their weekend vacations at home, enabling the therapists to observe whether transference has occurred from the therapeutic environment to the natural environment. It was found that the higher their level of awareness of their attention deficits, the greater the participants' ability was to implement the principles that were taught, thus improving their integration back into society.

Learning Strategies

Kandel (1998) stated that the ability to learn serves as the foundation for treatment and the individual's ability to change. There are various ways to learn, but first we discuss declarative academic learning. The basic components of learning include cognitive and the higher cognitive functions abilities. Stuss (1999, cited in Marlowe, 2000) suggested that cognitive skills develop before metacognitive skills do. He defined *cognitive skills* as "the learning of how." Cognitive skills are supported by information-processing strategies, which include how to perceive, gather, organize, and accumulate information for future use. In fact, information-processing strategies represent organizing strategies considered to be the most effective components that contribute to learning. The cognitive abilities needed for information processing are based on strategies that enhance the ability to perform objective, systematic, consistent, and abstract yet flexible thinking (Flavell, Miller, & Miller, 2002). Efficient learning requires the development of strategies for understanding and perceiving important and meaningful information. Information-processing ability depends in part on thinking operations, the main components of which are

1. *Optional–creative thinking:* The ability to be aware of various alternatives, even if not all of them are immediately applicable.
2. *Thinking processes based on assumptions:* The ability to consider what is and is not possible, as well as which alternatives are good and which are better, in any situation.
3. *Future planning:* The ability to plan ahead for the future.
4. *Metacognitive abilities:* The ability to think about our own thoughts and cognitive processes and to be aware of them.
5. *Self-criticism:* The ability to think beyond the boundaries of time, or abstract thinking.

We have drawn a model for intervention designed to systematically develop learning strategies. The first step of this model involves the development of categorization skills, which refer to one's ability to gather information and to conceptualize it. To do so, the client must first acquire strategies of efficient and systematic scanning and the ability to recognize which of the features of this are the same or different, main or subordinate. Once this has been accomplished, the individual needs to acquire the ability to form a hierarchical order of the information gathered so as to decide which information is needed first. This is what occurs if we examine the features of objects that we wish to categorize.

As was mentioned previously, to relay the significance and components of categorization or classification, training begins with the examination of neutral everyday objects. Only when the client has acquired classification strategies can we introduce training with texts or other more complicated material. Another important strategy used for the teaching of categorization is to train the client to shift flexibly between groups of objects, then between different possible solutions to a given problem until, ultimately, the client's acquired ability for flexible thinking will help him or her develop the ability to choose.

To categorize, one also must be able to identify mistakes. Therefore, when learning categorization, clients are also taught strategies for the development of the precision and self-inspection this skill requires. To deal with academic material, the client must first develop the ability to ask preliminary questions regarding the presented text, recognize his or her main goals, choose the best strategies and, finally, integrate the desired information. Sequencing is another meaningful and important skill needed for learning. To teach the client how to sequence, we must use several remediation strategies: forming a chronological sequence, understanding cause and effect, consistency, repetition of rules, organization of material in different ways, induction, and deduction.

In addition, the client is taught to develop awareness of and strategies for planning, prediction, the use of feedback (including self-inspection of performance), self-regulation, intention, planning, and consideration of his or her performance. These strategies for categorization, sequencing, and organization allow the client to learn and memorize information in a better and more efficient way. By adding strategies of awareness and executive functions like self-inspection, initiation, planning, judging, and use of feedback, we provide the client with the flexibility he or she needs to make wise choices (see Chapter 1 for further discussion of awareness and executive functions).

For example, we apply these types of intervention to low-achieving students, according to their abilities, to broaden their capacity to learn. To investigate the contribution of these interventions, we designed a treatment consisting of 14 sessions (following the assessment of the participants). The treatment consisted of 3 primary content areas: categorization, sequencing, and integration. The sequence of the treatment sessions was tailored individually for each student; however, the general content is described in Table 4.2. Currently, we are conducting a study with 14–15-year-old students in a regular school to

T A B L E 4 . 2 . Sequence of Treatment Sessions

First Stage: Categorization—Strategies of . . .

1st session: *Gathering information and conceptualization*
Efficient and systematic scanning
Precision and self-inspection
Awareness

2nd session: *Exception, main and subordinate*
  (using different channels)
Emphasis of the main ideas in the text
Identification of mistakes
Self-questioning throughout a given text

3rd session: *The principles of classification*
Emotional reference
Flexibility–shifting
Initiation in choice of strategy

4th session: *The skill of classification*
Different methods of classification
Combination of different methods of classification
Summary of (short) texts

5th session: *Classification*
Practice of contents and learned strategies in academic material

Second Stage: Sequence—Strategies of . . .

6th session: *Chronological sequence*
Cause and effect
Directed search of contexts in the text
Planning, prediction, and feedback

7th session: *Regularity/ruling*
Development of standpoint/perspective
Organization—flow diagrams
Self-inspection of performance

8th session: *Thinking operation/thinking process*
Analysis of the problem—expression of opinion of the material
Self-regulation—intention planning and assessment
  of the activity

9th session: *Conclusion/concluding*
Concluding—induction and deduction

Third Stage: Integration and Reasoning—Strategies of . . .

10th Session: *Combination of channels* (visual and auditory)
One- and two-dimensional tables

11th Session: *Problem solving*
Problem—strategy
Choice of strategy—inspection—change of strategy

12th session: *Memory*
Methods of improving memory

13th session: *Integration*
Organization and conclusion/concluding

14th session: *Asking questions*
Types of questions for academic material

---

evaluate the effect of this intervention on their academic achievement.

Procedural Strategies

Some clients, such as those who have incurred severe frontal damage, may be incapable of using specific visual, spatial, thinking, or memory-based remedial strategies. Nevertheless, these clients can still be trained to perform routine daily tasks in a specifically adapted environment through the use of procedural strategies. This refers to training in which the client is taught all of the component procedures needed to perform specific tasks repeatedly until they are transformed into a routine behavior pattern.

For example, to teach such clients to perform basic ADLs, they are trained in each of the individual component procedures, one at a time. The client is first trained in one procedure, such as to use the toilet on awakening in the morning. Once this is accomplished, another procedure, such as brushing teeth, is added. Gradually the therapist teaches the client to perform additional procedures, such as washing hands and face, combing hair, and then dressing, all in a consistent and repeatable sequence.

This type of treatment is time consuming, but it will enable clients to perform the entire routine on their own. As a result of this type of treatment, the client's performance will depend on his or her ability to perform the procedures in the exact fashion in which they were taught, with the environment remaining constant and familiar. If the environment is changed or something changes in the situation, the client will be unable to cope with these changes or perform the tasks successfully. Thus, although the client is capable of performing these tasks, we cannot say that real independence has been achieved because he or she is completely dependent on the particular environment in which the tasks were taught. In this context, environment refers not only to the physical environment, such as work or home, but also to the human environment, including the caretakers who reinforce the client's procedures and routines and thereby enable the maintenance of performance ability.

In procedural strategy training, a routine is composed of a sequence of several procedural strategies, whereas a behavior is composed of several routines. The more a behavior is repeated, the more it is reinforced until gradually it becomes almost automatic and more efficient. Procedural training can even be used to train a client to perform specific work-related tasks, provided they are concrete and can be divided neatly into individual procedural components. If so, the client is taught how to perform each component of the task so that eventually he or she can perform it in its entirety.

For example, we discuss the treatment that we provided to M.G., a client who had incurred severe bilateral frontal damage. After 2 years of therapy, we successfully trained him to perform specific tasks in a hospital laboratory. Since then, he has continued to work at the same laboratory, performing the same job, for more than 25 years. He is satisfied with his work, as are his colleagues and supervisors, because he continues to perform his job well.

In another case example of the effectiveness of our intervention, we present S.M., a 23-year-old woman who had been in a coma for approximately 4 months following a severe car accident. S.M. had diffuse traumatic brain damage with severe cognitive deficits that resulted from substantial damage to the frontal lobe. She received procedural training for the purpose of retraining functional performance. Retraining of good performance in basic ADLs required approximately a year of therapy. S.M. was trained to wash and dress herself, which she was able to perform well; however, she needed someone to cue her as to when certain tasks should be performed, such as when it was time to take a bath and when she should change from a soiled to a fresh washcloth. S.M. was also trained in tasks such as how to prepare light meals and how to operate a washing machine in a constant daily and weekly schedule.

At her discharge from the hospital, her mother was instructed to arrange S.M.'s closet with different sets of outfits, each designated for a specific day of the week. The mother was instructed to remind S.M. that each set was to be worn for one day only and then to put it into the wash. In addition, she was to remind her daughter to wake up daily at a certain preset time and to maintain an unchangeable daily and weekly schedule.

As long as her schedule remained consistent and the situation remained constant, S.M. succeeded in her activities and attained a degree of independence. However, in the face of unexpected occurrences, such as when she dropped a container of milk on the floor while preparing a cup of coffee, she had no idea how to respond and had to ask her mother to intervene.

S.M. also was given training so that she could work at a day center operating a computer. First, she was trained how to cross the streets to get to the day center, mainly by crossing only where there was a traffic light, which she succeeded to do within a few weeks. At the day center itself she received the training she needed to operate the computer. Her family arranged for S.M. to be given a data-entry task on a specific computer in one of the day center offices. She was trained in a specific program until she was able to perform the task, but she still required assistance every time one job was completed and new material was introduced. After 3 years of intensive treatment she achieved this level of performance, although she remained entirely dependent on her family and on her unchangeable routines.

Despite the limitations, through our intervention she had attained a certain quality of life that provided her with the ability to appreciate that she was able to work like everybody else and that she too went to work at an office every day. In addition, given unchanging circumstances, she was able to independently perform ADLs. Currently, S.M. attends meetings with other clients with TBI, where she reports that she is more or less satisfied with her life.

TREATMENT EFFECTIVENESS/ EVIDENCE-BASED PRACTICE

What is cognitive rehabilitation? To examine the evidence supporting the effectiveness of cognitive rehabilitation, we refer to the accepted definitions found in the literature. For example, according to the National Institutes of Health (1998) consensus statement issued by the developmental panel on people with TBI, "the goals of rehabilitation of individuals with cognitive deficits are to enhance the person's capacity to process and interpret information and to improve the person's ability to function in all aspects of family and community life" (p. 978). Robertson (1999) defined *cognitive rehabilitation* as follows:

> the systematic use of instruction and structured experience to manipulate the functioning of cognitive systems such as to improve the quality or quantity of cognitive processing in a particular domain. . . . The domain of cognitive rehabilitation is that of cognition, namely attention, memory, perception, gnosis, praxis, reasoning, and executive control. (p. 703)

Sohlberg and Mateer (1989) originally defined cognitive rehabilitation as "the way to increase or improve individual's capacity to process and use incoming information so as to allow increased functioning in everyday life" (p. 3). However, in 2001, they reconsidered this definition, stating that the use of the term resulted in too narrow a focus on remediation or compensation. Instead, they suggested using the term *rehabilitation of individuals with cognitive impairment,* which better captures the emphasis on the individuals that have, and always will be, the target of cognitive rehabilitation. It was their belief that this revised conceptualization could broaden the scope of such intervention to include a much wider range of targeted components and techniques.

Meta-analysis and Reviews on Evidence-Based Cognitive Rehabilitation

Cicerone and colleagues (2000) published a thorough analysis of 171 (out of 655) studies on cognitive rehabilitation. Their analysis included a qualification of the inclusion criteria used by the various researchers. They classified the studies into three levels of evidence according to the strength of their methodology (29 in Class I, 35 in Class II, 107 in Class III). They concluded that support exists for some techniques related to the remediation of language in patients with left-hemisphere strokes; perception in patients with right-hemisphere strokes; and for the remediation of attention, memory, functional communication, and executive functions in patients with TBI. On the basis of the strength of the evidence, the authors developed a three-tiered system of treatment recommendations to guide clinical decision making. The system refers to *practice standards, practice guidelines,* and *practice options.* For example, remediation of attention is recommended as a practice guideline for recovery of patients with moderate to severe TBI or stroke patients in the post-acute stage, but it was not found to significantly contribute to their recovery in the acute stage.

In contrast, they recommended as a practice standard training in visual scanning to improve compensation for visual neglect after right-hemisphere stroke on the basis of the high level of evidence found for its effectiveness in the treatment of visual–spatial deficits. In addition, the evidence demonstrated that training on more complex tasks appeared to enhance performance and facilitate generalization to other functional areas as well. Furthermore, as a result of this analysis, they stated that, although computer-based intervention on its own was not found to be effective for people with multiple areas of cognitive impairments, it could be recommended as a beneficial technique if included as part of a multimodal intervention.

Further support for these recommendations is provided in an European Federation of Neurological Societies Task Force report (Cappa et al., 2003), which states that cognitive rehabilitation is beneficial for the treatment of neglect and apraxia after stroke and recommends attention training for patients with TBI in the post-acute stage and memory compensatory training for patients with mild amnesia. Both reviews emphasized the importance of rigorous single-subject methodology in this area of research because the randomized controlled trials methodology is difficult to implement. Furthermore, most of the studies reviewed did not investigate outcomes at the disability level and long-term functional gains.

A recent systematic review of occupational therapy effectiveness in stroke rehabilitation included 32 studies that were divided into 7 categories of intervention (Steultjens et al., 2003). According to this review, comprehensive occupational therapy intervention demonstrated a small significant effect size for ADL, IADL, and social participation. Evidence for specific interventions was limited, with only a few studies examining the effectiveness of training in cognitive functions, although efficacy was revealed in visual–perceptual skills training similar to what had been reported in the general reviews discussed previously. However, the category of training of skills is confusing as it focuses on strategy training to overcome cognitive dysfunctions, which is part of cognitive rehabilitation. Unfortunately these studies used weak methodology and thus did not show significant results. The authors emphasized the need for more research to establish evidence-based occupational therapy intervention.

Studies in Progress

Because unilateral spatial neglect—which accompanies right-hemisphere stroke, resulting in poor rehabilitation outcomes—is one of the most devastating phenomena (Katz et al., 1999), it is vital to determine which intervention methods are optimal for each of the various stages of the condition. Bowen, Lincoln, and Dewey (2003) reviewed the evidence for the efficacy of various treatment methods for unilateral spatial neglect. They concluded that, although there is evidence of improvement according to results of impairment assessment, much less evidence exists for increased functional performance at the disability level. With this in mind, we are currently performing a randomized control trial in which we are comparing the treatment outcome of Phasic Alerting (Robertson, Mattingley, Rorden, & Driver, 1998) during a computer scanning task with the outcome of two alternative treatments in which one control group uses the same scanning task as the experimental group without the auditory alert and a second control group treated primarily through the use of leisure planning without direct cognitive training. In addition, all of the participants receive passive and active limb activation. Outcome measures include pre- and post-treatment and 5-week post-treatment assessments of attention and neglect, as well as functional measures. Recovery is assessed behaviorally as well as through imaging using functional magnetic reasonance imaging (Bar-Haim Erez & Katz, 2003). The results of the comprehensive cognitive-training approach described in this chapter is the gold standard against which the different treatment methods are compared, thus a fourth group that receives the retraining protocol is currently being studied within the same design. Findings of this study will provide valuable evidence for further treatment protocols.

Virtual reality (VR) is another promising new method used in rehabilitation (Rizzo, 2002; Rizzo, Schultheis, Kerns, & Mateer, 2004; Weiss & Katz, in press; Weiss, Kizony, Feintuch, & Katz, in press). Two studies are currently under way in which a new, innovative VR technology treatment method is applied to patients after right-hemisphere stroke with attention and neglect deficits. In the first study, a VR street-crossing program with successively graded levels of difficulty was developed for use on a desktop computer. The VR program is used to train patients to look to the left and scan the entire virtual scene before deciding to cross the street, the same way they would do on a real street (Katz et al., 2004). Actual street crossing is performed and videotaped before and after a 4-week treatment program for the VR group, as well as a control group that receives only basic computer scanning training. It was initially tested on 12 participants, including 6 stroke patients and 6 matched control patients (Naveh, Katz, & Weiss, 2000; Weiss, Naveh, & Katz, 2003). Results indicate that the program is suitable for patients with neurological deficits in terms of both its cognitive and motor demands.

Currently, the program is being used in a controlled clinical trial to train patients with right-hemisphere stroke and unilateral spatial neglect to improve their attention and ability to scan to the left. Measures include standard paper-and-pencil cancellation tests, as well as pre- and post-performance within the virtual environment and during actual street crossing. Initial results from 11 patients who used the virtual environment (VR street test) versus a control group of 8 patients who used non-VR computer-based scanning tasks demonstrated that the scores of both groups improved with respect to the number of correctly cancelled items on the Star Cancellation and Mesulam

symbol cancellation test. However, the VR group completed the tests in significantly less time than the control group, which may be considered to be an indicator of superior performance (Katz et al., 2004). The performance of the VR group in the VR street test showed training effects, as all patients improved in looking to the left, pre–post significant at $p < .05$, and most of them had fewer accidents during the virtual street crossing at posttest, whereas the majority of the control group did not change their performance from pre- to post-test on the VR street test. In the actual street crossing, the VR group improved in the number of times participants looked left, whereas the control group did not. The study continues at this stage with clients in day treatment, for whom it may be more directly relevant.

The Gesture Xtreme video capture VR system has recently been investigated to determine its potential for the remediation of cognitive and motor deficits (Kizony, Katz, & Weiss, 2003). In this system, the individuals see themselves on the screen as in a mirror and control the VR program through their movements. Various programs have been used, and three have been adapted for use in rehabilitation (Kizony et al., 2003). The feasibility of the system was investigated with healthy participants as well as with patients following spinal cord injury and stroke (Kizony, Raz, Katz, Weingarden, & Weiss, 2003).

Kizony and colleagues (2003) described the effects of such treatment on a patient with attention deficits 6 months after a right-hemisphere stroke. During VR treatment he was required to pay attention to the entire visual space and to move his affected arm within the neglected space. The patient played the role of a soccer goalkeeper whose task was to deflect balls that came toward him from all directions. During the game, he saw himself within the virtual environment and received immediate visual and auditory feedback to help him improve his performance. The patient expressed enjoyment and motivation to continue with this kind of treatment. The adaptations applied to these VR environments enable the treatment of visual–spatial attention and unilateral spatial neglect by controlling the direction, number, and color of stimuli and by adding distracters to the scenario (Kizony et al., 2003). A study is now under way to investigate the effect of training with this VR system to remediate attention and unilateral spatial neglect deficits in patients with right-hemisphere stroke, as well as to examine its transfer to daily activities. The study uses few single-subject designs, and outcome measures will include the assessment of attention and neglect, ADL and IADL.

Both the street-crossing environment as well as the video-capture VR system are examples of the application of VR technology in the treatment of stroke patients with attention deficits and unilateral spatial neglect. Whereas the desktop VR system focuses mainly on visual scanning to judge when a street can be safely crossed, the video-capture system combines visual scanning with motor activation and motor planning, all of which have been shown to be components of important rehabilitation goals. The advantage of using VR technology is that it enables clinicians to train patients in a safe environment in which many repetitions can be performed prior to attempting real street crossing. Furthermore, VR is fun for most people at any age and appears to provide patients with strong motivation to become engaged in the treatment process (Kizony et al., 2003).

REVIEW QUESTIONS

1. On which theoretical rationale is the intervention based?
2. What instruments are used for assessment, how are they selected, and how reliable and valid are they?
3. What treatment methods are used? With whom and when are they applied?
4. Think of another case and plan a treatment program based on this model.
5. How strong is the evidence that supports the model?
6. What kind of research is needed to support the treatment methods used?

ACKNOWLEDGMENTS

Many thanks to Dorit Hafner, Mishel Yaakobi, and Roni Barnea, occupational therapists at Loewenstein Rehabilitation Hospital, for their help and contributions to this chapter. Many thanks to Sarina Goldstand, MSc, OTR, from the School of Occupational Therapy, Hebrew University and Hadassah, for her major editorial contribution to this chapter.

REFERENCES

Alderman, N., Burgess, P. W., Knight, C., & Henman, C. (2003). Ecological validity of a simplified version of the multiple errands shopping test. *Journal of the International Neuropsychological Society, 9,* 31–44.

Annes, G., Katz, N., & Cermak, S. A. (1996). Comparison of younger and older healthy adults on the Loewenstein Occupational Therapy Cognitive Assessment. *Occupational Therapy International, 3,* 157–173.

Averbuch, S., & Katz, N. (1991). Age-level standards of the Loewenstein Occupational Therapy Cognitive Assessment (LOTCA). *Israel Journal of Occupational Therapy, Special Issue,* E1–E15.

Bar-Haim Erez, A., & Katz, N. (2003, June). *Treatment effectiveness and recovery pattern of stroke patients with unilateral spatial neglect on functional outcomes.* Paper presented at the American Occupational Therapy Association Conference, Washington, DC.

Bar-Haim Erez, A., & Katz, N. (in press). Cognitive profiles of individuals with dementia and healthy elderly: The Loewenstein Occupational Therapy Cognitive Assessment (LOTCA–G). *Physical and Occupational Therapy in Geriatrics.*

Bourne, L. E., Dominski, R. L., & Loftus, E. F. (1979). *Cognitive processes.* Englewood Cliffs, NJ: Prentice Hall.

Bowen, A., Lincoln, N. B., & Dewey, M. (2003). Cognitive rehabilitation for spatial neglect following stroke (Cochrane review). *The Cochrane Library, 4.*

Cappa, S. F., Benke, T., Clarke, S., Rossi, B., Stemmer, B., & Van-Heugten, C. M. (2003). EFNS guidelines on cognitive rehabilitation: Report of an EFNS task force. *European Journal of Neurology, 10,* 11–23.

Cermak, S. A., Katz, N., McGuire, E., Greenbaum, S., Peralta, C., & Maser-Flanagan, V. (1995). Performance of Americans and Israelis with cerebrovascular accident on the Loewenstein Occupational Therapy Cognitive Assessment (LOTCA). *American Journal of Occupational Therapy, 49,* 500–506.

Cicerone, K. D., Dahlberg, C., Kalmar, K., Langenbahn, D. M., Malec, J. F., Bergquist, T. F., et al. (2000). Evidence-based cognitive rehabilitation: Recommendations for clinical practice. *Archives of Physical Medicine and Rehabilitation, 81,* 1596–1615.

Clark, O., & O'Caroll, R. E. (1998). An examination of the relationship between executive functions, memory, and rehabilitation status in schizophrenia. *Neuropsychological Rehabilitation, 8,* 229–241.

Cockburn, J., & Smith, T. P. (1989). *The Rivermead Behavioral Memory Test supplement 3: Elderly people.* Titchfield, England: Thames Valley Test Company.

De Wall, C., Wilson, B. A., & Baddeley, A. D. (1994). The Extended Rivermead Behavioral Memory Test: A measure of everyday memory performance in normal adults. *Memory, 2,* 149–166.

Dvir, O. (2003). *The Test of Everyday Attention (TEA) in a population following brain injury ages 20–50 in Israel.* Unpublished master's thesis, Hebrew University and Hadassah, Jerusalem.

Dvir, O., Avni, N., Bor, B., Tamir, A., Naveh, Y., & Felzen, B. (2003). Performance profile of the Behavioral Assessment of Dysexecutive Syndrome (BADS) in healthy Israeli population. *Israel Journal of Occupational Therapy, 12,* H207–H223. (In Hebrew; English abstract, p. E139)

Elazar, B., Itzkovich, M., & Katz, N. (1996). *LOTCA–G manual.* Wayne, NJ: Maddak.

Evans, J. J., Chua, S. E., McKenna, P. J., & Wilson, B. A. (1997). Assessment of the dysexecutive syndrome in schizophrenia. *Neuropsychological Medicine, 27,* 635–646.

Flavell, J. H., Miller, P. H., & Miller, S. A. (2002). *Cognitive development* (4th ed.). Upper Saddle River, NJ: Prentice Hall.

Fleming, J., & Strong, J. (1999). A longitudinal study of self-awareness: Functional deficits underestimated by persons with brain injury. *Occupational Therapy Journal of Research, 19,* 3–17.

Fleming, J. M., Strong, J., & Ashton, R. (1996). Self-awareness of deficits in adults with traumatic brain injury: How best to measure? *Brain Injury, 10,* 1–15.

Fleming, J. M., Strong, J., & Ashton, R. (1998). Cluster analysis of self-awareness levels in adults with traumatic brain injury and relationship to outcome. *Journal of Head Trauma Rehabilitation, 13,* 39–51.

Folstein, M. F., & Folstein, S. E. (1975). Mini Mental State: A practical method for grading the cognitive state of patients for clinician. *Journal of Psychiatric Research, 12,* 189–198.

Ginsburg, H., & Opper, S. (1979). *Piaget's theory of intellectual development.* Englewood Cliffs, NJ: Prentice Hall.

Goldberg, S., & Katz, N. (1994). The validity of the Rivermead Behavioral Memory Test for assessing everyday memory of elderly Israeli CVA patients and a normal control group. *Israel Journal of Occupational Therapy, 3,* H149–H168. (In Hebrew)

Golden, C. J. (1984). Rehabilitation and the Luria–Nebraska Neuropsychological Battery. In B. A. Edelstein & E. T. Couture (Eds.), *Behavioral assessment and rehabilitation of the traumatically brain-damaged* (pp. 1–18). New York: Plenum.

Granger, C. V., Cotter, A. C., Hamilton, B. B., & Fiedler, R. C. (1993). Functional Assessment Scales: A study of persons after stroke. *Archives of Physical Medicine and Rehabilitation, 74,* 133–138.

Halligan, P. W., Cockburn, J., & Wilson, B. A. (1991). The Behavioural Assessment of Visual Neglect. *Neuropsychological Rehabilitation, 1,* 3–5.

Hartman-Maeir, A., & Katz, N. (1995). Validity of the Behavioral Inattention Test (BIT): Relationships with functional tasks. *American Journal of Occupational Therapy, 49,* 507–516.

Inhelder, B., & Piaget, J. (1964). *The early growth of logic in the child.* New York: W. W. Norton.

Itzkovich, M., Elazar, B., Averbuch, S., & Katz, N. (2000). *LOTCA Manual* (2nd ed.). Wayne, NJ: Maddak.

Kandel, E. R. (1995). Cellular mechanisms of learning and memory. In E. R. Kandel, J. H. Schwartz, & T. M. Jessell (Eds.), *Essentials of neural science and behavior* (pp. 667–694). East Norwalk, CT: Appelton & Lange.

Kandel, E. R. (1998). A new intellectual framework for psychiatry. *American Journal of Psychiatry, 155,* 457–469.

Kandel, E. R., & Pittenger, C. (1999). The past, the future, and the biology of memory storage. *Philosophical Transactions B, 354,* 2027–2052.

Katz, N., Champagne, D., & Cermak, S. A. (1997). Comparison of younger and older adults on three versions of a puzzle reproduction task. *American Journal of Occupational Therapy, 51,* 562–568.

Katz, N., Elazar, B., & Itzkovich, M. (1995). Construct validity of a geriatric version of the Loewenstein Occupational Therapy Cognitive Assessment (LOTCA) Battery. *Physical and Occupational Therapy in Geriatrics, 13,* 31–45.

Katz, N., Elazar, B., & Itzkovich, M. (1996). Validity of the Neurobehavioral Cognitive Status Examination (Cognistat) in assessing patients post CVA and healthy elderly in Israel. *Israel Journal of Occupational Therapy, 5,* E185–E198.

Katz, N., Fleming, J., Keren, N., Griffen, J., & Hartman-Maeir, A. (2002). Unawareness and/or denial of disability: Implications for occupational therapy intervention. *Canadian Journal of Occupational Therapy, 69,* 281–292.

Katz, N., Hartman-Maeir, A., Ring, H., & Soroker, N. (1999). Functional disability and rehabilitation outcome in right-hemispheric-damaged patients with and without unilateral spatial neglect. *Archives of Physical Medicine Rehabilitation, 80,* 379–384.

Katz, N., Hartman-Maeir, A., Ring, H., & Soroker, N. (2000). Relationship of cognitive performance and daily function of clients following right hemisphere stroke: Predictive and ecological validity of the LOTCA battery. *Occupational Therapy Journal of Research, 20,* 3–17.

Katz, N., Hartman-Maeir, A., Weiss, P., & Armon, N. (1997). Comparison of cognitive status profiles of healthy elderly persons with dementia and neurosurgical patients using the neurobehavioral cognitive status examination. *Neurorehabilitation, 9,* 179–186.

Katz, N., Hefner, D., & Ruben, R. (1990). Measuring clinical change in cognitive rehabilitation of clients with brain damage: Two cases, traumatic brain injury and cerebral vascular accident. *Occupational Therapy in Health Care, 7,* 23–43.

Katz, N., & Heimann, N. (1990). Review of research conducted in Israel on cognitive disability instrumentation. *Occupational Therapy in Mental Health, 10,* 1–15.

Katz, N., Itzkovich, M., Averbuch, S., & Elazar, B. (1989). Loewenstein Occupational Therapy Cognitive Assessment (LOTCA), battery for brain injured clients: Reliability and validity. *American Journal of Occupational Therapy, 43,* 184–192.

Katz, N., Kizony, R., & Parush, S. (2002). Cross-cultural comparison and developmental change of Ethiopian, Bedouin and mainstream Israeli children's cognitive performance. *Occupational Therapy Journal of Research, 22,* 1–10.

Katz, N., Parush, S., & Traub Bar-Ilan, R. (2004). *Dynamic Occupational Therapy Cognitive Assessment for Children (DOTCA–Ch).* Pequannock, NJ: Maddak.

Katz, N., Ring, H., Naveh, Y., Kizony, R., Feintuch, U., & Weiss, P. L. (2004, September). *Interactive virtual environment training for safe street crossing of right hemisphere stroke patients with unilateral spatial neglect.* International

Conference on Disability, Virtual Reality, and Associated Technologies, Oxford, England.

Kizony, R., Katz, N., & Weiss, P. L. (2003). Adapting an immersive virtual reality system for rehabilitation. *Journal of Visualization and Computer Animation, 14,* 261–268.

Kizony, R., Raz, L., Katz, N., Weingarden, H., & Weiss, P. L. (2003). Using a video projected VR system for patients with spinal cord injury. In G. C. Burdea, D. Thalmann, & J. A. Lewis (Eds.), *Proceedings of the 2nd International Workshop of Virtual Rehabilitation* (pp. 82–88). Rutgers, NJ: Rutgers University Press.

Knight, C., Alderman, N., & Burgess, P. W. (2002). Development of a simplified version of the multiple errands test for use in hospital settings. *Neuropsychological Rehabilitation, 12,* 231–255.

Kolb, B., & Gibb, R. (1999). Neuroplasticity and recovery of function after brain injury. In D. T. Stuss, G. Winocur, & I. H. Robertson (Eds.), *Cognitive neurorehabilitation* (pp. 9–26). Cambridge, MA: Cambridge University Press.

Lezak, M. (1995). *Neuropsychological assessment* (3rd ed.). New York: Oxford University Press.

Logue, P. E., Tupler, L. A., D'amico, C., & Schmitt, F. A. (1993). The Neurobehavioral Cognitive Status Examination: Psychometric properties in use with psychiatric inpatients. *Journal of Clinical Psychology, 49,* 80–89.

Luria, A. R. (1973). *The working brain.* London: Penguin Books.

Luria, A. R. (1980). *Higher cortical functions in man.* New York: Basic Books.

Marlowe, W. B. (2000). An intervention for children with disorders of executive functions. *Developmental Neuropsychology, 18,* 445–454.

Merzenich, M. M., Recanzone, E. G., Jenkins, W. M., Allard, T. T., & Nudo, R. J. (1988). Cortical representational plasticity. In P. Rakic & W. Singer (Eds.), *Neurobiology of neocortex* (pp. 41–67). New York: John Wiley & Sons.

Mesulam, M. (2000). Behavioral neuroanatomy. In F. Plum, J. R. Baringer, & S. Gilman (Eds.), *Principles of behavioral neurology* (pp. 1–61). Philadelphia: F. A. Davis.

Mysiw, W. J., Beegan, J. G., & Gatens, P. F. (1989). Prospective cognitive assessment of stroke patients before inpatient rehabilitation. *American Journal of Physical Medicine and Rehabilitation, 68,* 168–171.

Najenson, T., Rahmani, L., Elazar, B., & Averbuch, S. (1984). An elementary cognitive assessment and treatment of the craniocerebrally injured client. In B. A. Edelstein & E. T. Couture (Eds.), *Behavioral assessment and rehabilitation of the traumatically brain-damaged* (pp. 313–338). New York: Plenum.

National Institutes of Health. (1998). Consensus development panel on rehabilitation of persons with traumatic brain injury. *Journal of the American Medical Association, 282,* 974–983.

Naveh, Y., Katz, N., & Weiss, P. L. (2000). *The effect of interactive virtual environment training on independent safe street crossing of right CVA patients with unilateral spatial neglect.* Proceedings of the 3rd International Conference on Disability, Virtual Reality, and Associated Technology, Oxford, England.

Neisser, U. (1976). *Cognition and reality.* New York: W. H. Freeman.

Neistadt, M. E. (1992). The Rabideau Kitchen Evaluation–Revised: An assessment of meal preparation skill. *Occupational Therapy Journal of Research, 12,* 242–253.

Norris, G., &. Tate. R. L. (2000). The Behavioural Assessment of the Dysexecutive Syndrome (BADS): Ecological, concurrent, and construct validity. *Neuropsychological Rehabilitation, 10,* 33–45.

Northern California Neurobehavioral Group (1995). *Cognistat: The Neurobehavioral Cognitive Status Examination Manual.* Fairfax, CA: Author.

Osmon, D. C., Smet, I. C., Winegarden, B., & Gandhavadi, B. (1992). Neurobehavioral Cognitive Status Examination: Its use with unilateral stroke patients in a rehabilitation setting. *Archives of Physical Medicine, 73,* 414–418.

Parente, R., & Herrmann, D. (1996). *Retraining cognition: Techniques and applications.* Gaithersburg, MD: Aspen.

Park, N. W., & Ingles, J. L. (2001). Effectiveness of attention rehabilitation after an acquired brain injury: A meta-analysis. *Neuropsychology, 15,* 199–210.

Parush, S., Sharoni, C., Hahn-Markowitz, J., & Katz, N. (2000). Perceptual, motor and cognitive performance components of Bedouin children in Israel. *Occupational Therapy International, 7,* 216–231.

Rahmani, L. (1982). The intellectual rehabilitation of brain-damaged clients. *Clinical Neuropsychology, 4,* 44–45.

Rahmani, L., Geva, N., Rochberg, J., Trope, I., & Bore, B. (1987). Issues in neurocognitive assessment and treatment. In E. Vakil, D. Hoofien, & Z. Groswasser (Eds.), *Rehabilitation of the brain injured* (pp. 43–60). London: Freund.

Rizzo, A. A., (2002). Virtual reality and disability: Emergence and challenge. *Disability and Rehabilitation, 24,* 567–569.

Rizzo, A. A., Schultheis, M. T., Kerns, K., & Mateer, C. (2004). Analysis of assets for virtual reality in neuropsychology. *Neuropsychological Rehabilitation, 14,* 207–239.

Robertson, (1999). Setting goals for cognitive rehabilitation. *Current Opinion in Neurology 12,* 703–708

Robertson, I. H., Mattingley, J. B., Rorden, C., & Driver, J. (1998). Phasic alerting of right-hemisphere neglect patients overcome their spatial deficit in visual awareness. *Nature, 395,* 165–172.

Robertson, I. H., Ward, T., Ridgeway, V., & Nimmo-Smith, I. (1994). *The Test of Everyday Attention manual.* England: Tames Valley Test Company.

Robertson, I. H., Ward, T., Ridgeway, V., & Nimmo-Smith, I. (1996). The structure of normal human attention: The Test of Everyday Attention. *Journal of International Neuropsychological Society, 2,* 525–534.

Rosch, E. (1978). Principles of categorization. In E. Rosch & B. Lloyd (Eds.), *Cognition and categorization* (pp. 213–295). Hillsdale, NJ: Lawrence Erlbaum.

Rosch, E., & Mervis, C. B. (1975). Family resemblances: Studies in the internal structure of categories. *Cognitive Psychology, 7,* 573–605.

Rosenblum, S., Katz, N., Hahn-Markowitz, J., & Parush, S. (2000). Environmental influences on perceptual and motor skills of Ethiopian immigrant children. *Perceptual and Motor Skills, 90,* 587–594.

Schwamm, L. H., Van Dyke, C., Kierman, R. J., Merrin, E. L., & Mueller, J. (1987). The Neurobehavioral Cognitive Status Examination: Comparison with the cognitive capacity screening examination and the Mini-Mental State Examination in a neurosurgical population. *Annals of International Medicine, 107,* 486–490.

Shiel, A., & Wilson, B. A. (1992). *The relationship between unilateral neglect and dependence in activities of daily living.* Paper presented at the Occupational Therapy Conference, Dublin, Ireland.

Sohlberg, M. M., & Mateer, C. A. (1989). Remediation of executive function impairments. In M. M. Sohlberg & C. A. Mateer (Eds.), *Introduction to cognitive rehabilitation: Theory and practice* (pp. 233–263). New York: Guilford.

Sohlberg, M. M., & Mateer, C. A. (2001). *Cognitive rehabilitation: An integrative neuropsychological approach.* New York: Guilford.

Steultjens, E. M. J., Dekker, J., Bouter, L. M., van de Nes, J. C. M., Cup, E. H. C., & van den Ende, C. H. M. (2003). Occupational therapy for stroke patients: A systematic review. *Stroke, 34,* 676–687.

Toglia, J. P. (1994). *Toglia Categorization Assessment (TCA).* Wayne, NJ: Maddak.

Toglia, J., & Kirk, U. (2000). Understanding awareness deficits following brain injury. *Neurorehabilitation, 15,* 57–70.

Van Balen, H. G. G., Westzaan, P. S. H., & Mulder, T. (1996). Stratified norms for the Rivermead Behavioral Memory Test. *Neuropsychological Rehabilitation, 6,* 203–217.

Vygotsky, L. S. (1962). *Thought and language.* Cambridge, MA: MIT Press.

Wechsler, D. (1981). *Wechsler Adult Intelligence Scale.* New York: Psychological Corporation.

Weiss, P. (1994). The occupational therapist's role in assessment of patients with suspected normal pressure hydrocephals as predictor of good shunt outcome. *Israel Journal of Occupational Therapy, 3,* E33–E42.

Weiss, P. L., & Katz, N. (in press). The potential of virtual reality for rehabilitation. [Editorial]. *Journal of Rehabilitation Research and Development.*

Weiss, P. L., Kizony, K., Feintuch, U., & Katz, N. (in press). Virtual reality in neurorehabilitation. In M. E. Selzer, L. Cohen, F. H. Gage, S. Clarke, & P. W. Duncan (Eds.), *Textbook of neural repair and neurorehabilitation.* Cambridge, MA: Cambridge University Press.

Weiss, P. L., Naveh, Y., & Katz, N. (2003). Design and testing of a virtual environment to train stroke patients with unilateral spatial neglect to cross a street safely. *Occupational Therapy International, 10,* 39–55.

Wilson, B., Cockburn, J., & Baddeley, A. (1985). *The Rivermead Behavioral Memory Test: Manual.* London: Thames Valley Test Company.

Wilson, B., Cockburn, J., & Baddeley, A. (1986). *The Rivermead Behavioral Memory Test: Second supplement.* London: Thames Valley Test Company.

Wilson, B. A., Alderman, N., Burgess, P. W., Emslie, H., & Evans, J. J. (1996). *Behavioral assessment of dysexecutive syndrome.* St. Edmunds, UK: Thames Valley Test Company.

Wilson, B. A., Cockburn, J., & Halligan, P. W. (1987a). *Behavioural Inattention Test Manual.* Fareham, England: Thames Valley Test Company.

Wilson, B. A., Cockburn, J., & Halligan, P. W. (1987b). Development of a behavioral test of visuospatial neglect. *Archives of Physical Medicine and Rehabilitation, 68,* 98–102.

Wilson, B. A., Evans, J. J., Alderman, N., Burgess, P. W., & Emslie, H. (1997). Behavioral assessment of dysexecutive syndrome. In P. Rabbit (Ed.), *Methodology of frontal and executive functions* (pp. 239–250). London: Psychology Press.

Wilson, B. A., Evans, J. J., Emslie, H., Alderman, N., & Burgess, P. (1998). The development of an ecologically valid test for assessing patients with a dysexecutive syndrome. *Neuropsychological Rehabilitation, 8,* 213–228.

World Health Organization. (2001). *International Classification of Functioning, Disability, and Health (ICF).* Geneva, Switzerland: Author.

Gordon Muir Giles, PhD, OTR, FAOTA

A Neurofunctional Approach to Rehabilitation Following Severe Brain Injury

This chapter describes the neurofunctional approach to rehabilitation of clients with severe cognitive impairments (Giles & Clark-Wilson, 1993, 1999). The approach is applicable to people with traumatic brain injury (TBI, both penetrating and nonpenetrating, focal and diffuse), anoxic damage and other metabolic imbalances or poisonings causing neurological damage (e.g., diabetic coma, carbon monoxide poisoning), infections (e.g., encephalitis, meningitis), and some types of vascular events (e.g., aneurysms). In the World Health Organization (WHO) classification of impairment, abilities, and participation, the neurofunctional approach emphasizes the enhancement of abilities and participation (WHO, 2001). In terms of the Occupational Therapy Practice Framework, the neurofunctional approach emphasizes the modification of activity demands and contexts and the development of habits and routines (performance patterns) as key focuses of rehabilitation (American Occupational Therapy Association [AOTA], 2002).

The neurofunctional approach considers the constraints placed on client functioning by the injury. The approach is evidence-based, drawing from cognitive neuroscience and learning theory in the design and implementation of intervention programs. Although the approach addresses cognitive functioning, its focus is not retraining cognitive processes (client factors) but retraining real-world skill (occupational performance). Behavioral automaticity (habits and routines) and environmental dependency (context) are central concerns of the approach. These factors are explicitly recognized in the *Occupational Therapy Practice Framework* (AOTA, 2002).

RATIONALE

Most people with acute neurological injury show improvement in the early post-injury period. The rapid nature of the early recovery implicates a neurophysiological process or processes not reducible to learning. The human brain reorganizes in response to highly structured practice (Harding, Paul, & Mendl, 2004), and therapists have attempted to enhance the process by the provision of focused stimulation (Robertson, Ridgeway, Greenfield, & Parr, 1997). In the early acute period, coma stimulation is viewed as an important component of intervention by many therapists (Giles & Clark-Wilson, 1993, 1999). Occupational therapists have attempted to stimulate later recovery by exposing clients to increasing task demands in various cognitive, behavioral, and physical domains (Soderback & Normell, 1986a, 1986b). Activities typically involve paper-and-pencil tasks, computer retraining, or simulated functional tasks (Toglia, 1998). It has been suggested that the earlier that clients can be exposed to rehabilitation, the greater the recovery (Cope & Hall, 1982; Mackay, Bernstein, Chapman, Morgan, & Milazzo, 1992).

Acute rehabilitation could affect the rapidity or extent of improvement. Attempts to study the benefits of early inpatient rehabilitation (Cope & Hall, 1982; Mackay et al., 1992) have been methodologically problematic (Giles, 2001). However, reports of clients provided only minimal intervention, who were later admitted to rehabilitation and showed rapid improvement, suggests that some stimulation is necessary to ensure that clients function at the level permitted by their neurological recovery (Bell & Tallman, 1995; Shaw, Brodsky, & McMahon, 1985). There is little evidence that any specific form of acute intervention is more effective in promoting recovery than another (Giles, 2001).

In the post-acute recovery period, therapists also have attempted to address directly the cognitive substrata of perception, attention, memory, judgment, reasoning, and so on. Approaches may be general stimulation or process specific (Stablum, Umilta, Monentale, Carlan, & Guerrini, 2000). The advantage of these "top-down" interventions, were they to be effective, would be improvement in skills that depend on this function (e.g., improved attention would improve motor control and functional skills). The disadvantage of attempting to remediate basic cognitive functioning is that, although improvement has been demonstrated on the practiced tasks that are hypothesized to involve basic cognitive skills, these effects may not generalize to unpracticed tasks (Newell & Rosenbloom, 1981). If the tasks that are practiced are not functionally relevant to the individual's life (such as having patients play memory games or use computer attention tasks), then the opportunity to improve the individuals real-world functioning is lost.

Instead of addressing basic cognitive deficits, some therapists have attempted to train clients with brain injury in higher-order compensatory approaches to cognitive deficits (e.g., internal problem-solving and reasoning strategies), with the goal that clients will be able to generalize the application of these compensatory strategies to novel circumstances (Wilson & Moffat, 1984). Unfortunately, clients often are taught techniques without adequate consideration to whether the likely improvement in quality of life warrants the effort required to learn the strategy. Clients must be able to transfer a compensatory strategy to novel situations encountered in the real world. Several authors have noted that individuals with brain injury often learn strategies but are unable to apply them to novel circumstances. The most successful compensatory behaviors are those that the individual may practice to the point of automaticity. Compensatory techniques that, despite extensive practice, remain effortful (e.g., visualization strategies as a compensatory memory aid) may be too demanding to be used routinely. In addition to the general stimulation and the use of compensatory routines, a third approach is to train clients in highly specific compensatory strategies (behavioral routines) in which there is little expectation of generalized application.

A fourth approach is to assist clients to perform a specific functional behavior (specific task training). In specific task training, the therapist attempts to teach an actual functional task. The intervention is directed to a behavior of clinical importance. The author has suggested that, to be successful, training must be complete enough to be self-sustaining (i.e., used spontaneously and habitually) by the time the client is discharged from the intervention setting. By addressing basic skills, this "bottom-up" training may be able to improve client insight, mental efficiency, and organization, resulting in continued cognitive improvements. As a result of limitations in the "top-down" approaches, considerable research has been focused on developing methods to assist in compensatory skill training (Evans et al., 2000; Wilson, Baddeley, Evans, & Shiel, 1994).

The neurofunctional approach incorporates the third and fourth strategies while considering environmental context and client metacognitions in terms of addressing the client's willingness to engage in the therapeutic endeavor.

THEORETICAL BASE

Neurofunctional retraining considers the person's learning characteristics in the design and implementation of programs. Because memory, attention, and frontal-lobe-related impairments are central to many clients' problems in readapting to community independence, these areas must be considered in the development of retraining programs. They are not here considered as targets of direct intervention but instrumentally in the design of functional skills programs. A theoretical framework for considering these deficits is discussed before an outline of neurofunctional retraining is described.

Memory

Remembering and executing any skilled behavior probably involves multiple memory systems that may be differentially impaired by brain damage. Understanding effects of injury on different memory systems offers opportunities to improve rehabilitation effectiveness.

Long-term memory can be conceptualized under the headings *declarative* and *nondeclarative*. Declarative memory is available to introspection (i.e., the individual knows that they know) and may be divided into episodic and semantic subtypes. *Episodic memory* relates to discrete events that retain temporal and sensory associations. *Semantic memory* is organized knowledge about the world that is not context specific and includes the majority of information learned in institutional education (e.g., facts and dates; Tulving, 1983). Episodic memory appears to be dependent on the hippocampus and is the memory system most vulnerable to impairment after TBI. Although deficits in acquiring new semantic information probably occur in tandem with episodic memory deficits, semantic memory stores may still be accessed and learning may take place via frequent repetition of to-be-remembered information (Murre, 1997). Episodic memory requires the participation of the hippocampus as well as other neocortical areas in the storage process. With very frequent repetition of material, access to semantic memory—absent participation of the hippocampus—may be possible, such that the individual knows that they know but remains unable to recall the specific details of knowledge acquisition.

Nondeclarative memory can be thought of as the store of acquired patterns of behavior not necessarily mediated by cognitive learning. Nondeclarative "knowledge" is not available to introspection: Information is accessed through performance. Under the category of nondeclarative are multiple memory systems, including classical conditioning, various types of priming, habituation, sensitization, evaluative conditioning, and motor learning. Learning may occur without the client being aware that learning has taken place.

Nissen and Bullemer (1987) examined the attentional requirements of procedural learning to determine whether attention is an essential precondition of procedural learning as it is for introspectively available forms of knowledge acquisition. A computerized serial reaction time task was used. A light appeared at one of four locations. Participants pressed one key out of a set of four located directly below the position of the light. Learning was evaluated by measuring facilitation of performance on a repeating 10-trial stimulus sequence to which the participants were naïve. Non-neurologically impaired participants improved considerably in performance when this was the only task; however, when given in a dual-task condition (a condition reducing the participants' ability to attend to the task), learning of the sequence (as assessed by verbal report and performance measures) was minimal (Nissen & Bullemer, 1987). Clients with alcohol dementia also were able to learn the sequence in the single-task condition despite their lack of awareness of the repeating pattern. Nissen and Bullemer (1987) concluded that improved performance in the task required attention from the participant. Other workers using similar research paradigms have demonstrated that the material learned may be far more complex than the relatively simple motor tasks usually associated

with procedural learning (Lewicki, Czyzenska, & Hoffman, 1987; Lewicki, Hill, & Bizot, 1988).

Attention

Posner and Peterson (1990) highlighted three principles central to the understanding of attention: (a) the attentional system is separate from the more basic systems to which attention is allocated, (b) the attentional system depends on the interaction of different anatomical areas, and (c) the areas involved in attention are specific and distinct from one another and the rest of the brain (i.e., attention is the property of neither a single center nor the brain as a whole). Posner and Peterson described three attentional processes with their anatomical locations: orienting, target detection, and tonic arousal. The ability to orient to visual stimuli in space is associated with the posterior parietal lobe, thalamic nuclei, and the superior colliculi. Target detection (and response activation) is associated with midline frontal areas, including the anterior cingulate gyrus and supplementary motor area. Damage to medial prefrontal structures tends to diminish both the speed and the amount of human activity. The medial sagittal areas also are part of a system that includes brainstem structures responsible for tonic arousal. Tonic arousal appears to be mediated by pathways originating in the locus coeruleus and terminating in frontal areas with the function predominantly lateralized to the right.

The distinction between conscious (explicit) and automatic (implicit) processes may reflect the participation of different neural mechanisms mediated by different neuroanatomical systems. The participation of the attentional system in conscious processing may be analogous to the functioning of midline temporal structures in the declarative memory system.

Automatic and Control Processing

Cognitive Control

Shiffrin and Schneider (1977) described attention in terms of attention-dependent controlled processing and attention-independent automatic processing (Schneider, Dumais, & Shiffrin, 1984; Shiffrin & Schneider, 1977). Controlled processing is capacity limited and is required for new learning to occur. During the learning phase of an activity, the unskilled individual relies heavily on feedback about performance and devotes conscious attention to the activity (controlled processing). This focused attention continues during the practice stage of response acquisition. Once the action is learned, the individual's performance is controlled by a series of prearranged instruction sequences or schemas that act independently of feedback (automatic processing), leaving the individual free to concentrate on other aspects of the same or different tasks. Automatic processing occurs without conscious control and places only limited demands on the information-processing system. Following TBI, activities that were previously automatic may be disrupted by brain injury (Levin, Goldstein, High, & Williams, 1988). The development of automatic processing has been demonstrated to occur in people following severe TBI (Schmitter-Edgecombe & Rogers, 1997). Shiffrin and Schneider (Schneider & Shiffrin, 1977; Shiffrin & Schneider, 1977) have described two types of attentional system breakdown: divided attentional deficits and focused attentional deficits.

Divided Attentional Deficit

A divided attentional deficit (Schneider et al., 1984) indicates a failure of the capacity-limited attention system to accommodate all the information necessary for optimum task performance. For example, during gait retraining a client may be able to ambulate with standby assistance unless a person walks across their visual field or says "Good morning," whereupon the client may lose his or her balance. This failure constitutes a divided attentional deficit because the client had insufficient attention capacity to walk and attend to other information. Stuss and colleagues (1989) confirmed the existence of divided attentional deficit among clients with brain injury using a complex reaction-time task (Stuss et al., 1989). Clients are slow in tasks that require consciously controlled information processing and demonstrate an inability to process multiple pieces of information rapidly. Stuss and colleagues found this to be so even of people with mild TBI.

Focused Attentional Deficit

A focused attentional deficit typically occurs if an unfamiliar response is required to a stimulus that already has an overlearned response linked to it (Schneider et al., 1984). Continuous attention from the individual may be required to suppress this automatic behavior. Stuss and colleagues (1989) developed a series of computer tasks designed to assess this deficit; the central feature of the focused attentional deficit to be analyzed was the inability to suppress a previously learned complex level of processing when a simpler level of processing was demanded. A complex reaction-time computer program task that required multiple discrimination (shape, internal line orientation, color) was followed by a task that resembled the complex task in surface features but that required far less complex discrimination. Although both clients and control participants were informed of the change, the clients were less able than the control participants to inhibit redundant processing.

It should be recognized that the control–automatic processing distinction is an interactive one and that probably all complex human behaviors involve decision points to a greater or lesser degree (i.e., they are not completely automatic; Stuss & Alexander, 2000).

Selectivity

Task performance is influenced by the presence of competing demands on attention (Kewman, Yanus, & Kirsch, 1988). The ability to selectively attend depends on discriminating task-relevant information from background stimuli. For example, following TBI, individuals have difficulty in filtering out distracting from relevant verbal information (Kewman et al., 1988).

Alternating Attention

The ability to alternate attention in rapid succession between tasks is an important attention capacity. The ability to suppress a response tendency and shift sets is an ability that can be disrupted by frontal-lobe impairment.

Frontal-Lobe Functions

The frontal lobes constitute approximately half of the cerebral cortex in humans. Disorders that have been observed to follow damage to frontal areas have been termed *frontal-lobe syndrome, executive disorders,* or the *dysexecutive syndrome* (Baddeley & Wilson, 1988; Burgess, 2000; Wilson, Alderman, Burgess, Emslie, & Evans, 1996). The present focus is clinical and relates to frontal-brain-process relationships so that the terms *frontal* and *executive* are used interchangeably except where more specificity is used. Executive functions appear to be dissociable (i.e., reducible to more specific processes in which one process is impaired and another is not), suggesting that there are multiple executive functions (Bechara, Damasio, Tranel, & Anderson, 1998; Burgess & Shallice, 1996; Stuss & Alexander, 2000; Stuss & Levine, 2002). The neuroanatomical substrate of executive functions may involve the frontal lobes and more posterior areas working in functional systems. A single frontal area may be involved in many functional systems. Despite the dissociability of frontal functions, the functional manifestations of frontal impairment are likely to be disorders of control and regulation of more basic and relatively unimpaired behavioral routines mediated by subcortical and posterior brain areas (Stuss & Alexander, 2000).

In a now classic paper, Norman and Shallice (1986) proposed that two systems are involved in the selection and control of action: the supervisory attentional system and contention scheduling. *The supervisory attentional system* provides conscious attentional control of novel actions and selects automatic behaviors by modulating the level of activation and inhibition of automatic behavioral sequences (schemas). The supervisory attentional system is therefore responsible for conscious decision making, planning, and monitoring of behavior. The supervisory attentional system may involve distinct subprocesses, but all are involved in management of novelty and managing contention scheduling (Shallice & Burgess, 1996). By contrast, *contention scheduling* operates without conscious awareness or effort and is automatic. Activation (or inhibition) of action schemas occurs without awareness, and the behavior is initiated and executed automatically (potentially entering awareness after the fact). The supervisory attentional system is thought to be a frontal-lobe function and the contention scheduling to be a subcortical function. Impairments in conscious decision making and control of automatic behaviors may partially account for the increased environmental dependency that may follow frontal impairments (Lengfelder & Gollwitzer, 2001b).

Problem Solving, Planning, and Initiation

Neuropsychologists have noted the failure of office-based neuropsychological tests to reliably capture self-regulatory functions that may be readily evident in daily activities such as meeting deadlines, complex decision making, and prioritizing and performing complex tasks such as financial planning or organizing an event. These tasks have been described as "ill-structured" because the problem and its solution are not completely specified prior to the development of a task solution (Goel & Grafman, 2000). Tasks that involve planning and goal–subgoal hierarchies such as the Tower of Hanoi (Simon, 1975) may show deficits in these patients, although none indicate impairment in all patients with the disorder.

The problem has been termed *strategy application disorder* (Shallice & Burgess, 1991), *self-regulatory disorder* (Stuss & Levine, 2002), and *multitasking* (Burgess, 2000; Burgess, Veitch, Costello, & Shallice, 2000). These terms appear to focus on one element of a complex problem. People with frontal deficits are, for example, known to apply strategies less frequently than control partici-

pants (Burgess & Shallice, 1996), but impaired strategy application fails to account for all the observed deficits. The term multitasking appears to emphasize the rapid task switching required in dual or multiple-task paradigms. Although task switching may be a component of the deficit, it again fails to provide a full account of the disorder (Giles & Clark-Wilson, 1993; Reason, 1984; Shallice & Burgess, 1991; see also the discussion of planning and implementation intentions). Whatever term is selected to describe the real-world deficits observed in clients, it is most likely a midlevel explanatory label: Rather than hypothesizing a "planning deficit," the ability to plan is probably dependent on multiple dissociable frontal functions (Goel, Grafman, Tajik, Gana, & Danto, 1997). Evidence for multiple potentially dissociable functions comes from the observed low correlation on tasks that load on frontal functions (Shallice & Burgess, 1996), and the test, that are most likely to show deficits in patients with real-world deficits are tests designed to tax multiple frontal functions (Burgess et al., 2000).

Many individuals with frontal impairment appear not to prepare responses in anticipation of reasonably foreseeable task demands. Using a conditioning paradigm (a shuttlebox-analog avoidance task), Freedman, Bleiberg, and Freedland (1987) examined the ability of people with TBI to plan ahead. In comparison to a group of clients with stroke, the clients with TBI demonstrated decreased anticipatory behavior despite the fact that the TBI group performed equivalent or better on neuropsychological testing. Clarification of the instruction, additional trials, and enhancement of the warning cue failed to improve anticipatory behavior. The authors suggested that clients with anticipatory behavior deficits would show deficits in situations in which current behavior should be regulated on the basis of expected future consequences.

Vilkki (1988), using a task similar to the token test but with more ambiguity, found clients with frontal–lobe deficits fail to identify the appropriate sorting categories. Cicerone, Lazar, and Shapiro (1983) found that participants with frontal-lobe lesions failed to systematically explore a hypothesis (general concept formation) and failed to discard inappropriate hypotheses. Shallice and Evans (1978) observed that clients with frontal-lobe impairment demonstrated an inability to accurately answer questions that tapped areas of knowledge that most people possess but that require material to be accessed and manipulated in novel ways. Adequately answering such questions requires the selection of an appropriate plan to answer the question and checking potential answers mentally for error. Examples of the questions included "On average, how many TV programs are shown on one TV channel between 6:00 p.m. and 11:00 p.m.?" and "What is the length of an average man's spine?" To answer the latter question, one must compare the spontaneous estimate of an average person's height with the percentage of an individual's height accounted for by his spine. Clients with frontal lesions performed considerably worse than either clients with posterior lesions or uninjured control participants. The authors interpreted this finding as a deficit, checking answers against multiple types of data for bizarreness and inconsistency (Shallice & Evans, 1978).

Bechara, Damasio, Damasio, and Anderson (1994) developed a gambling task to describe a syndrome of insensitivity to future consequences in which patients with ventromedial frontal-lobe damage respond only to immediate, not deferred, consequences of action. Patients may have intact intellect and problem-solving ability, and deficits are evident in the patients "ecological niche," predominantly in personal and social arenas. Damasio, Tranel, and Damasio (1991) have accounted for the deficit as an impairment in "marking" an expected outcome with a negative or positive emotional value acquired through previous experience (the somatic marker hypothesis). According to this hypothesis, decision-making processes are normally assisted by the automatic activation of a somatic signal that indicates expected future affective states associated with a course of action. If this process is impaired, automatic arousal in response to stimuli and decision making may be impaired (Damasio et al., 1991).

Shallice and Burgess (1991) examined 3 people with TBI primarily to the frontal lobes who experienced severe problems in organizing everyday activities. The participants failed to show impairment on standard measures of neuropsychological and frontal-lobe impairment. Shallice and Burgess hypothesized that the patients' difficulty in real-life tasks stemmed from impairment in the performance of open-ended multiple, subgoal situations that standard neuropsychological tests fail to capture. Shallice and Burgess described two new tests designed to assess this hypothesis. The Multiple Errands Test assessed the behavior of the participants in task performance in a pedestrian shopping precinct. Participants were given simple tasks that were to be completed according to rules set by the researchers. Participants were given money and an instruction sheet and asked to find certain information, purchase certain items, and be at a certain location at a prespecified time, all while conforming to certain rules such "No shop should be entered other than to buy something." All participants performed significantly worse, both quantitatively and qualitatively, than control participants. The

second test, the Six Elements Test, required the participants to carry out three subtasks, each split into two sections. Participants were instructed that they were not permitted to carry out the first section of the subtask followed by the second section of the same task and that earlier items within a subtask are weighted more heavily than later items. Participants were instructed that otherwise they were free to structure their activities as they saw fit, with the overall goals being to maximize their score within the allotted time. All participants performed significantly below the "normal" range as compared with control participants.

People with TBI may not engage in the internal behaviors necessary for planning and subsequently executing complex dependent action sequences without environmental cues (e.g., budgeting, getting to an across-town appointment, preparing a dinner for guests; Shallice, 1982). To successfully execute complex behaviors that require the initiation of sequences of actions, one needs to (a) develop a plan that will achieve the goal and (b) to initiate and check, an "act–wait cycle" (Reason, 1984).

Planning is a multistage process based on integration of a generally specified goal and knowledge of constraints to goal achievement requiring goal revision (e.g., one of the dinner guests is a vegetarian). Components of plan development can be identified as the following:

- Problem specification
- Preliminary problem solution (strategy selection)
- Plan–constraint adjustment, a reiterative process often with multiple stages of constraint recognition and plan adjustment (Is the store open? Can I afford the ingredients?)
- Plan review (checking)
- Plan implementation timeline development, where individuals may work backward from an imagined goal-state and generate internal-markers for stage completion.

The process may not always be linear. Planning involves many frontal executive processes that may fail separately or in combination so that there may be many routes to inadequate performance of complex, real-world tasks.

Once the plan is developed, the individual compares "plan time" with real time to determine whether a plan component should be initiated or deferred. For example, to get to an appointment across town, time-dependent markers for behavioral implementation are generated (e.g., check that the address is correct, make sure funds are available, call a cab), and the individual intermittently checks the time throughout the day. Each time the person looks at the clock, a decision must be made to act or wait.

As the time for leaving approaches, the person looks at the clock with greater frequency and also begins to adjust other activities so as facilitate timely departure. Failure may occur at any stage, including failure to develop a plan that will meet the goal, failure to access and integrate known constraints, or failure to initiate act–wait cycles. I found it instructive to observe some clients with severe brain injury doing laundry. Many were unable to check to see if their laundry was washed and ready to move to the dryer. The absence of checking behavior could be accounted for by neither memory impairment (when questioned clients were aware that their clothes were in the washing machine), lack of knowledge about the laundry procedures involved, nor lack of motivation. Clients nonetheless required an external cue to enable them to initiate retrieving their laundry and placing it in the dryer.

Some more recent experimental work has supported clinical observation-based theorizing as to the nature of these disorders. Burgess, Veitch, Costello, and Shallice (2000) attempted to identify the contribution of task learning and remembering, planning, plan following, and remembering one's actions to performance of a task involving multiple subgoal scheduling. Burgess (2000) and colleagues found that a three-factor structural equation model best fit their observed results. The factors involved were (a) retrospective memory, or the ability to learn and remember the task rules; (b) planning, or the ability to form an appropriate plan; and (c) intentionality, or the ability to follow the plan established and to constrain actions on the basis of the task rules (the initiation of delayed intentions; Burgess, 2000; Burgess et al., 2000). Both planning and following the plan components depended on retrospective memory. Each factor has an associated neuroanatomical site implicated in impaired functioning; remembering involves anterior and posterior cingulate and forceps major; planning, right dorsolateral prefrontal cortex; and plan initiation, left frontal Brodman's area 10 and parts of 8 and 9.

Goel and Grafman (2000) have reported the difficulties experienced by an architect with a lesion to the right prefrontal cortex in a real-world, ill-structured planning task. Although functioning on basic neuropsychological testing was within normal limits, when faced with a real-world architectural design task, he was unable to organize and refine his solution on the basis of knowledge from different sources. Goel and Grafman described this as a problem of "lateral transformation" in which a plan is revisited and changed to incorporate what in our terms would be called constraining information.

Many therapists attempt to have clients practice problem-solving and reasoning skills to overcome this type of deficit. A range of constructs can be used to characterize behavior, but it is unclear that these are anything other than useful constructs and that "initiation" or "termination" can be practiced separated from the activity in which the clients is evidencing impaired initiation or termination (see discussion of practice below). The clients' problem is rather that they are unable to spontaneously develop and monitor a novel dependent sequence of actions that require later implementation in the absence of obvious environmental cueing. Rather than have clients attempt to improve their responses to novelty, an alternative approach is to have clients practice needed behavioral sequences so that they can become automatic (e.g., how to do the laundry). Some types of novelty can be accommodated by training clients in metacognitive control strategies such as the use of a diary or other form of external memory aid (Giles & Clark-Wilson, 1993, 1999; Giles & Shore, 1989a). However clients must have adequate self-awareness and adequate metacognitive control. The overlearning of the metacognitive control strategy also must be part of the training.

So-called frontal-lobe rehabilitation, whether it has a behavioral (Alderman & Ward, 1991) or a cognitive process focus (Stablum et al., 2000), is about practice of responses that were hitherto novel so that they become routine and are mediated by different anatomical systems.

Self-Awareness

The term *anosognosia* was initially used to describe denial of hemiplegia and has since been extended to include many types of failure to recognize limitations. Various theories have been proposed to explain the clinically observable phenomena, but they do not capture the full range of client behaviors, suggesting that they are not completely adequate. The more concrete the limitations, the more likely they are to be recognized by the person (physical deficits are more readily acknowledged than cognitive deficits, or personality change).

Individuals develop a sense of self over time, and it may be this sense of self remains stable despite the changes produced by TBI. A combination of deficits of attention, memory impairment, and impairments in the integration of the new information into a revised view of "self" may result in what clinicians label denial. The client may refuse to believe information presented about the client's "new self," preferring to use conventional or "common-language" explanations (people do not normally account for performance failures by reference to neurological dysfunction). Some researchers suggest that there is a distinction between motivated lack of awareness and organic lack of awareness (McGlynn & Schacter, 1989). However, the two types of denial may be viewed as overlapping, not mutually exclusive phenomena (Giles, 1999). Admission of errors in activities that should be within the individual's capability is embarrassing, and clients may not believe the feedback about their performance. That this part of the response is a human phenomenon rather than a neurological deficit is indicated by a similar response pattern being common among the family members of people with TBI.

Metacognitive Functioning

The term *metacognition* describes a person's understanding and use of his or her own basic cognitive and perceptual processes. Nelson and Narens (1994) described a two-level, two-process model of cognitive functioning. The two levels are the basic object level and the metalevel, and the two processes are *monitoring,* in which the flow of information is from the object level to the metalevel, and *control,* in which the flow of information is from the metalevel to the object level. Contained within the metalevel is a model of how the object level works. The model is necessarily imperfect. If, following TBI, there is no change in the model of object-level functioning, then individuals will have no ability to adjust their control functions to compensate for impairment. A readjustment of the model would, however, give the client the opportunity to engage in new object-level regulatory behaviors that could improve performance.

The client's memory, attentional skills, and frontal-lobe functioning constrain the interventions that can be used to assist the client. These limitations can be considered constraints on learning imposed by the injury. The neurofunctional approach considers these constraints in the development of retraining programs. Below, I discuss methods that can be incorporated into retraining to assist clients with these types of deficits and present a case study illustrating their use.

ASSESSMENT AND INTERVENTION

Severe TBI can result in the loss or disruption of patterns of adaptive behavior (habits and routines). In addition, the individual's ability to reacquire adaptive patterns of behavior is impaired. The frequency of disruption of basic self-care skills has been estimated at 5% to15% (Jacobs, 1988; Jennett & Teasdale, 1981), and the disruption of more complex skills is more common (Jacobs, 1988). The extent and location of brain damage places constraints on

learning, but new skills (concrete behavioral sequences and routines, not abstract mental processes) can be reacquired to some degree in all but the most profoundly impaired, provided the to-be-learned-information is presented in an appropriate format.

Assessment

Neurofunctional assessment uses a range of evaluation techniques, including standardized assessments, questionnaires, checklists, rating scales, and observation. The most important technique is observation. Occupational therapists typically assess clients' abilities in sensory, perceptual, motor, cognitive, affective, functional, and behavioral domains. A nonexhaustive list of factors to be considered on initial assessment is provided in Exhibit 5.1. Observation of real-life functioning is the primary mode of assessment, as there is rarely a one-to-one correspondence between component skills and functional skills. Observational techniques can be described as falling into two categories: naturalistic and structured.

In *naturalistic observation,* environmental demands are not specifically manipulated, allowing the therapist to develop an understanding of the client's natural behavioral repertoire. It is important to establish what the client does unconstrained by external cues or demands. Clients with TBI often have problems with initiation, so it is important to assess habitual performance rather than best performance in a structured testing environment. The therapist can evaluate whether the client produces any compensatory behaviors (appropriate or inappropriate).

Structured observations can be divided into two categories. First, specific areas of functioning can be cued and observed (e.g., washing and dressing behavior, transfers, street crossing). Second, specific behaviors can be evaluated for frequency of occurrence and environmental or situational cueing factors: frequency baselining or antecedent–behavior–consequence recordings. This second type of recording often is used to describe and measure inadequate behavioral control or social skills deficits (Giles & Clark-Wilson, 1999). Despite careful observation, the origin of some functional skills deficits can remain unclear. In those instances, the occupational therapist may use standardized testing to attempt to elicit the true cause of the problem so that an adequate intervention plan can be developed.

The functional skills assessed by occupational therapists are most often low-frequency behaviors (e.g., bathing, eating) that require observations to be scheduled. It should be remembered that this necessarily affects the

EXHIBIT 5.1. Initial Screening for Neurofunction

Sensation	**Perception**	Neuromuscular
Vision	Visual	Ataxia
Acuity	Visual neglect	Tremor
Visual fields	Visual suppression	Apraxia
Diplopia	Form discrimination, constancy	Spasticity
Depth perception	Visual agnosia	Akinesia
Color		Bradykinesia
	Tactile	Rigidity
Hearing	Tactile neglect	
	Tactile suppression	**Cognitive**
Touch	Stereognosis	Orientation (person, place, time)
Superficial		Attention
Deep	**Motor Skill**	Memory (for current ongoing information)
Sustained pressure	Biomechanical	Frontal-lobe functioning
	Fractures	Planning
Temperature	Contractures	Initiation (level of spontaneously occurring behavior)
	Heterotopic ossification	Self-awareness
Pain	Peripheral nerve injuries	Metacognitive functions
	Strength	
Proprioception	Endurance	**Affect**
Position sense		Depressed (tearful, psychomotor retardation)
Kinesthetic sense		Euphoric
		Labile
		Anger, irritability
		Flat or constricted affect

client's behavior. For example, a client may show adequate performance if prompted to wash and dress but does not engage in either behavior spontaneously. Central to the assessment of function is not what the client can do but what he or she actually does on a day-to-day basis.

Consider as an example assessing street crossing. Initially the therapist makes a determination of how safe it is to assess this behavior (i.e., a client whose behavior is erratic, aggressive, or confused and given to impulsive behavior might have this aspect of his or her assessment deferred). A purposive route (e.g., to the coffee shop) may be selected. The client is told that the purpose of the trip is to see if he or she can get to the store safely and find his or her way back (i.e., a general rather than a specific safety cue). The therapist then walks with (but a little behind) the client so as not to give nonverbal cues. The first street to be crossed should be quiet so as to give the therapist an opportunity to estimate performance in a relatively safe environment. The therapist should be ready to stop the client if he or she is unsafe. If the client is safe in crossing quiet streets, the therapist may progress with the client to busier streets both with and without crossing lights. The therapist should also assess the client's ability to maintain safety if distracted by conversation (as is natural when walking with others). If the client is initially unsafe (e.g., he or she does not check for traffic, inadequately checks for traffic, or checks but nonetheless be-

haves unsafely), the therapist's task is to determine what additional cues are required to elicit safe behavior. For some clients, a simple instruction to pay attention to how they cross the street may be adequate. Others may need additional opportunities to practice focusing on safe street-crossing behaviors as outlined by the therapist. Where there is a marked deficit, an identifiable perceptual deficit, or where the individual is unable to respond to general street-crossing stimulation, a more structured approach should be considered. The therapist should determine the most appropriate techniques, type of prompts, frequency of practice, and types of reinforcers, if indicated. Similarly, an appropriate measure of task acquisition should be selected. Progress in assessment is the same for all functional domains, from least structured to most structured.

Neurofunctional assessment determines current level of functioning and assists in the determination of optimal forms of retraining. The neurofunctional assessment is central to the selection of goals and target behaviors required for the rehabilitation team's integrated intervention plan. Neurofunctional assessments should be conducted under conditions as close as possible to those the person will experience following rehabilitation. Neurofunctional assessment therefore differs from other types of testing that demand highly standardized conditions. The rigorous control of variables is sacrificed in favor of ecological validity.

Standardized Assessment

In some instances, observation alone will not indicate why a person's performance breaks down. Standardized testing may assist in determining the origin of a performance deficit. Recently, several tests have been developed that claim to be ecologically valid in that subtests mimic real-world tasks and that these tests are more predictive of real-world functioning. Tests designed to be ecologically valid include the Behavioral Inattention Test (BIT), the Rivermead Behavioral Memory Test (RBMT), the Test of Everyday Attention (TEA), and the Behavioral Assessment of the Dysexecutive Syndrome (BADS), as well as numerous lesser known tests.

Behavioral Inattention Test

The BIT was designed to be an ecologically valid test of unilateral visual neglect (Wilson, Cockburn, & Halligan, 1987). The BIT is a test battery divided into two parts. Part 1—referred to as the *conventional tests*—is made up of 6 paper-and-pencil tests (Line Cancellation, Letter Cancellation, Star Cancellation, Figure and Shape Copying, Line Bisection, and Representational Drawing). Part 2 consists of 9 "behavioral tests." Picture Scanning has the participant list items in three large photographs: a meal on a plate, a washstand with toilet items, and a room with objects. Further subtests include Telephone Dialing, Menu Reading, Article Reading, Telling the Time, and Address and Sentence Copying, all of which are self-explanatory. Coin Sorting requires the participant to pick out from an array coins of various denominations, and Map Navigation requires the participant find a series of points on a line-drawn figure. Card Sorting requires the participant to pick out an array of various cards from a conventional card deck.

Individuals whose score falls below a total cutoff point or score below the cutoff on any of the conventional tests are administered the behavioral tests. Results from the latter can be used to provide a picture of how a person's neglect manifests itself in everyday life. A score below a certain cutoff score on the behavioral subtests suggests that the individual is likely to have problems in everyday activities.

Rivermead Behavioral Memory Test

The RBMT attempts to assess memory skills necessary for normal life functioning rather than performance on experimental materials and paradigms. The RBMT consists of 12 subtests that assess the participant's ability to remember a person's first and last name, remember the existence and location of a hidden belonging, remember an appoint-ment, recognize pictures, recognize faces, remember a short passage (immediate and delayed), remember a route and deliver a message (immediate and delayed), and state orientation information. There are two scoring methods: a screening score and a standardized profile score. Both allow for categorization on a 4-point scale from normal to severely impaired. The RBMT has four parallel forms (A–D) to reduce potential practice effects. Participants in the validation study included individuals with TBI, left and right stroke, and other diagnoses. Perfect interrater agreement is reported for the RBMT, and parallel form reliability is also high. The RBMT correlates moderately well with therapist ratings of memory lapses. Obtained correlations between lapses and the RBMT were greater than for any of the laboratory tests of memory given (Wilson, Cockburn, & Baddeley, 1991) and correlated with staff, patient, and family member ratings of everyday memory functioning (Malec, Zweber, & DePompolo, 1990; Schwartz & McMillan, 1989).

Test of Everyday Attention

The TEA was developed to reflect contemporary theories of attention (Robertson, Ward, Ridgeway, & Nimmo-Smith, 1994). The TEA measures selective attention, sustained attention, attentional switching, and the ability to divide attention. The TEA uses relatively familiar everyday materials and is plausible and acceptable to participants (Robertson et al., 1994). Participants are asked to imagine that they are on vacation in Philadelphia, where they are required to perform several activities.

Subtest 1, Map Search (a test of visual selective attention), is a timed visual search task in which the participant has to circle symbols found on the map within 2 min. In Subtest 2, Elevator Counting (a measure of sustained attention), the participant has to count strings of tones on an audiotape. Subtest 3, Elevator Counting With Distraction, is similar to Subtest 2 and also is presented on an audiotape. It differs from the previous subtest by the presence of a distracter tone, which participants must ignore, while paying attention to the original tone, to give the correct answer. Subtest 4, Visual Elevators, is a measure of switching attention and flexibility. Participants count a series of pictures of elevator doors interspersed with upward or downward pointing arrows. An upward arrow cues the participants to count forward, and a downward arrow cues the participants to count backward. Each trial may involve multiple switching. Subtest 5 is an auditory analogue of Subtest 4 and is not presented to severely impaired participants, as it is too difficult. Subtest 6 requires the participant to search a stylized telephone directory for symbols, whereas Subtest 7 is the same task with a distracter task superimposed on it, allowing a measure of divided attention. Subtest 8, Lottery, has the participant pick out certain number and letter strings from an extensive set of aurally presented distracters. It is a measure of sustained attention. The TEA has four parallel forms (A–D) to address potential practice effects. Test–retest reliability on Forms A and B are between .59 and .90 for the control participants and .41 and .90 for the stroke patients (Robertson et al., 1994). Preliminary validation data have been reported on a control, stroke, and TBI sample. Factor analysis of the standardization sample ($N = 154$) identified 4 factors: Visual Selective Attention and Speed, Attentional Switching, Sustained Attention, and Auditory–Verbal Working Memory.

Behavioral Assessment of the Dysexecutive Syndrome

Executive functioning may be an important predictor of real-world functional capacity (Hanks, Rapport, Millis, & Deshpande, 1999). The BADS is a battery of 6 tests plus a questionnaire designed to assess problems in organization, problem solving, setting priorities, and following rules that are believed to be central to the dysexecutive syndrome (Wilson et al., 1996). The Rule Shift Card test uses 21 spiral-bound, nonpicture playing cards to examine the participant's ability to follow a rule and to shift from one rule to another. The Action Program test requires the participant to use objects provided to them in a nonobvious way to solve a puzzle. The solution is constrained by specific rules. In the Key Search test, participants are presented with a piece of paper with a 100-mm square in the middle and are instructed to imagine that they have lost their keys in the field and that they have to develop a search strategy. They are asked to draw a line starting from a specified starting point to represent their search strategy. The efficiency of the strategy is evaluated. The Temporal Judgment test comprises 4 short questions concerning the duration of commonplace events. The Zoo Map test requires participants to show how they would visit a series of locations on a map of a zoo while respecting a set of rules. There are two trials of the test (a high-demand and a low-demand version). The Modified Six-Elements test involves the participants being given instructions to do three tasks (dictation, arithmetic, and picture naming), each of which is divided into two parts, A and B. The participants are required to attempt at least something from each of the 6 subtests within a 10-min period without progressing from one to the other part of the same subtest consecutively. In addition to the 6 subtests, the BADS includes a Dysexecutive Questionnaire that is not included in computation of the overall score. The authors have reported that the overall BADS profile differentiated between the performance of a healthy control group and a group of 78 patients with neurological disorders, most with TBI.

Ecological tests do seem to offer some advantages over standard laboratory tests. Ecological tests have face validity and appear to be well tolerated by participants.

Intervention

Having discussed some of the factors that lead to the disruption of functional behaviors, it is time to consider how to retrain a cognitively impaired person with brain injury to perform a functional task. Continuing with the example of street crossing, let us consider how an individual with severe memory impairment might be trained to cross the street. During assessment, it is determined that the client has no perceptual deficits but that he or she walks across intersections without checking for traffic. Having performed a task-analysis, one determines that crossing the street safely consists of stopping at the curbside, looking in both directions, and then walking directly across the street when there are no motor vehicles within a certain distance (depending on the client's speed of ambulation and so forth). Having performed the task-analysis, one can develop a program of prompts, the purpose of which is to elicit from the client safe street crossing. There are several mandatory activities and decision points, and it is the therapist's task to direct the client's attention to these key factors determining success or failure in task performance.

The first time the client practices street crossing is an "episode." It is processed, and the specific to-be-learned activity is associated with the specific street intersection, the passing traffic, and other incidental information. This episode may not be available later for introspection, but a certain priming effect will have occurred. On the second occasion, only certain aspects of the situation will have remained constant, for instance, the specific instructions given. As this street-crossing routine is repeated, always using the same prompts, the street-crossing episodes are not retained. The street-crossing activity becomes an abstraction of many specific behavioral memory traces, all slightly different, that eventually produces the generalized memory structure of "crossing streets." This experience becomes prototypical, and the client develops a habit of crossing the street in the way practiced. In optimum cases, the client no longer chooses to cross the street in a certain manner, the client just crosses the street in this way (i.e., the client develops automaticity). Initially during intervention there is an attempt to minimize errors by cue saturation (see the discussion of errorless learning below). As automaticity develops and performance improves, cues are faded. The task practiced must be ultimately performable given the fixed aspects of the client's deficits.

The role of the therapist is to negotiate with the client the functional skill to be trained, develop methods that allow the client to perform the task with the minimum amount of new learning, and develop a method that directs the client's attention to the central components of the task. Figure 5.1 shows the routes to the development of automaticity and its consequences for task performance in terms of reduced effortful initiation and reduced need for environmental cueing.

Metacognitive Control and Skills Training

Intervention may be thought to exist on a behavioral to cognitive–behavioral continuum. All intervention aims to modify the client's previous responses (Giles & Clark-Wilson, 1988, 1993, 1999) and replace them with new

and more adaptive ones via practice (see below). Clients who are able to develop a new and more accurate model of their own basic cognitive functioning can learn new metacognitive control strategies and engage in self-initiated learning. Interventions on metacognitive control involve learning a new language or way to think about the post-injury self. Functional skills that require the client to cope with novelty require a complex set of cognitive abilities. For example, complete functional use of a day planner or personal digital assistant involves decisions about what information to enter. Practice in how to make entries and what information to record reduces the difficulty of these tasks, and this decision-making process may itself become more automatic. However, for practice to produce automaticity, the client must be capable of categorizing a particular event as one of the classes of events that should be recorded and then initiate the recording.

Training programs may include the following three stages:

1. A *cognitive overlearning element* to focus the client's attention on the behavior or area of skills deficit and to develop a verbal label for the behavior. The therapist

FIGURE 5.1. Routes to the development of automaticity.

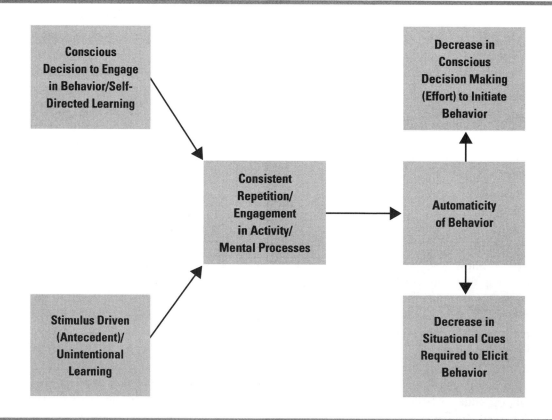

discusses the long-term consequences of the behavior or skill deficit with the client. Hayes and Gifford (1997) noted that behavior and its verbal representation are connected and that both are viewed either positively or negatively (Hayes & Gifford, 1997). For example, if an individual relabels a behavior as *impulsive* rather than *assertive,* the positive associations of that behavior are replaced by negative associations (Hayes & Gifford, 1997). This type of relabeling can theoretically affect the client's desire to engage in the behavior (Hayes & Gifford, 1997; Hayes & Hayes, 1992). The therapist emphasizes the current behavior's inconvenience and the benefits likely to accrue to the client from replacing it with a more adaptive behavior. If the client has severe deficits, this cognitive component may need to be reviewed one or more times per day and may continue throughout or beyond the other program elements. This aspect of a program can be usefully done in a group format, such as in a goals-setting group in which goals for each client are reviewed.

2. *With sessional practice of required behaviors* the client practices the behavior for a short period of time in an environment controlled by the therapist. The client must be able to produce the behavior with only moderate effort in this controlled environment before progressing to Stage 3.

3. In Stage 3, there is an attempt to target *each instance of the behavior* throughout the day. This type of intervention requires the client to have good self-monitoring skills or an interdisciplinary team with a high level of staff training. In the latter case, each time the client exhibits the target behavior, a staff member responds in a predetermined manner so as to have the client attend to the behavior or categorize it as an instance of the target behavior and suppress and replace it with an alternative or incompatible behavior.

The degree to which a behavior becomes automatic influences its durability. Behaviors that develop to a high degree of automaticity, such as washing and dressing (and which are practiced repeatedly), are extremely durable (Lloyd & Cuvo, 1994). Behaviors that must be consciously initiated by the participant and that have more variable cues to implementation, such as use of a day planner, require more specific and ongoing environmental support.

Intervention Components

Reinforcement and Skill Building

A reinforcer is an event that increases the likelihood of the behavior that it follows being repeated. Reinforcers may be primary or secondary. There is some evidence that reinforcement aids learning (Dolan, 1979; Lashley & Drabman, 1974). The reason that reinforcement increases learning is unknown but may be related to the ability of reinforcement to direct attention toward the to-be-learned aspects of the practiced behaviors.

Task Analysis

Task analysis involves a process of dividing tasks into component parts that can be taught. The task analysis provides a method of organizing behaviors to make them easier to learn. The components of a task analysis may be converted to verbal, visual, or tactile cues. If using a task analysis to develop a set of verbal cues, the number of cues is related to the client's ability to control behavior. For example, in developing a washing and dressing program, some clients require only a few cues such as "wash your face" to produce complex behavioral chains. Other clients require several cues, for example, "pick up the wash cloth," "put soap on the wash cloth," "wash your face," and "rinse the wash cloth."

Chaining

Functional tasks can be thought of as complex stimulus–response chains in which the completion of each activity acts as the stimulus for the next step in the chain (Kazdin, 1994). Three chaining options are available for training functional tasks: (a) *backward chaining,* in which the last step of the task is trained first, followed by the second-to-last step and the last step and so on, progressing backward through the chain; (b) *forward chaining,* in which the first step of the chain is trained first, followed by the first and second step and so on, progressing forward through the chain; and (c) *whole-task method,* in which each step of the chain is trained on each presentation. Basic operant researchers have preferred backward chaining on theoretical grounds (G. L. Martin, Koop, Turner, & Hanel, 1981; Skinner, 1938), whereas clinicians have focused on the practical advantages of the whole-task method. Contemporary studies have found the whole-task method to be equivalent or superior to backward chaining (D. J. Martin, Garske, & Davis, 2000; McDonnell & Laughlin, 1989; Spooner, 1984).

Cues

Events that facilitate the production of a behavior are called cues (or prompts). In many instances, cues are available in the environment, but they are no longer sufficient to guide behavior, or they have lost their meaning entirely (e.g., arriving at a busy junction no longer cues safe street-crossing routines). The therapist adds additional cues to those already available in the environment (saying "stop" when the client arrives at the curb). Therapists can facilitate the learning of skills with a range of differing types of cues. Two types of cueing systems have been evaluated in teaching chained tasks: the system of least prompts (SLP) and time-delay procedures. The system of least prompts (sometimes referred to as the increasing assistance procedure) involves the presentation of a cue hierarchy that is arranged from most general to most specific. The individual is cued progressively through the hierarchy of cues available for each step in the chain until a correct response is produced. The time-delay cueing system typically involves two training stages: (a) a cue designed to elicit the next step in the chain is delivered so as to coincide with the stimulus (i.e., the completion of the previous step in the chain) and (b) a defined interval is introduced between the occurrence of the stimulus and the response-eliciting cue. Two types of time-delay procedures are used clinically: progressive time delay (PTD), in which progressively longer intervals are inserted between the occurrence of the stimulus and the cue, and constant time delay (CTD), in which a fixed-response interval is inserted between stimulus and cue (Wolery, Griffen, Ault, Gast, & Doyle, 1990).

Although the system of least prompts has been used with individuals with TBI (McMillan, Papadopoulos, Cornall, & Greenwood, 1990; O'Reilly & Cuvo, 1989), the majority of reports of functional interventions using chained tasks have used CTD (Giles & Clark-Wilson, 1988, 1993; Giles, Ridley, Dill, & Frye, 1997; Katzman & Mix, 1994). No studies comparing SLP with time-delay methods with people with TBI have been conducted. However, in studies comparing these methods in people with mental retardation, both CTD and PTD have been shown to be superior to SLP (McDonnell, 1987; Wolery et al., 1990). In most circumstances, CTD procedures may be preferred because they require less attention from the therapist to the cueing itself (Wolery et al., 1990). Some therapists may prefer to begin with CTD and use PTD as a fading technique. However, PTD should be used only if the client has already developed the skill to the point at which he or she can be 80% to 90% correct, as otherwise they are likely to "practice" the propagation of incorrect responses, with potentially detrimental effects on learning (see discussion of errorless learning below). Telling the individual to "go ahead" or "do what comes next" also can help the individual initiate the activity and decrease dependence on cues.

Practice

The development of performance skills results from practice (Newell & Rosenbloom, 1981). Practice is essentially the repetition of the same behavior: An identical response is provided to an identical stimulus (Newell & Rosenbloom, 1981). The repetition of invariant behavioral responses to invariant stimuli is referred to in the literature as consistent mapping (CM) because the stimulus–response relationship is constant (Schmitter-Edgecombe & Rogers, 1997; Shiffrin & Dumais, 1981). CM practice results in improved performance skills and may lead to automaticity. In contrast to CM tasks, tasks that lack consistent stimulus–response relationships are referred to as varied mapping (VM) tasks. In VM training conditions, automatization of behavior does not occur, and performance skills show little improvement (Schmitter-Edgecombe & Rogers, 1997). Tasks with changing relationships between stimulus and response (VM) cannot be practiced to automaticity. In complex functional tasks that include both CM and VM components, only CM components will develop automaticity.

As discussed earlier, the development of automaticity also requires that the learner allocate attention resources to the task (required for the transition from automatic to controlled processing). Laboratory studies from various theoretical perspectives (E. Miller, 1980; Schmitter-Edgecombe & Rogers, 1997) and reports of functional skills training (Giles & Morgan, 1989; Giles et al., 1997) demonstrate that, after TBI, performance skills may become automatic with practice. In laboratory studies of development of either cognitive or perceptual motor skills (E. Miller, 1980; Schmitter-Edgecombe & Rogers, 1997), clients with TBI begin with performance that is substantially inferior to that of control participants and develop automaticity more slowly than control participants (Schmitter-Edgecombe & Rogers, 1997). However, when people with TBI are provided with extensive practice, the skill level achieved often approximates the skill levels of the unimpaired control group and, once achieved, automaticity may be robust and enduring.

Overlearning refers to the practice of a skill beyond the point at which mastery has been achieved so as to make it less susceptible to forgetting. Overlearning increases the chances that a skill is consolidated in the individual's repertoire of skills and reduces the effort required for performance of the skill (Giles & Clark-Wilson, 1993). When a skill becomes automatic, it becomes the easiest behavior to initiate from an array of possible behaviors (i.e., the possibility of an interference error is reduced). For example, a street-crossing program should not be terminated on meeting the functional criteria but on meeting criteria plus a certain number of practice sessions designed to make the behavior automatic. It has been suggested that continuing overlearning more than 50% of trials to criteria yields diminishing returns (Krueger, 1929), although others suggest that loss can still be significantly diminished after this point (Postman, 1962). The amount of overlearning in clinical populations is a function not only of memory alone but also of the frequency with which behavioral intrusion errors occur (see Case Example 5.2, below, for an extreme example). The number of additional sessions required to develop automaticity cannot be defined across individuals or behaviors. Automaticity is assessed by ongoing monitoring of the client's behavior in conjunction with distractions.

Errorless Learning

The training method of errorless learning was first proposed by Terrace (1963) and has subsequently been used widely with clinical populations (Kern, Liberman, Kopelowicz, Mintz, & Green, 2002; Komatsu, Minimua, Kato, & Kashima, 2000; O'Carroll, Russell, Lawrie, & Johnstone, 1999; Parkin, Hunkin, & Squires, 1998), including individuals with TBI (Evans et al., 2000; Wilson et al., 1994). In trial-and-error learning, errors are corrected; in errorless learning, errors are prevented. The greatest benefits of errorless learning accrue to people with the most severe memory impairments (i.e., people who are unable to suppress a behavior on the basis of knowledge of the behavior's prior failure). When a profoundly amnesic person propagates an error, that error may, as a result of priming, become the behavior that is most available (attached to the stimulus). So, if prompted to produce the behavior again, the patient (who has no conscious knowledge of performing the behavior before and of the response failure) repeats the error (i.e., the patient learns the error). Indeed, clinical observations underline the tendency for amnesic patients to get "stuck" with early response errors. In errorless learning, the therapist provides sufficient support (e.g., cueing, implicit guidance) to prevent the propagation of errors. By preventing errors, the priming effect may be used to "jumpstart" the learning that occurs through time as a result of sheer repetition (Murre, 1997). As a practical matter, it may be very difficult to completely prevent all errors; however, errors can be kept to a minimum. My reports of washing and dressing training are examples of what are essentially errorless learning techniques applied to real clinical practice. Detailed descriptions of their application can be found in the original reports and may be used as treatment guides (Giles et al., 1997).

Control of a Behavior by Antecedents

Antecedent interventions alter the chances that a behavior will occur by changing the cueing events in the environment (discriminative antecedents; Giles, 1999; Yuen & Benzing, 1996; Zencius, Wesolowski, Burke, & McQuade, 1989) or by changing the reinforcement effectiveness of an object or event (motivational antecedents). Discriminative antecedent techniques offer an indirect way to initiate a desired behavior if a direct approach has been ineffective (Zencius et al., 1989) and a way to avoid eliciting unwanted behaviors (Fluharty & Glassman, 2001). Directly cueing a behavior (e.g., "Please take a shower") presupposes that the client shares the same background information as the person making the request (Whittington & Wykes, 1996) or assumes that the client is spontaneously acquiescent (i.e., they do what people ask whether or not it makes sense to them). Discriminative antecedent approaches have been successfully incorporated in interventions for clients with challenging behaviors (Burke, Wesolowski, & Lane, 1988; Manchester, Hodgkinson, Pfaff, & Nguyen, 1997; Rothwell, LaVigna, & Willis, 1999) and who are nonresponders to straightforward operant approaches (Zencius et al., 1989).

Motivational antecedents, also called *establishing operations,* include states of deprivation and other nonobvious antecedents that may alter responses to environmental events. Establishing operations often are temporally distant events that alter the reinforcing effectiveness of another event and can increase or decrease the amount of behavior directed toward obtaining a reinforcer. For example, individuals who are receiving high levels of attention are less likely to engage in attention-seeking behaviors (Mace & Lalli, 1991; Smith & Iwata, 1997).

Zencius and colleagues (1989) compared the effect of altering antecedents with the effect of varying consequences in 3 clients with marked memory disorder following TBI. For one client, posting a sign regarding break times at the workstation drastically reduced the number of unauthorized breaks. For the second client, the most effective way to increase cane usage, a rehabilitation goal, was to provide the client with her cane during morning ADLs. This technique was found to be more effective than social praise, a contract for money, or someone to escort her to get her cane when she was found without it. For the third client, a map and a written daily schedule was more powerful than a contract for money in increasing therapy attendance. In each case, alteration of the antecedent produced behavioral improvement following attempts to alter behavior by consequences, which had proved to be only marginally successful (Zencius et al., 1989).

Therapeutic Alliance

A positive therapeutic alliance is predictive of positive outcome across therapeutic approaches (Castonguay, Goldfried, Wiser, Raue, & Hayes, 1996; Follette, Naugle, & Callaghan, 1996; Hovath & Symonds, 1991; Luborsky, McLellan, Woody, O'Brien, & Auerbach, 1985; D. J. Martin et al., 2000; W. R. Miller & Rollnick, 1991; Woody & Adessky, 2002) and predicts TBI rehabilitation outcome (Klonoff, Lamb, Henderson, & Shepherd, 1998). Bordin (1979) identified three components of the working alliance: (a) the emotional bond between client and therapist, (b) mutual agreement on goals, and (c) mutual agreement on the tasks that form the substance of the intervention. Subsequently, others have emphasized the negotiation of alliance components (Safran & Muran, 2000).

Motivational Interviewing and Goal Setting

Motivational interviewing provides a method to help clients develop a goal of self-change and a framework for a nonaversive approach to lack of insight. Five general principles of motivational interviewing are (a) express empathy, (b) develop discrepancy, (c) avoid argumentation, (d) roll with resistance, and (e) support self-efficacy (W. R. Miller & Rollnick, 1991).

Initially, the therapist attempts to understand the client's perspectives without judging, criticizing, or blaming. The therapist accepts the client's view as being one way of seeing the problem. Acceptance is not the same as agreement or approval. The crucial attitude is respectfully listening to the client with a desire to understand his or her perspectives. The client's ability to maintain self-esteem is an important condition for change, and attacking the client's position undermines the therapeutic alliance and puts the client in a position of self-justification. Clients may not recognize how their current behavior impedes their ability to meet their long-term goals (Bechara, Damasio, Damasio, & Anderson, 1994). Motivation for change is enhanced by helping clients recognize a disjunction between their short-term and long-term goals or between their goals and their current behavior (Manchester & Wood, 2001). It is nonetheless important for the therapist to avoid argumentation and not to trap clients into defending a position that is unhelpful to them. It is important to support the client's sense of self-efficacy, recognizing the need for clients to see themselves as progressing and to have achievable goals. (For a more detailed discussion of the application of these methods to TBI rehabilitation, see Giles & Clark-Wilson, 1999; Manchester & Wood, 2001.)

Goal Statements and Implementation Intentions

Explicit goals are important because the consequence of having formed a goal is a sense of commitment that obligates the individual to strive to reach the goal. The likelihood of goal attainment is affected by how people frame their goals: Better performances are observed when people set themselves challenging specific goals as opposed to challenging but vague goals. Once a goal is selected, achievement of the goal is facilitated by making decisions about how the goal is to be implemented: Decisions about the circumstances under which the individual is to engage in specific behaviors related to the achievement of a goal are termed *implementation intentions* (Lengfelder & Gollwitzer, 2001a).

The steps in the achievement of the goal have to be defined specifically. For example, a goal of losing weight might be partially met by increasing the amount of physical activity: Increasing physical activity can be achieved by exercising at a gym. To increase the likelihood of success, however, making decisions about what gym to go to and when to go to the gym will cue gym attendance. Making decisions both about how and when to implement a specific behavior associated with the goal and about the stimulus conditions that will cue the new behavior have been found to be helpful in goal attainment. By placing the implementation of the new goal-related behavior under the control of environmental stimuli (by creating an external marker for behavioral initiation) makes the implementation of the goal-related behavior automatic (i.e., the action does not require conscious decision making to be performed). Implementation intentions are hypothesized to cause the mental representations of the anticipated situation to become highly activated and thus easily accessible (Gollwitzer, 1993, 1996). This activation has perceptual, attentional, and mnemonic consequences that help to overcome problems in action initiation.

Lengfelder and Gollwitzer (2001b) tested the hypothesis that people with impaired deliberative ability from frontal-lobe impairment would preferentially benefit from interventions that place behaviors under environmental control (Lengfelder & Gollwitzer, 2001a, 2001b). In a test requiring participants to plan, sequence, and solve goal–subgoal conflicts (called the Tower of Hanoi), patients with frontal lesions with weak performance (Simon, 1975) were found to have particularly poor performance on a task involving deliberative processes and to be preferentially helped by the use of implementation intentions in responding on a computer task. By forming an action plan ahead of time and determining the cues that will trigger the plan, the initiation of the plan becomes reflexive, obviating the need for decision making once the behavior is cued by the environment. Individuals with more severe frontal-lobe impairments (i.e., those people with the most impaired deliberative ability) were the most assisted by the use of implementation intentions (Lengfelder & Gollwitzer, 2001a, 2001b).

Intervention Using Metacognitive Control Strategies

Metacognitively oriented intervention should involve consideration of the learning factors already discussed but, in addition, should maximize use of the client's own retained, self-directed learning ability. The therapist's role is to supervise clients in setting their own goals and developing their own strategies to perform functional tasks based on knowledge of their own limitations. For example, a client who has been working on improving community mobility might set him- or herself the task of finding the way to a specific novel location. The client would then develop, with the assistance of the therapist, knowledge of the parameters involved in the task, (e.g., available means of transportation, time requirements, cost, route-finding methods). As the client shows increasing competencies, longer periods of time and more complex tasks can be set for the client. Intervention becomes the client pursuing his or her own goals and periodically checking in with the therapist who can support critically self-awareness and a positive attitude focused on recovery. The therapist's goal is to set tasks and direct the client's attention on how his or her current experience can be used to improve future task performance. The client is encouraged to learn about his or her own cognitive abilities and to develop effective metacognitive control strategies.

Evidence-Based Research Supporting the Model

Single-case or small-group studies have demonstrated the efficacy of functional task training following TBI in the areas of continence (Cohen, 1985), self-feeding (Hooper-Row, 1999), transfers (Hooper-Row, 1999), personal hygiene (Giles & Clark-Wilson, 1999; Giles et al., 1997), mobility and community skills (Giles & Clark-Wilson, 1993), and social skills (Brotherton, Thomas, Wisotzek, & Milan, 1988; Gajar, Schloss, Schloss, & Thompson, 1984; Giles, Fussey, & Burgess, 1988). Lloyd and Cuvo (1994) reviewed results of behavioral interventions, concluding that treatment effects are robust and enduring. Several follow-up studies have examined the effectiveness of post-acute brain injury programs. Even when cog-

nitive skills are directly addressed, it is often functional skills that improve (Mills, Nesbeda, Katz, & Alexander, 1992). Follow-up of 42 patients treated at an outpatient postacute cognitive rehabilitation found that cognitive measures were not significantly affected by treatment but that there was significant improvement in clients' functional performance and that this was maintained at 18-month follow-up (Mills et al., 1992). Johnston and Lewis (1991b) assessed 1-year outcome of 82 patients treated at post-acute community re-entry programs and found that there were enduring improvements in independent living and productive activities, with patients' requirements for supervision showing substantial decline. Although improved independent living and household skills were the most frequent dimension of actual benefit, they were seldom documented as goals (Johnston & Lewis, 1991a).

Harrick, Krefting, Johnston, Carlson, and Minnes (1994) reported a 3-year outcome of clients treated at a transitional living center for people with post-acute TBI. The participants were the first 21 people who completed the program of a single transitional living center and were available for 3-year follow-up. Participants in the study had all sustained severe TBI (M = 28.1 days, range 3–90, SD = 24.7). Participants were an average of 37.1 months post-injury (range 30–168, SD = 42.1), with many having participated in inpatient medical rehabilitation prior to admission to the transitional living center. Mean length of stay was 25.5 weeks (range 8–56, SD = 11.2). Treatment included behavior management, activities of daily living retraining, counseling, and academic and vocational retraining, all provided in the context of a group residential facility with a community-living focus. Guiding concepts included the importance of self-awareness to adapting to community life and the use of compensatory strategies and modification of the physical and social environment so as to reduce disability. Functional status was measured by participation in productive activity, need for financial support, place of residence, and level of supervision required. Improvements observed at 1-year follow-up remained stable or had improved at 3-year follow-up. Loneliness and depression increased over time to become the problems reported most frequently at follow-up.

Other workers have found that functional performance may continue to improve following the end of a program of functional retraining, even in patients who are significantly post-injury (Fryer & Haffey, 1987). Willer, Button, and Rempel (1999) compared the outcomes of individuals with severe TBI treated in a post-acute residential rehabilitation program (n = 23) with a matched sample of individuals receiving limited services in their homes or on

During the final year of an undergraduate course in electrical engineering, Client 1 developed herpes simplex encephalitis. The course of the client's acute illness is reported elsewhere (Greenwood, Bhalla, Gordon, & Roberts, 1983). Following acute recovery, Client 1 was found to be amnesic (with an inability to remember new material for more than 30 s), hyperoral, sullenly uncooperative, and aggressive. Remote memory was impoverished in content and sequential organization. Client 1 also had a category-specific knowledge deficit about food and food-related items (he was unable to distinguish food from nonfood items).

One-year post-onset, Client 1 was living with his mother, who was providing extensive supervision. Early in Client 1's recovery, it had been suggested that he keep a diary. Unfortunately, this had become a focus for obsessional behavior such that Client 1 was obsessed by recording everything "before I forget." The recording had no functional value, as Client 1 was unable to select relevant aspects of his environ-ment (recording largely irrelevant, idiosyncratic, and repetitive themes) and because he wrote in but never referred to his diary.

Increasing resistance to ADLs and escalating physical aggression led to psychiatric hospital admission, where his behavior was managed with antipsychotic medication alone. Following a 1-month trial period, admission was arranged to a specialized behavior disorder program (Eames & Wood, 1985a, 1985b) in which the intervention described here took place.

FIGURE 5.2. Response of Client 1 to a washing and dressing training program.

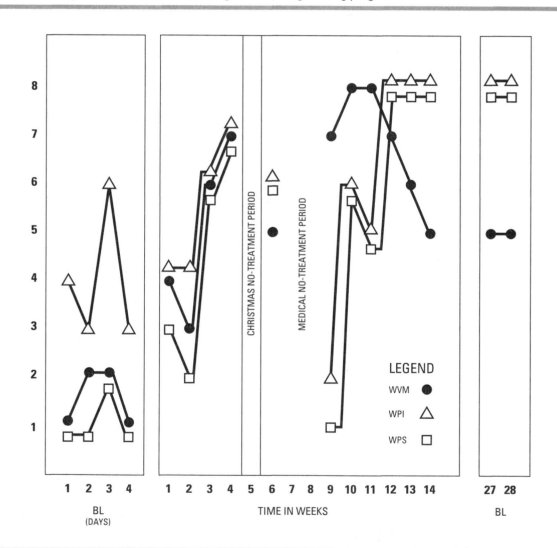

Note. WVM = acts of washing verbally mediated, WPI = acts of washing performed independently, WPS = acts of washing performed in sequence, BL = baseline.

(continued)

On admission, Client 1 was constantly angry, pacing incessantly with pen and diary in hand. Any frustration was construed as persecutory and frequently resulted in dangerously aggressive outbursts (Client 1 had been an Olympic-class swimmer and was 6 f. 3 in. tall, making his outbursts quite threatening). Client 1 maintained a constant stream of repetitive questions particularly related to his stated desire to die, stating "all I need is a driver's license" and asking for "suicide pills." Client 1 would approach staff, stand 6 in. away, glare down at them, and ask "How long does it take for a pointless place to admit they can't help your illness?"

Client 1 rarely bathed and smelled continuously of sweat and stale soap. He was constantly hungry and believed that staff were trying to starve him; however, he remembered that he was given medication and referred to his "constant pill diet."

Observation revealed that Client 1 would attempt to use environmental cues and to verbally regulate his behavior; unfortunately, his attempts were mostly inappropriate. For example, Client 1 would not wash under his arms because "it is cold outside so I cannot have been sweating." Client 1 had some insight into his circumstances and a paranoid and negative attitude toward himself, his environment, and those around him, particularly staff. It was recognized that, if intervention were to be effective, changes meaningful to Client 1 would have to take place. It was hoped that this would allow an improved therapeutic alliance. Occupational therapy–related goals for Client 1 were improved personal hygiene, increased positive social interaction, and independence in meal preparation.

Personal hygiene was selected partly because Client 1's unpleasant odor significantly affected his social acceptability. Baseline observations indicated that Client 1 could manage functions such as washing his face or brushing his teeth but that he could not put these units together nonrepetitively into a coherent sequence. For example, he might wash his face, brush his teeth four times, and then stop.

A behavioral program using verbal mediation was selected because Client 1 spontaneously attempted to verbally regulate his own behavior. Staff performing the program ignored any inappropriate verbalizations. The program is described in detail elsewhere (Giles & Morgan, 1989). Client 1 was told a phrase that linked the act performed to the one that immediately followed it (e.g., "Teeth cleaned, now shave. Say after me . . ."); he was rewarded (with chocolate) and praised when he stated the link phrase and then again for initiating the behavior. Eight mediating phrases were used to link the 9 activities of the program together. Failure to perform the activity—which was rare—lead to 30 s of noninteraction followed by regrouping by the therapist. The program was carried out twice per day, 5 days a week. As learning occurred, reinforcement was made increasingly intermittent. It was hoped that Client 1 would learn to verbally mediate his own behavior in the sequence that he was being taught.

Figure 5.2. shows his progress over the 14 weeks of intervention. There was an unexpected reduction in "Acts of washing verbally mediated" toward the end of the program because Client 1 consolidated part of the sequence into "Wash the body from top to bottom." At 3-months follow-up, the client continued to be independent in basic ADLs and continued to use the same behavioral sequence. When followed up 7 years later, the client had no recollection of the therapist or of the training program but continued to use the behavioral sequence independently, claiming "I have always washed and dressed this way."

Social interaction was addressed using a shaping procedure. When not escorted to a specific location, Client 1 would pace in an agitated state. The goal of the intervention was to encourage him to sit with others and engage in appropriate conversation. Initially, the therapist would stand by the doorway to the day room and give Client 1 praise and a cookie for approaching the doorway. Later, Client 1 was rewarded for entering the room and provided with additional reinforcement for each 30 s he stayed in the room. Later he was reinforced only when he was sitting down, and still later only for sitting quietly or when engaged in socially appropriate conversation. Inappropriate behaviors were timed-out on-the-spot. The intervention was rapidly effective, with Client 1 attending the day room independently during scheduled breaks.

Despite the ongoing success of the interventions described above, Client 1 remained preoccupied by the idea that staff were attempting to starve him and keeping him on "a pointless pill diet." Physical confrontations with staff were often about access to food. Staff hypothesized that, if Client 1 could be taught to prepare a meal for himself, he would be less likely to believe that he was being starved. Teaching Client 1 to prepare a meal was complicated by the fact that he was amnesic and had a category-specific loss of information for food and objects in the kitchen. Client 1 could not distinguish food from nonfood items; did not know what color toast should be; did not know what boiling meant; and could not recognize an oven, a grill, or basic kitchen implements.

Client 1 was observed for 1 week attempting to make a breakfast consisting of two slices of toast with a can of baked beans and sausages (his selection). A program of written instructions was developed and modified in response to difficulties Client 1 experienced in carrying them out (cue experimentation). Client 1 was prompted with "check instructions" on entering the kitchen. All food items were set out with a copy of the instructions and a pen for Client 1 to check off each item as it was completed. For the first 2 weeks, Client 1 continued to require verbal instructions as well as the written instructions, but after 3 weeks, he was independent with the instruction sheet and supervision was withdrawn. After performing the program every morning for 6 weeks, the instruction sheet was withdrawn, food was left in the cupboard, and Client 1 continued to make his breakfast independently. Nonetheless, for another 6 weeks, Client 1 had to be escorted to the kitchen each morning as he protested that he could not cook.

One day about 14 weeks after the beginning of the program, Client 1 greeted every person who entered the unit with a broad smile of excitement and the statement "I can make my own breakfast!" (see Figure 5.3). Client 1's protests that he was being starved ceased, and his level of cooperation with subsequent interventions improved. He was subsequently discharged to a board-and-care home and participated in a sheltered work program.

FIGURE 5.3. Response of Client 1 to a cooking program.

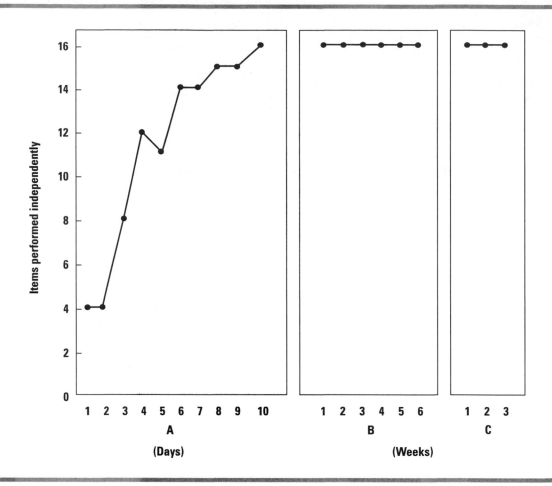

Note. A = food and instruction sheet on counter and with additional verbal prompts when necessary (primarily "check instructions"); B = food and instruction sheet on counter; C = food left in cupboards, no instruction sheet.

an outpatient basis. The treatment groups included all people admitted consecutively over a 3-year period. None had coma duration of less than 3 days, and 18 of the 23 had coma duration of more than 21 days. The control group was obtained from the local brain-injury support group. The treatment and the control group were matched for gender, length of coma, time since injury, and level of disability. Participants in the treatment group improved more significantly in community integration, cognitive, and motor skills than the control group.

Wood, McCrea, Wood, and Merriman (1999) attempted to assess the clinical and cost-effectiveness of intervention with a group of 76 individuals treated at various sites who underwent social rehabilitation for a minimum of 6 months and in whom cognitive and behavioral problems had previously prevented community living. Most participants were young adults (average age, 27 years), were 12 months or more post-injury, and were injured in motor vehicle

accidents, with a mean posttraumatic amnesia of 23.5 days ($SD = 41.2$, range 3–168). Clients were divided into three groups according to time from injury to admission; group 1, 0–2 years ($n = 18$); group 2, 2–5 years ($n = 30$); and group 3, 5 years or more ($n = 28$). Interventions used both behavioral and cognitive–behavioral approaches. Outcome was assessed by examining changes in living situation, employment status, hours of care, persistence and intrusiveness of neurobehavioral problems, and projected cost of care. There was significant reduction in the percentage of clients in high-dependency living situations. More than 60% of clients were in some type of vocational or educational placement post-rehabilitation, in contrast to 4% prior to rehabilitation. Behavior problems were reduced in frequency and severity, although 13.6% of clients continued to have problems that made it difficult to retain in-home support workers. Many clients continued to improve after discharge and were performing more independently at fol-

Case Example 5.2. ADL Retraining in a Client With Profound Bilateral Frontal-Lobe Impairment

Thanks are due to the clients and staff of Crestwood Treatment Center in Fremont, California, and to the *Journal of Clinical and Experimental Neuropsychology* for permission to reprint material previously published in "Training Functional Skills Following Herpes Simplex Encephalitis: A Single Case Study," by G. M. Giles and J. H. Morgan, 1989, *Journal of Clinical and Experimental Neuropsychology, 11,* 311–318.

Client 2 was a 35-year-old computer programmer of above-average intelligence with ongoing depression. He was married with one daughter, and his wife was having an extramarital relationship. Client 2 took his daughter, drove to the apartment of his wife's boyfriend, shot his wife and her boyfriend (both nonfatally), then drove home with his daughter, shot her (fatally), then shot himself in the right temporal lobe. Coma duration is unknown; he was treated with right parietal craniotomy and repair of the cribriform plate.

When first seen by the present authors, he was 11 years post-injury and had been in continuous institutional care. CT showed severe right dorsolateral and ventral prefrontal cortex damage and left ventral prefrontal damage with associated subcortical damage. He had experienced multiple treatment failures, moving from one psychiatric treatment facility to another as a result of highly repetitive verbal, physical, and sexual assaultiveness; incontinence; and fecal smearing. Ongoing functional deficits in addition to the incontinence included extensive assistance for bathing and dressing, with refusal to change himself after incontinence and inability to get out of bed for meals. He showed repetitively physically assaultive behavior, including biting. He was unable to sit still or remain in any activity, requiring constant cueing to sit.

Client 2 experienced frequent falls resulting from poor motor planning and impulsivity. He experienced delusions that he would be released "next week" and that people have raped him particularly at night ("someone is sleeping with me, but I do not know who it is"). Despite the fact that he knew that his wife now lived out of state, he also believed that she worked in another part of the hospital and was planning to harm him (possibly a delusion or reduplicative paramnesia). Memory functioning was moderately impaired. Results of cognitive testing are provided in Table 5.1.

Functionally, Client 2's behavior was marked by gross disinhibited behavior (public nudity, attempted grooming behavior on unwilling peers and staff, slapping and biting others), impulsivity, and inability to organize and plan behavior. His behavior was chaotic and marked by motor impersistence (e.g., attempts to tie his shoelaces would be abandoned midway with the statement "They just don't want to be tied"). There was very poor behavioral self-monitoring, self-awareness, or insight into the behavioral difficulties.

Intervention directed toward reducing assaultiveness is to be reported elsewhere. Here, we comment briefly on the application of a washing and dressing program. Basic ADL functioning was selected because much of the assaultive behavior occurred during ADLs (possibly due to the demand characteristics of the event and possibly due to physical proximity) and because the fecal smearing appeared to be associated with a chaotic response to incontinence and utilization behavior (manipulation) of the feces.

The ADL retraining program implemented was the procedure described by Giles and colleagues (Giles & Clark-Wilson, 1988; Giles et al., 1997; Giles & Shore, 1989b) and is an errorless learning procedure that in itself reduces the likelihood of eliciting avoidance behaviors.

Although considered the best available, the intervention was believed to have limited *(continued)*

TABLE 5.1. Standardized Test Scores for Client 2

Rivermead Behavioral Memory Test
Standardized Profile Score 11 (Moderately impaired)
Screening Score 4 (Moderately impaired)

Cognitive Estimation Test
Deviation Score 0 (Unimpaired)

Behavioral Assessment of the Dysexecutive Syndrome

Scores	Raw	Mean	(*SD*)	*SD* below mean
Rule Shift Cards	0	3.56	(0.78)	4.5
Action Program	3	3.77	(0.52)	1.2
Key Search	1	2.60	(1.32)	1.1
Temporal Judgment	1	2.15	(0.91)	1.1
Zoo Map	2	2.44	(1.13)	0
Modified Six Elements	1	3.52	(0.8)	3.0
Age corrected total	48	100	15.0	>3

Multiple Errands Test	Scores	Mean	(*SD*)	*SD* below mean
Inefficiencies	6	1.6	(1.3)	3.6
Rule breaks	4	1.4	(1.1)	2.3
Interpretation failures	1	0.4	(0.7)	<1
Task failures	4	1.1	(1.4)	2.0
Total errors	15	4.6	(2.1)	4.9

Note. During testing, Client 2 attempted to hug unfamiliar young children.

Case Example 5.2. ADL Retraining in a Client With Profound Bilateral Frontal-Lobe Impairment *(Continued)*

chances of success due to the client's profound frontal discontrol and chaotic and impulsive behaviors and therefore represented a major test of the approach.

Our standard approach is to obtain baseline behavior when prompted to wash and dress and then to develop a task analysis and series of cues that can reliably result in the patient producing a functionally equivalent behavior each time the cue is provided. Because of the profoundly impulsive and chaotic behavior demonstrated by Client 2, the period required to establish the cue program was protracted (30 days), and the cue program itself was detailed. To reliably get the same response, the "behavioral load" of each cue had to be small, resulting in an initial program of 93 cues but not requiring any physical assistance to perform the behaviors. As Client 2 learned the ADL routine, he could perform certain behavioral sequences to single as opposed to

multiple cues so that the number of cues could be reduced. Major program revisions occurred at 3 months (57 cues) and at 6 months (35 cues). At various periods in the program, time-based or other performance-based reinforcers were provided. The program continued daily for a total of 28 months until he could reliably perform daily ADLs independently with weekly monitoring. Period program retaining is required.

After the initial period of establishing the program, the time it required was comparable to the time required to bathe and dress Client 2. Major advantages for Client 2 are his increased sense of independence and the fact that on those rare occasions when he is incontinent, he can implement this behavioral routine and take care of himself without anxiety and distress (smearing has essentially been eliminated).

Staff providing routine ADL assistance had of course not affected the client's behavioral competencies. The client's behavior prior to the implementation of the program had failed to produce ADL independence because it had been essentially random, resulting in no practice effects. Each attempt at self-care was essentially novel problem solving, with a high risk of distraction and significant demands placed on the client's capacity for response inhibition. By providing a highly structured situation and an errorless approach that controlled his responses, stimulus–response relationships were established, and overlearning resulted in increasing automaticity as the new responses became the most available response. In a sense, the client's impersistance then becomes an advantage because performance errors are not be easily sustained, and behavior "defaults" back to the overlearned program.

low-up than at the time of discharge. Wood and colleagues concluded that community-oriented neurobehavioral intervention is effective in ameliorating the social and behavioral skills deficits of clients with TBI (Wood et al., 1999).

CONCLUSION

Interventions for people with TBI should aim to improve real-world functioning or quality of life. Attention should be paid to what needs to change to reduce the client's dependency in his or her environment. This chapter emphasizes attention, memory, and frontal-lobe processes and describes and integrates these elements into a model of rehabilitation. Rather than attempt to address the elusive "underlying cause" of a functional impairment, this chapter highlights the advantages of a direct approach to functional impairments that uses the development of implicit and automatic knowledge structures (habits, routines, and the adaptive use of context). A range of interventions can assist clients in the development and implementation of automatic adaptive behaviors. Activation of adaptive behavioral schemas can be increased through the following:

1. *Cognitively mediated processes and conscious decision making.* Multiple mechanisms can support goal-

setting and the motivation of individuals to meet goals (e.g., motivational interviewing).
2. *Increasing habit strength through the use of practice.* Practice may have short-term priming effects and long-term effects through the development of automaticity. Effective habits cued by environmental regularity may partially offset client problems in novel decision making and planning. Training techniques such as errorless learning may be helpful in people with profound memory impairments.
3. *Assessing and establishing links between the cueing environment (context) and the behavior.* Altering the environment and changing antecedents are powerful techniques to use with individuals with severe impairments. The use of implementation intentions may be helpful in clients with impaired decision-making ability.

REVIEW QUESTIONS

1. Describe the advantages and disadvantages of a skill-based intervention approach such as the neurofunctional approach (a top-down approach) compared with cognitive remediation approaches (a bottom-up approach).
2. Describe the types of behaviors that are practicable and the types of behavior that do not improve with practice.

3. Describe the methods and purpose of neurofunctional assessment. Describe when standardized assessments are used in the neurofunctional approach.

4. Describe the process by which clients with episodic memory deficits can develop new implicit knowledge structures (habits and routines) using neurofunctional intervention methods.

5. Explain the concept of self-awareness and how and when therapists should address self-awareness in clients following TBI.

6. Describe the influence of context under the headings of discriminative and motivational antecedents. Describe how this understanding indicates intervention strategies to be used in skill training.

REFERENCES

Alderman, N., & Ward, A. (1991). Behavioral treatment of the dysexecutive syndrome: Reduction of repetitive speech using response cost and cognitive overlearning. *Neuropsychological Rehabilitation, 1,* 65–80.

American Occupational Therapy Association. (2002). Occupational therapy practice framework: Domain and process. *American Journal of Occupational Therapy, 56,* 609–639.

Baddeley, A., & Wilson, B. A. (1988). Frontal amnesia and the dysexecutive syndrome. *Brain and Cognition, 7,* 212–230.

Bechara, A., Damasio, A. R., Damasio, H., & Anderson, W. S. (1994). Insensitivity to future consequences following damage to human prefrontal cortex. *Cognition, 50,* 7–15.

Bechara, A., Damasio, A. R., Tranel, D., & Anderson, S. W. (1998). Dissociation of working memory from decision making within the human prefrontal cortex. *Journal of Neuroscience, 18,* 428–437.

Bell, K. R., & Tallman, C. A. (1995). Community re-entry of long-term institutionalized brain injured patients. *Brain Injury, 9,* 315–320.

Bordin, E. S. (1979). The generalizability of the psychoanalytic concept of the working alliance. *Psychotherapy, 16,* 252–260.

Brotherton, F. A., Thomas, L. L., Wisotzek, I. E., & Milan, M. A. (1988). Social skills training in the rehabilitation of patients with traumatic closed head injury. *Archives of Physical Medicine and Rehabilitation, 69,* 827–832.

Burgess, P. W. (2000). Strategy application disorder: The role of the frontal lobes in human multitasking. *Psychological Research, 63,* 279–288.

Burgess, P. W., & Shallice, T. (1996). Response suppression, initiation and strategy use following frontal lobe lesions. *Neuropsychologia, 34,* 263–273.

Burgess, P. W., Veitch, E., Costello, A., & Shallice, T. (2000). The cognitive and neuroanatomical correlates of multitasking. *Neuropsychologia, 38,* 848–863.

Burke, W. H., Wesolowski, M. D., & Lane, I. (1988). A positive approach to the treatment of aggressive brain injured clients. *International Journal of Rehabilitation Research, 11,* 235–241.

Castonguay, L. G., Goldfried, M. R., Wiser, S., Raue, P. J., & Hayes, A. M. (1996). Predicting the effect of cognitive therapy for depression: A study of unique and common factors. *Journal of Consulting and Clinical Psychology, 64,* 497–504.

Cicerone, K. D., Lazar, R. M., & Shapiro, W. R. (1983). Effects of frontal lobe lesions on hypothesis sampling during concept formation. *Neuropsychologia, 21,* 513–524.

Cohen, R. E. (1985). Behavioral treatment of incontinence in a profoundly neurologically impaired adult. *Archives of Physical Medicine and Rehabilitation, 67,* 833–834.

Cope, D. N., & Hall, K. (1982). Head injury rehabilitation: Benefits of early rehabilitation. *Archives of Physical Medicine and Rehabilitation, 63,* 433–437.

Damasio, A. R., Tranel, D., & Damasio, H. (1991). Somatic markers and the guidance of behavior. In H. S. Levin, H. Eisenberg, & A. Benton (Eds.), *Frontal lobe function and dysfunction* (pp. 217–229). New York: Oxford University Press.

Dolan, M. P. (1979). The use of contingent reinforcement for improving the personal appearance and hygiene of chronic psychiatric inpatients. *Journal of Clinical Psychology, 35,* 140–144.

Eames, P., & Wood, R. L. (1985a). Rehabilitation after severe brain injury: A follow-up study of a behavior modification approach. *Journal of Neurology, Neurosurgery, and Psychiatry, 48,* 613–619.

Eames, P., & Wood, R. L. (1985b). Rehabilitation after severe brain injury: A special-unit approach to behavior disorders. *International Rehabilitation Medicine, 7,* 130–133.

Evans, J. J., Wilson, B. A., Schuri, U., Andrade, J., Baddeley, A., Bruna, O., et al. (2000). A comparison of "errorless" and "trial-and-error" learning methods for teaching individuals with acquired memory deficits. *Neuropsychological Rehabilitation, 10*(1), 67–101.

Fluharty, G., & Glassman, N. (2001). Use of antecedent control to improve the outcome of rehabilitation for a client with frontal lobe injury and intolerance for auditory and tactile stimuli. *Brain Injury, 15,* 995–1002.

Follette, W. C., Naugle, A. E., & Callaghan, G. M. (1996). A radical behavioral understanding of the therapeutic relationship in effecting change. *Behavior Therapy, 27,* 623–641.

Freedman, P. E., Bleiberg, J., & Freedland, K. (1987). Anticipatory behaviour deficits in closed head injury. *Journal of Neurology, Neurosurgery, and Psychiatry, 50,* 398–401.

Fryer, L. J., & Haffey, W. J. (1987). Cognitive rehabilitation and community readaptation: Outcomes from two program models. *Journal of Head Trauma Rehabilitation, 2,* 51–63.

Gajar, A., Schloss, P. J., Schloss, C., & Thompson, C. K. (1984). Effects of feedback and self-monitoring on brain trauma youth's conversational skills. *Journal of Applied Behavioral Analysis, 17,* 353–358.

Giles, G. M. (1999). Management of behavioral disregulation and non-compliance in the post-acute severely brain injured adult.

In G. M. Giles & J. Clark-Wilson (Eds.), *Rehabilitation of the severely brain injured adult: A practical approach* (2nd ed., pp. 81–96). Cheltenham, England: Stanley Thornes.

Giles, G. M. (2001). The effectiveness of neurorehabilitation. In R. L. Wood & T. M. McMillan (Eds.), *Neurobehavioural disability and social handicap following traumatic brain injury* (pp. 231–255). Hove, England: Psychology Press.

Giles, G. M., & Clark-Wilson, J. (1988). The use of behavioral techniques in functional skills training after severe brain injury. *American Journal of Occupational Therapy, 42,* 658–665.

Giles, G. M., & Clark-Wilson, J. (Eds.). (1993). *Brain injury rehabilitation: A neurofunctional approach.* San Diego, CA: Singular.

Giles, G. M., & Clark-Wilson, J. (Eds.). (1999). *Rehabilitation of the severely brain injured adult: A practical approach.* Cheltenham, England: Stanley Thornes.

Giles, G. M., Fussey, I., & Burgess, P. (1988). The behavioral treatment of verbal interaction skills following severe head injury: A single case study. *Brain Injury, 2,* 75–81.

Giles, G. M., & Morgan, J. H. (1989). Training functional skills following herpes simplex encephalitis: A single case study. *Journal of Clinical and Experimental Neuropsychology, 11,* 311–318.

Giles, G. M., Ridley, J., Dill, A., & Frye, S. (1997). A consecutive series of brain injured adults treated with a washing and dressing retraining program. *American Journal of Occupational Therapy, 51,* 256–266.

Giles, G. M., & Shore, M. (1989a). The effectiveness of an electronic memory aid for a memory impaired adult of normal intelligence. *American Journal of Occupational Therapy, 43,* 409–411.

Giles, G. M., & Shore, M. (1989b). A rapid method for teaching severely brain-injured adults to wash and dress. *Archives of Physical Medicine and Rehabilitation, 70,* 156–158.

Goel, V., & Grafman, J. (2000). Role of the right prefrontal cortex in ill-structured planning. *Cognitive Neuropsychology, 17,* 415–436.

Goel, V., Grafman, J., Tajik, J., Gana, S., & Danto, D. (1997). A study of the performance of patients with frontal lobe lesions in a financial planning task. *Brain, 120,* 1805–1822.

Gollwitzer, P. M. (1993). Goal achievement: The role of intentions. In W. Stroebe & M. Hewstone (Eds.), *European Review of Social Psychology* (Vol. 4, pp. 141–185). Chichester, England: Wiley.

Gollwitzer, P. M. (1996). The volitional benefits of planning. In P. M. Gollwitzer & J. A. Bargh (Eds.), *The psychology of action: Linking cognition and motivation to behavior* (pp. 287–312). New York: Guilford

Greenwood, R., Bhalla, A., Gordon, A., & Roberts, J. (1983). Behavioral disturbance during recovery from herpes simplex encephalitis. *Journal of Neurology, Neurosurgery, and Psychiatry, 46,* 809–817.

Hanks, R. A., Rapport, L. J., Millis, S. R., & Deshpande, S. A. (1999). Measures of executive functioning as predictors of functional ability and social integration in a rehabilitation sample. *Archives of Physical Medicine and Rehabilitation, 80,* 1030–1037.

Harding, E. J., Paul, E. S., & Mendl, M. (2004). Changes in grey matter induced by training. *Nature, 427,* 311–312.

Harrick, L., Krefting, L., Johnston, J., Carlson, P., & Minnes, P. (1994). Stability of functional outcomes following transitional living programme participation: 3-year follow-up. *Brain Injury, 8,* 439–447.

Hayes, S. C., & Gifford, E. V. (1997). The trouble with language: Experiential avoidance, rules and the nature of verbal events. *Psychological Science, 8,* 170–173.

Hayes, S. C., & Hayes, L. J. (1992). Verbal relations and the evolution of behavior analysis. *American Psychologist, 47,* 1383–1395.

Hooper-Row, J. (1999). Rehabilitation of physical deficits in the post-acute brain injured: Four case studies. In G. M. Giles & J. Clark-Wilson (Eds.), *Rehabilitation of the severely brain injured adult: A practical approach* (pp. 153–163). Chichester, England: Stanley-Thornes.

Hovath, A. O., & Symonds, B. D. (1991). Relationship between working alliance and outcome in psychotherapy: A meta-analysis. *Journal of Counseling Psychology, 38,* 139–149.

Jacobs, H. E. (1988). The Los Angeles head injury survey: Procedures and initial findings. *Archives of Physical Medicine and Rehabilitation, 69,* 425–431.

Jennett, B., & Teasdale, G. (1981). *Management of head injuries.* Philadelphia: F. A. Davis.

Johnston, M. V., & Lewis, F. D. (1991a). Outcomes of community re-entry programmes for brain injury survivors. Part 1: Independent living and productive activities. *Brain Injury, 5,* 141–154.

Johnston, M. V., & Lewis, F. D. (1991b). Outcomes of community re-entry programs for brain-injury survivors. Part 2: Further investigations. *Brain Injury, 5,* 155–168.

Katzman, S., & Mix, C. (1994). Improving functional independence in a patient with encephalitis through behavior modification shaping techniques. *American Journal of Occupational Therapy, 48,* 259–269.

Kazdin, A. (1994). *Behavior modification in applied settings.* Pacific Grove, CA: Brooks/Cole.

Kern, R. S., Liberman, R. P., Kopelowicz, A., Mintz, J., & Green, M. F. (2002). Application of errorless learning for improving work performance in persons with schizophrenia. *American Journal of Psychiatry, 159,* 1921–1926.

Kewman, D. G., Yanus, B., & Kirsch, N. (1988). Assessment of distractibility in auditory comprehension after traumatic brain injury. *Brain Injury, 2,* 131–137.

Klonoff, P. S., Lamb, D. G., Henderson, S. W., & Shepherd, J. (1998). Outcome assessment after milieu-oriented rehabilitation: New considerations. *Archives of Physical Medicine and Rehabilitation, 79,* 684–690.

Komatsu, S., Minimua, M., Kato, M., & Kashima, H. (2000). Errorless and effortful processes involved in the learning of face-name associations by patients with alcoholic Korsakoff's syndrome. *Neuropsychological Rehabilitation, 10,* 113–132.

Krueger, W. C. F. (1929). The effect of overlearning on retention. *Journal of Experimental Psychology, 12,* 71–78.

Lashley, B., & Drabman, R. (1974). Facilitation of the acquisition and retention of sight-word vocabulary through token reinforcement. *Journal of Applied Behavioral Analysis, 7,* 307–312.

Lengfelder, A., & Gollwitzer, P. M. (2001a). Implementation intentions and efficient action initiation. *Journal of Personality and Social Psychology, 81,* 946–960.

Lengfelder, A., & Gollwitzer, P. M. (2001b). Reflective and reflexive action control in patients with frontal brain lesions. *Neuropsychology, 15,* 80–100.

Levin, H. S., Goldstein, F. C., High, W. M., & Williams, D. (1988). Automatic and effortful processing after severe closed head injury. *Brain and Cognition, 7,* 283–297.

Lewicki, P., Czyzenska, M., & Hoffman, H. (1987). Unconscious acquisition of complex procedural knowledge. *Journal of Experimental Psychology: Learning, Memory, and Cognition, 13,* 523–530.

Lewicki, P., Hill, T., & Bizot, E. (1988). Acquisition of procedural knowledge about a pattern of stimuli that cannot be articulated. *Cognitive Psychology, 20,* 24–37.

Lloyd, L. F., & Cuvo, A. J. (1994). Maintenance and generalization of behaviors after treatment of persons with traumatic brain injury. *Brain Injury, 8,* 529–540.

Luborsky, L., McLellan, A. T., Woody, G. E., O'Brien, C. P., & Auerbach, A. (1985). Therapist success and its determinants. *Archives of General Psychiatry, 42,* 602–611.

Mace, F. C., & Lalli, J. S. (1991). Linking descriptive and experimental analyses in the treatment of bizarre speech. *Journal of Applied Behavioral Analysis, 24,* 553–562.

Mackay, L. E., Bernstein, B. A., Chapman, P. E., Morgan, A. S., & Milazzo, L. S. (1992). Early intervention in severe head injury: Long-term benefits of a formalized program. *Archives of Physical Medicine and Rehabilitation, 73,* 635–641.

Malec, J., Zweber, B., & DePompolo, R. (1990). The Rivermead Behavioral Memory Test, laboratory neurocognitive measures, and everyday functioning. *Journal of Head Trauma Rehabilitation, 5,* 60–68.

Manchester, D., Hodgkinson, A., Pfaff, A., & Nguyen, F. (1997). A non-aversive approach to reducing hospital absconding in a head-injured adolescent boy. *Brain Injury, 11,* 271–277.

Manchester, D., & Wood, R. L. (2001). Applying cognitive therapy in neurobehavioral rehabilitation. In R. L. Wood & T. M. McMillan (Eds.), *Neurobehavioral disability and social handicap following traumatic brain injury* (pp. 157–174). Hove, England: Psychology Press.

Martin, D. J., Garske, J. P., & Davis, M. K. (2000). Relationship of the therapeutic alliance with outcome and other variables: A meta-analytic review. *Journal of Consulting and Clinical Psychology, 68,* 438–450.

Martin, G. L., Koop, S., Turner, G., & Hanel, F. (1981). Backward chaining versus total task presentation to teach assembly tasks to severely retarded persons. *Behavior Research of Severe Developmental Disabilities, 2,* 117–136.

McDonnell, J. (1987). The effect of time delay and increasing prompt hierarchy strategies on the acquisition of purchasing skills by students with severe handicaps. *Journal of the Association for the Severely Handicapped, 12,* 227–236.

McDonnell, J., & Laughlin, B. (1989). A comparison of backward and concurrent chaining strategies in teaching community skills. *Education and Training in Mental Retardation, 24,* 230–238.

McGlynn, S. M., & Schacter, D. L. (1989). Unawareness of deficits in neuropsychological syndromes. *Journal of Clinical and Experimental Neuropsychology, 11,* 143–205.

McMillan, T. M., Papadopoulos, H., Cornall, C., & Greenwood, R. J. (1990). Modification of severe behavior problems following herpes simplex encephalitis. *Brain Injury, 4,* 399–406.

Miller, E. (1980). The training characteristics of severely head injured patients: A preliminary study. *Journal of Neurology, Neurosurgery, and Psychiatry, 43,* 525–528.

Miller, W. R., & Rollnick, S. (1991). *Motivational interviewing.* New York: Guilford.

Mills, V. M., Nesbeda, T., Katz, D. I., & Alexander, M. P. (1992). Outcomes for traumatically brain-injured patients following post-acute rehabilitation programs. *Brain Injury, 6,* 219–228.

Murre, J. M. J. (1997). Implicit and explicit memory in amnesia: Some explanations and predictions by the trace link model. *Memory, 5,* 213–232.

Nelson, T. O., & Narens, L. (1994). Why investigate metacognition. In J. Metcalf & P. Shimamura (Eds.), *Metacognition: Knowing about knowing* (pp. 1–26). Cambridge, MA: MIT Press.

Newell, A., & Rosenbloom, P. S. (1981). Mechanisms of skill acquisition and the law of practice. In J. R. Anderson (Ed.), *Cognitive skills and their acquisition* (pp. 1–55). Hillsdale, NJ: Lawrence Erlbaum.

Nissen, M. J., & Bullemer, P. (1987). Attentional requirements of learning: Evidence from performance measures. *Cognitive Psychology, 19,* 1–32.

Norman, D. A., & Shallace, T. (1986). Attention to action: Willed and automatic control of behavior. In R. J. Davidson, G. E. Schwartz, & D. Shapiro (Eds.), *Consciousness and self-regulation: Advances in research and theory* (Vol. 4, pp. 1–18). New York: Plenum.

O'Carroll, R. E., Russell, H. H., Lawrie, S. M., & Johnstone, E. C. (1999). Errorless learning and the cognitive rehabilitation of memory impaired schizophrenic patients. *Psychological Medicine, 29,* 105–112.

O'Reilly, M. F., & Cuvo, A. J. (1989). Teaching self-treatment of cold symptoms to an anoxic brain injured adult. *Behavioral Residential Treatment, 4*, 359–375.

Parkin, A. J., Hunkin, N. M., & Squires, E. J. (1998). Unlearning John Major: The use of errorless learning in the reacquisition of proper names following herpes simplex encephalitis. *Cognitive Neuropsychology, 15*, 361–375.

Posner, M. I., & Peterson, S. E. (1990). The attentional system of the human brain. *Annual Review of Neuroscience, 13*, 25–42.

Postman, L. (1962). Retention as a function of degree of over-learning. *Science, 135*, 666–667.

Reason, J. (1984). Absent-mindedness and cognitive control. In J. E. Harris & P. E. Morris (Eds.), *Everyday memory actions and absent mindedness* (pp. 113–132). London: Academic Press.

Robertson, I. H., Ridgeway, V., Greenfield, E., & Parr, A. (1997). Motor recovery after stroke depends on intact sustained attention: A 2-year follow-up study. *Neuropsychology, 11*, 290–295.

Robertson, I. H., Ward, T., Ridgeway, V., & Nimmo-Smith, I. (1994). *The Test of Everyday Attention.* Bury St. Edmund's, England: Thames Valley Test Company.

Rothwell, N. A., LaVigna, G. W., & Willis, T. J. (1999). A non-aversive rehabilitation approach for people with severe behavior problems resulting from brain injury. *Brain Injury, 13*, 521–533.

Safran, J. D., & Muran, J. C. (2000). *Negotiating the therapeutic alliance: A relational treatment guide.* New York: Guilford.

Schmitter-Edgecombe, M., & Rogers, W. A. (1997). Automatic process development following severe closed head injury. *Neuropsychology, 11*, 296–308.

Schneider, W., Dumais, S. T., & Shiffrin, R. M. (1984). Automatic and control processing and attention. In R. Parasuraman & D. R. Davis (Eds.), *Varieties of attention* (pp. 1–27). London: Academic Press.

Schneider, W., & Shiffrin, R. M. (1977). Controlled and automatic human information processing: I. Detection, search, and attention. *Psychological Review, 84*, 1–66.

Schwartz, A. F., & McMillan, T. M. (1989). Assessment of everyday memory after severe head injury. *Cortex, 25*, 665–671.

Shallice, T. (1982). Specific impairments of planning. In D. E. Broadbent & L. Weiskrantz (Eds.), *The neuropsychology of cognitive function* (pp. 199–209). London: Royal Society.

Shallice, T., & Burgess, P. W. (1991). Deficits in strategy application following frontal lobe damage in man. *Brain, 114*, 727–741.

Shallice, T., & Burgess, P. W. (1996). The domain of supervisory processes and temporal organization of behavior. *Philosophical Transactions of the Royal Society of London. Series B, 351*, 1405–1402.

Shallice, T., & Evans, M. E. (1978). The involvement of the frontal lobes in cognitive estimation. *Cortex, 14*, 294–303.

Shaw, L., Brodsky, L., & McMahon, B. T. (1985). Neuropsychiatric intervention in the rehabilitation of head injured patients. *Psychiatric Journal of the University of Ottawa, 10*, 237–240.

Shiffrin, R. M., & Dumais, S. T. (1981). The development of automatism. In J. R. Anderson (Ed.), *Cognitive skills and their acquisition* (pp. 111–140). Hillsdale, NJ: Lawrence Erlbaum.

Shiffrin, R. M., & Schneider, W. (1977). Controlled and automatic information processing: II. Perceptual learning, automatic attending, and a general theory. *Psychological Review, 84*, 127–190.

Simon, H. A. (1975). The functional equivalence of problem solving. *Cognitive Psychology, 7*, 268–288.

Skinner, B. F. (1938). *The behavior of organisms.* New York: D. Appleton-Century-Crafts.

Smith, R. G., & Iwata, B. A. (1997). Antecedent influences on behavior disorder. *Journal of Applied Behavioral Analysis, 30*, 343–375.

Soderback, I., & Normell, L. A. (1986a). Intellectual function training in adults with acquired brain damage: Evaluation. *Scandinavian Journal of Rehabilitation Medicine, 18*, 147–153.

Soderback, I., & Normell, L. A. (1986b). Intellectual function training in adults with acquired brain damage: An occupational therapy method. *Scandinavian Journal of Rehabilitation Medicine, 18*, 139–146.

Spooner, F. (1984). Comparison of backward chaining and total task presentation in training severely handicapped persons. *Education and Training of the Mentally Retarded, 19*, 15–22.

Stablum, F., Umilta, C., Monentale, C., Carlan, M., & Guerrini, C. (2000). Rehabilitation of executive deficits in closed head injury and anterior communicating artery aneurysm patients. *Psychological Research, 63*, 265–278.

Stuss, D. T., & Alexander, M. P. (2000). Executive functions and the frontal lobes: A conceptual view. *Psychological Research, 63*, 289–298.

Stuss, D. T., & Levine, B. (2002). Adult clinical neuropsychology: Lessons from studies of the frontal lobes. *Annual Review of Psychology, 53*, 401–433.

Stuss, D. T., Stethem, L., Hugenholtz, H., Picton, T., Pivik, J., & Richards, M. T. (1989). Reaction time after head injury: Fatigue, divided attention, and consistency of performance. *Journal of Neurology, Neurosurgery, and Psychiatry, 52*, 742–748.

Terrace, H. S. (1963). Discrimination learning with and without "errors." *Journal of the Experimental Analysis of Behavior, 6*(1), 1–27.

Toglia, J. P. (1998). A dynamic interactional model to cognitive rehabilitation. In N. Katz (Ed.), *Cognition and occupation in rehabilitation: Cognitive models for intervention in occupational therapy* (pp. 5–50). Bethesda, MD: American Occupational Therapy Association.

Tulving, E. (1983). *Elements of episodic memory.* Oxford, England: Clarendon Press.

Vilkki, J. (1988). Problem solving after focal cerebral lesions. *Cortex, 24,* 119–127.

Whittington, R., & Wykes, T. (1996). Aversive stimulation by staff and violence by psychiatric patients. *British Journal of Clinical Psychology, 35,* 11–20.

Willer, B., Button, J., & Rempel, R. (1999). Residential and home-based postacute rehabilitation of individuals with traumatic brain injury: A case control study. *Archives of Physical Medicine and Rehabilitation, 80,* 399–406.

Wilson, B. A., Alderman, N., Burgess, A. W., Emslie, H., & Evans, J. J. (1996). *Behavioral assessment of the dysexecutive syndrome.* Bury St. Edmund's, England: Thames Valley Test Company.

Wilson, B. A., Baddeley, A., Evans, J. J., & Shiel, A. (1994). Errorless learning in the rehabilitation of memory impaired people. *Neuropsychological Rehabilitation, 4,* 307–326.

Wilson, B. A., Cockburn, J., & Baddeley, A. (1991). *The Rivermead Behavioral Memory Test.* Bury St. Edmund's, England: Thames Valley Test Company.

Wilson, B. A., Cockburn, J., & Halligan, P. W. (1987). *Behavioral inattention test manual.* London: Thames Valley Test Company.

Wilson, B. A., & Moffat, N. (1984). *Clinical management of memory problems.* London: Croom Helm.

Wolery, M., Griffen, A. K., Ault, M. J., Gast, D. L., & Doyle, P. M. (1990). Comparison of constant time delay and the system of least prompts in teaching chained tasks. *Education and Training in Mental Retardation, 25,* 243–257.

Wood, R. L., McCrea, J., Wood, L. M., & Merriman, R. (1999). Clinical and cost effectiveness of post-acute neurobehavioral rehabilitation. *Brain Injury, 13,* 69–88.

Woody, S. R., & Adessky, R. S. (2002). Therapeutic alliance, group cohesion, and homework compliance during cognitive–behavioral group treatment of social phobia. *Behavior Therapy, 33,* 5–27.

World Health Organization. (2001). *International classification of functioning, disability, and health (ICF).* Geneva, Switzerland: Author.

Yuen, H. K., & Benzing, P. (1996). Guiding of behavior through redirection in brain injury rehabilitation. *Brain Injury, 10,* 229–238.

Zencius, A. H., Wesolowski, M. D., Burke, W. H., & McQuade, P. (1989). Antecedent control in the treatment of brain injured clients. *Brain Injury, 3,* 199–205.

PART

Mental Health

6

Naomi Josman, PhD, OTR

The Dynamic Interactional Model in Schizophrenia

The pathology and sequelae of schizophrenia are well-documented and, over the past
20 years, major efforts have been devoted to
research and treatment of cognitive disabilities of people with schizophrenia. Within the
study of schizophrenia, cognitive deficits are
the focus of much recent research and theoretical writings. Weickert and colleagues
(2000) argued that executive function and attention deficits may constitute a core cognitive
impairment in schizophrenia, independent
from variations in intelligence level. The
presence of various cognitive deficits in patients with schizophrenia has been established in many studies (Bellack, Gold, &
Buchana, 1999; Binks & Gold, 1998; Bustini
et al., 1999; Evans, Chua, McKenna, & Wilson,
1997; Green, Kern, Braff, & Mintz, 2000; Katz
& Tolchinsky-Landsmann, 1991; Lysaker,
Bell, & Beam-Goulet, 1995; Pantelis et al.,
1999). These cognitive disabilities manifested
by people with schizophrenia are markedly
similar to those of people with brain injury. A
few cognitive models for the intervention of
people with schizophrenia have been developed in occupational therapy; the majority of
them focus on specific cognitive components,
yet most do not incorporate a metacognitive
perspective.

The dynamic interactional model as developed by Toglia (1989, 1998; see Chapter
2, this volume) for intervention with people
experiencing brain injury, specifically addresses both metacognitive and cognitive
components. The purpose of this chapter is
to describe the adaptation of the dynamic
interactional model for people with schizophrenia. A comprehensive review of the literature on cognitive and metacognitive disabilities in schizophrenia is followed by a
conceptual model and a proposal for implementing the dynamic interactional model in
occupational therapy. A case study is provided to demonstrate the potential utility of
this model. Finally, I describe some evidence-
based research, mainly for the assessment instruments.

THEORETICAL BACKGROUND

Recent literature has examined cognitive deficits in schizophrenia (Corrigan & Calabrese,
2004). Research has shown that most discrete
cognitive functions, such as attention, short-
term memory, recognition, consolidation, long-
term memory, and decision making are diminished in schizophrenia. Some researchers
proposed that some cognitive demands (such
as memory and attention tasks) overwhelm
the limited capacity of people with schizophrenia (Nuechterlein & Dawson, 1984). This
model is one example of information processing; however, more recent approaches use parallel distributed processing paradigms (Cohen
& Servan-Schreiber, 1992). Parallel distributed processing models represent the complex events of human cognition as concurrent,
and sometimes independent, processes. These
models have been applied to understand cognitive deficits associated with schizophrenia
(Cohen & Servan-Schreiber, 1992). Other conceptualizations have framed cognitive deficits
in schizophrenia as reflecting a failure of
cognitive systems to process data in an integrated fashion (Green & Nuechterlein, 1999;
Spaulding & Poland, 2001).

Researchers have, in recent years, begun to explore the similarities in neuropsychological deficits in people with chronic brain injuries and those with schizophrenia (Davalos, Green, & Rial, 2002). Thus, the dynamic interactional approach, initially developed for people with brain injuries, may be adapted for use with people diagnosed with schizophrenia.

Neuropsychological Disabilities

Increasing evidence in psychiatry supports neurological explanations for the manifested functional disorders in schizophrenia (Weinberger, 1995, 1996; Weinberger & Lipska, 1995). There is accumulating evidence that clients with schizophrenia are unable to fully activate their frontal lobes during cognitive tasks requiring sustained frontal-lobe activation (Meltzer, 1994). They also show clinical signs of frontal-lobe dysfunction, including blunted affect, difficulty with problem solving, and impoverished thinking (Weinberger, Aloia, Goldberg, & Berman, 1994). Binks and Gold (1998), although focusing on issues of measurement, found major neuropsychological deficits in their sample of clients with schizophrenia. The treatment of these symptoms also has long been the target of various therapeutic approaches and interventions (Josman, 1998). Cognitive or neuropsychological deficits in schizophrenia include problems of attention, concentration, and memory, as well as impairment in abstraction and concept formation abilities. Abundant literature documents the presence of significant neuropsychological impairments in schizophrenia (David & Cutting, 1994), but only in the past decade have these impairments emerged as targets for research and treatment (Clark & O'Carroll, 1998; Davalos et al., 2002; Levine et al., 2000; Stuve, Erickson, & Spaulding, 1991; Wykes, Reeder, Corner, Williams, & Everitt, 1999).

Clients with schizophrenia experience everyday difficulties that are characteristic of cognitive disabilities (Allen, 1992). These impairments also are similar to those disabilities manifested by people with other diagnoses, including brain injuries. Moreover, these people exhibit common learning difficulties, which may be attributed to the component parts of brain function, such as apraxia, impairment of perception, attention, memory, and orientation.

Memory Disorders

Memory impairments in schizophrenia have been well documented (Clare, McKenna, Mortimer, & Baddley, 1993; Kuperberg & Heckers, 2000; So, Toglia, & Donohue, 1997). According to Calev and Edelist (1993), these impairments represent the most significant neuropsychological problem in schizophrenia. More recent studies have found that memory deficits in schizophrenia, unlike the classical amnesic syndrome observed after brain injury, involve both episodic and semantic memory, as well as impairments in general knowledge of concepts, categories, and meanings (Chen, Wilkins, & McKenna, 1994; Clare et al., 1993; Duffy & O'Carroll, 1994; Kuperberg & Heckers, 2000).

As a major memory process, *encoding* refers to a mental activity or type of strategy that a learner uses when studying material to be remembered. Several studies link memory recall deficits in clients with schizophrenia to ineffective encoding of to-be-remembered verbal materials (Calev, Venables, & Monk, 1983; Harvey, Earle-Boyer, Wielgus, & Levinson, 1986). For example, people with schizophrenia require more trials than normal participants to organize sets of words consistently on a sorting task; however, after accomplishing this task, recall for words and categorical order was equal to normal participants' recall (Larsen & Fromholt, 1976). Thus, it is apparent that induced affective or semantic encoding strategies attenuate the encoding deficit in schizophrenia. Additional studies have shown that the process of making meaningful sentences out of to-be-remembered words (Koh, Marusarz, & Rosen, 1980), or an increase in the level of semantic processing (Koh, Grinker, Marusarz, & Forman, 1981), have similar normalizing effects in recall of clients with schizophrenia.

There is evidence that these encoding memory deficits may be related to an inefficient use of mnemonic strategies by these clients rather than to irreversible structural defects (Koh & Peterson, 1978). Although they demonstrate the potential to use mnemonic organizational properties, they may fail to do so at the encoding stage (Calev et al., 1983). The impaired capacity to form meaningful and efficient associations—functions that constitute the fundamentals of memory—may be attributable to overinclusive thinking. Gray, Feldon, Rawlins, Hemsley, and Smith (1991) proposed that the basic problem in schizophrenia may be a weakening of the ability to use and incorporate past experiences in current learning. Duffy and O'Carroll (1994) hypothesized further that the cognitive mechanisms involved in the formation and retention of association networks in general may be markedly dysfunctional in schizophrenia. Schwartz, Rosse, and Deutsch (1993) have suggested an alternate hypothesis accordingly, whereby clients with schizophrenia may have difficulty in using conceptual or organizational processes in performing tasks that require explicit retrieval of contextual information.

Hutton and associates (1998) tested people with schizophrenia on several functions and found that the participants had shorter spatial spans, suggesting that they had difficulty in maintaining a sequence of moves in memory over a short period of time. They also were impaired on the spatial working memory test (Hutton et al., 1998). Clark and O'Carroll (1998) reported on a study that demonstrated that episodic memory dysfunction (as measured by the Rivermead Behavioral Memory Test) was the only cognitive variable associated with poor psychosocial outcome in schizophrenia.

Executive Functions

Executive functions describes the way information is controlled and processed (Wykes et al., 1999) and consist of a variety of skills, including volition, planning, concept formation, purposive action, and effective performance (Lezak, 1995). Goal management is another ability that relies on executive functions (Levine et al., 2000). Researchers suggest that people with schizophrenia exhibit cognitive impairment in the realm of executive functions that is considered debilitating to the individual's ability to function effectively in the world (Levine et al., 2000).

A variety of tests have been used to assess executive functions in patients with schizophrenia (Clark & O'Carroll, 1998; Davalos et al., 2002; Hutton et al., 1998; Wykes et al., 1999). Green and Nuechterlein (1999), in their review of neurocognitive deficits and functional outcomes, found card sorting to be associated with community daily activities. In a further meta-analysis, Green and colleagues (2000) found highly significant but small-to-medium effect size over pooled samples of 1,002 participants for card sorting. As the authors stated, these general findings suggest that a relationship exists between this construct card-sorting–executive function and functional outcomes. They further raise issues of neurocognitive deficits and their relationships to functional outcomes, suggesting that they are probably mediating variables, like learning potential, between more basic neurocognitive processes and functional outcomes. To better understand the relationships of cognitive abilities and functional outcomes, it was suggested that general functional outcomes, as analyzed by Green and colleagues (2000), are global insofar as any daily activity requires a combination of many cognitive abilities (Josman & Katz, in press).

In one study, one aspect of executive functions, concept formation, was a target for intervention (Kurtz, Moberg, Gur, & Gur, 2001). Another study reported a cognitive intervention used to treat people with schizophrenia with identified deficits in executive functions (Davalos et al., 2002). This intervention emphasized the establishment of routines, the development of well-rehearsed strategies, and the acquisition of compensatory techniques. Individuals were taught organization principles and the application of these strategies to make plans, as well as how to simplify information to deal more easily with problems. Self-awareness, goal-setting, and generalization of acquired skills were addressed as well. The results of this study suggest that a well-delineated cognitive rehabilitation approach that addresses executive functions could demonstrate efficacy.

The main categorization-sorting test used in the clinic and in research is the Wisconsin Card Sorting Test (WCST; Heaton, Chelune, Talley, Kay, & Curtiss, 1983). It is viewed as a measure of executive functions for mental flexibility and the ability to shift set (Pantelis et al., 1999) as the main indicator of prefrontal deficit (Goldberg, Weinberger, Berman, Pliskin, & Podd, 1987; Green, Satzm, Ganzell, & Vaclav, 1992) and as a measure of problem solving (Bustini et al., 1999). The performance of clients with schizophrenia on the WCST is found to be inferior to that of participants without schizophrenia, and the deficit is resistant to neuroleptic treatment (Meltzer, 1994). Teaching the test in intervention studies did not result in sustained improvement (Green et al., 2000), but a more recent review and meta-analysis show that remediation of WCST performance yielded a fairly substantial effect regardless of method of instructional remediation (Kurtz et al., 2001).

In general, two issues remain in the studies about the WCST: durability is typically not tested beyond 24 hours, and generalization effects have not typically been examined. Bellack and colleagues (1999), for example, have demonstrated an improvement in the performance of clients with schizophrenia on the WCST following a one-day training procedure. Furthermore, the authors claim for a moderate generalization of the training procedure to the performance on the Tower of Hanoi, another test of problem solving and hypothesis testing. However, it is important to note that the authors have found performance improvements 24 hours after the training procedure and did not examine the preservation of this improvement in the long run (Josman & Katz, in press).

Other researchers studied the relationship among executive functions, visuospatial problem solving, and measures of occupational functioning among men with schizophrenia or schizoaffective disorder (Secrest, Wood, & Tapp, 2000). The WCST was used to measure executive functions, abstract reasoning, and problem solving abilities; the Allen Cognitive Level (ACL; Allen, Earhart, & Blue, 1992) measured learning, problem solving, and visuospatial abilities; and the Routine Task Inventory (RTI; Allen et al, 1992) measured performance level in activities of daily living. The WCST and the ACL were both found to be sensitive to similar domains of functioning and to predict task performance (Secrest et al., 2000).

Awareness

A lack of awareness of deficit has been documented for a broad range of neuropsychological syndromes, including schizophrenia. This phenomenon has significant implications for treatment and management. Clients who are unaware of their problems are unlikely to cooperate with treatment plans or accept help from concerned family members (Katz, Fleming, Keren, Lightbody, & Hartman-Maier, 2002; McGlynn & Kaszniak, 1986). Furthermore, these clients may attempt to perform activities that are entirely unrealistic, considering their given disabilities. Greenfield (1985) claimed that clients who lack awareness of their mental illness, insisting that they have no illness or symptoms requiring treatment, are virtually inaccessible to treatment. Katz and colleagues (2002) discussed implications for occupational therapy for people with schizophrenia, concluding that it is very difficult to distinguish between unawareness and denial with this population because psychological factors are an integral part of the disease and no clear neurological factors can be determined. According to Toglia (2003a), an individual's lack of understanding of his strengths and limitations prevents him or her from choosing realistic, attainable goals. Toglia and Kirk (2000) suggested that breaking down the client's unrealistic goals into more realistic subgoals by using structured methods can help him or her target current strengths and limitations. Katz and colleagues (2002) presented a case study that supports this suggestion (see also Chapters 1 and 2, this volume).

Delusions have been considered, by definition, to be outside the realm of patients' awareness. Kihlstrom and Hoyt (1988) viewed delusions as part product of disordered perceptual and attentional processes. According to this view, clients with schizophrenia are entirely unaware of their most fundamental cognitive deficit: a perceptual–attentional disorder. As a consequence, they search for some explanation for their anomalous experiences, not realizing their own role in constructing the bizarre experiences. Schizophrenia with negative symptoms, however, provides evidence that brain dysfunction is restricted primarily to subcortical structures and the frontal lobes (Kihlstrom & Hoyt, 1988).

Stuss and Benson (1986) discussed the possible contribution of frontal-lobe damage to the pathogenesis of anosognosia. The role of frontal damage in unawareness of deficits is further indicated by the extensive literature on people following head injuries, who often exhibit symptoms of frontal-lobe damage with unawareness of deficits (McGlynn & Kaszniak, 1986).

Amador and colleagues (1994) conducted a study to assess insight into multiple aspects of mental disorder using a standardized measure. Their sample of 412 patients included clients with psychotic and mood disorders. Their results indicate that poor insight is a prevalent feature of schizophrenia. Moreover a variety of self-awareness deficits were found to be more severe and pervasive in participants with schizophrenia than in clients with schizoaffective or major depressive disorders, with or without psychosis.

Toglia (2003b; Toglia, Abreu, & Allen, 2001) defined self-awareness as self-knowledge and beliefs (regarding abilities, limitations, and functioning) and self-monitoring and appraisal. She suggested using processing strategies to produce efficient and effective occupational performance. Several studies support the association between awareness and functional outcome (LaBuda & Lichtenberg, 1999; Malec & Moessner, 2000; Prigatano & Wong, 1999; Sherer et al., 1998; Tham, Ginsberg, Fisher, & Tegner, 2001).

DYNAMIC ASSESSMENT AND INTERVENTION IN SCHIZOPHRENIA

Occupational therapy had focused on five cognitive models in the intervention of individuals with schizophrenia: cognitive disabilities (Allen, 1985; Allen & Blue, 1998); the model of human occupation's cognitive perspective (Keilhofner, 1995); cognitive organization, Piagetian framework (Katz & Ziv, 1992); dynamic interactional multicontext treatment (Josman, 1998; Toglia, 1992, 1998); and dynamic–cognitive modifiability (Hadas-Lidor & Katz, 1998).

Katz and Hadas-Lidor (1995) suggested that the abovementioned models fall into two major approaches: remedial and adaptive–functional. The target of remedial approaches is the individual's impaired capabilities, whereas the functional approaches aim at the assets or strengths of the individual for functioning; however, they proposed a third category, dynamic–cognitive approach. The authors examined the efficacy of dynamic cognitive treatment in the rehabilitation of clients with schizophrenia over 1 year. The study group showed significant gains on tests of memory, thought processes, functional outcomes, and work and residence status at posttest, in comparison to the control group. These findings supported the use of long-term dynamic cognitive intervention for clients with schizophrenia (Hadas-Lidor & Katz, 1998; Hadas-Lidor, Katz, Tyano, & Weizman, 2001; see Chapter 15, this volume).

Wiedl (1999) reported on pilot studies conducted with the aim of developing a formula for classifying participants according to cognitive modifiability or learning capacity. The WCST was used in these studies to estimate the classification's validity. Results indicated that people with schizophrenia could be classified according to modifiability in concept formation using a dynamic assessment design that includes the WCST in the various phases (pretest, training, and posttest). The author concluded that the WCST may be a useful tool for rehabilitation planning for clients with schizophrenia by helping to classify them according to cognitive modifiability (Wiedl, 1999).

This same author later investigated dynamic assessment, again using the WCST and the Auditory Verbal Learning Test (Wiedl, Schottke, & Garcia, 2001). Specific verbal mediation was used during administration to increase performance. Wiedl found excellent predictive validity results, vis-a-vis proficiency in a clinical training with participants diagnosed with schizophrenia, by using dynamic tools, as compared to static test scores.

According to Toglia (1992), the remedial approaches for cognitive–perceptual impairments are further divided into those that aim at cognitive remediation of deficit-specific skills and those that use a dynamic interactional model. The multicontext treatment approach as part of the dynamic interactional model within the remedial approach assumes that transfer and generalization will occur from the treatment context to other areas and activities.

In the following section, I propose using the dynamic interactional model to further our understanding and to enhance our ability to intervene with clients with schizophrenia.

Main Concept of the Dynamic Interactional Model

Toglia's model (1992, 1998; see also Chapter 2, this volume) uses a broad definition of *cognition* encompassing information-processing skills, learning, and generalization. Moreover, the model does not merely divide cognition into distinct entities but rather analyzes cognitive abilities and deficiencies according to underlying processes, strategies, and potential for learning. Awareness is a major component already acknowledged by rehabilitation professionals. Toglia and Kirk (2000) offered a comprehensive model of awareness to guide the development of assessment tools and interventions. In essence, cognition is viewed as an ongoing product of the dynamic interaction among the individual, the task, and the environment.

Metacognition components of the individual are emphasized in this model. *Metacognition* refers to knowledge and regulation of one's own cognitive processes and capacities. It includes two interrelated aspects: awareness of one's own cognitive processes and capacities and the ability to monitor performance (Flavell, 1985). Clinical application of this model will provide essential information about an individual's potential for change as well as help to answer the following questions: How is he or she aware of his or her difficulties? How promptly does an individual learn new material? How well does he or she retain it? How does he or she go about organizing new information? How does he or she proceed with decisions in response to environmental demands? How orderly and comprehensive are the client's problem-solving strategies? (Erickson & Binder, 1986).

The dynamic interactional model addresses learning potential, analyzes individual processing strategies and style, and provides important guidelines for treatment. Implementing this elaborate method with clients with schizophrenia may significantly advance both our understanding of the disorder and enhance the capacity for effective therapeutic intervention. This model is based on the assumption that direct practice of the impaired skill or, as termed by Toglia (2003a), "specific skill training," with multicontext and different modalities promotes recovery or reorganization of that skill. It provides a framework for simultaneously using and integrating remedial and functional approaches.

Evaluation Process and Instruments

The initial step in evaluating clients with schizophrenia should be based on the use of static assessments, such as standardized cognitive screening instruments that are not developed within the dynamic interactional model. The results of such an evaluation will define a client's "here-and-now" performance baseline. Objectives of the static assessment are the identification and quantification of cognitive deficits, information essential for diagnosis, monitoring progress, discharge planning, and client or caregiver education regarding expected behaviors (Toglia, 1989).

Dynamic interactional assessment (DIA) methods and instruments were developed and studied by Toglia (1992, 1993, 1994). Therapists should use the DIA at the next step of evaluation. DIA consists of three components that are integrated during assessment: awareness questions, cueing and task grading, and strategy investigation (Toglia, 1993). The main contribution of the DIA is that, at the conclusion of the evaluation process, a therapist is able to provide answers to three questions: Can performance be facilitated or changed? What conditions increase or decrease client symptoms? What is the client's potential for learning? Moreover, the DIA of occupational performance needs to carefully consider the conditions of the activity and environment. The conditions under which the activity is performed need to be specified (see Chapter 2).

Instruments

The following section briefly describes three of the instruments developed by Toglia: the Contextual Memory Test (CMT; Toglia, 1993), the Toglia Category Assessment (TCA; Toglia, 1994), and the Deductive Reasoning Test (DR; Toglia, 1994). All three instruments are in use in both treatment and research with clients with schizophrenia.

The CMT was designed to objectively investigate awareness of memory capacity, performance recall, and strategy use. Two different picture cards with 20 line drawings of items from the same theme are included, as well as 40 cards of each theme in which 20 are the same pictures that are drawn on the card and the other 20 are similar pictures (for recognition testing). The test can be used as a static test, by using only Part 1, or as a dynamic test by using both parts. If recall performance is not facilitated with cues, then recognition will be tested (Toglia, 1993). The following are the CMT test components:

1. *Awareness of memory capacity:* general questioning, prediction of memory capacity prior to task performance, and estimation of memory capacity following task performance
2. *Recall of line-drawn objects:* both immediate and delayed recall
3. *Strategy use:* the ability to describe the use of strategy and the ability to benefit from a strategy provided by the examiner.

The CMT is a reliable and valid test, and norms have been provided on the basis of 375 adults ranging in age from 18–86 years (Toglia, 1993; for more information, see Chapters 2 and 10, this volume). In addition, the CMT has been studied in Israel on a group of 217 adults without dis-

ability divided into three age groups parallel to the American age groups (Josman & Hartman-Maeir, 2000). Highly similar levels of performance for Israelis and Americans on the various test components were obtained. Statistically significant differences between American and Israeli participants' performance levels were evident in three memory components among the elderly groups (Group 3) and only in two memory components among the young group (Group 1). In addition, within-sample comparisons of the three Israeli age groups yielded significant age effects for recall, recognition, strategy use, and general awareness.

This study confirmed discriminant validity for the CMT. The tool appears to be highly appropriate for use by occupational therapists in assessing memory and metamemory with American and Israeli adult participants.

The TCA was designed to examine the ability of adults to establish categories and switch conceptual sets. An investigation of awareness is included prior to and following task performance. The evaluator investigates the relationship between the individual's prediction and estimation and his or her actual TCA score. The test uses 18 plastic utensils that can be sorted according to size, color, and type of utensil. The test objectively examines the client's ability to profit from cues and task modification. The TCA is a reliable and valid test. The test manual describes administration, scoring, interpretation, and research done with this test both with clients following brain injury (Toglia, 1994) as well as with clients with schizophrenia (Toglia & Josman, 1994; for more information, see chapters 2 and 10, this volume).

The DR is a continuation of the TCA, uses the same plastic utensils, and can be administered as the next step immediately after administration of the TCA. A questioning game is introduced, wherein the client is instructed to guess which utensil the examiner is thinking of. The client can respond with only "yes" or "no" questions in trying to guess the correct utensil. The examiner does not actually think of an item but answers "no" uniformly to all questions until only one possibility remains. The correct answer should be attained with five questions (Toglia, 1994). A person can have difficulty with this task for several reasons, including failure to keep track of previous questions or their answers, failure to use feedback, failure to discard an inappropriate hypothesis, decreased ability to attend to the relevant attribute, impulsivity, and so forth (Toglia, 1994). The interrater reliability and discriminant validity of the DR test was established in a sample of 42 people with brain injury and 51 people without disabilities ranging in age from 18–84 years (Goverover

& Hinojosa, 2004; for more information, see Chapters 2 and 10, this volume).

A first study designed to establish construct-related validity of the DR with typically developed children was conducted by Josman and Jarus (2001). The results of the study indicate statistically significant differences in the average performance of children in various age groups on the DR assessments but do not show differences among all the groups. The findings of this study provide evidence to support the suitability of the DR for use with children. For more information on this study, please see Chapter 10, this volume.

Intervention Principles

In dynamic interactional assessment, individuals are not classified as having a deficit in separate cognitive areas or in one component of cognition. An individual may have difficulties on a memory task, a visual-processing task, and a problem-solving task; however, DIA focuses on the common behaviors that influence task performance. For example, difficulty in considering all aspects of a situation can interfere with performance on a memory task and a visual-processing task. DIA provides a starting point for treatment. It specifies the task parameters under which cognitive–perceptual symptoms are most likely to emerge. These task parameters represent the starting point for treatment activities. In addition, those behaviors or symptoms observed on a wide range of tasks and most responsive to cues are targeted for intervention using the multicontext approach. Moreover, the individual's self-awareness of his or her own abilities and disabilities is evaluated, and problem-solving strategies used for task performance are recorded and examined. It is important to note that the areas most responsive to cues do not always exhibit the most observable deficits. They represent weakened skills that lie just below the surface and emerge inconsistently and with guidance (Toglia, 1998).

Multicontext Treatment Approach

It should be noted that the multicontext treatment approach does not apply to every client with schizophrenia. The individual's self-awareness and ability to learn are evaluated in the DIA. If the conclusion of this evaluation is that the client's ability to learn or his or her self-awareness is very poor, then different approaches such as adaptation, functional skill training, or compensation should be applied. Moreover, the occupational therapist needs to be aware of the clinical work setting and context and the overall purposes of the setting. In light of the contemporary practice policy of many health services, most clients with schizophrenia are admitted to psychiatric hospitals in an acute stage, where efforts are aimed at stabilizing psychotic symptoms and expediting transfer to a rehabilitation center. In light of this situation, the main purposes of occupational therapy intervention are evaluation, treatment goal setting, and production of a clear report. Most frequently, the client is discharged before having a chance to undergo a DIA. However, for those occupational therapists working in a long-term rehabilitation center or in home services, it is recommended that both the DIA and the multicontext treatment approach be applied.

The multicontext approach simultaneously integrates both compensatory and remedial strategies with awareness-training techniques. There is an emphasis on changing the person's use of strategies and self-monitoring skills within tasks and environments that may need to be adapted to meet the information-processing level of the client. The components of the multicontext approach include an emphasis on processing strategies, task analysis, establishment of criteria for transfer, practice in multiple environments, metacognitive training, and consideration of learner characteristics (Toglia, 1991, 1998).

Following is a list of the main multicontext treatment principles for clients with schizophrenia. A full description of this method is presented in Toglia (1989, 1991, 1992, 1998; see Chapter 2, this volume).

- The sequence of treatment is not predetermined but rather is developed step-by-step according to the client's achievements.
- During all treatment sessions, the therapist analyzes the processing strategies used by the client and determines whether the task may be performed in a more efficient way.
- Determining client motivation is crucial for this kind of treatment; when planning and selecting treatment activities, the therapist needs to consider learner characteristics, including motivation and individual personality characteristics.
- Treatment usually begins at the level at which performance breaks down, or the point at which the client is able to successfully complete the task with the aid of only 1–3 cues.
- Treatment should use activities that meet the abilities of the individual.
- Task complexity is not increased until evidence of generalization is observed at all levels of transfer.
- The underlying strategy or conceptual characteristics remain the same in all treatment tasks, whereas

the surface characteristics of the task change gradually as treatment moves from near transfer to far transfer (Toglia, 1991).

- The therapist should define the goals of each activity in clear, concrete terms comprehensible to the client.
- The therapist can use a variety of computer, gross motor, tabletop, and functional tasks in treatment; the therapist avoids the use of one exclusive type of activity to ensure that, although the instruction may have been embedded in one context, the learned skills may be accessible not exclusively in relation to that specific context (Toglia, 1991).
- Metacognitive training to promote awareness and self-monitoring skills should be incorporated into each treatment session, as well as in different situations.
- To help the client adapt to different environments, both individual and group activities should be used.

CASE STUDY

Susan is a 25-year-old single woman who was hospitalized 9 months ago in an acute psychotic state at a psychiatric hospital. The oldest of three siblings, Susan's father is a cognitive psychologist who has been out of work for the past 18 years, while her mother is an active clinical psychologist. Her parents describe Susan as having been a normal child with intact skills, and all her developmental stages were comparably similar to those of the other children in the family.

Susan related that her problems began at age 10 years, when the family moved to a new residential area. Her first bout of depression occurred at age 15. As a result, she began to miss school days, her school grades deteriorated rapidly, and she eventually completely withdrew from school. Susan received both psychotherapy and drug treatment for her condition. At age 17, she started exhibiting an eating disorder—she began to be extremely concerned with her body weight and shape, and she experienced dramatic weight loss. Despite her unstable emotional state, she succeeded in completing high school at age 18 with fair matriculation grades.

Susan experienced binge eating—frequent episodes of eating large quantities of food in short periods of time—and a psychotic crisis with confusional contents and psychosomatism. She had a few psychotic attacks with accompanying highly regressive behavior, including a neglect of personal hygiene. At the same time, she maintained a relationship with a boyfriend for a year and also was able to keep a job at a store. A psychiatrist

treated her by focusing on rebalancing her with antipsychotic drugs.

At age 24, she was accepted to study fashion design at a higher technical school and commenced her first year of studies while living with her grandmother. A short while later, she stopped taking her medications. Her psychiatrist had great difficulty trying to balance her condition and subsequently referred her to the psychiatric hospital. The purpose of her hospitalization was to reset her balance with medication while also implementing a target rehabilitation program. All previous efforts to remove her from her parents' home had precipitated psychotic attacks. Thus, the ultimate goal of the rehabilitation program was to enhance Susan's ability to live independently outside of her parents' home.

At the time of her admission to the psychiatric wing, Susan behaved negatively: She was unable to accept department boundaries, failed to wake in the morning with everybody else, exhibited tension, and expressed anger toward her parents and therapists. She felt she was not receiving appropriate treatment, made numerous somatic complaints, became markedly anxious as a result of her medication, and was unable to care for her personal hygiene. She was diagnosed as having unspecified schizophrenia with disorganized components, psychosomatism, affective components, and dysphoric states. After receiving medication with Olanzapine and a mood stabilizer, her condition showed some improvement.

In the occupational therapy department, Susan was highly impulsive when performing arts and crafts work; she failed to plan her steps and ignored any advice from her therapist. She exhibited attention and concentration difficulties, was critical of other clients and department staff, and voiced her complaints about virtually everything. Susan was, however, oblivious to her emotional condition as well as her performance difficulties. She professed to be able to work as a fashion designer; however, the quality of her sewing was essentially very poor. She performed her work in short spurts, taking many breaks and frequently falling asleep both outside as well as while working in occupational therapy.

At the initial evaluation, Susan took the Allen Cognitive Level (ACL–90) test and scored at level 5.2, the *exploratory actions* level, defined by Allen (1992) as "the level where the participant can learn through inductive reasoning; the major disability at this level is that costly, imprudent, or dangerous errors must be prevented by someone else" (p. 58). A dynamic assessment was subsequently introduced. A battery of DIA instruments was chosen, including the CMT, the TCA, and the DR, to identify deficits as well as conditions that might maximize performance.

Findings of the DIA

Contextual Memory Test

Awareness

Prior to performing the CMT, Susan was quite aware of her memory difficulties and attributed them to her medication. She underestimated her memory abilities and predicted that she would remember only 7 pictures out of 20, whereas she actually remembered 11 pictures. Immediately after task performance, Susan reported the memory task to be quite difficult for her and claimed that she remembered about half of the card items; her performance awareness proved to be accurate. She also accurately rated the sorting task as being difficult.

Task Performance

Susan was able to recall only 11 items in the immediate recall and 11 in the delayed recall. The recognition part of the test also was administered, but this strategy did not increase her recognition of more items. Susan recognized 16 true positive items but missed 6 other false items, resulting in an overall score of 10. It should be noted that the norm score for her age group on the CMT has a mean of 15.2, with a 2.3 standard deviation for the immediate recall, and a mean of 15.03 and a 2.35 standard deviation for delayed recall (Josman & Hartman-Maeir, 2000). The norm recognition score has a mean of 17.84, with a 2.09 standard deviation. Given that Susan obtained scores of 1 to 2 standard deviations below the norm for both immediate and delayed recall, one might conclude that Susan has mild memory difficulties. Her score on the recognition part of the CMT, however, ranged between 3–4 standard deviations below the normal score, and therefore it appears that recognition did not constitute a viable method for helping Susan to remember items.

Strategy Use

When asked to describe how she studied the items, Susan responded, "I created a story while looking at the items"; when prompted further about the story content, she answered that it was "a restaurant." Her order of recall showed a clustering or grouping of associated items; for example, she said, "knife, fork, and spoon" consecutively. Susan was able to use the contextual strategy in both immediate and delayed recalls. This appears to indicate that the contextual strategy may be effective for use with Susan in her treatment.

Toglia Category Assessment

Awareness

Prior to performing the TCA, Susan refuted any notions of changes in her thinking skills and predicted that the task would be easy to perform. Immediately following task performance, she claimed the task to be of moderate difficulty and then added that "lately I've stopped reading books, and it does not help my thinking skills."

Task Performance

Susan had no difficulty sorting the utensils according to type and, on the second sort, according to color, but she needed a cue to sort them according to size. This seems to indicate that her categorization skills were intact and could be depended on in her treatment.

Deductive Reasoning

Awareness

Prior to performing the DR, Susan reported no change in her thinking skills and professed her familiarity with games of deductive reasoning, such as "Guess Who." On completing the test, she felt the task was easy for her yet noted, quite accurately, that she was able to improve her performance from the first to the second trial.

Task Performance

Susan started the game by asking the evaluator whether the item he thought of was "sharp"; the evaluator in turn asked her to clarify what she meant, to which she replied that both the knives and forks were sharp. This kind of question seems to underline Susan's intact ability to classify to a broader category (sharpness), compared with those that are based visibly on the utensils used in the test. Susan was apparently able to understand the game quite well and attempted to ask fewer questions. She required only one cue to give the correct answer; she did, however, jump to a conclusion one step before really having all the information needed. On the second and third trials, she was able to attain the correct answer with a minimum of 5 questions. Her final score for the DR test was 20 out of 21.

Summary

Susan evidenced mild recall deficits but demonstrated an increase in her ability to estimate the quality of her performance, as well as in her use of strategies. Performance in both categorization and deductive reasoning was very close to normal for her age group. Susan's performance demonstrated a clear learning curve for both tests, as well as a "carry-over" generalization effect in the use of strategies. Susan thus appears to qualify as a suitable candidate for metamemory training and cognitive training in other areas.

Intervention

The goals of the intervention were

1. To define a clear framework and activity-based program to assist Susan's organizing and perseverance skills
2. To enhance cognitive skills associated with attentional functions with the goal of performing continuous and uninterrupted activities, with only minimal work breaks
3. To increase her work attention span and enhance her concentration abilities
4. To improve metacognitive abilities by increasing awareness of her thought processes and difficulties and her sense of product outcome and quality
5. To provide metamemory training to address memory processes and awareness thereof and the associated executive functions
6. To improve activities of daily living skills in preparation for her living independently.

Intervention Plan

The intervention plan tailored to Susan's needs included the following:

1. A work plan was arranged for Susan in occupational therapy, clearly defining required time of arrival at the activity room, the amount of work to be accomplished, and mandatory participation in groups.
2. Susan was provided cognitive and metacognitive training for performing tasks that demand continuous and sustained attention, feedback on performance, and increased awareness of work outcomes and methods of planning. In her work in occupational therapy, Susan preferred sewing activities because of her goal to resume studying fashion design. This area served both global and multiple-stage activities. Given such activities as designing and sewing, Susan was free to work using strategies that tapped into executive functions of planning, performing, and checking work performance. At the outset, Susan claimed her work to be faultless and that she was ready to return to her former college. She picked up sewing tools, cut materials, and attempted to work the sewing machine without any planning or attention to whether she was doing so efficiently; she also became frustrated very quickly and had trouble remembering how to correctly operate the sewing machine. We experimented in finding ways for Susan to remember the required operating steps, such as jotting down the steps, drawing a scheme, and so forth, with an immediate effect of her marked calming down. The next stage involved getting her to stop and plan before commencing any work: This included determining what were required materials, locating them, and then drawing up a plan. After showing her plan to the therapist, she was encouraged to begin sewing.
3. As part of the departmental program, Susan was obliged to rise on time and maintain her personal hygiene. She began to partake in a kitchen activity group in preparation for independent living. Susan made numerous manipulative attempts to avoid having to participate in the group, claiming the group to be inappropriate because of her past eating problems. Despite her protestations, she attended sessions regularly, although she initially experienced difficulties in working independently, was unable to work according to a plan, and required significant assistance. Her work showed a high degree of impulsivity and an inability to follow steps; on several occasions, she spoiled her dish. With mediation, she gradually learned how to read a recipe, plan, and follow through on required steps. Susan is now practically independent in this area and has progressed significantly in her organizing skills.
4. Following the marked improvement in her condition, Susan was transferred to the hospital's unit for evaluation and rehabilitation to assess her vocational preferences in advance of an ambulatory follow-up arrangement.

EVIDENCE-BASED RESEARCH OF THE DIA

The research to date emanating from this model in schizophrenia related only to the DIA instruments and has been described previously (Josman, 1998). However, I repeat it here because of its importance for new readers.

Using the tools developed in the DIA, three studies are reported in this section: (a) a study using the TCA with both clients with schizophrenia and clients with brain injury (Toglia & Josman, 1994); (b) a study of differences in metamemory in participants with chronic schizophrenia and control participants, using the CMT (Josman, 1997); and (c) a study of memory functions in participants with chronic schizophrenia using the CMT (So et al., 1997).

Josman's (1993) study was designed to examine categorization skills in participants with schizophrenia and those with brain injury, and compare the performance of these two populations. A total of 70 hospitalized adults was examined, including 35 participants with schizophrenia and 35 with brain injury. The population with schizophrenia included participants with paranoid schizophrenia, simple-type schizophrenia, residual schizophrenia, and schizoaffective disorders. Participants with active hallucinations or delusions were excluded from the study. The mean age for the participants with schizophrenia was 39 years ($SD = 12$), whereas the mean age for the participants with brain injury was 54 years ($SD = 19$). The age difference between the two groups reflected differences between the two populations. In general, the average age at onset of schizophrenia is in the mid-20s, while cerebral vascular accidents are more commonly seen in the elderly population. In this study, the population with brain injury was generally more educated than the population with schizophrenia. A positive correlation of $r = .59$ ($p < 0.001$) between level of education and the TCA was found. The higher education level of the population with brain injury may partially account for the higher scores obtained by this population as compared to the population with schizophrenia. It should be noted that the population with brain injury constituted an acute population, whereas the population with schizophrenia had been in treatment for an average of 12.48 years, with a standard deviation of 9.5 (Toglia & Josman, 1994).

Categorization Performance

The mean performance score of the participants with schizophrenia on the TCA was 23.08 ($SD = 7.60$), whereas the score of the participants with brain injury on the TCA was 25.17 ($SD = 6.3$). Overall, the population with brain injury scored slightly higher than the population with schizophrenia, but the difference was not significant. This indicated that the TCA should not be used to discriminate between adults with schizophrenia and with brain injury. This finding is not surprising, because there is evidence that participants with chronic schizophrenia show decline in cognition and are assumed to have structural neurological changes located in the frontal lobe (Weinberger et al., 1994). Most neuropsychological tests are unable to differentiate chronic schizophrenia (Lezak, 1995). The TCA was not designed with the purpose of differential diagnosis or discrimination between organic and psychiatric illnesses but rather to provide information that may be helpful for treatment planning.

Awareness Performance

In this study, questions pertaining to awareness were included immediately following task performance. There were significant differences between the mean awareness scores: The participants with brain injury obtained poorer estimation scores than their counterparts with schizophrenia. In addition, there was a significant correlation between the total TCA score and the awareness score for the participants with schizophrenia ($r = .40$) but not for the participants with brain injury. Participants with brain injury, however, demonstrated an interesting crossover pattern: Those who estimated the task to be easy tended to have more difficulty than those who estimated the task to be difficult, whereas participants who estimated the task to be difficult tended to perform better than they had estimated.

This finding is consistent with other studies, which have found that a similar failure to recognize the difficulty of a task in relation to one's own abilities results in impaired performance (McGlynn & Kaszniak, 1986). Results also indicate that questions pertaining to awareness may be sensitive in differentiating between populations with schizophrenia and brain injury.

Using the CMT

In a recent study, Josman (1997) compared the performance of participants with chronic schizophrenia to healthy control participants. A total of 89 participants was examined, including 30 clients with chronic schizophrenia hospitalized within three psychiatric hospitals in Israel and 59 healthy control clients. The mean age for the participants with chronic schizophrenia was 35.6 ($SD = 8.94$) and for the control group was 37.3 ($SD = 14.3$). All other demographic variables were similar for both groups and showed no significant differences. The CMT (Toglia, 1993) was used to measure three aspects of memory: (a) awareness (general, prediction, and estimation), (b) recall (immediate and delayed), and (c) strategy use. The test was administered uniformly to all participants without the provision of any interventions or cues during administration. The restaurant version was administered to half the participants, and the morning version was administered to the remainder of the participants.

Memory Performance

Significant differences were obtained on both immediate and delayed recall between participants with schizophrenia and healthy control participants. The mean score of recall performance of the healthy participants (immediate = 14.6, delayed = 14.3) fell within normal limits, according to the CMT manual (Toglia, 1993), whereas that of the participants with schizophrenia (immediate = 10.1, delayed = 8.6) fell into the mild category of memory ability. The mean scores of the participants with schizophrenia (x(mean) = 22.3, SD = 5.3) were significantly lower (t = 3.85, $p <$ 0.001) than the scores of the healthy participants (x = 25.8, SD = 3.2). The prediction scores before immediate recall were very similar for both healthy participants (x = 11.9) and those with schizophrenia (x = 11.3). However, the participants with schizophrenia overestimated the number of pictures to be remembered, whereas the healthy participants underestimated them. The mean estimation scores directly following the immediate recall of both the participants with schizophrenia (x = 10.8) and the healthy participants (x = 14) were more reflective of their true recall scores: Only the mean estimation scores of the healthy participants were statistically significant with the true recall score obtained but not for the participants with schizophrenia. The estimation scores after the delayed recall for both groups were more reflective of actual recall scores and statistically significant. This finding indicates that the participants with schizophrenia's awareness of their memory ability differed from the awareness of the healthy participants. It should be noted that the participants with schizophrenia overestimated their recall ability before task performance, but their estimation was more accurate immediately after recall performance.

Strategy Use

A significant difference between the participants with schizophrenia and healthy participants was found in reference to their strategy use. The healthy participants used higher-order strategies such as restaurant or association and group, whereas a third of the participants with schizophrenia used a visualization strategy. Most of the participants with schizophrenia did not report the use of any strategy. In response to this finding, So and colleagues (1997) studied the memory performance of adult participants with chronic schizophrenia in terms of (a) awareness of memory capacity, (b) immediate and delayed recall, and (c) strategy use and ability to use contextual information using the CMT (Toglia, 1993). Twenty-three participants with chronic schizophrenia with a mean age of 38.3 years (SD = 6.5) residing in a state hospital in New Jersey were included in the study. The study consisted of 18 men and 5 women, with the mean number of years of education of 11.7 (SD = 2). The mean duration of inpatient stay was 38.6 months (SD = 54.1). The

mean number of years since either the onset of illness or the participants' first admission was 15.87 (SD = 7.4). The primary diagnosis of the participants included 11 (47.8%) with chronic paranoid schizophrenia and 12 (52.2%) with chronic undifferentiated schizophrenica. Among the 23 participants, 14 (60.9%) indicated a history of alcohol abuse, drug abuse, or both. All participants were being treated with neuroleptic medication.

In Part I of the test, each participant was assessed without the aid of any cueing. In Part II, each participant was provided with cueing through being told the theme prior to viewing the objects. This is the usual sequence of directions for the CMT. Part II was administered at least 3 days after the presentation of Part I to minimize the learning effect. This study investigated whether the cue of providing the theme or context facilitated recall. The Brief Psychiatric Rating Scale–Anchored (BPRS–A; Woerner, Mannuzza, & Kane, 1988) and the Scale for the Assessment of Negative Symptoms (SANS; Andreasen, 1989) were used and scored on the basis of the information derived from the interview with the investigator, from chart review of nursing notes, and from consultations with other medical staff. A quasiexperimental design using a one-group, pretest–posttest design format was used. In Part I, but not in Part II, the participant had to estimate his or her own memory capacity.

Immediate and Delayed Recall

In Part II (with a cue providing the theme), the participants achieved higher mean scores in both immediate (19.7) and delayed (9.2) recall than in Part I (without cue) immediate (8.5) and delayed (7.5) recall. The differences between the two mean scores in immediate recall was 2.08 (SD = 2.72; t = −3.67, $p <$ .001). the differences between the two mean scores for delayed recall was 1.65 (SD = 3.11; t = −2.55, $p <$ .05).

Recall and Positive and Negative Symptoms

All participants manifested negative-symptom schizophrenia as classified by Andreasen (1982, 1985, 1989). Participants showed varying degrees of severity of negative symptoms, indicating a range of chronicity. The mean score of the BPRS–A was 31.21 (SD = 8.1). Pearson correlations were computed between the scores of the BPRS–A and immediate and delayed recall in both parts of the CMT. The results reveal significant inverse correlations between the scores of the BPRS–A and the scores of recall (r ranging from −.65 to −.83, $p <$ .01). The mean scores of the SANS items was 61.6 (SD = 29.9). Pearson correlations were computed between the sum scores of the SANS and the scores of recall on CMT (r ranging from $-.64$ to $-.77$, $p < .01$). An analysis of variance was performed between the global rating of each individual category of the SANS and the CMT recall scores. The categories of alogia and attentional impairment showed a significant correlation with the recall scores, whereas the other three categories showed no consistent significant correlations.

Recall and Strategy Use

The sum of the scores on Questions 15 and 16 was calculated. These two questions asked the participants what they did to recall the items (Toglia, 1993). Pearson correlations were then computed between the scores of strategy use and the scores of recall. The correlation coefficient of immediate recall increased from $r = .61$ in Part I to $r = -.63$ ($p < .01$) in Part II. The correlation coefficient of delayed recall increased from $r = .60$ in Part I to $r = .69$ ($p < .01$) in Part II.

Recall and Awareness of Memory Capacity

The participants were only asked to estimate their own memory capacity on Part I of the CMT. Of these participants, 65.2% rated their memory capacity in the 51%–100% range in reference to their performance before illness, whereas 30.4% of the participants rated themselves within a 0–50% range. Participants reported experiencing a lower frequency of forgetting things. The participants were required to estimate how many items out of 20 they could remember, and following the recall task, to estimate how many items they did remember. Correlations between prediction and recall ranged from $r = .08$ to $r = .32$, and those between recall and estimation ranged from $r = .31$ to $r = .75$ ($p < .01$).

A post hoc question was raised as to whether a difference could be observed between paranoid and undifferentiated participants in their CMT performance. In 3 out of the 4 memory tests, paranoid participants achieved mean scores 40% higher than the undifferentiated participants with schizophrenia.

Recent Study

The focus on occupational performance represents a change that has taken place during recent years in the dynamic interactional model to cognitive rehabilitation, concomitant with a re-emphasis and change in general occupational therapy perspectives. A major question emerging from this emphasis is whether occupational therapists should evaluate memory, categorization, visual processing and related components—defined as *bottom-up*—or rather conduct evaluations of actual task performance—or *top-down*. Correlations between evaluations of memory abilities, for example, and their relatedness to a person's everyday memory are still suspect and unconvincing. To pursue this issue, we conducted a study to explore the relationships of categorization on tests and daily tasks in clients with schizophrenia, post-stroke clients, and a control group of people without cognitive problems (Josman & Katz, in press). The purpose of this study was to explore the relationships between performance on formal categorization-sorting tests and daily tasks that require sorting skills among individuals with schizophrenia, as compared with post-stroke and control groups. Furthermore, the relationships among the different tests' performances of clients with schizophrenia were studied.

The study included 70 participants: 37 clients with schizophrenia treated at a community day center, 18 post-stroke clients, and 15 healthy control clients. Participants were evaluated on four categorization tests, including the Wisconsin Card Sorting Test (Heaton, 1993), the Short Category Test (Wetzel & Boll, 1992), Categorization from the Loewenstein Occupational Therapy Cognitive Asessment (Itzkovich, Elazar, Averbuch, & Katz, 2000), and Riska Object Classification (Williams Riska & Allen, 1985), and on five functional daily tasks that require categorization abilities, such as sorting laundry, organizing bills, and sorting food utensils into drawer. Results showed significant differences between performance of clients and control participants on both tests and daily tasks. Spearman correlations within the group with schizophrenia between test scores showed moderate significant correlations, and between-tests and daily tasks scores showed low to moderate significant correlations. These findings may suggest that test scores may not explain the full daily task performance capacity of individuals with schizophrenia. Further research is needed to clarify the underlying components of categorization and their relation to daily task performance of individuals with schizophrenia (Josman & Katz, in press). In line with such research are the *International Classification of Functioning, Disability, and Health* (World Health Organization, 2001), which provides categories for Body Functions (e.g., cognitive skills and higher-level cognitive functions) and Activity and Participation (e.g., occupational performance), components that also are part of the *Occupational Practice Therapy Framework: Domain and Process* (American Occupational Therapy Association, 2002).

SUMMARY AND RECOMMENDATIONS FOR FUTURE RESEARCH

In this chapter I have proposed adopting the dynamic interactional model—a model initially developed by Toglia for use with clients following brain injuries (Toglia, 1992, 1998)—for evaluating and treating people with schizophrenia. The rationale for this idea is that both populations have very similar cognitive and neuropsychological disorders, although for different causes. The dynamic interactional model requires further exploration with clients with schizophrenia, specifically research investigating the therapeutic efficacy of this cognitive intervention. However, in the absence of much research evidence demonstrating the therapeutic efficacy of other cognitive approaches, I suggest that the dynamic interactional model should be used by clinicians. However, it is strongly recommended that researchers study the effectiveness of this intervention method with individuals with schizophrenia.

SUMMARY QUESTIONS

1. What kinds of cognitive problems do people with schizophrenia experience?
2. What kinds of questions does clinical application of the dynamic interactional model help to answer with this population?
3. What kinds of information can be gleaned by implementing the dynamic interactional model and assessment tools?
4. Which of the assessment tools have been adapted and tested for use with a population of people with schizophrenia, what do they examine, and what outcomes resulted from studies of the tools?
5. When is the dynamic interactional model inappropriate for application with people with schizophrenia?

ACKNOWLEDGMENT

The case study discussed in this chapter comes from Ayelet Reizberg, occupational therapist.

REFERENCES

Allen, C., & Blue, T. (1998). Cognitive disabilities model: How to make clinical judgments. In N. Katz (Ed.), *Cognition and occupation in rehabilitation: Cognitive models for intervention in occupational therapy* (pp. 225–279). Bethesda, MD: American Occupational Therapy Association.

Allen, C. K. (1985). *Occupational therapy for psychiatric diseases: Measurement and management of cognitive disabilities.* Boston: Little, Brown.

Allen, C. K. (1992). Cognitive disabilities. In N. Katz (Ed.), *Cognitive rehabilitation model for intervention in occupational therapy* (pp. 1–21). Stoneham, MA: Butterworth-Heinemann.

Allen, C. K., Earhart, C. A., & Blue, T. (1992). *Occupational therapy treatment goals for physically and cognitively disabled.* Rockville, MD: American Occupational Therapy Association.

Amador, F. X., Flaum, M., Andreasen, N. C., Strauss, D. H., Yale, S. A., Clark, S. C., et al. (1994). Awareness of illness in schizophrenia and schizoaffective and mood disorders. *Archives of General Psychiatry, 11,* 826–836.

American Occupational Therapy Association. (2002). Occupational therapy practice framework: Domain and process. *American Journal of Occupational Therapy, 56,* 609–639.

Andreasen, N. C. (1982). Negative symptoms in schizophrenia: Definition and reliability. *Archives of General Psychiatry, 39,* 784–788.

Andreasen, N. C. (1985). Positive and negative schizophrenia: Acritical evaluation. *Schizophrenia Bulletin, 3,* 380–389.

Andreasen, N. C. (1989). The Scale for the Assessment of Negative Symptoms (SANS): Conceptual and theoretical foundation. *British Journal of Psychiatry, 155,* 49–52.

Bellack, A. S., Gold, J. M., & Buchana, R. W. (1999). Cognitive rehabilitation for schizophrenia: Problems, prospects, and strategies. *Schizophrenia Bulletin, 25,* 257–274.

Binks, S. W., & Gold, J. M. (1998). Differential cognitive deficits in the neuropsychology of schizophrenia. *Clinical Neuropsychologist, 12,* 8–20.

Bustini, M., Stratta, P., Daneluzzo, E., Pollice, R., Prosperini, P., & Rossi, A. (1999). Tower of Hanoi and WCST performance in schizophrenia: Problem-solving capacity and clinical correlates. *Journal of Psychiatric Research, 33,* 285–290.

Calev, A., & Edelist, S. (1993). Affect and memory in schizophrenia: Negative emotion words are forgotten less rapidly than other words by long-hospitalized schizophrenics. *Psychopathology, 26,* 229–235.

Calev, A., Venables, P. H., & Monk, A. F. (1983). Evidence for distinct verbal memory pathologies in severely and mildly disturbed schizophrenics. *Schizophrenia Bulletin, 9,* 247–264.

Chen, E. Y., Wilkins, A. J., & McKenna, P. J. (1994). Semantic memory in both impaired and anomalous in schizophrenia. *Psychological Medicine, 24,* 193–202.

Clare, L., McKenna, P. J., Mortimer, A. M., & Baddley, A. D. (1993). Memory in schizophrenia: What is impaired and what is preserved? *Neuropsychologia, 31,* 1225–1241.

Clark, O., & O'Carroll, R. E. (1998). An examination of the relationship between executive function, memory, and rehabilitation status schizophrenia. *Neuropsychological Rehabilitation, 8,* 229–241.

Cohen, J. D., & Servan-Schreiber, D. (1992). A neural network model of disturbances in the processing of context in schizophrenia. *Psychiatric Annals, 22,* 131–136.

Corrigan, P. W., & Calabrese, J. D. (2004). Cognitive therapy and schizophrenia. In M. A. Reinecke & D. A. Clark (Eds.), *Cognitive therapy across the lifespan* (pp. 315–332). New York: Cambridge University Press.

Davalos, D. B., Green, M., & Rial, D. (2002). Enhancement of executive functioning skills: An additional tier in the treatment of schizophrenia. *Community Mental Health Journal, 38,* 403–412.

David, A. S., & Cutting, J. C. E. (1994). *The neuropsychology of schizophrenia.* Hillsdale, NJ: Lawrence Erlbaum.

Duffy, L., & O'Carroll, R. (1994). Memory impairment in schizophrenia: A comparison with that observed in the alcoholic Korsakoff syndrome. *Psychological Medicine, 24,* 155–165.

Erickson, R. C., & Binder, L. M. (1986). Cognitive deficit among functionally psychotic patients: A rehabilitative perspective. *Journal of Clinical and Experimental Neuropsychology, 3,* 257–274.

Evans, J. J., Chua, S. E., McKenna, P. J., & Wilson, B. A. (1997). Assessment of the dysexecutive syndrome in schizophrenia. *Psychological Medicine, 27,* 635–646.

Flavell, J. H. (1985). *Cognitive development* (2nd ed.). Englewood Cliffs, NJ: Prentice Hall.

Goldberg, T. E., Weinberger, D. R., Berman, K. F., Pliskin, N. H., & Podd, M. H. (1987). Further evidence for dementia of the prefrontal type in schizophrenia. *Archives of General Psychiatry, 44,* 1008–1014.

Goverover, Y., & Hinojosa, J. (2004). Interrater reliability and discriminant validity of the deductive reasoning test. *American Journal of Occupational Therapy, 58,* 104–108.

Gray, J. A., Feldon, J., Rawlins, J. N. P., Hemsley, D. R., & Smith, A. D. (1991). The neuropsychology of schizophrenia. *Behavioral and Brain Science, 14,* 1–14.

Green, M. F., Kern, R. S., Braff, D. L., & Mintz, J. (2000). Neurocognitive deficits and functional outcome in schizophrenia: Are we measuring the "right stuff"? *Schizophrenia Bulletin, 26,* 119–136.

Green, M. F., & Nuechterlein, K. H. (1999). Should schizophrenia be treated as a neurocognitive disorder? *Schizophrenia Bulletin, 25,* 309–319.

Green, M. F., Satzm, P., Ganzell, S., & Vaclav, J. F. (1992). Wisconsin Card Sorting Test performance in schizophrenia: Remediation of a stubborn deficit. *American Journal of Psychiatry, 149,* 62–67.

Greenfield, D. (1985). *The psychotic patient.* New York: Free Press.

Hadas-Lidor, N., & Katz, N. (1998). A dynamic model for cognitive modifiability: Application in occupational therapy. In N. Katz (Ed.), *Cognition and occupation in rehabilitation* (pp. 281–304). Bethesda, MD: American Occupational Therapy Association.

Hadas-Lidor, N., Katz, N., Tyano, S., & Weizman, A. (2001). Effectiveness of dynamic cognitive intervention in rehabilitation of clients with schizophrenia. *Clinical Rehabilitation, 15,* 349–359.

Harvey, P. D., Earle-Boyer, E. A., Wielgus, M. S., & Levinson, J. C. (1986). Encoding, memory and thought disorders in schizophrenia and mania. *Schizophrenia Bulletin, 12,* 252–261.

Heaton, R. K. (1993). *Wisconsin Card Sorting Test manual.* Odessa, FL: Psychological Assessment Resources.

Heaton, R. K., Chelune, G. J., Talley, J. L., Kay, G. G., & Curtiss, G. (1983). *Wisconsin Card Sorting Test manual, revised and expanded.* Los Angeles: Western Psychological Services.

Hutton, S. B., Puri, B. K., Duncan, L. J., Robbins, T. W., Barnes, T. R. E., & Joyce, E. M. (1998). Executive function in first-episode schizophrenia. *Psychological Medicine, 28,* 463–473.

Itzkovich, M., Elazar, B., Averbuch, S., & Katz, N. (2000). *LOTCA Manual* (2nd ed.). New Jersey: Maddak.

Josman, N. (1993). *Assessment of categorization skills in brain-injured and schizophrenic persons: Validation of the Toglia Category Assessment (TCA).* Unpublished doctoral dissertation, New York University.

Josman, N. (1997). *Study of differences in metamemory in chronic schizophrenic participants and controlling the CMT.* Unpublished manuscript.

Josman, N. (1998). Dynamic interactional model in mental health. In N. Katz (Ed.), *Cognition and occupation in rehabilitation: Cognitive models for intervention in occupational therapy* (pp. 151–164). Bethesda, MD: American Occupational Therapy Association.

Josman, N., & Hartman-Maeir, A. (2000). Cross-cultural assessment of the Contextual Memory Test (CMT). *Occupational Therapy International, 7,* 246–258.

Josman, N., & Jarus, T. (2001). Construct-related validity of the Toglia Category Assessment and the Deductive Reasoning Test with children who are typically developing. *American Journal of Occupational Therapy, 55,* 524–530.

Josman, N., & Katz, N. (in press). Relationships of categorization on tests and daily tasks in patients with schizophrenia, post-stroke patients and healthy controls. *Psychiatry Research.*

Katz, N., Fleming, J., Keren, N., Lightbody, S., & Hartman-Maier, A. (2002). Unawareness and/or denial of disability: Implications for occupational therapy intervention. *Canadian Journal of Occupational Therapy, 69,* 281–292.

Katz, N., & Hadas-Lidor, N. (1995). Cognitive rehabilitation: Occupational therapy models for intervention in psychiatry. *Psychiatric Rehabilitation Journal, 19,* 29–37.

Katz, N., & Tolchinsky-Landsmann, L. (1991). A Piagetian framework as a basis for the assessment of cognitive organization in schizophrenia: A comparison of adolescent and adult patients to a normal control group. *Israeli Journal of Psychiatry and Related Sciences, 28,* 1–18.

Katz, N., & Ziv, N. (1992). Cognitive organization: A Piagetian framework for occupational therapy in mental health. In N. Katz (Ed.), *Cognitive rehabilitation: Models for intervention in occupational therapy* (pp. 77–100). Boston: Butterworth-Heinemann.

Kielhofner, G. (1995). *A model of human occupation: Theory and application* (2nd ed.). Baltimore: Williams and Wilkins.

Kihlstrom, J. F., & Hoyt, I. P. (1988). Hypnosis and the psychology of delusions. In T. F. Oltmanns & B. A. Maher (Eds.), *Delusional beliefs* (p. 66–109). New York: Wiley.

Koh, S. D., Grinker, R. R., Marusarz, T. Z., & Forman, P. (1981). Affective memory and schizophrenic anhedonia. *Schizophrenia Bulletin, 7,* 292–307.

Koh, S. D., Marusarz, T. Z., & Rosen, A. J. (1980). Remembering of sentences by schizophrenic young adults. *Journal of Abnormal Psychology, 87,* 303–313.

Koh, S. D., & Peterson, R. A. (1978). Encoding orientation and the remembering of schizophrenic young adults. *Journal of Abnormal Psychology, 89,* 291–294.

Kuperberg, G., & Heckers, S. (2000). Schizophrenia and cognitive function. *Current Opinion in Neurobiology, 10,* 205–210.

Kurtz, M. M., Moberg, P. J., Gur, R. C., & Gur, R. E. (2001). Approaches to cognitive remediation of neuropsychological deficits in schizophrenia: A review and meta-analysis. *Neuropsychology Review, 11,* 197–210.

LaBuda, J., & Lichtenberg, P. (1999). The role of cognition, depression and awareness of deficit in predicting geriatric rehabilitation patient's IADL performance. *Clinical Neuropsychologist, 13,* 258–267.

Larsen, S. F., & Fromholt, P. (1976). Mnemonic organization and free recall in schizophrenia. *Journal of Abnormal Psychology, 85,* 61–65.

Levine, B., Robertson, I., Clare, L., Carter, G., Hong, J., Wilson, B. A., et al. (2000). Rehabilitation of executive functioning: An experimental–clinical validation of goal management training. *Journal of the International Neuropsychological Society, 6,* 299–312.

Lezak, M. D. (1995). *Neuropsychological assessment* (3rd ed.). New York: Oxford University Press.

Lysaker, P., Bell, M., & Beam-Goulet, J. (1995). Wisconsin Card Sorting Test and work performance in schizophrenia. *Psychiatry Research, 56,* 45–51.

Malec, J. F., & Moessner, A. M. (2000). Self-awareness, distress, and postacute rehabilitation outcome. *Rehabilitation Psychology, 45,* 227–241.

McGlynn, S. M., & Kaszniak, A. W. (1986). Unawareness of deficits in dementia and schizophrenia. In G. P. Prigatano (Ed.), *Neuropsychological rehabilitation after brain injury* (pp. 84–110). Baltimore: Johns Hopkins University Press.

Meltzer, H. Y. (1994). Frontal and non-frontal lobe neuropsychological test performance and clinical symptomatology in schizophrenia. In J. A. Talbott (Ed.), *The yearbook of psychiatry and applied mental health* (pp. 247–261). St. Louis, MO: Mosby.

Nuechterlein, K. H., & Dawson, M. E. (1984). Vulnerability and stress factors in the developmental course of schizophrenic disorders. *Schizophrenia Bulletin, 10,* 158–159.

Pantelis, C., Barber, F. Z., Barnes, T. R. E., Nelson, H. E., Owen, A. M., & Robbins, T. W. (1999). Comparison of set-shifting ability in patients with chronic schizophrenia and frontal lobe damage. *Schizophrenia Research, 37,* 251–270.

Prigatano, G. P., & Wong, J. L. (1999). Cognitive and affective improvement in brain dysfunctional patients who achieve inpatient rehabilitation goals. *Archives of Physical and Medical Rehabilitation, 80,* 77–84.

Schwartz, B. L., Rosse, R. B., & Deutsch, S. I. (1993). Limits of the processing view in accounting for dissociation among memory measures in clinical population. *Memory and Cognition, 21,* 63–72.

Secrest, L., Wood, A. E., & Tapp, A. (2000). A Comparison of the Allen Cognitive Level Test and the Wisconsin Card Sorting Test in adults with schizophrenia. *American Journal of Occupational Therapy, 54,* 129–133.

Sherer, M., Bergloff, P., Levin, E., High, W. H., Oden, K. E., & Nick, T. G. (1998). Impaired awareness and employment outcome after traumatic brain injury. *Journal of Head Trauma Rehabilitation, 13,* 52–61.

So, Y. P., Toglia, J., & Donohue, M. V. (1997). A study of memory functioning in chronic schizophrenic patients. *Occupational Therapy in Mental Health, 13,* 1–23.

Spaulding, W. D., & Poland, J. S. (2001). Cognitive rehabilitation for schizophrenia: Enhancing social cognition by strengthening neurocognitive functioning. In P. W. Corrigan & D. L. Penn (Eds.), *Social cognition and schizophrenia* (pp. 217–247). Washington, DC: American Psychological Association.

Stuss, D. T., & Benson, D. F. (1986). *The frontal lobes.* New York: Oxford University.

Stuve, P., Erickson, R. C., & Spaulding, W. (1991). Cognitive rehabilitation: The next step in psychiatric rehabilitation. *Psychosocial Rehabilitation Journal, 1,* 9–26.

Tham, K., Ginsberg, E., Fisher, A., & Tegner, R. (2001). Training to improve awareness of disabilities in clients with unilateral neglect. *American Journal of Occupational Therapy, 55,* 46–54.

Toglia, J. (1991). Generalization of treatment: A multicontext approach to cognitive perceptual impairment in adults with brain injury. *American Journal of Occupational Therapy, 45,* 505–516.

Toglia, J. (2003a). Interventions to improve personal skills and abilities. In E. S. Crepeau, E. S. Cohn, & B. A. B. Schell (Eds.), *Willard and Spackman's occupational therapy* (10th ed., pp. 607–629). Philadelphia: Lippincott Williams & Wilkins.

Toglia, J. (2003b). The multicontext approach. In E. S. Crepeau, E. S. Cohn, & B. A. B. Schell (Eds.), *Willard and Spackman's occupational therapy* (10th ed., pp. 264–267). Philadelphia: Lippincott Williams & Wilkins.

Toglia, J., Abreu, B., & Allen, C. (2001, May). *The multicontext approach to cognitive rehabilitation.* Paper presented at the meeting of the American Occupational Therapy Association, Philadelphia.

Toglia, J., & Kirk, U. (2000). Understanding awareness deficits following brain injury. *NeuroRehabilitation, 15,* 57–70.

Toglia, J. P. (1989). Approaches to cognitive assessment of the brain-injured adult: Traditional methods and dynamic investigation. *Occupational Therapy Practice, 1,* 36–57.

Toglia, J. P. (1992). A dynamic interactional approach to cognitive rehabilitation. In N. Katz (Ed.), *Cognitive rehabilitation: Models for intervention in occupational therapy* (pp. 104–143). Boston: Andover Medical.

Toglia, J. P. (1993). *Contextual Memory Test manual.* Tucson, AZ: Therapy SkillBuilders.

Toglia, J. P. (1994). *Dynamic assessment of categorization: TCA—The Toglia Category Assessment.* Pequannock, NJ: Maddak.

Toglia, J. P. (1998). A dynamic interactional model to cognitive rehabilitation. In N. Katz (Ed.), *Cognition and occupation in rehabilitation* (pp. 5–50). Bethesda, MD: American Occupational Therapy Association.

Toglia, J. P., & Josman, N. (1994). Preliminary reliability and validity studies on the TCA. In J. P. Toglia (Ed.), *Dynamic assessment of categorization: TCA—The Toglia Category Assessment.* Pequannock, NJ: Maddak.

Weickert, T. W., Goldberg, T. E., Gold, J. M., Bigelow, L. B., Egan, M. F., & Weinberger, D. R. (2000). Cognitive impairments in patients with schizophrenia displaying preserved and compromised intellect. *Archives of General Psychiatry, 57,* 907–913.

Weinberger, D. (1995). Neurodevelopmental perspectives on schizophrenia. In F. E. Bloom & D. J. Kupfer (Eds.), *Psychopharmacology: The fourth generation of progress* (pp. 1171–1183). New York: Raven Press.

Weinberger, D. (1996). On the plausibility of "the neurodevelopmental hypothesis" of schizophrenia: A new understanding—Neurological basis and long-term outcome of schizophrenia. *Neuropsychopharmacology, 14,* 1–11.

Weinberger, D., & Lipska, B. (1995). Cortical maldevelopment, antipsychotic drugs, and schizophrenia: A search for common ground. *Schizophrenia Research, 16,* 87–110.

Weinberger, D. R., Aloia, M. S., Goldberg, T. E., & Berman, K. F. (1994). The frontal lobe and schizophrenia. *Journal of Neuropsychiatry and Clinical Neuroscience, 6,* 419–427.

Wetzel, L., Boll, T. J. (1992). *Short Category Test, Booklet Format.* Los Angeles: Western Psychological Services.

Wiedl, K. H. (1999). Cognitive modifiability as a measure of readiness for rehabilitation. *Psychiatric Services, 50,* 1411–1419.

Wiedl, K. H., Schottke, H., & Garcia, M. D. C. (2001). Dynamic assessment of cognitive rehabilitation potential in schizophrenic persons and in elderly persons with and without dementia. *European Journal of Psychological Assessment, 17,* 112–119.

Williams Riska, L., & Allen, C. K. (1985). Research with a nondisabled population. In C. K. Allen (Ed.), *Occupational therapy for psychiatric diseases: Measurement and management of cognitive disabilities* (pp. 315–338). Boston: Little Brown.

Woerner, M. G., Mannuzza, S., & Kane, J. M. (1988). Anchoring the BPRS: An aid to improved reliability. *Psychopharmacology Bulletin, 24,* 112–117.

World Health Organization. (2001). *International classification of functioning, disability and health (ICF).* Geneva, Switzerland: Author.

Wykes, T., Reeder, C., Corner, J., Williams, C., & Everitt, B. (1999). The effects of neurocognition remediation on executive processing in patients with schizophrenia. *Schizophrenia Bulletin, 25,* 291–307.

7

Linda Duncombe, EdD, OTR, FAOTA

The Cognitive–Behavioral Model in Mental Health

LEARNING OBJECTIVES

By the end of this chapter, readers will
1. Understand the theoretical underpinnings of the cognitive–behavioral model in psychotherapy and appreciate the model's compatibility with occupational therapy's philosophical and theoretical foundation and intervention models
2. Be aware of a variety of assessment tools that provide information relevant to selecting and using cognitive–behavioral principles, strategies, and techniques in occupational therapy intervention
3. Be familiar with the variety of cognitive–behavioral principles, strategies, and techniques that might be used effectively in occupational therapy interventions in mental health
4. Be aware of the current evidence related to the cognitive–behavioral model in occupational therapy intervention
5. Value the importance of accessing and adding to evidence-based literature to support the use of cognitive–behavioral principles and strategies.

The cognitive–behavioral model is perhaps most frequently practiced in occupational therapy in the form of psychoeducational groups. In addition, some of the many cognitive–behavioral techniques are incorporated into individual intervention sessions or when working on individual goals within a group context.

To help readers understand the theoretical background of the cognitive–behavioral frame of reference, the development of cognitive therapy, the beginnings of behavior therapy, and their synthesis are presented. Next, I discuss the relevance of this model to occupational therapy. A section on intervention includes a discussion of appropriate assessments and ways in which occupational therapists have used cognitive–behavioral techniques and strategies in intervention. Psychoeducational groups, specifically, are highlighted. Three cases exemplify application of cognitive–behavioral techniques and strategies in occupational therapy intervention in different occupational therapy practice contexts: Case 1 describes a client in an acute inpatient program who is discharged to a partial-day program, Case 2 focuses on a resident in a group home where the occupational therapist is a consultant, and Case 3 illustrates a group intervention in a wellness program. Finally, I discuss research, especially the use of outcome measures, and implications for use of this model in the context of trends in health care.

DEVELOPMENT OF COGNITIVE–BEHAVIORAL THERAPY

Cognitive Therapy

Departing from the psychoanalytic traditions in which they had been trained, early cognitive therapists proposed that behavior could be changed through alterations in an individual's thoughts (Beck, 1970; Ellis, 1985; Frankl, 1985; Glasser, 1965). In fact, some historians write, cognitive therapy really began in 1911 when Sigmund Freud and Alfred Adler agreed to disagree and parted ways (Werner, 1982). Adler had difficulty accepting Freud's belief that all psychological problems were the result of intrapsychic conflict. It was Adler's belief, instead, that each individual's personality functioned as a unified whole, and conflicts in people resulted from distorted thinking about the world around them and their place (competency–function) within that world. Thinking, not unconscious drives, shapes behavior. Adler's Law of Compensation, which suggests that an organism can and does change its behavior to compensate for personal deficits that interfere with *adaptation to the environment,*[1] provided the rationale for his later addition of cognition to his earlier theoretical constructs about feelings of inferiority and the striving for mastery (Shulman, 1985).

Adler had many followers in the 1920s and 1930s, but after his death in 1937, interest in his work declined until about 1956, when excerpts of his writings were republished (Werner, 1982). Since then, interest in his partially cognitive approach and in other forms of cognitive therapy have been steadily increasing. The Adlerian therapist, however, does not think of him- or herself entirely as a cognitive therapist. The goal of therapy, in large part, is to change the way one thinks about the world and reacts to it; in addition, the individual is asked to use

---

[1]Italics denotes relevance to occupational therapy philosophy.

his or her insights to make changes in emotions and behavior as well.

At least one more aspect of Adler's theory relates to cognitive therapy. Adler placed great importance on the *uniqueness of each person*. This leads to the individuality of each intervention plan for each client. A variety of techniques are used, depending on the individual's needs and capacities. These include the "as–if" method (instructing the client to act "as if" he or she could), "creating images" of what one wants to happen, "the push-button technique" in which the client pushes the happy or sad button to indicate his or her emotional tone, the "paradoxical technique . . . to create cognitive dissonance," and "confrontation" (Shulman, 1985, p. 254).

Albert Ellis, whose work also derives from the psychoanalytic tradition, suggested that insight alone was not enough to change the behaviors of his clients. He believed that we say sentences to ourselves that affect our behavior. We can control the content of those sentences cognitively and thus change, in a positive direction, both emotion and behavior (Ellis, 1958). Mentally healthy people have accurate perceptions of themselves, the primary contexts in which they function, and their behavior in relation to those contexts. They then are acting on an accurate understanding of reality. If they do not have a realistic view of their world and their place in the world, it is the therapist's role to clarify reality.

Ellis attempted to do this by systematically convincing clients of the fallacy of their internalized assumptions, distorted perceptions, and illogical thinking. The goal was "cognitive restructuring." The client had to accept what the therapist considered to be rational in an effort to change emotions and behaviors (Hoffman, 1984). In Ellis's own words, which build on the work of Adler, one tenet of rational–emotive therapy is that "humans are purposeful, or goal-seeking creatures and . . . they bring to A (Activating events or Activating experiences) general and specific goals (G)" (Ellis, 1985, p. 314). Rational or irrational beliefs (rBs or iBs) help or get in the way of these goals. $A \times B = C$ (cognitive, emotional, or behavioral Consequences). This is quite simplistic, as Ellis explains, but can serve as a starting place for understanding the relationship among one's thinking, emotions, and behaviors (Ellis, 1985, p. 314). There are many types of Bs, or beliefs. Some examples are self-concept, images, assumptions, and internal scripts (McMullin, 2000).

Therefore, in addition to being a framework for intervention with individuals who are dysfunctional, it "also is a personality theory that shows how people largely create their own normal or healthy (positive and negative) feel-

ings and how they can change them if they wish to and work at doing so" (Ellis, 1985, p. 322). One final note about rational–emotive therapy is the use of homework. Clients are asked to continue the work of therapy during the week, between appointments. For some situations, standard homework sheets are given. At other times, individuals are given specific tasks, for example, participating in a feared social event. This is part of altering one's consciousness about how one is currently thinking, acting, and feeling. The use of homework in today's psychoeducational groups may stem from this aspect of Ellis's theory.

William Glasser published *Reality Therapy: A New Approach to Psychiatry* in 1965. This approach was quite different from the approaches discussed above. Proposed was a way of changing thinking and emotions by first changing behavior. The major tenet of reality therapy was that one has the responsibility to meet one's own needs without infringing on the rights of others to meet their needs. The first question asked by a reality therapist is not "How are you feeling?" but rather "What are you doing?" Next, the therapist points out that what the client is doing is obviously not helping if he or she is feeling bad enough about him- or herself that he or she has sought counseling. Therapy then proceeds through the arrangement of a daily schedule of client activities chosen for their success potential. Emphasis is placed on taking small steps over short periods of time. If there is success in small things, it is hypothesized, the client can then progress toward success in larger things. As the success experiences increase in number, self-esteem improves, and thinking and feeling have been changed in a positive direction through doing. Glasser's approach may be considered a cognitive therapy in that there is no time spent on the search for insight or on an analysis of intrapsychic conflict.

A theorist whose name has become almost synonymous with cognitive therapy is Aaron Beck. He added to Adler's belief that *thinking shapes behavior* in noting that *thinking shapes emotion* and *behavior*:

> In a broad sense, any technique whose major mode of action is the modification of faulty patterns of thinking can be regarded as cognitive therapy. . . . However, cognitive therapy may be defined more narrowly as a set of operations focused on a client's cognitions (verbal or pictorial) and on the premises, assumptions, and attitudes underlying these cognitions. (Beck, 1970, p. 187)

The basic concepts of cognitive therapy include the underlying theory of cognitive therapy, strategies for working in the cognitive sphere, and specific techniques for use in the therapy process. More specifically, Beck identified the central processing abilities of individuals as necessary for survival. That processing includes receiving information from the environment, synthesizing it with what has already been processed, and planning and acting on the results of the processing (Beck & Weishaar, 1994). On the basis of his belief that one's thinking about events leads to emotional reactions, the goal of therapy is to "reshape the erroneous beliefs which produce inappropriate emotions and behavior" (Werner, 1982, pp. 19–20). The strategies used to produce this *cognitive shift* are *collaborative empiricism*, in which the client and therapist work together to use the exploratory principles of scientific thinking to determine "dysfunctional interpretations" (Beck & Weishaar, 1994, p. 286), and *guided discovery*, in which misperceptions of the past are identified as being similar to those in the present. Clients are asked to take note of the experiences in their lives and identify what they believe to be the associated dysfunctional thought processes (Vallis, 1991). Although this sounds like Ellis's rational–emotive therapy, the techniques of Beck's form of cognitive therapy are less teacherlike (no homework sheets; homework is more experientially based) and involve more discussion about questions raised by the therapist. These interventions are considered less forceful; greater emphasis is placed on learning while doing. Beck's cognitive therapy focuses on empowering the individual to change thought processes from dysfunctional to functional, enhancing one's ability to cope (Beck & Weishaar, 1994).

Aspects of cognition that are emphasized in cognitive therapies are automatic thoughts, underlying assumptions, and cognitive distortions (Freeman, Pretzer, Fleming, & Simon, 1990). *Automatic thoughts* are immediate interpretations of events. Everyone has automatic thoughts, but in psychopathology these may be distorted, mistaken, or unrealistic. *Underlying assumptions* are the beliefs of an individual that shape his or her perceptions and interpretations of events. Similar beliefs or beliefs entrenched over a period of time are frequently called *schemas*. These are usually unspoken and may not be in the immediate awareness of the individual until discovered in diagnostic interviews or during empirical data gathering. *Cognitive distortions* are also referred to as *errors in logic* (Beck, 1970). Distortions in one's thinking can have a positive or negative effect on underlying assumptions.

Intervention in the cognitive model is focused on changing any or all of the above aspects of cognition. A feedback loop is envisioned in which beliefs and assumptions (internally generated), external events, responses of others to one's interpersonal behavior, and emotional reactions based on perception and memory all contribute to the automatic thoughts that direct behavior. Therapy, then, is geared toward breaking this cycle and modifying automatic thoughts. This should improve one's mood and contribute to a change in behavior. As emotions and behavior change, so will the feedback to the system, diminishing the negative impact of the cycle (Freeman et al., 1990). The *goal* in cognitive therapy is "to achieve greater self-esteem, improved functioning at work and school and more satisfying personal relationships" (Burns, 1989b, p. ix).

In the 1970s, there was a burgeoning of literature from behaviorists who were beginning to wonder if the positive results they were attributing to behavior therapy were actually due to cognitive aspects of therapy, such as a client's expectation of positive results (Hoffman, 1984). As the basis of behavior in learning theory was further examined, some began to identify various cognitive processes as being responsible for the changes effected by behavioral therapy (Hoffman, 1984; Seiler, 1984).

Behavior Therapy

The *classical conditioning* techniques of Ivan P. Pavlov, with contributions by John B. Watson, Mary Cover Jones, Knight Dunlap, Orval Hobart Mowrer and later, Joseph Wolpe, Richard S. Lazarus, Valerie Reyna, Dianne S. Salter, and Hans Eysenck, provided the foundation from which behavior therapy emerged (Mahoney, 1984). As interest in the *operant conditioning* of B. F. Skinner (1953) and other pioneers grew stronger in the 1950s and 1960s, behaviorists began to use behavior modification strategies such as *token economies* and *shaping*. During this time, two developments were identified as historical antecedents for the movement toward a combined cognitive–behavioral approach (Mahoney, 1984). These are Skinner's (1953) reference to behavioral self-control and the description by Homme and Cautela of "coverants: the operants of the mind" (as cited in Mahoney, 1984). Self-control refers to the ability of the individual to have some influence in the direction his or her life will take (Bruce & Borg, 2002). Coverants refer to thoughts and thought processes that follow the principles of operant conditioning. For example, a therapist might instruct a client to picture him- or herself performing a desired behavior and then have him or her imagine a pleasant event as the result (coverant reinforcer) of that behavior (Hoffman, 1984). Bandura (1985) later elaborated on these notions of self-control and coverant thought in describing the importance of the central nervous system processes in behavior modification in 1969.

By the 1970s, there were two behaviorist schools of thought: the cognitive and the noncognitive. Beck is an example of a cognitive therapist who, although taking behavior therapy techniques into account, did not attempt to integrate the tenets of behavior therapy with cognitive therapy (Semmer & Frese, 1984). Seiler (1984), however, documented the appearance of cognitive interpretations for what had been the domain of behavioristic research. Positive results from behavior therapy techniques were potentially explained in cognitive therapy terms. Skinner and his followers, conversely, rejected any attempt at explaining behavior therapy through cognitive descriptions, for example, with references to "the inner man" (Hoffman, 1984, p. 54). There were, however, enough behaviorists who were interested in the cognitive components of behavior to form a special interest group for cognitive–behavioral research within both the Association for the Advancement of Behavioral Therapy and the Association for Behavioral Analysis. These groups studied the inner person within the confines of behavior therapy, and the result of this was what is now known as cognitive–behavioral psychology (Bruce & Borg, 2002).

CONTEMPORARY COGNITIVE–BEHAVIORAL THERAPY

> Cognitive–behavioral interventions . . . [include] . . . behavior therapists' increasing concern with mediational (mental/cognitive) therapeutic approaches and cognitive therapists' growing recognition of methodological behaviorism. (Kendall & Hollon, 1979, p. 2)

Thus, as contemporary cognitive–behavioral therapy has evolved, practitioners acknowledge both the mediating impact of thoughts on behavior and the importance of behavioral methodology in changing how one thinks and feels about oneself. In addition, when cognitive and behavioral intervention methods are combined, they must include both verbal intervention procedures for cognitive change and contextual or activity manipulations to encourage behavioral change (Hollon & Kendall, 1979).

Much of current cognitive therapy has been influenced by behavior analysis and therapy. For example, Dobson's (1988) covert conditioning models included the covert conditioning of Cautela (1967) and the thought-stopping techniques of Wolpe (1958). Bandura's (1985) social learning theory incorporated observational learning as well as other nonbehavioral constructs such as *self-*

efficacy. Meichenbaum developed self-instructional training, D'Zurilla and Goldfried wrote about problem-solving intervention using cognitive restructuring, and Rehm developed self-control therapy (cited in Vallis, 1991). These forms of cognitive therapy were highly structured, didactic, and educational; little attention was paid to the development of a therapeutic relationship.

In considering the intertwining of cognitive and behavioral therapies, it is important to trace theoretical underpinnings of each. Beck (1976) described behavior therapy as being a subset of cognitive therapy but articulated how similar they are in comparison to psychoanalytic theory. Commonalities are a structured therapeutic interview, description of the presenting problem in cognitive or behavioral terms, and determination of an intervention plan, including identification by the therapist of the expected response or expected goal of intervention (Beck, 1976). Kendall and Hollon (1979) identified four threads, or influences, that are relevant to understanding the relationship between cognitive and behavioral psychology. The first is that thoughts are subject to the same laws of learning as are overt behaviors. Second, "attitudes, beliefs, expectancies, attributions, and other cognitive activities are central to producing, predicting, and understanding psychopathological behavior and the effects of therapeutic intervention" (Kendall & Hollon, 1979, p. 5). The third influence comes from social learning theorists such as Kanfer and Bandura, who used behavioral paradigms to look at self-efficacy and self-regulation. The last thread proposes that the combination of cognitive interventions with behavioral management results in an outcome that is both expected and meaningful.

The *principles of traditional cognitive therapy* that must be reflected in a cognitive–behavioral approach are phenomenology, collaboration, activity, empiricism, and generalization. The following set of descriptors relies on the work of Vallis (1991).

- *Principle 1: Phenomenology* is a critical aspect of cognitive therapy in that information gathered about the individual, and how important that background information is to the individual, must be confirmed by the client. A series of diagnostic interviews are conducted to obtain a detailed description of the client's subjective experience. This forms the basis for the intervention plan. How this information is used—that is, how the intervention plan is established or how much emphasis is placed on various aspects of cognition (e.g., content, process, structure)—varies with the conceptual model. As first identified by Adler, the individual is the unique piece in the puzzle.

- *Principle 2: Collaboration* is another cornerstone of cognitive therapy. The therapist and the client together decide on the path to take, then work in concert toward their goals. The knowledge that one is participating in the planning and working through of the intervention plan affirms the ability of the individual to shape his or her own destiny. Participation in the planning optimizes the client's commitment to change and decreases resistance and opposition.
- *Principle 3: Activity,* not just verbal interactions between therapist and client, is necessary to change behavior. Attention is paid to the ways in which different behaviors affect mood and to how thinking can set the stage for satisfying interpersonal interactions. The strategic use of activity in the therapeutic context clearly differentiates the cognitive therapists from the psychoanalysts.
- *Principle 4: Empiricism* emphasizes the importance of a scientific or rational approach to understanding cognition, behavior, and emotion. In some cases, the client is asked to collect data that the therapist and the client can look at together as part of understanding where to go next with the intervention plan. The collaboration between the client and the therapist in this systematic discovery process ensures that the intervention process and outcomes are not imposed on the client.
- *Principle 5: Generalization* refers to guaranteeing that therapeutic changes will benefit the individual beyond as well as within the therapy sessions. The homework given to clients is one way of ensuring that some activity takes place in the intended context.

The *principles of behavior therapy* that must be included in a cognitive–behavioral model are the use of a behavioral assessment, intervention aimed at specific behaviors or components of behaviors, and specific intervention strategies that are individualized to attend to the specific behaviors in the unique context of that person (Wilson, 1994). These principles are based on a learning theory model in which behavior (response) is believed to be the result of an event (stimulus). In addition, "behavior is learned when it is immediately reinforced" (Stein & Cutler, 1998, p. 123).

There is agreement about the importance of the scientific method (empiricism) within the principles of cognitive and behavioral therapy. The other principles are combined throughout intervention.

TECHNIQUES AND STRATEGIES OF COGNITIVE–BEHAVIORAL THERAPY

There are many more intervention techniques and strategies used in cognitive–behavioral therapy than can be presented here, but some examples have been selected to illustrate what this form of intervention might include. Freeman and colleagues (1990) have provided a structure for classifying these intervention techniques and strategies. Primarily cognitive techniques involve "thinking" as the strategy for changing cognitions or behavior, and behavioral techniques primarily include "action strategies" for cognitive or behavioral change.

Cognitive techniques can be described in the following six categories:

1. *Techniques for challenging automatic thoughts:* An example of this is *challenging absolutes.* In this technique the therapist asks questions that help the client discover the lack of logic in his or her thinking. The Socratic method of questioning frequently used with this technique is a hallmark of Beck's cognitive therapy (Beck & Weishaar, 1994).
2. *Techniques for eliminating cognitive distortions: Decatastrophizing,* also referred to as the "what-if" technique (Beck & Weishaar, 1994, p. 309), is an example of this. The therapist requests that the client think of the opposite of what he or she fears, thus directly counteracting the cognitive distortion of catastrophic exaggeration.
3. *Techniques for challenging underlying assumptions:* Assumptions tend to surface as underlying themes in the automatic thoughts that guide one's behavior. One way to challenge them is to have the client *write an alternative assumption.* This is frequently done through the medium of a journal. First, the client is asked to write down his or her worst emotions and what he or she thought instigated the feelings. Next, the client is to record his or her interpretation of the situation. For example, a neighbor does not say hello as he walks by. The client might feel rejected, and the interpretation might be that "I am not liked or lovable." The next assignment is for the client to think of three or four additional interpretations for why the neighbor might not have spoken. Each interpretation is examined for how plausible it might be, being as objective as possible. Finally, one is selected as being the most probable. In the example, the client might decide that the neighbor was deeply engrossed in thought and did not see him or her standing there. The client and therapist can continue examining other underlying assumptions until the process becomes automatic for the client (McMullin, 2000).
4. *Mental imagery techniques: Replacement imagery* and *flooding imagery* are two ways to enable clients to

alter the mental scenes they have conjured up in response to events or perceived events. Clients frequently report visual images associated with anxiety or fears (Beck & Weishaar, 1994). If one is instructed to visualize something in place of the feared event, replacement imagery is being used. Flooding imagery is an example of desensitization in which the client imagines the feared scene and identifies the concurrent irrational thoughts. As the image becomes more and more real, the client's feelings build and build until they eventually go away (McMullin, 2000). Another example in this category of techniques is *cognitive rehearsal,* in which clients rehearse, in their thoughts only, what they need to say before it has to be done in real life.

5. ***Techniques for controlling recurrent thoughts:*** *Thought stopping* is a method in which, in a relaxed state, the therapist yells "Stop" at the point at which the client identifies the beginning of an obsessional thought (Salkovskis & Kirk, 1989). The client is taught to do this for him- or herself eventually. A less immediate approach is *refocusing,* in which the therapist first asks the client to focus on the troublesome emotion and the event that triggered that emotion. Then the client is asked to identify situations similar to the antecedent event that did not result in the negative emotion and to practice replacing or refocusing on the more positive feelings.

6. ***Techniques for changing and controlling behavior:*** *Self-instructional training* results in a series of instructions that the individual uses as self-talk to carry out a task or to perform an activity that would otherwise be difficult or impossible. For example, an individual might learn to say to oneself "Relax and take a deep breath" prior to a situation that is seen as anxiety-provoking (Meichenbaum & Asarnow, 1979).

Behavioral techniques are described as follows:

1. ***Techniques for behavioral change:*** *Graded task assignments* are simply sequenced tasks and subtasks that an individual must perform to increase the probability for success. Generally, they are organized from simple to complex or "least demanding to most demanding" (Hollon & Beck, 1979, p. 185). Glasser (1965) explained the use of this technique in *reality therapy.* Occupational therapists use graded occupations throughout intervention, frequently in a growth-facilitating context (Mosey, 1972). Outcomes of intervention can be determined from graded task assignments because of the specificity of the task definition. *Activity scheduling* is a continuation of graded task assignments in that the client's entire day is scheduled, hour by hour. This has

been noted as especially helpful with clients with depression (Hollon & Beck, 1979). *Social skills training* and *assertiveness training* also are examples of action-oriented techniques for behavioral change. In both of these techniques, specific skills are taught to clients using tangible and intangible (or social) reinforcers, usually in a group setting, so that clients can learn the specific skills necessary for participation in their expected contexts. Both techniques require practice of the skills being learned. The practicing is a form of *behavioral rehearsal.* However, any skill or interaction can be rehearsed before the actual event happens.

2. ***Techniques to achieve cognitive change:*** *Behavioral experiments,* or trying different ways of acting in a particular situation, provide information that the client can think about in terms of each behavior's effectiveness and the emotional response connected to it. *Role-playing* and *role reversal* are used to give the client insight into both how he or she might act and how he or she is perceived. These techniques provide behavioral information that can be explored cognitively (see Exhibit 7.1). In some cases, the client is asked to take a role opposite one he or she usually plays and to convince the therapist, who is playing the role of the client, that his or her thoughts are irrational (McMullin, 2000).

EXHIBIT 7.1. Cognitive and Behavioral Techniques

Primarily Cognitive Techniques	Primarily Behavioral Techniques
For Challenging Automatic Thoughts ● Challenging absolutes	For Behavioral Change ● Graded task assignments ● Activity scheduling ● Social skills training ● Assertiveness training ● Behavioral rehearsal
For Eliminating Cognitive Distortions ● Decatastrophizing	
For Challenging Underlying Assumptions ● Writing an alternate assumption	To Achieve Cognitive Change ● Behavioral experiments ● Role-playing ● Role reversal
Mental Imagery ● Replacement imagery ● Flooding imagery ● Cognitive rehearsal	
For Controlling Recurrent Thoughts ● Thought stopping ● Refocusing	
For Changing and Controlling Behavior ● Self-instructional training	

Vallis (1991) identified educational techniques as an additional category of techniques for changing behavior and cognition. Lecture, reading assignments, and homework are examples of these techniques.

It is important to note that frequently, in practice, these techniques may be combined for an effective and meaningful intervention. For example, in stress management groups, lectures and assigned reading may be used to educate individuals about stress and stress management. This knowledge may be combined with mental imagery, cognitive rehearsal, and self-instructional training to modify stress-producing thoughts and behavior. Adding the action-oriented techniques of role-playing and graded task assignments may provide skill learning to support the cognitive and behavioral change. When this type of group is offered in a mental health setting, it is frequently referred to as a *psychoeducational group.*

Given the many strategies and techniques available to the cognitive–behavioral therapist, one might wonder how to select the appropriate strategy. Freeman and his colleagues (1990) have identified two guiding principles: the more verbal the client, the more cognitive the strategy, and the more anxious the client, the more behavioral the strategy. In addition, the different techniques, with emphasis on education, cognition, and behavior, each play a different role in working on changing one's thinking, feeling, and behavior. If one wants to change an individual's thinking through knowledge, then an educational approach might be the strategy of choice. If one wants to attack the distorted thinking directly, a more cognitive approach might be best. For techniques that focus on behavior, the goal is to change the individual's cognitions and affect through the feedback from the activity.

Occupational therapy practice literature describes the use of the cognitive–behavioral principles and the educational, cognitive, and behavioral techniques described above. Therefore, the next section discusses the compatibility of the cognitive–behavioral model with occupational therapy and its congruence with the *Occupational Therapy Practice Framework.*

COGNITIVE–BEHAVIORAL INTERVENTION AND THE *OCCUPATIONAL THERAPY PRACTICE FRAMEWORK*

In the first stated philosophy of occupational therapy, Meyer (1922) spoke of *habits,* which he described as organized patterns of behavior *and* thinking. Meyer believed that people with mental illness could be helped by altering their milieu and modifying their habits of thinking (Lidz, 1985).

Ergasia (from the Greek, meaning *work*) was a term created by Meyer that referred to "mentally integrated activity" (Lidz, 1985, p. 44). Meyer believed that, to help a client solve or resolve a problem, one needed to focus on those personal and contextual aspects of the individual to which one had access. Therefore, Meyer's perspective suggests that intervention options are changing the context and altering habit patterns (behaviors) and ways of thinking (cognition). It is relevant to note that these also are the underlying tenets of the cognitive–behavioral therapists.

The *Occupational Therapy Practice Framework* states that "engagement in occupation to support participation in context is the focus and targeted end objective of occupational therapy intervention" (American Occupational Therapy Association [AOTA], 2002, p. 611). In cognitive–behavioral therapy, purposeful activities are explored. Then contextual feedback is given, and intrinsic feedback occurs to help the individual effect changes in thinking and future behaviors so he or she will be better able to participate in his or her context of choice. In addition, Burns (1989b) defined the goal of cognitive–behavioral therapy as achieving "greater self-esteem, improved functioning at work and school, and more satisfying personal relationships" (p. viii). The meaningful occupation, the occupational therapy intervention and change process, and the occupational performance and participation outcomes identified in the *Framework* (AOTA, 2002) are strikingly similar to the exploration of purposeful activity described in cognitive–behavioral therapy. This congruity of the *Framework* with the process and desired outcomes of the cognitive–behavioral model along with the previously identified philosophical and theoretical compatibility between occupational and cognitive–behavioral therapies provide further rationale for occupational therapists to incorporate cognitive–behavioral strategies and techniques into their practice.

COGNITIVE–BEHAVIORAL THERAPY IN OCCUPATIONAL THERAPY

Throughout the occupational therapy literature are many examples that describe behavior therapy as consistent with occupational therapy practice (e.g., Diasio, 1968; Giles, 2003; Levy, 1993; Sieg, 1974; Stein, 1982; Stein & Cutler, 1998) and others that describe it as effective in specific occupational therapy interventions (e.g., Giles, Ridley, Dill, & Frye, 1997; Jodrell & Sanson-Fisher, 1975; Sieg, 1974; Smith & Tempone, 1968; Zschokke, Freeberg, & Erickson, 1975). Some have felt, however, that the reliance on external reinforcement in behavior therapy is incompatible with the occupational therapist's belief in the inherent motivation of valued occupation (AOTA, 2002; Barris, Kielhofner, & Watts, 1983; Bruce & Borg, 2002).

The principles of cognitive therapy—phenomenology, collaboration, activity, empiricism, and generalization—are more than compatible with the beliefs of occupational therapy. Both place emphasis on the following:

1. The phenomenological experience of the individual, or client-centered practice;
2. The collaborative interaction between client and therapist regarding outcomes and intervention;
3. The use of rational thinking to solve problems and increase cognitive awareness of behavior; and
4. The importance of ensuring the generalizing of therapy to an individual's performance in his or her context of choice.

More specifically, the therapeutic use of meaningful occupation, one of the hallmarks of occupational therapy, is also what is said to set cognitive therapists apart from psychoanalytic (verbal) therapists. Just as the cognitive–behavioral therapist believes that a change in one's thinking can change behavior and that a positive experience can change one's thinking about oneself, occupational therapists have long believed that "Man is an active being whose development is influenced by the use of purposeful activity" (AOTA Representative Assembly, 1979, p. 785) and that "When individuals engage in occupations, they are committed to performance as a result of self-choice, motivation, and meaning" (AOTA, 2002, p. 611). Fidler (1969) stated it well in relation to task-oriented groups:

> The intent of the task-oriented group is to provide a shared working experience wherein the relationship between feeling, thinking, and behavior; their impact on others; and task-accomplishment and productivity can be viewed and explored. (p. 45)

The biopsychosocial model (Mosey, 1974) was suggested to the occupational therapy community as an alternative to either the medical model, with its focus on pathology, or a health model, which primarily emphasizes an individual's assets. More recently, in discussing schizophrenia, Fine (1993) referred to the relevance of the biopsychosocial model for all disabilities. The cognitive–behavioral model is similar to the biopsychosocial model in that the latter "directs attention to the body, mind, and environment of the client" (Mosey, 1974, p. 138). As in most other occupational therapy models, the biopsychosocial model focuses on the teaching and learning process that takes place during a client-centered, occupational

therapist-planned activity, on the outcome of adaptive performance in an individual's context of choice, and on the use of specific behavioral objectives. It is interesting to note that the *International Classification of Function, Disability, and Health,* on which the occupational therapy practice framework is based, is classified as a biopsychosocial model (Arthanat, Nochajski, & Stone, 2004).

The role of occupational therapists when using the cognitive–behavioral model is multifaceted. They facilitate learning, model a scientific attitude, question generalizations, form a collaborative relationship, assess performance areas through the use of occupations, and create an intervention tailored to the client (Bruce & Borg, 2002). Cole (1998) described how cognitive–behaviorism may be used by occupational therapists in psychoeducational groups, such as stress management, assertiveness, social skills, and other skill training. Further, she refers to the role of the occupational therapist as educator–facilitator, helping clients to change their distorted thinking. "We can teach our group members to challenge each other and to encourage their use of rational thinking to solve problems" (Cole, 1998, p. 154).

Cognitive–behavior therapy, which combines activity with the cognitive awareness for change, provides a model of intervention for treating and preventing psychosocial dysfunction. Although the cognitive–behavioral model of intervention is not an occupational therapy model, its use by occupational therapists is recommended in the occupational therapy literature (e.g., DeMars, 1992; Henderson, 1998; Jao & Lu, 1999; Johnson, 1987; Mitchell, 2000; Taylor, 1988; Yakobina, Yakobina, & Tallant, 1997).

In their book *Cognitive Therapy With Inpatients,* Wright, Thase, Beck, and Ludgate (1993) also discussed the appropriateness and benefits of collaboration between the occupational and the cognitive therapist:

> Occupational therapists who work in a psychiatric setting are primarily concerned with teaching skills to promote self-reliance and independence. These therapists . . . are probably better prepared than most psychiatrists, psychologists, or social workers to teach adaptive skills to persons with significant handicaps. Occupational therapists can augment the cognitive therapy program in a number of ways. First, they can provide a detailed assessment of functional capacity. This evaluation often gives more practical information than does extensive psychological testing. Can the patient manage daily activities of living, handle financial matters, or complete job-related tasks? . . . During the treatment phase of occupational therapy, there is a natural partnership between the occupational and cogni-

tive therapist. Both are interested in reducing symptoms and improving coping skills. The occupational therapist uses psycho-educational procedures, demonstrations, and *in vivo* rehearsal to build functional ability and self-esteem. Socratic questioning may also be used to uncover the patient's cognitive responses to the occupational therapy exercises. The cognitively oriented occupational therapist will be able to point out maladaptive cognitions and help the patient to develop more balanced thinking. In addition the occupational therapist can assist the patient in carrying out specific assignments from individual or group cognitive therapy. (p. 79)

Several similarities between occupational therapy and cognitive–behavioral therapy have been identified. A literature review revealed that many occupational therapists have used the principles of cognitive–behavioral therapy in their practice with a variety of populations, and still others have led psychoeducational groups that are based on the principles of cognitive–behavioral therapy (e.g., Cox & Findley, 1998; Crist, 1986; Goldstein, Gershaw, & Sprafkin, 1979; Greenberg et al., 1988; Henderson, 1998; Jao & Lu, 1999; Luboshitzky & Gaber, 2000; Mitchell, 2000; Yakobina et al., 1997). Criteria for including articles as cognitive–behavioral were the presence of the five cognitive principles of phenomenology, collaboration, activity, empiricism, generalization, and the presence of behavioral methodology. Some psychoeducational programs were identified as being based on behavioral or learning theory principles. However, if in the presentations of these programs a discussion was described in which clients were expected to think about their behavior and identify feelings connected with the behaviors or skills being learned or practiced, that discussion was considered to be a cognitive component to what had been described as a behavioral approach. It should be noted that the use of a cognitive–behavioral technique or referring to an intervention as psychoeducational does not mean that the therapy has been carefully designed as cognitive–behavioral therapy. This is discussed further in the "Intervention" section below. We first look at the types of assessments used by occupational therapists, then the different cognitive–behavioral interventions are described and the populations and diagnoses treated are identified.

Evaluation

One purpose of an initial evaluation is for the occupational therapist and the client to collaborate in identifying the client's current occupational performance and, based on

the client's values, interests, and priorities, how current performance compares with the individual's goals (AOTA, 2002; Law et al., 1994). Another purpose is to determine if the cognitive–behavioral model of intervention is appropriate for a client. The more cognitively oriented strategies and techniques require the ability to "think about one's thinking" and to monitor one's behavior. The Allen Diagnostic Battery, which consists of the Allen Cognitive Level Scale (ACLS–90), the Allen Diagnostic Module, and the Routine Task Inventory, is designed to evaluate cognitive abilities, including the ability to use symbolic thought and logical reasoning (Allen & Reyner, 1996). Cole (1998) suggested that clients with an Allen Level of 5 or above have the reasoning abilities to learn and benefit from cognitive–behavioral interventions. However, if the cognitive–behavioral approach is conceptualized as a continuum, then the strategies and techniques can be graded so that the more cognitively capable the client, the more cognitive the intervention, and the less cognitively capable the client, the more behavioral the intervention. For more behaviorally oriented aspects of therapy, it also is important for the evaluation to identify appropriate types of reinforcers, preferred methods of feedback, and aspects of the expected context that are relevant to the behavioral aspect of the therapy. It is also important to evaluate a client's motivation, a complex combination of "readiness" to change, goals, values, contextual factors, and cognitive abilities. Finally, to identify targeted outcomes, the current occupational performance of the individual must be determined.

Twenty-five articles referring to psychoeducation or cognitive–behavioral intervention in occupational therapy were reviewed for assessment techniques. Six of those articles did not mention evaluation (Cox & Findley, 1998; Eilenberg, 1986; Friedlob, Janis, & Deets-Aron, 1986; Goldstein et al., 1979; Johnson, 1986; Nickel, 1988). The remaining 19 articles yielded 21 assessments relevant to the cognitive–behavioral model. Two categories of assessments emerged: those that yielded information about the cognitive abilities of clients and those that identified the presence or absence of performance skills necessary for performance in one's context of choice. Most practitioners who described the evaluation process identified more than one method of assessment that provided relevant information.

Formal, but Nonspecific Assessments

An *interview* was mentioned most frequently (Courtney & Escobedo, 1990; DeMars, 1992; Giles & Allen, 1986; Luboshitzky & Gaber, 2000; Maslen, 1982; Salo-

Chydenius, 1996; Taylor, 1988; Yakobina et al., 1997). During the interview, the therapist attempted to elicit an individual's cognitive abilities, such as memory, attention, concentration, and judgment, as well as motivation to participate and identification of goals and needs from the client's perspective. This addresses the *phenomenological* perspective of the individual, required in a cognitive–behavioral approach, as well as initiating shared *collaboration* around intervention outcomes. The occupational profile, as recommended by the *Occupational Therapy Practice Framework* (AOTA, 2002), includes the client's history and priorities. Several articles mentioned the use of *questionnaires,* which may have been given in interview format as well (Crist, 1986; Maslen, 1982; Yakobina et al., 1997). Four articles referred to the use of a self-assessment (Greenberg et al., 1988; Luboshitsky & Gaber, 2000; Mitchell, 2000; Salo-Chydenius, 1996).

Observations of clients in structured and unstructured *activities* were helpful in identifying skills and problem-solving strategies (Fine, 1993). More specifically, Salo-Chydenius (1996) used role-playing and videotaping during which observations were made and shared with clients after their self-assessment. A collage activity was suggested to provide information about knowledge and feelings of self and self-esteem (Lindsay, 1983). Two authors referred to the need to evaluate the cognitive levels and abilities of clients but did not describe how this was, or should be, done (Courtney & Escobedo, 1990; Kaseman, 1980). The *Framework* recommends an analysis of actual occupational performance in context (AOTA, 2002).

Standardized Assessments Yielding Information About Cognitive Abilities

Four occupational therapy evaluations provide valuable information about cognition for individuals with mental illness. The Allen Diagnostic Battery (Allen & Reyner, 1996) identifies levels of cognitive abilities. The Cognitive Performance Test uses everyday occupations such as dressing, making toast, and using the telephone to identify the cognitive abilities of individuals with Alzheimer's disease or dementia (Burns, Mortimer, & Merchak, 1994); this test is described in Chapter 15. The Bay Area Functional Performance Evaluation (BaFPE; Bloomer & Williams, 1982) evaluates the cognitive components of memory for written or verbal instructions, organization of time and materials, attention span, evidence of thought disorder, and ability to abstract. In addition, there are opportunities for the therapist to observe qualitative signs that might indicate organic involvement interfering with

participation in everyday performance. The BaFPE requires 30 to 45 minutes to administer and must be given individually. Those working in an acute–care setting might have difficulty using it as a basic screening for all clients Luboshitzky and Gaber (2000) found the Assessment of Motor and Process Skills (Fisher, 1995) useful in identifying difficulties in a client's ability to use knowledge, temporal organization, space, and objects.

Three additional occupational therapy evaluations, although not developed specifically for use with individuals with mental illness, yield information about cognitive abilities that can be helpful in deciding whether or not to use a cognitive–behavioral approach and in selecting appropriate intervention strategies and techniques. The Loewenstein Occupational Therapy Cognitive Assessment, although widely used to test the cognitive abilities of individuals post–cerebral vascular accident (CVA) and those with traumatic brain injuries (TBI), is valuable in assessing the "thinking operations" of individuals with mental illness (Itzkovich, Elazar, Averbuch, & Katz, 2000). The Cognitive Assessment of Minnesota is a standardized screening tool of 17 subtests assessing such areas as memory, money skills, and concrete problem solving. It, too, was standardized for use with individuals with cognitive deficits resulting from CVAs and TBI but might be useful for individuals with mental illness who also have cognitive deficits (Rustad et al., 1993). The dynamic investigative approach, applied by Toglia (1992) to assess the learning potential of adults with brain injury, is important to mention. Using this assessment method, the therapist first provides the client with opportunities for problem solving. Then the therapist varies the task, the environment, or the cues for problem solving and task performance as a way to determine the best strategies to facilitate learning. This assessment is presented in depth in Chapter 2 of this volume.

In addition, the Woodcock Johnson Psycho-Educational Battery (Woodcock & Johnson, 2000), although not specifically designed for use by occupational therapists, also yields information relevant to cognitive abilities. Finally, Jao and Lu (1999) recommended the Means–Ends Problem-Solving Procedure (Platt & Spivack, 1977) as an assessment of one's ability to work toward a goal.

Formal or Standardized Assessments That Focus on Ability to Perform Everyday Life Activities

- Basic Living Skills Battery (Skolaski & Broekema, cited in Crist, 1986)

- Kohlman Evaluation of Living Skills (KELS; Crist, 1986; Lillie & Armstrong, 1982; Thomson, 1992)
- Living Skills Evaluation (Ogren, 1983)
- Phillips's Social Skills Criterion Scale (Crist, 1986; Phillips, 1978)
- Scorable Self-Care Evaluation (Clark & Peters, 1984; Crist, 1986)
- Stress Management Questionnaire (Stein, 2003)
- Task Check List (Lillie & Armstrong, 1982)
- Self-Evaluation Form for Patient A (for evaluating social skills; Salo-Chydenius, 1996)
- Self-Evaluation Form for Patient B (for evaluating social skills and how one learns social skills; Salo-Chydenius, 1996).

These suggested assessments are useful in initial data-gathering, but evaluation is an ongoing process (AOTA, 2002; Bruce & Borg, 2002; Giles, 1985; Yakobina et al., 1997) and provides the opportunity to scientifically examine the cognitive, affective, and behavioral barriers to performance. Ongoing evaluation and generation of alternate hypotheses is part of the *empirical focus* of this frame of reference.

Finally, one needs to ascertain the client's view of his or her context and current and expected contextual demands (AOTA, 2002). This provides information about *generalization,* without which intervention is merely an exercise.

To summarize, when performing an evaluation in the cognitive–behavioral frame of reference, one needs to identify the following:

- Cognitive components
  - Ability to think and process information (concrete, abstract, metacognition)
  - Ability to communicate thinking through words
  - Attention span and concentration
  - Memory functions
  - Problem solving and judgment
  - Learning style
  - Awareness of disability
- Behavioral components
  - Appropriate reinforcement (tangible and intangible)
  - Feedback—client's preferred form
  - Specific adaptive and maladaptive behaviors
- Cognitive and behavioral components combined
  - Interest in participating in intervention
  - Outcomes/identified needs.

The *Occupational Therapy Practice Framework* (AOTA, 2002) recommends that the evaluation process should include an interview, observation of the occupational performance, and a standardized or formal assessment that can be the basis for evaluating intervention outcomes and for demonstrating that change has taken place after intervention has ended. In conclusion, it is important to acknowledge the art of assessment. "Clearly, the art of assessment requires the capacity to narrow the focus and magnify particular components of performance without losing sight of the bigger psychosocial picture" (Fine, 1993, p. 94).

The results of the evaluation must be shared with the client, after which the client and the therapist can collaborate and identify the desired outcomes of intervention. These outcomes also should be based on the client's cognitive abilities and current adaptive and maladaptive performance skills. The intervention phase, during which there is ongoing evaluation and collaboration, then commences.

Intervention

A good intervention plan starts with specific targeted outcomes (AOTA, 2002). Four areas for change use the cognitive–behavioral model: the context, thoughts and attitudes, knowledge, and skills (Bruce & Borg, 2002). Just as one has to include both cognitive and behavioral aspects as part of a cognitive–behavioral evaluation, the same is true for intervention. In this process, it is useful to keep in mind that, the more cognitively capable the individual, the more cognitive the approach can be and, the less cognitively capable the person, the more behavioral the approach may need to be. Flexibility in adapting and grading strategies and techniques to changes in a client's level of function also is important. Cognitive–behavioral strategies must be carefully selected to effect change in relevant cognitive and behavioral aspects of the individual (Johnson, 1987; Yakobina et al., 1997).

The ultimate outcome of all occupational therapy intervention, regardless of the theoretical model or techniques being used, is "improved client performance" (AOTA, 2002, p. 614) in his or her context of choice. In the cognitive–behavioral model, the general outcome is self-regulation through improved cognitive function (Bruce & Borg, 2002). Cognitive behaviorists believe that one's thoughts, feelings, and beliefs can, and do, affect one's behavior or ability to function in context. Also, feedback about how one acts, from both the nonhuman and the human context, can alter one's thinking, beliefs, and feelings about one's capabilities. This, in turn, will affect behavior. As occupational therapists work toward targeted outcomes, they use their role as teacher and collaborator, role-modeling problem solving and meaningful occupations to increase performance skills and to provide feedback and cognitive awareness necessary for a change in one's cognitive beliefs.

Occupational therapists use a variety of cognitive–behavioral principles, strategies, and techniques to achieve occupational therapy outcomes with clients. Bruce and Borg (2002) listed several strategies and techniques, including homework tasks, bibliotherapy, process task groups such as assertiveness and social skills groups, films, modeling and role-play, physical guidance during motor acts, teaching problem solving, identifying cognitive distortions, testing cognitions (reality testing), and providing knowledge in an educational format. Occupational therapists participating in a qualitative study revealed that "In the task-based sessions, activity was identified as a means to promote development of cognitive skills (e.g., concentration, organization, problem solving)" (Moll & Cook, 1996, p. 666). Social skills and life skills groups and stress management and relaxation groups are examples of psychoeducational groups that have been successful in helping clients meet their goals. These groups are described below.

Because cognitive–behavior therapy requires some ability to reflect on one's thinking and on the contextual feedback from one's behavior, it is not surprising that occupational therapists have reported success using cognitive–behavioral strategies and techniques with clients whose cognitive abilities are less likely to be limited or impacted by their symptoms and diagnosed condition. More specifically, occupational therapists have identified cognitive–behavioral therapy as effective in working with clients who have been diagnosed with alcoholism (Lindsay, 1983; Moyers, 1988; Stoffel, 1994), eating disorders (Giles, 1985; Giles & Allen, 1986; Henderson, 1998), depression (Eilenberg, 1986; Johnson, 1986; Stein & Smith, 1989; Yakobina et al., 1997), and chronic pain (Engel, 1991; Engel & Rapoff, 1990). For clients whose symptoms and diagnostic condition have a much greater long-term and disabling impact on cognitive function, the intervention strategies and techniques often need to be more behavioral to accommodate their cognitive limitations and impaired metacognitive abilities. Specific strategies, techniques, and programs using modified or graded cognitive interventions and a more behavioral approach have been identified for clients with schizophrenia (Luboshitsky & Gaber, 2000; Stein & Nikolic, 1989), in acute care (Bradlee, 1984; Fine & Schwimmer, 1986; Greenberg et al., 1988; Ogren, 1983), in outpatient care (Tang, 2001), and in long-term care settings (Campbell

& McCreadie, 1988; Drouet, 1986; Friedlob et al., 1986; Jao & Lu, 1999; Nickel, 1988; Salo-Chydenius, 1996).

The next section of this chapter presents three case studies that illustrate various psychoeducational groups and programs using cognitive–behavioral approaches in different settings with different populations and involving different role expectations for the occupational therapist. Case Example 7.1 exemplifies the role of an occupational therapist working in inpatient, outpatient, and partial-day intervention programs with a woman who is depressed and suicidal. Case Example 7.2 describes the use of a more behaviorally oriented approach by an occupational therapist functioning as a consultant to a group home. Social skills training for a client with serious and persistent schizophrenia is highlighted in this case. Finally, psychoeducational coping skills groups offered in a wellness context are described in Case Example 7.3. A couples' communication group led by an occupational therapist illustrates this type of cognitive–behavioral intervention.

Cognitive–Behavioral Techniques in a Traditional Psychiatric Setting

Occupational therapists use a variety of cognitive–behavioral principles, strategies, and techniques, including psychoeducational groups in both short- and long-term work with clients. This is illustrated in numerous descriptions of programs for inpatients (Bradlee, 1984; Courtney & Escobedo, 1990; Fine & Schwimmer, 1986; Giles, 1985; Giles & Allen, 1986; Greenberg et al., 1988; Heine, 1975; Jao & Lu, 1999; Klein, 1988; Luboshitzky & Gaber, 2000; Ogren, 1983; Stein & Smith, 1989) and in day and community programs (Campbell & McCreadie, 1988; Courtney & Escobedo, 1990; Crist, 1986; Johnson, 1986; Kaseman, 1980; Mitchell, 2000; Nickel, 1988; Salo-Chydenius, 1996; Stein & Nikolic, 1989; Tang, 2001).

Case Example 7.1 illustrates an occupational therapy intervention in the context of a cognitive–behavioral therapy approach in acute inpatient and partial-day programs as part of a community mental health center.

Social Skills and Life Skills

Many descriptions of social or life skills groups include behavior therapy as their underlying theoretical base, but in reality, there is the expectation of cognitive awareness and of the individual participating in the groups for the intrinsic value or meaning of the occupation, not merely for an external reinforcement (Drouet, 1986; Liberman, Massel, Mosk, & Wong, 1985).

Case Example 7.1. Intervention in an Acute Inpatient and Partial-Day Program

Edna is a 57-year-old widow with two married daughters. She was admitted to the acute inpatient psychiatric unit following a suicide attempt 4 months after the unexpected death of her husband. At the time of her hospital admission, her daughter reported that her mother's participation in self-care and home maintenance routines and in work, leisure, social, family, and community interests and activities had declined greatly since her husband's death. Her daughter also shared that Edna frequently talked about feeling her life was over and that everyone would be better off without her.

Inpatient Occupational Therapy Evaluation

The Allen Cognitive Level Screen (ACLS–90), the Canadian Occupational Performance Measure (COPM; Law et. al., 1994), and a semistructured interview were used to develop Edna's occupational profile. The COPM explored Edna's needs, concerns, priorities, and goals. The interview focused on identifying thoughts and behaviors that hindered or facilitated engagement in occupations meaningful to Edna. The ACLS–90 evaluated her cognitive-reasoning abilities. In analyzing Edna's occupational performance patterns, it became clear that Edna's sense of meaning and purpose in life had been centered on the very satisfying, active, and involved lifestyle she and her husband enjoyed together during their 40 years of marriage. Without him, she was at a loss as to what to do with her time and could not imagine finding meaning in resuming past or potentially new routines, interests, and occupations. In her words, Edna explained, "My husband was my life. We did everything for or with each other. He paid the bills and took care of the house, the yard, and the cars. I cooked, shopped, cleaned, and planned our social activities. We both worked hard and participated together in family, church, and community activities. Together, we enjoyed gardening, bowling, travel, and spending time with our daughters' families." She reported that she used to be a creative and fun-loving person who enjoyed quilting and crafts as well as

her work as a postal clerk, where she had recently been honored for her 30 years of excellence of service. Regarding her work, Edna confessed that she had tried to return to work but was unable to concentrate and felt overwhelmed by the expectations of coworkers and customers. She and her work supervisor decided that she should take a medical leave of absence. Although Edna confirmed her supervisor's assurances that she was a valued employee and would be welcomed back to her job when she felt up to it, she expressed fear that she would never be able to work again and that she would likely be fired for incompetence if she tried to return.

In discussing her current functioning and plans for the future, Edna sadly lamented, "My life is over. I can't do anything. I'm useless. My family would be better off without me." However, with some reluctance, she tearfully admitted that, although she couldn't imagine life being worth living without her husband, she would rather live than die if she could feel better and be a more worthwhile person again.

On the ACLS–90, Edna scored ACL 5.2. Although her performance indicated slowed cognitive processing with difficulty concentrating, attending to details, and imagining a future different from the present, she was able to use inductive reasoning and a trial-and-error approach for problem solving. This suggested that Edna had sufficient cognitive ability to use more cognitively oriented strategies for coping with her loss and lifestyle changes and for exploring occupational choices and options that might support renewed participation in the activities and occupations she valued, as well as bring renewed meaning to her life.

Inpatient Intervention, Including Occupational Therapy

Edna and the occupational therapist collaboratively decided that her occupational therapy goals while in the hospital would focus on establishing a daily routine of self-care and leisure activities and exploring

ways to help her feel better through participation in activities that might contribute to her feelings of worth as a person. The occupational therapist explained that engaging in a structured daily routine was an important step to begin reversing the experience of hopelessness and helplessness that Edna described. Along with setting up a routine for self-care, meals, and rest, the occupational therapist encouraged Edna to participate in the following daily group activities:

1. *Morning and evening exercise groups:* participation in a structured exercise class along with exploration of various types of exercise (e.g., walking, aerobics, stretching, and education about the positive effects of exercise for health, stress reduction, and relieving symptoms of depression).
2. *Occupational therapy task group:* participation in various leisure activities, crafts, games, and so forth, structured to promote social interaction, successful task performance, leisure exploration and engagement, and improved concentration and problem solving.
3. *Coping-skills group:* education about the relationship among thoughts, feelings, and behaviors and exploration of various cognitive–behavioral techniques and strategies for decreasing negative thoughts and behaviors and increasing positive thoughts and behaviors as a way to feel better and experience more satisfaction in daily life (e.g., thought stopping, role-playing, identifying and reframing thought distortions, and assertiveness skills).
4. *Healthy-living group:* education about the importance of sleep, nutrition, exercise, social participation, and stress and anger management for decreasing depression and improving overall health and feelings of well-being and exploration of various healthy-living activities and ways to incorporate them into a daily routine after discharge.

Edna met with the occupational therapist to begin to plan a daily routine for self-care,

(continued)

household management, and social and leisure activities to put in place when she resumed living at home. As a way to encourage Edna to begin participating in some of the interests she enjoyed, the occupational therapist urged Edna to have her daughter bring in a quilting project that she had begun for her new granddaughter. The occupational therapist also supported Edna in using the cognitive–behavioral strategies she was learning about in other groups to identify thoughts, feelings, and behaviors that made it difficult for her to engage in her previous routines and occupations or to explore new ones. For example, she encouraged Edna to record her thoughts and feelings before and after engaging in activities and taught her the TIC-TOC technique (Burns, 1989a). This technique helped Edna identify "Task-Interfering Cognitions" and to reframe them as "Task-Oriented Cognitions." The following example illustrates how Edna used this technique when she felt like skipping her morning grooming routine:

- *Task-Interfering Cognition:* "Now that my husband is gone, it doesn't matter what I look like, so why bother?"
- *Task-Oriented Cognition:* "Even though my husband is gone, I might feel better about myself if I took care of my health and appearance."

After completing her grooming routine, Edna then evaluated whether her reframed thoughts were helpful in following through with her planned routine and whether or not she did feel better.

Inpatient Progress

After 6 days with antidepressant medication, participation in a structured daily routine, social support, and cognitive–behavioral education and therapy, Edna appeared less withdrawn and anxious. She attended and participated in all scheduled groups and activities without needing to be reminded. She commented

that, although she still found it difficult to participate in self-care, group, and social activities, the recording of her thoughts and feelings helped her to realize that she felt better after participating. She noted that the TIC-TOC technique was helpful and might be something she also could share with her grandchildren to help them do chores and schoolwork when they didn't want to or felt their efforts weren't valued or worthwhile. Edna concurred with her intervention team's perception that she was sufficiently safe and in control of her thoughts and actions to be discharged home and to attend the partial hospital day program for 2 weeks.

Partial-Day Program, Including Occupational Therapy

In the partial-day program, Edna continued to participate in cognitive–behavioral therapy and in a structured daily routine of self-care, social, leisure, and therapeutic activities and groups similar to those she attended as an inpatient. She added three additional groups that met twice a week:

1. *Leisure participation group:* exploration of leisure opportunities in the community planned by the group members with staff support and consultation.
2. *Structured-learning group:* psycho-educational "classes" and homework related to topics such as coping with mental illness, medication side effects, community resources, communication skills, assertiveness skills, anger management, time management, vocational readiness, techniques for managing negative self-talk, and relapse prevention.
3. *Life choices and options group:* led by an occupational therapist and other professional team members; group members help each other identify choices and options for solving problems, fears, and doubts that interfere with their health, occupational and role performance, and

life satisfaction. Members give each other feedback on their thoughts, behavior, and feelings and support each other in using various cognitive–behavioral strategies such as role-playing, modeling, and problem solving to decrease and modify maladaptive thoughts and behaviors and increase adaptive thoughts and behaviors. In this group, Edna focused on reality testing and modifying her perceptions that her life was over, that there was nothing worth doing without her husband, that she was a burden to everyone, and that she would be fired from her job. She explored options and choices to fill the void left by her husband's death and located community activities and resources for support.

Edna continued to work with an occupational therapist in planning a daily routine with time use and motivational strategies to support her recovery and prevent relapse. Her plan included working in her garden, taking community classes in rubber-stamp art and yoga, and joining a quilting group at her church. She decided to try walking with a neighbor for exercise and to gradually return to her volunteer work at church and to spending more time with her grandchildren. She set up a plan for managing her finances; bills; and house, yard, and car upkeep. In collaboration with the occupational therapist, Edna decided to ask for an additional month's leave of absence from work to give herself time to take care of herself and adjust to her changed lifestyle.

After 14 days in the partial-day program, Edna reported feeling less discouraged and more able to cope with her loss and reach out to others for support. She chose to attend a weekly grief and loss support group offered by the community mental health center and made a commitment to turn her Task-Interfering Cognitions into Task-Oriented Cognitions to help her participate in her redesigned lifestyle plan.

When one examines the procedure used in a social skills approach (Hayes, 1989; Hewitt, Wishart, & Lambert, 1981; Kaseman, 1980; Salo-Chydenius, 1996), it includes the five principles of cognitive therapy (individualization, collaboration, activity, problem solving, and generalization). One early occupational therapist described a group, clearly using cognitive–behavioral techniques, without identifying it as such (Heine, 1975). Another practitioner created a social skills game that incorporated cognition, behavioral skills, and self-awareness (Love, 1988). Although some programs used tangible reinforcements (Drouet, 1986; Hayes, 1989), all other requirements of cognitive–behavioral therapy were met. More recently, Salo-Chydenius (1996) documented the effectiveness of a social skills program based totally on a cognitive–behavioral model for individuals with long-term mental illness.

Because these groups are based on cognitive–behavioral therapy principles, the groups must be organized around the needs or prioritized goals of the individuals in the groups. Case Example 7.2 provides an example of the intervention process using cognitive–behavioral therapy with social skills and life skills groups.

Stress Management and Relaxation Training

These groups have been documented for individuals with schizophrenia (Stein & Nikolic, 1989), depression (Stein & Smith, 1989), alcoholism (Moyers, 1988; Stoffel, 1994), and eating disorders (Giles, 1985) for caregivers of individuals with dementia (Mitchell, 2000) and for a well population (Burns, 1989a). There is generally an educational component to these groups in which the "students" learn about stress and then are asked to identify how they know when they are feeling stress, how they feel stress in their bodies, and how they act when they are feeling under stress. Homework sheets usually help group members begin to identify stress and their own coping or noncoping strategies on a daily basis. Once the stress factors have been identified, individuals are asked to problem-solve and identify stress management or relaxation techniques that might be helpful. Next, they practice the techniques, first in the group and then as homework, and give feedback to themselves and the group about the effectiveness of the techniques. Generalization, making sure that the group members continue to use the stress management techniques after they leave the intervention facility, is probably the most difficult part in the strategy. Examples of other coping-skills groups are anger management (Tang, 2001) and communication skills.

The three case examples in this chapter illustrate the use of cognitive–behavioral therapy within the context and philosophy of occupational therapy. It is important to note that, although the occupational therapy philosophy is relatively stable, the context of occupational therapy is ever changing. For that reason, the cases are described in four different settings. The roles of the occupational therapist in direct intervention, both in- and outpatient; consultation; and community education were meant to reflect the changes in health care.

Evidence-Based Research

The value of any intervention method based on one or many theoretical rationales must be determined through research. One difference between cognitive therapy and psychoanalytic therapy has been identified as the researchability of cognitive therapy. "Outcome studies are easily conducted because the principles of cognitive therapy can be systematized within a relatively uniform set of therapeutic procedures" (Beck, 1976, p. 318). "Cognitive therapy has been extensively tested since the first outcome study was published in 1977" (Beck, 1995, p. 2). (For references on intervention efficacy for depression, anxiety, panic disorders, phobias, substance abuse, eating disorders, and couples' problems, see Beck, 1995.) Although descriptions abound of occupational therapists using cognitive–behavioral techniques, the research on the efficacy of these techniques for occupational therapy is sparse.

In reviewing the literature for effectiveness of intervention with individuals with schizophrenia, Hayes (1989) found four intervention methods most often mentioned. Two of these, social-skills training and living-skills training, have a cognitive component even though they are frequently considered more behavioral than cognitive. This places them in the realm of cognitive–behavioral therapy. However, because of methodological flaws, one cannot infer that the intervention described would have the same effect in other settings and with other clients (Hayes, 1989). Two outcome studies did add statistical support to the use of social-skills training with clients with mental illness (Campbell & McCreadie, 1983; Friedlob et al., 1986). They were limited, however, to small numbers of clients. A 1991 study found that social-skills training was effective in increasing the social behavior of clients with schizophrenia but not in transferring those skills to their community settings (Hayes, Halford, & Varghese, 1991). Salo-Chydenius (1996) described an occupational therapy social-skills training program based on cognitive–behavioral theory and documented the effectiveness of

Case Example 7.2. A Group Home With an Occupational Therapist Consultant

Bob is a 70-year-old resident in a group home. His diagnosis is serious and persistent schizophrenia. He was hospitalized in a state hospital until the facility was closed 5 years ago. He was selected for inclusion in a group home because he was well-maintained on his medication, had no history of violence, and currently had no active hallucinations. Because he has been hospitalized for most of his life, he is very dependent on staff to take care of all of his daily needs. He is mostly independent in activities of daily living (ADL), needing reminders about shaving and not wearing dirty clothes. He is dependent on staff for the maintenance of his clothes (laundry) and for shopping, preparing, and cleaning up after his meals. He can read but generally does not choose to. He mostly sits, head down, and waits for something to do. He participates in group activities but never suggests one. He greets staff but does not talk to fellow residents unless it is in the context of a group activity or he is asked by a staff member to elicit information from another resident.

The occupational therapist is a consultant to his group home and routinely evaluates group members and identifies programs run by the staff that are appropriate for selected members to attend. The occupational therapist also participates in staff training and supervision in leading a variety of groups, including leisure skills, gardening, cooking, exercise, reminiscence, and others that incorporate interests of the staff or are suggested by residents.

Bob was given two formal assessments, the Bay Area Functional Performance Evaluation (BaFPE; Bloomer & Williams, 1982) and the Kohlman Evaluation of Living Skills (KELS; Thomson, 1992).

The BaFPE was administered on March 18. This standardized assessment consists of five tasks that differ in degree of complexity and structure and yield scores in three component areas (cognitive, performance, and affective) as well as qualitative indicators of possible organic involvement. Bob scored 1 standard deviation (SD) below the norm in 7 out of 12 functional areas.

Cognitive Component

Bob scored more than 1 SD below the norm in memory for written and verbal instructions, organization of time and materials, and attention span. Primarily because of these areas, he also performed below the norm in the total cognitive score. He scored within normal limits in ability to abstract, and there was no evidence of thought disorder.

Performance Component

Bob's scores were within normal limits for 2 of the 3 areas tested, task completion and efficiency. He scored 1 SD below the norm in errors.

Affective Component

He scored more than 1 SD below the norm in frustration tolerance, self-confidence, and general affective impression. His scores were within normal limits for motivation.

Structure and Complexity

Bob scored more than 1 SD below the norm in money and marketing, a cognitively oriented task involving several steps; in a home drawing, in which there was some structure and some choice; and in the block design, a visual memory task. In both the money and marketing and the home drawing tasks, although he was able to give some idea of what he was expected to do before he began, he appeared to not know what was expected during the actual task. It is unclear whether he forgot the instructions, had intervening thoughts or preoccupations that interfered with his remembering, never really comprehended what he was to do, or was unable to act on what he heard and could verbalize having heard. He scored within normal limits for the structured task of sorting shells and for the least structured task, the kinetic person drawing. His total score for this task-oriented assessment was more than 1 SD below the norm for the sample group with which he was compared. (This client's scores were compared with norms from a population of people with chronic mental

illness whose demographics resemble those of this particular client.)

The KELS is currently a nonstandardized assessment. Although research on validity and reliability has been conducted, more is needed (Thomson, 1992). Scores are available in 17 living skills. In addition, there are many opportunities to assess the client's cognitive abilities such as "orientation, attention span, and memory . . ." (Thomson, 1992, p. 40). On March 25, Bob was given 11 areas that were considered relevant to his living situation. Under *self-care*, he needed assistance in appearance, specifically in hair care and shaving. He was dressed appropriately in street clothes, but the cleanliness of the clothes was questionable. He reported daily performance of some activities, like toothbrushing, but not of washing and shaving. In the *safety and health* category, he was aware of dangerous household situations but not what to do about them; he had some idea of appropriate action for sickness but not for accidents. He had no knowledge of emergency phone numbers or of availability of medical and dental facilities. He reported being totally dependent in the area of *money management*. He bought coffee regularly and always got the same change back but, using real money and store items, he was unable to determine how much change he should receive from a $1 bill. Likewise, he was dependent on others for his *transportation* needs and had no knowledge of the transit system. Although he said he knew how to use the telephone book, he said he had no need to do so. Finally, for *work and leisure*, he had no plans to seek employment and listed only three activities that he liked to do in his spare time: go on trips (especially out to eat), watch television, and read the newspaper.

General Observations

Bob was compliant throughout. He slowly attempted every task presented. He spoke in a low, quiet monotone and displayed no affect toward the examiner or to anything she did or said. When it was time to end each session, the examiner said, "Thank you for your cooperation," to which he

(continued)

Case Example 7.2. A Group Home With an Occupational Therapist Consultant *(Continued)*

replied, without emotion, "It was a pleasure." Throughout all tests and tasks, he seemed to have the most difficulty following directions. In some cases, he thought he understood the directions when he did not. In other cases, he began to work before the examiner finished giving the directions. In still other situations, directions needed to be repeated for every item in the category. Finally, psychomotor retardation and lack of initiative were apparent throughout the evaluation sessions.

On the basis of the results of these assessments, social and life skills training in the cognitive–behavioral frame of reference seemed appropriate. Bob's motivation was high, and the presence of the cognitive ability to abstract indicated the potential for self-awareness. His other cognitive abilities, although low, seemed adequate to work on the skills suggested as lacking in the KELS: ADL, safety, money management, and leisure.

The results of the evaluation were explained to Bob with some ideas of areas in which he might be able to perform better in his structured living situation. He was asked what he would like to be able to do better. He said he had concern about what he would do if his roommate started choking. (When asked why he was concerned about this, he responded that his roommate often ate in their room, even though this was not allowed, and he, Bob, had never learned any first aid.) He would like to manage his money better. He is frustrated with the staff at the group home in the lack of activities and feels the members need to take more charge of this. He enjoys going out on trips and realizes that to be more acceptable to people he meets, he needs to be more consistent about his physical appearance.

With this in mind, Bob and the therapist created the following activities and outcome goals:

1. In a safety skills group, Bob will
   a. Be able to dial 911 and state his name, address, telephone number, and a description of the emergency to the person on the other end of the line
   b. Keep a card that indicates the information for the 911 operator by the phone near his room
   c. Demonstrate the Heimlich maneuver
   d. Consistently carry a card with personal emergency information in his wallet
   e. Successfully exit his home within 1 min during a fire drill.
2. During a 3-week money management course, Bob will
   a. Demonstrate ability to count change for $1, $5, $10, and $20
   b. Recognize when he has been given incorrect change
   c. Demonstrate what to say and do if he believes he has been given incorrect change
   d. List weekly items he would like to buy and activities he would like to participate in that cost money, compare this with his weekly allowance, and create a personal budget.
3. In an ongoing leisure skills group, Bob will
   a. Give at least one suggestion at every discussion for possible events
   b. Participate in either preparation or cleanup of the activity once every other week
   c. Start at least one conversation with another group member each time the group meets
   d. Participate in making weekly schedule posters for the house members.
4. Bob and his resident advisor will make a chart of ADL tasks to be done and when they should be done. Bob will check off when he has done the listed activities. After 2 weeks, the chart can be modified or the frequency of Bob's checked responses on the chart can be changed as Bob and his resident advisor see progress. After all morning ADL activities are completed, Bob will be asked how he thinks he looks, and he will write that in the appropriate space on the chart.

Bob participated in three groups or classes: one on safety, one on money management, and one on leisure activities. They were all psychoeducational groups with homework, practical tasks built into the groups, role-playing, printed information, and instructional videotapes. At the end of each group, the group leader elicited from each participant his or her thoughts and feelings about the content of the group and how he or she might change

his or her behavior because of the group. The occupational therapist met weekly with staff concerning supervision of the groups. Bob also worked with his resident advisor on ADLs. This endeavor was mostly behavioral, with a slight cognitive component built into it.

Does this fit for the cognitive–behavioral frame of reference? In terms of phenomenology, the interview included Bob's concerns and goals and what he thought some of the problems were. Both the outcomes and the intervention plan were created collaboratively with Bob. All interventions included activity (occupation). In terms of empiricism, Bob was asked to help problem-solve why he felt anxious about safety situations, and his identification of a lack of knowledge of safety led to a group for all interested members in his house. This procedure was carried out for all outcomes. Because Bob's outcomes and occupations were being carried out in the context in which they were expected to occur, generalization was expected to take place. The reinforcement schedule for his ADL needed to be changed so that Bob was aware that he had made these changes and so that his involvement in them would become self-reinforcing.

Three Months Later

In a follow-up session with Bob, the occupational therapist asked how things were going. He was well-dressed, clean-shaven, and sat upright. He reported that he was pleased with his "courses." He was no longer worried about the safety of his roommate. The class on safety and first aid had decided to do follow-up safety drills, such as fire drills, once in a while to keep people "on their toes." He felt more competent with his money, and the food servers where he occasionally bought coffee had complimented him on his appearance during a money transaction. The one area he was still concerned about was leisure activities. There had been recent turnover of weekend staff, and he did not yet feel comfortable enough with the new people to voice his opinions. After problem-solving around this concern, he decided to suggest the idea of a planning group at a group home meeting.

Case Example 7.3. A Wellness Group

A *couples communication group* offered by a health maintenance organization is advertised as a health and wellness group for people who want to improve their communication skills with a significant other. (No singles are permitted to attend the group.) The group meets for 6 weeks, one evening a week. An occupational therapist is the group leader. She identifies herself as an occupational therapist and defines the expected outcome: that everyone in the group will function optimally in his or her context, specifically, in the area of communication with another person. Although they have arrived as couples, individuals in the group introduce themselves and identify their goals and why they have chosen to attend this group.

Because this is not an intervention situation, there are no clinical evaluations. Instead, each person is asked to take a pretest identifying areas of concern or potential conflict, such as competition, workload, cultural backgrounds, relationships with his or her partner's family, need for emotional space, and willingness to change the current communication style (Cohen-Kaplan, 1991). Then, in psychoeducational format, a lecture or discussion about communication styles and skills starts the classes. Each participant receives his or her own booklet of handouts, which includes a bibliography of lay people's books on the subject, several of which are recommended as "texts" for the course.

During the 6 weeks, couples learn about their own communication style and practice different styles. A homework log, in which they record when they use different styles and what the results are, is brought back to class and discussed. Assertiveness is defined, discussed, practiced, and discussed again. The participants learn through role-playing how to listen and respond in a nondefensive way to their partner as they learn about conflict resolution. The group explores anger and how to handle it. They write their life scripts and share them with their partners. To focus on the real issues for each couple, the therapist devotes much of the time to role-playing actual conversations that the couples have chosen as a focus. The group gives the

couple feedback, and they are encouraged to change their behavior. There is no follow-up after the couples' communication group is over, but several groups of couples have spontaneously organized support groups to carry on the work of the group.

This is the story of Peter and Valerie, who had been married for a little more than 2 years. They both worked and had no children. They were saving for a house and had been spending much time on househunting in the recent past. They felt they had a healthy relationship in that they had maintained their own interests and friends as well as doing things together. However, something was wrong. They both recognized it. Valerie would go out on a Friday evening with her friends from work, and Peter felt that he was OK with that and found ways to occupy his time. Then on Saturday mornings, Peter would frequently play golf with his brother or father. He could not understand why Valerie would be so upset when he got home from these outings. It was identified, during the communication style exercise, that Peter tended to be compliant (passive) in his communication style and that Valerie tended to be passive-aggressive. Thus, Peter had responded to this situation by saying nothing, yet silently wondering and worrying about what was wrong. Valerie, in a passive-aggressive style, and had been unpleasant and sarcastic until her mood wore off.

Each person was committed to identifying the problem and had been reading the texts and doing the homework faithfully. They participated in the role-play, accepting feedback and discussing the group's reaction to their styles. They also provided excellent feedback to other members. The night arrived for them to role-play a real situation in their lives. Each had selected a different scenario to role-play and had received permission from the other person to share that with the group. Peter went first and described the interaction with Valerie after his return from a golf game with his father. When Valerie appeared passive-aggressive, the group identified that for

her, and she tried to be more assertive. Peter was admonished for being passive. The re-enactment of their role-play progressed but seemed like acting, not like genuine change. Neither described any difference in thinking or feeling after their role-play. Valerie gave the background for the communication she wanted to examine. It took place at the home of her in-laws. During this description and role-play, it was evident that Valerie had a lot of feeling about her relationship with her husband when he was with his family. Valerie explained what she had observed, how she felt about it, and what she desired. Peter listened. When his turn came to report on what he had heard, an amazing thing happened. He had truly heard Valerie for the first time on this issue. Maybe she had communicated clearly about it for the first time; however, he realized that, rather than her being jealous of the time he spent with his family, she was reacting to the way he acted toward her when they were together with his family. She felt ignored and not respected as an equal individual. They both responded positively to their newfound knowledge about each other and the way in which they communicated their important concerns. They agreed to continue communicating in this style and reported in later sessions that this particular interaction was a major breakthrough for them. They had changed their thinking about themselves, about each other, and about how to communicate.

The cognitive–behavioral aspects of this group are seen more clearly, perhaps, because this group has more of the cognitive components in it than behavioral. Exercises are used throughout to identify the thoughts and feelings that group members have that are interfering with the ability to communicate with each other. The uniqueness of each person in the group is emphasized, and nothing is done without collaborating and problem-solving with the person involved. Many cognitive–behavioral techniques are used: bibliotherapy, role-playing, homework, role-modeling, cognitive rehearsal, identifying cognitive distortions, feedback from group members, and the use of an educational format.

the program with a single case study. Nonoccupational therapy literature has indicated that social-skills training increased client's skills (Liberman et al., 1985).

The presence of clients' money management skills was identified before and after they were included in a life skills program (Kaseman, 1980). Although only raw data were presented, the results indicated an increase of skills. Two other outcomes of living-skills groups for clients with mental illness have been described, one in an acute setting (Ogren, 1983) and one in a well population (DeMars, 1992). No statistics were included in these descriptions. Two studies have provided evidence on which to base treatment. Jao and Lu (1999) taught problem-solving skills to individuals with long-term schizophrenia (M age = 35.4 years) and found a significant increase in skills for those in the treatment group ($p > .007$) as compared with those in the control group ($p > .46$), as measured by the Means–Ends Problem-Solving Procedure (MEPA; Platt & Spivack, 1977, cited in Jao & Lu, 1999). This was based on a small number (treatment group, $n = 10$; control group, $n = 8$) and the research was conducted in Taiwan; therefore, generalizability is limited. Positive results were reported for an anger management program for individuals with mental illness (Tang, 2001). The majority of these participants were diagnosed with depression, and the mean age was 40 years (range = 18–65 years). Participants' responses on two questionnaires, pre- and post-treatment, were compared using two-tailed paired t tests. Fourteen of 16 scales on the Anger Control Inventory (ACI; Hoshmand & Austin, 1987, cited in Tang, 2001), and 5 of 8 scales of the State-Trait Anger Expression Inventory (STAXI; Spielberger, 1996, cited in Tang, 2001) showed that the participants had significantly more control over their angry feelings after treatment. There were 35 respondents to the ACI and 20 sets of data for the STAXI. There was, however, no control group for this study, and the authors listed many internal and external threats to the validity of this study.

From the research evidence thus far, it seems that several factors would facilitate our ability to document outcomes in the area of mental health. First, the number of clients we have assigned to groups and on whom we collect data has been limited. We need to find ways to combine data to increase our numbers rather than being isolative in our research efforts. Because the wide variety of diagnoses and medication may affect the intervention and provide uncontrollable variables (Hayes, 1989; Tang, 2001), combining data across clinics would help with increasing numbers in similar groups. In addition, occupational therapists are not always using standardized measures for pre- and post-testing.

Thien (1987) suggested that occupational therapists could provide outcome data on clients by assessing their progress toward goals using client satisfaction questionnaires and behavior-rating scales. These suggestions are appropriate in the cognitive–behavioral frame of reference. Behavioral rating scales could provide pre- and post-data for the specific behaviors identified in behavioral objectives, as was done in a documentation review system that was set up to look at outcomes (Thien, 1987). Because of the emphasis in cognitive–behavioral therapy on the individual taking responsibility for him- or herself through cognitive awareness, the use of client satisfaction questionnaires also is appropriate. This is an excellent way to determine whether the coping skills taught have generalized to the context in which the individual needs to use them (Thien, 1987).

The use of standardized measures for determining progress has been quite limited in occupational therapy outcome research. Several studies have used standardized measures outside of, but related to, occupational therapy such as the Simple Rathus Assertiveness Schedule (McCormick, 1984, cited in Hayes et al., 1991), the Tennessee Self-Concept Scale (Fitts, cited in Stoffel, 1993), the MEPA (Platt & Spivack, 1977, cited in Jao & Lu, 1999), the ACI (Hoshmand & Austin, 1987, cited in Tang, 2001), and the STAXI (Spielberger, 1996, cited in Tang, 2001). Several assessments mentioned earlier in the chapter are standardized and could be used for research purposes to show efficacy of intervention. Clearly we also need more standardized assessments, and work is currently progressing on providing data for sev-eral (e.g., KELS, ACLS–90). The recently standardized Stress Management Questionnaire (Stein, 2003) is recommended for occupational therapists leading stress management groups or working with a depressed population.

There is promise in these attempts to develop standardized assessments and to document outcomes. To further demonstrate the value of occupational therapy and of the use of specific methods in occupational therapy practice, we need to "clarify which clients respond to what particular forms of intervention, what behaviors and symptoms can be changed and whether specifically trained skills generalize to the home, and to the community" (Hayes, 1989, p. 151).

CHALLENGE OF THE FUTURE

The changes in health care toward cost containment through managed care have had a profound effect on how and where we function as occupational therapists. Just as a mechanic is expected to diagnose the problem, provide an estimate of costs, estimate the amount of time necessary to fix the vehicle, and determine the expected performance of the vehicle after repair, so are health care providers expected to inform clients regarding specific outcomes, the time needed to achieve these outcomes, and the effectiveness of the intervention they will receive. As reported above, our outcome measures are sorely lacking. An emotional belief that what we do is beneficial is not sufficient. Before we can validate our presence in *any* context, we need to document the effectiveness of what we do. In addition, as research becomes available, occupational therapists should base their evaluation and intervention methods on that evidence (Lloyd, Bassett, & King, 2004).

In addition, in the era of cost containment, management determines who does what best and in the least expensive way. We need to ask the question, What can occupational therapy add to a mental health team that is unique? Then we need to capitalize on that uniqueness. I propose that one of the unique aspects of occupational therapy is not the use of cognitive–behavioral techniques but the ability to identify the combination of a client's cognitive abilities coupled with the identification of performance skills needed for survival in his or her community. When this information is synthesized with contributions of other team members, the foundation for a holistic intervention plan is in place.

Our goal must be to document what we are doing and to provide the measures of effectiveness necessary for validation of our unique skills. Further, we are challenged to change the arena in which we have been working for so long and move to where managed care is placing our clients (Fidler, 1991).

The basic tenets of cognitive–behavioral therapy and the practice of occupational therapy have many commonalities. Occupational therapists have adopted many cognitive–behavioral strategies and techniques in conjunction with other occupational therapy frames of reference. The intent of this chapter has been to define the relationship of a cognitive–behavioral approach to occupational therapy and to provide an understanding of the theoretical antecedents of the cognitive–behavioral components of occupational therapy practice. Understanding the background of these cognitive–behavioral principles should prove useful to the occupational therapist as he or she creates a collaborative, client-centered, holistic intervention plan for an individual client.

It is often necessary to combine several schools of thought and draw from many resources when working with populations whose illness reflect biopsychosocial phenomena. Neither the client, or the course of a given illness, are unidimensional. Different intervention models can augment or jointly stimulate desired effects, and changing needs certainly may require different approaches. (Fine, 1989, cited in Ross, 1991, p. vii)

Finally, when occupational therapists use cognitive–behavioral principles, strategies, and techniques to meet occupational therapy intervention goals, it does not mean that they are cognitive–behavioral therapists. Furthermore, the technique is not the expected outcome of intervention. We are not specialists in stress management or coping or rational thinking. Our uniqueness as occupational therapists lies in our professional judgment and ability to identify clients' global cognitive assets and limitations and how they affect client performance. We use a variety of techniques and strategies, graded to the clients' cognitive abilities, to enable them to learn the performance skills and patterns necessary for meaningful lives and social participation in their context of choice.

SUMMARY QUESTIONS

1. What are the theoretical underpinnings of the cognitive–behavioral model?
2. What philosophical, theoretical, and intervention principles do cognitive–behavioral and occupational therapists have in common?
3. How does the cognitive–behavioral model fit with the *Occupational Therapy Practice Framework?*
4. Identify assessments that an occupational therapist might use to develop a client profile and an intervention plan incorporating cognitive–behavioral principles and strategies.
5. How might information from these assessments guide the selection and implementation of cognitive–behavioral strategies as part of an occupational therapy intervention?
6. Give examples of cognitive–behavioral principles, strategies, and techniques that might be appropriate to use in an occupational therapy intervention.
7. Review Case Example 7.1 about Edna. Describe two additional cognitive–behavioral techniques that might be appropriate to include as part of her occupational therapy intervention.
8. Review Case Example 7.2. Suggest a different cognitive or skills assessment to use with Bob.

9. A communication skills group was presented in Case Example 7.3. What other psychoeducational groups might an occupational therapist lead in a wellness context?

10. What is the current evidence supporting use of cognitive–behavioral principles, strategies, and techniques in occupational therapy practice?

11. Describe how an occupational therapist might approach the evaluation and intervention process with a client so that the outcome data could contribute to the efficacy of occupational therapy intervention.

ACKNOWLEDGMENT

The authors thank Deane McCraith for her support through providing Case Example 7.1, related material, and valuable suggestions and for reviewing earlier drafts of this manuscript.

REFERENCES

Allen, C., & Reyner, A.(1996). *How to start using the Allen Diagnostic Module* (2nd ed.). Colchester, CT: S & S Worldwide.

American Occupational Therapy Association. (2002). Occupational therapy practice framework: Domain and process. *American Journal of Occupational Therapy, 56,* 609–639.

American Occupational Therapy Association, Representative Assembly. (1979). Resolution 531-79. *American Journal of Occupational Therapy, 33,* 785.

Arthanat, S., Nochajski, S., & Stone, J. (2004). The international classification of functioning, disability, and health and its application to cognitive disorders. *Disability and Rehabilitation, 26,* 235–245.

Bandura, A. (1985). Model of causality in social learning theory. In M. Mahoney & A. Freeman (Eds.), *Cognition and psychotherapy* (pp. 81–99). New York: Plenum.

Barris, R., Kielhofner, G., & Watts, J. (1983). *Psychosocial occupational therapy.* Laurel, MD: RAMSCO.

Beck, A. T. (1970). Cognitive therapy: Nature and relation to behavior therapy. *Behavior Therapy, 1,* 184–200.

Beck, A. T. (1976). *Cognitive therapy and emotional disorders.* New York: International University Press.

Beck, A. T., & Weishaar, M. (1994). Cognitive therapy. In R. Corsini & D. Wedding (Eds.), *Current psychotherapies* (4th ed., pp. 285–320). Itasca, IL: Peacock.

Beck, J. (1995). *Cognitive therapy: Basics and beyond.* New York: Guilford.

Bloomer, J., & Williams, S. (1982). The Bay Area Functional Performance Evaluation. In B. Hemphill (Ed.), *The evaluative process in psychiatric occupational therapy* (pp. 255–308). Thorofare, NJ: Slack.

Bradlee, L. (1984). The use of groups in short-term psychiatric settings. *Occupational Therapy in Mental Health, 4*(3), 47–57.

Bruce, B., & Borg, B. (2002). *Psychosocial frames of reference: Core for occupation-based practice* (3rd ed.). Thorofare, NJ: Slack.

Burns, D. (1989a). *The feeling good handbook.* New York: Plume.

Burns, D. (1989b). Foreword. In J. Persons (Ed.), *Cognitive therapy in practice: A case formulation approach* (pp. vii–ix) New York: Norton.

Burns, T., Mortimer, J., & Merchak, P. (1994). The Cognitive Performance Test: A new approach to functional assessment in Alzheimer's disease. *Journal of Geriatric Psychiatry and Neurology, 7,* 46–54.

Campbell, A., & McCreadie, R. (1988). Occupational therapy is effective for chronic schizophrenic day clients. *British Journal of Occupational Therapy, 46,* 327–328.

Cautela, J. (1967). Covert sensitization. *Psychological Reports, 20,* 459–468.

Christiansen, C., & Baum, C. (1991). *Occupational therapy: Overcoming human performance deficits.* Thorofare, NJ: Slack.

Clark, E., & Peters, M. (1984). *Scorable self-care evaluation.* Thorofare, NJ: Slack.

Cohen-Kaplan, E. (1991). *Couples communication skills course.* Boston: Harvard Community Health Plan.

Cole, M. (1998). *Group dynamics in occupational therapy.* Thorofare, NJ: Slack.

Courtney, C., & Escobedo, B. (1990). A stress-management program: Inclient-to-outclient continuity. *American Journal of Occupational Therapy, 44,* 306–310.

Cox, D., & Findley, L. (1998). The management of chronic fatigue syndrome in an inpatient setting: Presentation on an approach and perceived outcomes. *British Journal of Occupational Therapy, 61,* 405–409.

Crist, P. (1986). Community living skills: A psychoeducational community-based program. *Occupational Therapy in Mental Health, 6,* 51–64.

DeMars, P. (1992). An occupational therapy life skills curriculum model for a Native American tribe: A health promotion program based on ethnographic field research. *American Journal of Occupational Therapy, 46,* 727–736.

Diasio, K. (1968). Psychiatric occupational therapy: Search for a conceptual framework in light of psychoanalytic ego psychology and learning theory. *American Journal of Occupational Therapy, 22,* 400–406.

Dobson, K. (1988). *Handbook of cognitive–behavioral therapies.* New York: Guilford.

Drouet, V. (1986). Individual behavioral programme planning with long-stay clients. Part 1: Programmes planned and followed in an occupational therapy department. Part 2: Social skills training. *British Journal of Occupational Therapy, 49,* 227–232.

Eilenberg, A. (1986). An expanded community role for occupational therapy: Preventing depression. *Physical and Occupational Therapy in Geriatrics, 5,* 47–57.

Ellis, A. (1958). Rational psychotherapy. *Journal of General Psychology, 59,* 35–49.

Ellis, A. (1985). Expanding the ABC's of rational–emotive therapy. In M. Mahoney & A. Freeman (Eds.), *Cognition and psychotherapy* (pp. 313–323). New York: Plenum.

Engel, J. (1991). Social validation of relaxation training in pediatric headache control. *Occupational Therapy in Mental Health, 11*(4), 77–90.

Engel, J., & Rapoff, M. (1990). Biofeedback-assisted relaxation training for adult and pediatric headache disorders. *Occupational Therapy Journal of Research, 10,* 283–299.

Fidler, G. (1969). The task-oriented group as a context for intervention. *American Journal of Occupational Therapy, 11,* 43–48.

Fidler, G. (1991). The challenge to change occupational therapy practice. *Occupational Therapy in Mental Health, 11*(1), 1–11.

Fine, S. (1993). Neurobehavioral perspectives on schizophrenia. In J. Van Deusen (Ed.), *Body image and perceptual dysfunction in adults* (pp. 83–115). Philadelphia: Saunders.

Fine, S., & Schwimmer, P. (1986). The effects of occupational therapy on independent living skills. *Mental Health Special Interest Section Newsletter, 9*(4), 2–3.

Fisher, A. (1995). *Assessment of motor and process skills.* Ft. Collins, CO: Three Star Press.

Frankl, V. E. (1985). Logos, paradox, and the search for meaning. In M. Mahoney & A. Freeman (Eds.), *Cognition and psychotherapy* (pp. 259–275). New York: Plenum.

Freeman, A., Pretzer, J., Fleming, B., & Simon, K. (1990). *Clinical applications of cognitive therapy.* New York: Plenum.

Friedlob, S., Janis, G., & Deets-Aron, C. (1986). A hospital connected half-way house program for individuals with long-term neuropsychiatric disabilities. *American Journal of Occupational Therapy, 40,* 271–277.

Giles, G. (1985). Anorexia nervosa and bulimia: An activity-oriented approach. *American Journal of Occupational Therapy, 39,* 510–517.

Giles, G. (2003). Behaviorism. In E. Crepeau, E. Cohn, & B. Schell (Eds.), *Willard and Spackman's occupational therapy* (10th ed., pp. 257–259). Philadelphia: Lippincott Williams & Wilkins.

Giles, G., & Allen, M. (1986). Occupational therapy in the rehabilitation of the client with anorexia nervosa. *Occupational Therapy in Mental Health, 6*(1), 47–66.

Giles, G., Ridley, J., Dill, A., & Frye, S. (1997). A consecutive series of adults with brain injury treated with a dressing retraining program. *American Journal of Occupational Therapy, 51,* 256–266.

Glasser, W. (1965). *Reality therapy: A new approach to psychiatry.* New York: Harper & Row.

Goldstein, A., Gershaw, N., & Sprafkin, R. (1979). Structured learning therapy: Development and evaluation. *American Journal of Occupational Therapy, 33,* 635–639.

Greenberg, L., Fine, S., Cohen, C., Larson, K., Michaelson-Bailey, A., Rubinton, P., et al. (1988). An interdisciplinary psychoeducation program for schizophrenic clients and their families in an acute care setting. *Hospital and Community Psychiatry, 39,* 277–282.

Hayes, R. (1989). Occupational therapy in the intervention of schizophrenia. *Occupational Therapy in Mental Health, 9,* 51–68.

Hayes, R., Halford, W., & Varghese, F. (1991). Generalization of the effects of activity therapy and social skills training on the social behavior of low functioning schizophrenic clients. *Occupational Therapy in Mental Health, 11*(4), 3–20.

Heine, D. (1975). Daily living group: Focus on transition from hospital to community. *American Journal of Occupational Therapy, 29,* 628–630.

Henderson, S. (1998). Frames of reference utilized in the rehabilitation of individuals with eating disorders. *Canadian Journal of Occupational Therapy, 66,* 43–51.

Hewitt, K., Wishart, C., & Lambert, R. (1981). Social skills training with chronic psychiatric clients. *British Journal of Occupational Therapy, 44,* 284–285.

Hoffman, N. (Ed.). (1984). *Foundations of cognitive therapy: Theoretical methods and practical approaches.* New York: Plenum.

Hollon, S., & Beck, A. (1979). Cognitive theory of depression. In P. Kendall & S. Hollon (Eds.), *Cognitive–behavioral interventions* (pp. 153–203) New York: Academic Press.

Hollon, S., & Kendall, P. (1979). Cognitive–behavioral interventions: Theory and procedure. In P. Kendall & S. Hollon (Eds.), *Cognitive–behavioral interventions* (pp. 445–454). New York: Academic Press.

Itzkovich, M., Elazar, B., Averbuch, S., & Katz, N. (2000). *Loewenstein Occupational Therapy Cognitive Assessment (LOTCA) manual* (2nd ed.). Pequannock, NJ: Maddak.

Jao, H.-P., & Lu, S.-J. (1999). The acquisition of problem-solving skills through instruction in Siegel and Spivack's problem-solving therapy for chronic schizophrenia. *Occupational Therapy in Mental Health, 14,* 47–63.

Jodrell, R., & Sanson-Fisher, R. (1975). Basic concepts of behavior therapy: An experiment involving disturbed adolescent girls. *American Journal of Occupational Therapy, 29,* 620–624.

Johnson, M. (1986). Use of cognitive–behavioral techniques with depressed adults in day intervention. In American Occupational Therapy Association (Ed.), *Depression: Assessment and intervention update—Proceedings* (pp. 49–61). Rockville, MD: American Occupational Therapy Association.

Johnson, M. (1987). Occupational therapists and the teaching of cognitive behavioral skills. *Occupational Therapy in Mental Health, 7,* 69–81.

Kaseman, B. (1980). Teaching money management skills to psychiatric outclients. *Occupational Therapy in Mental Health, 1,* 59–71.

Kendall, P., & Hollon, S. (1979). Cognitive–behavioral interventions: Overview and current status. In P. Kendall & S. Hollon (Eds.), *Cognitive–behavioral interventions* (pp. 1–9). New York: Academic Press.

Klein, J. (1988). Abstinence-oriented inclient intervention of the substance abuser. *Occupational Therapy in Mental Health, 8,* 46–49.

Law, M., Baptiste, S., Carswell, A., McColl, M., Polatajko, H., & Pollock, N. (1994). *Canadian Occupational Performance Measure* (2nd ed.). Toronto, Ontario: Canadian Occupational Therapy Association.

Levy, L. (1993). Behavioral frame of reference. In H. Hopkins & H. Smith (Eds.), *Willard and Spackman's occupational therapy* (8th ed., pp. 62–66). Philadelphia: Lippincott.

Liberman, R., Massel, H., Mosk, M., & Wong, S. (1985). Social skills training for chronic mental clients. *Hospital and Community Psychiatry, 36,* 396–403.

Lidz, T. (1985). Adolf Meyer and the development of American psychiatry. *Occupational Therapy in Mental Health, 5,* 33–53.

Lillie, M., & Armstrong, H., Jr. (1982). Contributions to the development of psychoeducational approaches to mental health service. *American Journal of Occupational Therapy, 36,* 438–443.

Lindsay, W. (1983). The role of the occupational therapist in the intervention of alcoholism. *American Journal of Occupational Therapy, 37,* 36–43.

Lloyd, C., Bassett, H., & King, R. (2004). Occupational therapy and evidence-based practice in mental health. *British Journal of Occupational Therapy, 67,* 83–88.

Love, H. (1988). Concept and use of the social skills game to facilitate group interaction: A case study. *Occupational Therapy in Mental Health, 8,* 119–133.

Luboshitzky, D., & Gaber, L. (2000). Collaborative therapeutic homework model in occupational therapy. *Occupational Therapy in Mental Health, 15,* 43–60.

Mahoney, M. (1984). Behaviorism, cognitivism, and human change processes. In M. Reda & M. Mahoney (Eds.), *Cognitive psychotherapies* (pp. 11–49). New York: Plenum.

Maslen, D. (1982). Rehabilitation training for community living skills: Concepts and techniques. *Occupational Therapy in Mental Health, 2,* 33–49.

McMullin, R. (2000). *The new handbook of cognitive therapy techniques.* New York: Norton.

Meichenbaum, D., & Asarnow, J. (1979). Cognitive–behavioral modification and metacognitive development: Implications for the classroom. In P. Kendall & S. Hollon (Eds.), *Cognitive–behavioral interventions* (pp. 11–36). New York: Academic Press.

Meyer, A. (1922). The philosophy of occupation therapy. *Archives of Occupational Therapy, 1,* 1–10.

Mitchell, E. (2000). Managing carer stress: An evaluation of a stress management programme for carers of people with dementia. *British Journal of Occupational Therapy, 63,* 179–184.

Moll, S., & Cook, J. (1996). "Doing" in mental health practice: Therapists' beliefs about why it works. *American Journal of Occupational Therapy, 51,* 662–670.

Mosey, A. (1972). *Three frames of reference for occupational therapy.* Thorofare, NJ: Slack.

Mosey, A. (1974). An alternative: The biopsychosocial model. *American Journal of Occupational Therapy, 28,* 137–140.

Moyers, P. (1988). An organizational framework for occupational therapy in the intervention of alcoholism. *Occupational Therapy in Mental Health, 8,* 27–46.

Nickel, I. (1988). Adapting structured learning therapy for use in a psychiatric adult day hospital. *Canadian Journal of Occupational Therapy, 55,* 21–25.

Ogren, K. (1983). A living skills program in an acute psychiatric setting. *Mental Health Special Interest Section Newsletter, 6,* 1–2.

Phillips, E. (1978). *The social skills bases of psychopathology.* New York: Grune & Stratton.

Platt, J., & Spivack, G. (1977). *Manual for Means-Ends Problem-Solving Procedure.* Philadelphia: Department of Mental Health Science, Hahnemann Community Mental Health/Mental Retardation Center.

Ross, M. (1991). *Integrative group therapy: The structured five-stage approach* (2nd ed.). Thorofare, NJ: Slack.

Rustad, R., DeGroot, T., Jungkunz, M., Freeberg, K., Borowick, L., & Wanttie, A. (1993). *The Cognitive Assessment of Minnesota.* San Antonio, TX: Therapy SkillBuilders.

Salkovskis, P., & Kirk, J. (1989). Obsessional disorders. In K. Hawton, P. Salkovskis, J. Kirk, & D. Clark, (Eds.), *Cognitive–behaviour therapy for psychiatric problems: A practical guide* (pp. 129–168). New York: Oxford University Press.

Salo-Chydenius, S. (1996). Changing helplessness to coping: An exploratory study of social skills training with individuals with long-term mental illness. *Occupational Therapy in Mental Health, 8,* 21–30.

Seiler, T. B. (1984). Developmental cognitive theory, personality, and therapy. In N. Hoffman (Ed.), *Foundations of cognitive therapy* (pp. 11–49). New York: Plenum.

Semmer, N., & Frese, M. (1984). Implications of action theory for cognitive therapy. In N. Hoffman (Ed.), *Foundations of cognitive therapy* (pp. 97–134). New York: Plenum.

Shulman, B. (1985). Cognitive therapy and the individual psychology of Alfred Adler. In M. Mahoney & A. Freeman (Eds.), *Cognition and psychotherapy* (pp. 243–258). New York: Plenum.

Sieg, K. W. (1974). Applying the behavioral model to the occupational therapy model. *American Journal of Occupational Therapy, 28,* 421–428.

Skinner, B. (1953). *Science and human behavior,* New York: Macmillan.

Smith, N., & Tempone, B. (1968). Psychiatric occupational therapy within a learning theory context. *American Journal of Occupational Therapy, 22,* 415–420.

Stein, F. (1982). A current review of the behavioral frame of reference and its application to occupational therapy. *Occupational Therapy in Mental Health, 2,* 35–62.

Stein, F. (1987). Stress and schizophrenia. *Alberta Psychology, 16,* 10–11.

Stein, F., & Cutler, S. (1998). *Psychosocial occupational therapy: A holistic approach.* San Diego, CA: Singular.

Stein, F., & Nikolic, S. (1989). Teaching stress management techniques to a schizophrenic client. *American Journal of Occupational Therapy, 43,* 162–169.

Stein, F. (2003). *Stress Management Questionnaire: Individual Version.* Clifton Park, NY: Thomson Delmar Learning.

Stein, F., & Smith, J. (1989). Short-term stress management programme with acutely depressed in-patients. *Canadian Journal of Occupational Therapy, 56,* 185–191.

Stoffel, V. (1993). Women's self-esteem issues in substance abuse and eating disorders. *Occupational Therapy Practice, 4,* 12–18.

Stoffel, V. (1994). Occupational therapists' roles in treating substance abuse. *Hospital and Community Psychiatry, 45,* 21–22.

Tang, M. (2001). Clinical outcome and client satisfaction of an anger management group program. *Canadian Journal of Occupational Therapy, 68,* 228–236.

Taylor, E. (1988). Anger intervention. *American Journal of Occupational Therapy, 42,* 127–155.

Thien, M. (1987). Demonstrating intervention outcomes in mental health. *Mental Health Special Interest Section Newsletter, 10*(4), 2–3.

Thomson, L. (1992). *The Kohlman Evaluation of Living Skills* (3rd ed.). Bethesda, MD: American Occupational Therapy Association.

Toglia, J. (1992). A dynamic interactional approach to cognitive rehabilitation. In N. Katz (Ed.), *Cognitive rehabilitation: Models for intervention in occupational therapy* (pp. 5–50). Boston: Andover Medical Publishers.

Vallis, T. M. (1991). Theoretical and conceptual bases of cognitive therapy. In T. Vallis, J. Howe, & P. Miller (Eds.), *The challenge of cognitive therapy: Applications to nontraditional populations* (pp. 3–21). New York: Plenum.

Werner, H. D. (1982). *Cognitive therapy: A humanistic approach.* New York: Free Press.

Wilson, G. (1994). Behavior therapy. In R. Corsini & D. Wedding (Eds.), *Current psychotherapies* (4th ed., pp. 241–282). Itasca, IL: Peacock.

Wolpe, J. (1958). *Psychotherapy by reciprocal inhibition.* Stanford, CA: Stanford University Press.

Woodcock, R., & Johnson, M. (2000). *Woodcock Johnson Cognitive Abilities Test.* Itasca, IL: Riverside.

Wright, J., Thase, M., Beck, A., & Ludgate, J. (1993). *Cognitive therapy with inpatients: Developing a cognitive milieu.* New York: Guilford.

Yakobina, S., Yakobina, S., & Tallant, B. (1997). I came, I thought, I conquered: Cognitive behavior approach applied to occupational therapy for the treatment of depressed (dysthymic) females. *Occupational Therapy in Mental Health, 13,* 59–73.

Zschokke, J., Freeberg, M., & Ericckson, E. (1975). Influencing behavior to improve attendance at occupational therapy in a psychiatric setting. *American Journal of Occupational Therapy, 29,* 625–627.

8

Ivelisse Lazzarini, OTD, OTR/L

A Nonlinear Approach to Cognition

A Web of Ability and Disability

LEARNING OBJECTIVES

By the end of this chapter, readers will
1. Recognize how approaches to cognition have evolved over time
2. Define *cognition* in nonlinear terms
3. Define and describe *self-organization* and *circular causality* as the terms relate to cognition throughout adulthood
4. Explain the importance and value of using a nonlinear dynamics approach to cognition as it relates to impairments and function in adult performance
5. Understand the role of the occupational therapist when applying a nonlinear dynamical cognitive framework
6. Understand and contrast the differences between functional and optimal ranges of stages and levels in adult performance.

In the past 20 years, there has been a tremendous increase in explorations of the mind and its by-product, cognition. Understanding the workings and connections of the brain–mind–body as a cognitive whole ranks high on the agendas of neuroscience and worldwide society. Cognitive science and neuroscience have developed into a new interdisciplinary field, conflating knowledge and skills from multiple scientific approaches to develop mathematical and nonmathematical explanations for the works of the mind. The umbrella term in which this work occurs is called the *nonlinear* or *dynamical systems approach* to cognition.

A *system* is a way of looking at the world, a theoretical construct that simplifies nature. A *dynamical system* is one that changes over time (Freeman, 1995; Kelso, 1999; Ward, 2002). Dynamical systems are characterized by complexity, randomness, and nonlinearity (Kelso, 1999; Thelen & Smith, 1994). The underlying assumption is that biological organisms are complex, multidimensional, interdependent, cooperative systems that exhibit *self-organization* (McLaughlin, Kennedy, & Zemke, 1996; Wright & Liley, 1996): the brain's ability to demonstrate pattern formation and change under nonspecific parametric influences, demonstrating self-control (Diebner, Druckrey, & Weibel, 2001; Kelso, 1999; Van Orden, Moreno, & Holden, 2003; Ward, 2002). Self-organization is the primary concept that helps one understand how the brain is shaped by development, learning, and disease (Bressler, 2003; Gibbs & Van Orden, 2002; Van Orden, Moreno, & Holden, 2003).

The brain is fundamentally a pattern-forming, self-organized system governed by potentially discoverable, nonlinear dynamical laws (Kelso, 1999). The goal of the nonlinear dynamics approach is to describe cognition in terms of brain dynamics (Freeman, 1995; Nuñez & Freeman, 1999; Thelen & Smith, 1994; van der Maas & Molenaar, 1992; van Geert, 1991; Van Orden & Holden, 2002; Van Orden, Holden, & Turvey, 2003); in other words, its goal is to explain how cognitive performance is conceived, planned, and executed in the brains of individuals. More specifically, actions such as intending, perceiving, acting, learning, and remembering arise as meta-stable spatiotemporal patterns of brain activity that are themselves produced by cooperative interactions among populations of neurons (Freeman, 1988a, 1995, 2000; Kelso, 1999; Llinas, 2002). Thus, nonlinear dynamics articulates human cognition as an intentional,[1] self-organizing process in which pattern formation (i.e., patterns of brain activity observed in electroencephalograms and that are based on prior knowledge and experiences) and neural organization develop through internal interactions (Freeman, 2000; Lazzarini, 2004), that is, without the intervention of external influences, such as a leader or agency, directing the process. Pattern formation is

---

[1] *Intention,* or *intentionality,* articulates the process by which human beings act in agreement with their own growth and maturation. An *intent* is the aiming of an action toward a future goal that is defined and selected by the individual (Lazzarini, 2004).

viewed as an emergent[2] property of the system itself rather than as a property imposed on the system by an external supervisory influence (Freeman, 1988a, 1995, 2000; Katagiri, Lazzarini, Singer, & Shen-Orr, 2003). Hence, the emphasis on the connectedness of elements is central to the study of cognition.

The approach I outline in this chapter draws from the concepts of nonlinear dynamics and chaos theory to explain a remarkably different approach to cognition. Learning, for example, is considered a psychological phenomenon. I might learn how to play the guitar or how to solve a differential equation and subsequently demonstrate my learning through my actions. In recent years, however, it has become increasingly clear that learning is mediated by the constant and ever-so-infinitesimal changes in the structure of brain's neurons at the *synapse,* the junction between cells, underscoring that learning has a dynamic neurobiological aspect (Freeman, 1997, 2000; Port & van Gelder, 1995; Ward, 2002). The neurobiological processes that mediate learning and cognition are always evolving and changing because of the brain's synaptic plasticity (Freeman, 1990; Kelso, 1999; Thelen & Smith, 1994, 1998). Assimilation of new learning or a change in habits, therefore, is not stored in any single neuron or any single area of the brain but rather in the patterns of activation of distributed arrays of neurons (Freeman, 1997, 2000). Thus, cognition is not only a psychological process in the brain but also a physiological, embodied process involving the body and populations of networks of neurons (Nuñez & Freeman, 1999).

VIEWS IN COGNITION

Theories of the brain or cognition have historically been described in terms of three kinds of theories of perception. The first and most accepted notion of perception is the passive Platonic view, which excludes intentional behavior (Gibbs & Van Orden, 2002; Juarrero, 2002). According to this view, perception is the passive inflow of information from the environment, which is used to make and process representations of objects and events (Freeman, 1997, 2000). This view maintains that the brain conducts information processing by using hierarchies of neural networks or reflexes. Actions begin in the senses and are driven primarily by the visual and tactile systems. Neurons respond to patterns of energy, such as a variety of textures

(rough/soft) and notions of light and dark (day/night), generating patterns of action potentials that carry and encode the forms of objects as input and information (Freeman, 2000; Llinas, 2002).

Through relays, action potentials carry the information transmitted from the sense organs into the higher cortex (Freeman, 2002). Once accumulated in the higher cortex, the information is refined in the sensory cortices, stored in the frontal lobes, retrieved, and compared with new information to classify fresh stimuli and select appropriate emotions and courses of action (Nuñez & Freeman, 1999). Actions as well as emotions are selected from a multitude of algorithms stored in the amygdala and basal ganglia, and movements are initiated by motor commands that descend into the brain stem and spinal cord to contract the muscle in response to the inputs (Freeman, 2000; Nuñez & Freeman, 1999). Models of behaviorism concerning brains, feedforward (input–output), artificial intelligence, neural networks, and industrial robotics using supervised learning are all products of the Platonic model (Nuñez & Freeman, 1999).

The second view, based on Aristotelian philosophy, depicts perception as an active search for information that is inherent in the environment and is extracted by tuned resonances in brain circuits (Juarrero, 2002; van Orden, Moreno, & Holden, 2003). According to this view, individuals learn by engaging in the manipulation of forms, textures, weights, and appearances of objects. Human behavior, in this view, is proactive, not reactive.

This model is central to a variety of cognitive approaches, such as Piagetian developmental psychology; existentialism; pragmatism; and Gestaltism and its by-product, ecological psychology. In these approaches, information and meaning are contained in the objects sought by the individual's brain (Juarrero, 2002). The brain creates a need that requires information from the environment to satisfy specific needs or goals. The brain instructs the sense organs to find relevant information from the world, using the cognitive map in the medial temporal lobe to direct the search (Freeman, 1995; Kay, Lancaster, & Freeman, 1996). At the same time, the brain prepares the sensory circuits by tuning them with copies of motor commands called *corollary discharges* (Freeman, 2001; Sperry, 1950), which selectively sensitize the cortices to the desired input. The information carried by objects is noticed by the senses, which send the information to the sensory cortices, where it is extracted by resonances in the neural circuits that are tuned just before the search takes place (Freeman, 2001; Nuñez & Freeman, 1999). These actions and the prior tuning represent the exercise of fore-

---

[2]*Emergent,* or *emergence,* refers to composition law, according to which the whole is more than the sum of its parts, the idea that a simple combination of the properties of the separate elements of a system does not describe the properties of the system itself.

sight and selective attention. The brain constrains the access of information to that which is desired, not to whatever forms or energies from irrelevant objects happen to enter the sense organs or be put there by a naïve experimenter or therapist. This is the unsupervised learning approach proposed by neural networks (the blind probing for structure), which obtain information by minimizing the errors in high-dimensional measurement spaces.

The third and last view comes from the philosophy of St. Thomas Aquinas. Perception, according to this view, creates information through chaotic dynamics by forming hypotheses about the environment and testing the sensory consequences of actions through which learning takes place (Freeman, 2000; Hendriks-Jansen, 1996; Llinas, 2002). *Chaotic dynamics,* as mentioned earlier, is the intentional process by which the brain–mind–body creates, destroys, and regulates its inflow of neural information expressing the *expectancy* and *readiness* of the system to move in any given direction. It alludes to the *flexibility* and *variability* of brain–mind–body states (Freeman, 1995, 1997, 2001; Juarrero, 2002; Lazzarini, 2004; Yan & Fischer, 2002). As a result, learning occurs through the assimilation of the sensory consequences of the actions experienced by individuals (Freeman, 1999; Lazzarini, 2004). This view is based on the *unity* of the self that is inherently present in the brain–mind–body trilogy (Freeman, 2000; Kelso, 1999; Lazzarini, 2004; Llinas, 2002). The concept of unity as proposed here is discovered in the system's ability to combine all sensory input into gestalts and its body-coordinated activities, both autonomic and musculoskeletal, into adaptive, flexible, variable, and yet focused and refined movements (Freeman, 2002; Kelso, 1999; Llinas, 2002).

The function of the brain is to formulate a hypothesis before action and thus learn from the result of the trial-and-error testing by assimilating the sensory consequences of these actions. This concept is not present in the Aristotelian view (Freeman, 2000; Juarrero, 2002). Perception has a unidirectionality, in which the forms captured by brain activity in the sensory cortices are privately and individually shaped, not merely imposed, by the form of stimuli (Aquinas, 1948, 1988; Freeman, 1995). The combined input is self-organized and flexible and has a high degree of variability, affording abstraction and generalization over new situations that are triggered by everyday activities. These processes of experience and generalization create information that assimilates the brain, mind, and body to the world. *Assimilation* is not the alteration of or change in brain structure and function by passive information processing; neither is it an accumulation of re-

TABLE 8.1. Comparison Between Classical and Nonlinear Dynamical Science

Classical Science	Nonlinear Science
Causality	Emergent properties
Linear	Nonlinear
Objective	Includes subjectivity
Isolates events	Emphasizes context
Matter	Process
Focuses on stability	Focuses on sensitivity
Logic	Deeper pattern
Closed system	Open system
Reductive	Complex
Predictability	Chaotic/stochastic
Explicit/observable	Implicit/hidden
Time is uniform	Sensitive to critical periods
Cause and effect	Positive feedback loops of autocatalysis
Sequential	Experience dependent
Mechanistic	Self-regulating
Fixed relations	Network interconnections
Objects/parts	Fields/relationships with parts
Particulate	Parallel

presentation by resonances[3] (Haken, 2002; Kelso, 1999; Llinas, 2002; Nuñez & Freeman, 1999). Aquinas (1948) and Piaget (1930) defined *assimilation* as the process by which the self comes to understand the world by adapting itself to the world. The goal of an action is a state of increased competence or actualization that Merleau-Ponty (1945/1962) called *maximum grip.* As a result, assimilation is the dynamic self-organizing process that facilitates the beginning of the creation for all knowledge (Freeman, 1997; Haken, 2002; Kelso, 1999).

LINEAR VS. NONLINEAR DYNAMICS AND COGNITION

It is important to explain the differences between what is meant by *linear* and *nonlinear* approaches to cognition (see Table 8.1). Linear approaches to cognition state that the behavior of a system is easily predictable from the behavior of individual neurons or brain structures. In a linear system, small changes produce small effects, and large changes produce large effects. In this view, intentional behaviors are representations that set into motion a causal

---

[3]*Resonance* in this context means reinforcing, repeating, or amplifying a given state (actions or occupation) because the frequency of the stimulus experienced resounds with the already-existing knowledge.

chain. Representations, according to linear models, function as internal causes of behavior (Markman & Dietrich, 2000; Wegner & Wheatley, 1999). As a consequence behavior, metaphorically speaking, is the end result of chains of billiard ball–type interactions among representations (Freeman, 1999; Kelso, 1999).

Most cognitive models, particularly information-processing approaches, use Newtonian efficient cause as a metaphor that largely defines the content and boundaries of discussion, thus restricting discoveries and the study of human cognition to cause-and-effect relationships (Juarrero, 2002; Van Orden & Holden, 2002). Some of the limitations of the assumptions of linear science are prediction, reduction, and inferential design and analysis methods of the research of stable systems. However, human beings are not stable, closed linear systems; they are open, variable, and complex systems that are far from a state of equilibrium (Prigogine, 1994). Humans are open in the sense that they can interact with their environment, exchanging information, energy, and matter, and they are far from equilibrium in the sense that, without these sources, humans and other animals cannot maintain their structure or function (Freeman, 1995; Prigogine, 1994). As a result, metaphors that are more inclusive are needed to understand purposeful behavior in occupation. Otherwise, intentional performance as an endogenous process remains forever unsubstantiated, vague, and inexplicable, even supernatural.

Nonlinear cognitive models, on the other hand, maintain that behavior arises from interactions between interdependent components that also may include feedback effects based on the constraints (variables that limit the degrees of freedom for interactions among the processes of the human brain–mind–body) of control parameters[4] (variables that lead the system through the variety of possible patterns or states but do prescribe or contain the code for emerging patterns; Freeman, 1988a, 1988b; Kay et al., 1996; Kelso, 1999). This kind of behavior is not easily predictable from the individual interaction of the parts, and it can be quite rich (Van Orden, Holden, & Turvey, 2003). In a nonlinear system it is possible that small changes may have large effects, and large changes may have only small effects (Prigogine & Stengers, 1984). This is what most people recognize as the *butterfly effect,* inspired by the meteorological experiments of Edward Lorenz in 1961. The butterfly effect implies that two states differing by imperceptible amounts may eventually evolve into two considerable dif-

ferent states. If, then, there is any mistake in observing the present state—and in any real dynamic system such error seems inescapable—then an acceptable prediction of the instantaneous state in the distant future may well be impossible. Thus, instead of making predictions about the future state of a system, nonlinear dynamics attempts a qualitative study of the system by concentrating on behavior that is unstable and aperiodic in an effort to better understand and describe the tendencies or fluctuations of the system over time.

Research using electroencephalograms has demonstrated that the brain has different *strange attractors*[5] for different activities (Bressler, 2003; Freeman, 2002; Guastello, 1995; Kelso, 1999; Llinas, 2002; Sheer, 1989). A healthy brain maintains a low level of chaos, which often self-organizes into a simpler order when presented with a familiar stimulus (Ward, 2002). *Low levels of chaos* refers to the brain's state of expectancy and flexibility from which hasty comparisons of the sensory-referred properties of the external world can be made, forming a self-organized internal pattern of brain activity (Freeman, 1995, 2002; Tsuda, 1991, 1996). Hence, purposeful activities and behaviors of living systems are viewed as self-organized and pattern forming and cannot be reduced to basic cause-and-effect assumptions. When researchers discuss *patterns,* they refer to the relations among things (Haken, 2002, 2003; Kelso, 1999; Ward, 2002). *Pattern formation* is the brain's basic means of storing information, and *pattern recognition* is the basic means of sharing it. At the genetic level, patterns contain the seed of who and what we are (Kelso, 1999; Ward, 2002). Repetition and variation of these patterns are the processes by which selections occur (Kelso, 1999). Patterns convey information about an individual's lifestyle, habits, rituals, and present situation; consequently, the interdependence of brain activity as a self-organizing whole demonstrates that pattern formation is at the heart of cognitive neuroscience.

Dynamical patterns of brain activity are constructed from a very large number of material components (Haken, 2002; Kelso, 1999). The brain has approximately 10^{10} neurons, each of which can have up to 10^4 connections with other neurons and 50-plus neurotransmitters (chemicals that are necessary for neurons to work; Freeman, 1995; Haken, 2002; Kelso, 1999). Thus, pattern formation is about not one specific pattern but many patterns produced to accommodate different circumstances. Human beings are multifunctional in that they use the same anatomical

---

[4]*Control parameter* refers to an arrangement of causal factors that yield emergent properties.

[5]The attractor of a chaotic function is called a *strange attractor* when the stable behavior is so strange that the function jumps around a limited region, never landing on the exact same point.

components for different behavioral functions, as for eating and speaking, or different components to perform the same function (e.g., using a pencil attached to one's toes). Thus, self-organization of pattern formation in cognition is ubiquitous.

Fluid convection serves as an example that helps explain the key concepts of pattern formation that provide a foundation for understanding the emergence of biological order and change. Although this example concerns nonliving systems, it introduces a different way of thinking about living systems (Depew & Weber, 1995; Kelso, 1999; Kugler & Turvey, 1987; Shaw, 2001; Ulanowicz, 1997). Convection depends on how interactions among molecules are situated within a larger system and not simply on the causal properties of molecules.

The following experiment demonstrates convection. Take a frying pan, add some cooking oil—enough to fry an egg—and place the pan onto the stove. As the pan heats, it also heats the oil. As the heat is conducted and the temperature gradient increases (hot/cold), a remarkable event called *instability* occurs. The oil begins to move as a coordinated whole, no longer randomly but in an orderly, rolling motion. The reason for the onset of this motion is that the cooler liquid at the top of the layer of oil is more dense and tends to fall, whereas the warmer and less dense oil at the bottom tends to rise. The resulting convection divides the oil into honeycombs of cells, which physicists call a *collective* or *cooperative effect.* The collective or cooperative effect arises from the interdependent interaction of the oil molecules and without any external instructions or agency.

The control parameter[6] encapsulates the status of the heated oil; in this case, the modeled system. The control parameter is an arrangement of causal factors that yield emergent properties. The honeycomb of cells formed in the convection rolls is a pattern of fluid motion displaying its emergent property. Convention, as a control parameter, conflates the amount of heat into and out of the oil, the friction among the oil molecules, and other particles in a ratio. The most important factor driving the changes in the system's states and, ultimately, marking the formation of patterns, is the difference between the amount of heat entering the oil versus the amount that leaves (the *critical value*). The parameter sits near a critical value right before the convection honeycomb rolls appear. At this point, the

amount of heat exiting the oil is significantly less than the amount coming in. This critical value determines the boundary between diffusion and convection—the *critical state.* On either side of the critical value the system shows evidence of one or the other kind of behavior: random, haphazard collisions versus honeycomb convection rolls. Convection rolls join together because of the interdependence movements of molecules.

The molecules change one anothers' dynamics as they interact. Near the critical state, interactions among molecules coordinate the behavior of these same molecules and greatly reduce their freedom of motion. Once convection rolls emerge, they subsequently control the flow of molecules and become self-perpetuating. Movements of molecules both cause, and are caused by, convection rolls, a process called *circular causality.*[7] As a result, the system self-organizes without necessitating an external agency, demonstrating that self-organizing systems exhibit self-control, and self-control is a quintessential aspect of purposeful behavior. Ultimately, the system chooses its unique patterns of rotation and macroscopically exhibits the orderly behavior we observe.

In a critical state, each molecule could move either clockwise or counterclockwise; both rotations are possible for every molecule in the system. A critical state, or *criticality,* is a global state that is extremely context sensitive, that depends exclusively on the circumstances in a given space and at a given time (Kelso, 1999). Competing rotations exist as balanced tendencies at the same time everywhere in the system. Across the critical state, molecules move in the same rotation inside the same convection roll. To be in a critical state means that there is balance among constraints; the tendency to answer "yes" or "no" to a questions holds an equal value. A difference in circumstances that favors one option over another, no matter how imperceptible or small, breaks the symmetry of equally poised options. Near the state of criticality, nearest neighbor interactions become correlated (Kelso, 1999). This coordinates the choice across the entire system and determines the behavior we as observers describe.

The sudden collapse of the critical state captures something essential to choice and self-organization in human behavior. The details of changing circumstances determine movements that are expressed, and local movements transition to a larger global configuration of movements,

---

[6]In this case, the temperature gradient serves as the control parameter. However, the control parameter can be quite unspecific in nature. It leads the system through different patterns, but it is not dependent on the patterns themselves. Control parameters bind the various formed patterns into one pattern of action.

[7]In *circular causality,* the global state is upwardly generated by microscopic molecules, and simultaneously the global state downwardly organizes the activities of the individual molecules. An order parameter is created by the coordination between the parts but in turn influences the behavior of the parts.

a product of global emergence. In convection, changing circumstances choose a global pattern of movement. Each molecule's trajectory is uniquely situated in these circumstances of the larger systems (Prigogine, 1997). Likewise, every movement of the human body also is uniquely situated. Even the act of scratching one's eye or swinging an ax follows a unique trajectory in each movement (Berkinblit, Feldman, & Fukson, 1986; Bernstein, 1967).

The example of convection affords physical metaphors for self-organization, self-control, and goal-directed actions, which are salient aspects of purposeful behavior. In living systems, criticality itself emerges spontaneously as self-organized criticality (Bak, 1993). Living systems self-organize to stay near critical states, at the brink of instabilities. The advantages and profits may be obvious. Criticality allows an attractive mix of creativity and constraint. It creates new options for actions and allows the choice of behavior to fit the specific circumstance at a specific time.

Concise, purposeful, goal-directed actions originate in self-organized criticality, and its intentional contents poise human beings near states of criticality (*instabilities;* Freeman, 1999; Juarrero, 2002). At any given time, the system can choose to go either way. Thus, the product of goal-directed actions depends on a critical state that is context sensitive, forming a boundary that is constrained by the present cognitive ranges and states. In the presence of a cognitive disability, the potential courses of action may be constrained because of limitations in the ability to perceive and assimilate subtle changes in circumstances. The observation of pervasive, habitual behaviors disconnected from real spatiotemporal circumstances will demonstrate the individual's failure to self-organize and actualize his or her actions according to the circumstance.

A physiological system, like that of humans, has innate variability. Loss of this variability signals an impaired system that loses its flexibility to respond to stimuli within the present context, constraints, and time. For example, cardiologists call this decrease in variability a decrease in the dynamics of the heart's *system oscillations* (changes in causal factors leading to emergence) that is due to changes in control parameters (Goldberg, 1996). The changes in control parameters explicate the decrease of heart rate and brain wave variability and the physiological changes leading to abnormal or pathological dynamics of the overall activity of the system.

Another example, which is at the heart of occupational therapy practice, is therapists' facilitation of an individual's ability to perform bathing, dressing, or grooming after a stroke. The goal is to facilitate change in an old, habitual, self-organized pattern of brain activity. For change to occur in the individual's ability to perform the activity, the pattern of brain activity guiding bathing, dressing, or grooming, which is context sensitive, needs to be poised at a critical (unstable) state, collapse, and give rise to a new global configuration of movements and, therefore, a new way of performing the activity. In this way, occupation serves as the vehicle of change in which self-controlled performance can be facilitated by the endogenous process of self-organization of the brain–mind–body embedded in its environment.

THEORIES OF LEARNING VS. THEORIES OF BRAIN PLASTICITY

The nonlinear approach to cognition is rather a different perspective and explanation of what takes places when one experiences and learns something new. Traditional theories of learning specify the cognitive and behavioral processes involved in acquiring a new skill or new information, whereas theories of synaptic plasticity, based on nonlinear dynamics, are concerned with what takes place in the brain while a person is engaged in the dynamic experience of being in the world.

Nonlinear brain dynamics relationships are vital for the practice of rehabilitation services, specifically in the area of occupational therapy. Occupational therapy addresses the nature of an individual's ability to function in an ever-changing world associated with changes in cognitive states. As an individual experiences a decline in cognitive function, higher cognitive abilities, as well as safety and independence, are often compromised. Cognitive skills are complex, and the processes by which they emerge, decline, or both, are found and expressed by chaotic destabilizations. Chaotic destabilizations become apparent when an individual is exposed to new learning experiences and demonstrates the ability, or lack of ability, to assimilate the new into the old. The therapist's role is to assess and recognize these chaotic states to begin to comprehend the meaningful patterns of brain activity—*tendencies*—from which therapeutic interventions may be facilitated and organized. Thus, nonlinear dynamics encompasses a natural subject matter for occupational therapy cognitive approaches.

COGNITION AS A SELF-ORGANIZED, EMBODIED, AND EMERGENT PHENOMENON

Approaches to cognition based on nonlinear dynamic systems theory underscore the importance of an ordinary sense of embodiment that embraces all our mundane experiences, emphasizing the primacy of the self-organization of the living and the resulting bodily experience it sustains (Freeman, 2001; Merleau-Ponty, 1945/1962; Nuñez, 1999). Thus this view, instead of dealing with static properties or the structure of organs, endorses cognition as a product of chaotic dynamics (instabilities). Chaotic dynamics has the property of creating, destroying, and regulating the sensory inflow of neural information, which is essential for the construction of new goals through the action–perception–assimilation cycle, emerging from ongoing action on the part of an individual, which is always immersed in a real-world environment, and with physical and real-time constraints (Freeman, 2002; Kelso, 1999). In this sense, cognition becomes the ebbs, eddies, and vortices of flexible neural processes that articulate the changes of mental states in space and in the course of time.

The common denominator of the nonlinear approach to cognition is a simple one: mind as a self-organizing and emergent process, that is, viewing adult nervous system functions as a dynamic self-organizing process and the modeling function as the emergent property of the assembly of infrastructure, none of which contain a prescription or command center (Skarda & Freeman, 1987; Szentagothai, 1984). Instead of describing the purely abstract structures of the mind, the nonlinear approach seeks to understand the emergence of a dynamic and neural flexible coupling (in which the influence between the two parts is gradual and not radical; Eoyang, 1997) between direct real-time processes and cognitive process that are less tightly coupled (i.e., have a high degree of influence on one another)[8] to the receiving input (Thelen & Smith, 1994). This view is shared by most, if not all, of the proponents of the dynamical systems approach to cognitive science (Freeman, 2000; Haken, 2002; Kelso, 1999; Guastello, 1995; Llinas, 2002; Thelen & Smith, 1994; Tschacher & Dauwalder, 2003; Port & van Gelder, 1995; Ward, 2002).

At present, contemporary work in physics, chemistry, biology, and psychology is weakening traditional resistance to the idea that the human brain can produce patterns of brain activity without prescription or agency (Haken, 2002; Kelso, 1999; Lazzarini, 2004; Thelen & Smith, 1994). The active fields of synergetics and nonlinear dynamics in physics and mathematics, for example, show in mathematically precise ways how a complex system may produce emergent order, that is, without a preexisting prescription for the pattern (Bressler, 2002; Freeman, 1995; Nuñez & Freeman, 1999; Haken, 2002; Prigogine, 1994). Consequently, the role of occupational therapists and other rehabilitation practitioners is to facilitate the process of self-organization and change within the dynamics and variability that comprise human performance throughout the course of rehabilitation services. Viewing occupation as a dynamic construction of webs facilitates an understanding of the complex patterns of adult development and learning.

GENERAL BACKGROUND OF THE CONCEPTUAL FRAMEWORK

Adult cognitive research indicates that an individual's development is complex, rich, and dynamic, perhaps even more so than in the early years of life (Van Orden, Holden, & Turvey, 2003). The conceptual framework presented here is based on a nonlinear dynamical cognitive approach that rejects the views of brain–mind–body as a computer and cognitive development as a linear metaphor. Instead, cognition is proposed as a developmental web that portrays adult cognitive development as a complex process of dynamic construction within multiple ranges and in multiple directions. In other words, cognition is a nonlinear, intentional, experiential, historical, and emergent process that is always changing. The overall principles guiding this framework are mind as self-organized, mind as an emergent property of bodies engaged in the world, and mind as action that is always under construction. As such,

- Cognition is *intentional, self-organized,* and *goal directed,* comprising the endogenous initiation, construction, and purpose of experiencing the world by which individuals decide their goals; plan their strategies; and choose when to begin, modify, and stop courses of action (Lazzarini, 2004). It is a weblike process, operating from single neurons to a network of neural populations working as a synergy (Haken, 2000; Kelso, 1999). All that brains can know are the hypotheses they formulate and the results of trial-and-error testing by acting in the environment and learning by assimilation from the sensory consequences of the individual's actions (Freeman, 2002; Llinas,

---

[8]A small change in one side of the boundary results in an immediate and radical change on the other side of the boundary (Eoyang, 1997).

[9]Circular causality expresses the interaction between levels in a hierarchy where a top-down macroscopic state simultaneously influences microscopic neural activity that functions in a bottom-up manner to create and sustain the macroscopic level of observation (Freeman, 1999).

FIGURE 8.1. Circular causality of self-organization and construction of new occupational experiences.

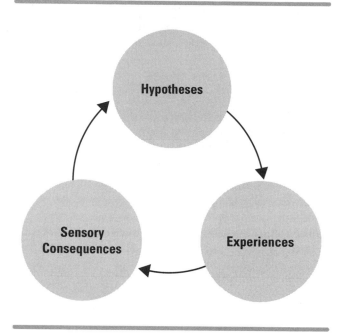

Hypotheses, intentional acts, and past meaningful occupations or experiences are used to elicit the construction of new occupational **experiences,** which by trial-and-error test the "experiential relevance" of the hypothesis. The **sensory consequences** of these experiences reformulate the initial **hypotheses.**

This process occurs by the trial and error of individuals' hypothesis testing, leading to the assimilation of the sensory consequences experienced, which in turn leads to the construction of new meanings. This is the nonlinear dynamical process of circular causality; a cause must produce an effect, which in turn changes its cause.

Individuals' intentional state and self-organized hypothesis testing is observed by therapists as an occupational experiential process that enhances therapeutic interventions and facilitates change.

Note. © 2004 Ivelisse Lazzarini. Used with permission.

2002). This process operates through the circular causality[9] of the action–perception–assimilation cycle (Figure 8.1). Thus, self-organization dynamics create information, and information modifies, actualizes, and directs the system's dynamics.

- Cognition is *embodied.* The body serves as the principal tool of the brain for cognitive development. This view requires a shift from predicting how individuals' brains react to objects in the environment to understanding their actions in terms of self-organized probabilities or tendencies; that is, of a body–mind–brain immersed in the environment, experiencing the sen-

sory consequences of goal-directed activities affords the individual the possibilities to change his or her history and, therefore, the essence of the neural patterns of brain dynamics. Thus, cognition can be understood only as a manifestation of the interactions among the individual's past, present, and expectancy of future patterns of activity performance. Cognition is therefore not an isolated, goal-directed action but rather an event that interconnects all other experiences in a particular way (Freeman, 2002; Haken, 2003; Guastello, 1995; Kelso, 1999). Hence, understanding the workings of the mind requires reconsideration of what one understands as *mind.* This framework articulates mind as brain and body and as a dynamic web of interrelated events in space and time.

- Cognition is *situated;* the mind is embedded in environmental constraints and is driven by energetic gradients. The structure of the environment constrains, and is constrained by, the actions of individuals seeking knowledge (Juarrero, 2002).

- Cognition operates in a fashion characterized by *circular causality.* It is not a single, basic attribute of the mind, which may be discovered in some specific location in the brain or pinned down as a special algorithmic model of higher cognitive skills. Instead, it is the hierarchical and heterarchical interrelation and complementarity that exist among microscopic, mesoscopic, and macroscopic[10] states. As such, cognition builds as successful and unsuccessful meaningful experiences develop. Consequently, in the language of dynamics, *cognition* refers to the meaning of the stimulus (i.e., occupations, habits, and rituals) that individuals experience in their everyday life as opposed to motivation. See Figure 8.2 for further explanation.

NONLINEAR RANGES IN ADULTS' COGNITIVE WEBS

Accumulated evidence shows that adult cognitive development is a complex process of dynamic construction within multiple ranges or levels and in multiple directions (Yan & Fischer, 2002). The dynamic skill theory scale (Fischer, 1980) is best suited to assess and

---

[10]A *microscopic state* represents the activity of individual neurons, it is sensory and bottom up; a *mesoscopic state* represents collective neural activity enveloping the part of the brain and expresses the meaning of a stimulus; and a *macroscopic state* exhibits the emergent patterns of actions or cognitive actions of the brain: top down (what one observes).

FIGURE 8.2. Relationship among macroscopic, mesoscopic, and microscopic states and intention, meaning, and perception.

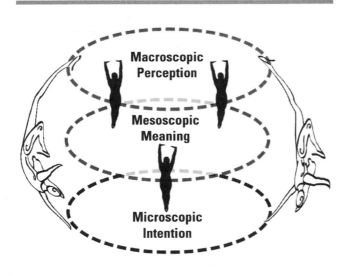

The microscopic (intentional) state shows a linear causality that disappears at the mesoscopic (meaning) state by the formation of wave packets (WPs) that later constrain the cortex at the macroscopic level (perceptual), ultimately renewing the old experiences and sending the new sensory consequences of actions back to microscopic level in a circular causality fashion.

Macroscopic activity of the whole forebrain is expressed by behavior and is perceptual. Awareness is the key state.

In mesoscopic activity formation of meaning, this level bridges the gap between microscopic and macroscopic in a nonlinear fashion by the formation of WPs. WPs are the resultant of microscopic sensory stimuli. They are hemisphere-wide, self-organized patterns of neural activity largely broadcast through the forebrain. WPs form when sensory-driven input destabilizes the primary receiving areas by local state transitions and are the precursors of awareness.

Microscopic activity expressed by action potential is sensory and intentional. Sensory-driven action potentials condense into mesoscopic WPs like molecules forming raindrops from vapor (Freeman, 2002). The major function is self-organization.

Note. © 2004 Ivelisse Lazzarini. Used with permission.

explain the complexity of the variability of cognitive structures in adult performance. The scale has been validated through extensive research and using a variety of methods for identifying levels of skill complexity (Commons, Trudeau, Stein, Richards, & Krause, 1998; Fischer, 1980; Fischer & Bidell, 1998; Fischer & Granott, 1995; Kitchener, Lynch, Fischer, & Wood, 1993). Viewed from the perspective of dynamic skill theory, adult cognitive development is nonlinear, with many factors acting together to produce systematic, dynamic variation (Fischer & Granott, 1995; Yan & Fischer, 2002). Variation as the principal concept envelops the idea that activities take place in specific contexts (Yan & Fischer, 2002) as opposed to a simple static correspondence between mental representations and physical objects (Freeman, 1995, 2002).

Studies of adult cognitive development also have demonstrated that assimilation of new cognitive skills occurs not by simple forward progression (input–output) but instead depends on the level of task complexity (Yan & Fischer, 2002). Moreover, adult cognitive growth means that individuals must assimilate, adapt, and integrate the challenges presented by everyday life situations with their emotional, social, cultural, physical, and technological dimensions. According to Yan and Fischer (2002), individuals, regardless of expertise, demonstrate regression in performance by moving down to lower levels and then constructing higher levels of cognitive skills. This process is referred to as *backward transition* (Yan & Fischer, 2002). Backward transition appears to challenge present views of cognition and addresses the complex dynamics behind the variability in adult cognitive development (Fischer, 1980; Fischer & Bidell, 1998; Valsiner, 1991; van Geert, 1994; Yan & Fischer, 2002). Each individual performs at diverse ranges or levels depending on task demands, background, domain, assistance provided (scaffolding), and capacity, showing asynchrony in level as opposed to simple linear consistency. Thus, individuals' activities or occupations vary widely in content and complexity as well as across long-term developmental periods and infinitely through time.

Consequently, understanding adult cognitive variations is crucial for illuminating the dynamic structure of the ways that individuals construct activities or occupations under the influence of multiple factors interacting in complex ways, in context and over time and in the presence of cognitive disabilities. Cognition portrayed as a weblike structure serves as a new metaphor to explain how adult cognitive development occurs in space and in real time. The concept of a cognitive weblike metaphor also provides a way to explain adult cognitive development as a series of dynamic choices, dynamic elements and populations of neurons, and dynamic constructions of patterns of brain activity (e.g., the example of convection provided earlier). Provided with this heterarchical view, one can begin to explain the ubiquity and complexity of adult cognitive improvements or limitations.

FORWARD PROGRESSION VS. WEBLIKE PROGRESSION

Metaphors have historically served to explain brain models and other scientific inquiry. Two examples are considering a spiral as the structure of DNA or viewing the earth as the center of the universe. However, the most powerful and insidious metaphor throughout the history of science, which has had a tremendous impact on scientific thinking, has been considering individuals' performance, as well as brains, as computers. The purpose of this view was to provide a precise, pervasive, and uniform paradigm and methodology for operationalizing and reproducing the essential aspects of the mind (not merely behavior) in an objective, transparent, and controllable manner. The mind as a rational calculating device served as a framework, and the rising field of computer technology provided the primary tools for making the concept of brain–mind as computer flourish.

The digital computer metaphor was the ideal platform on which researchers could understand many cognitive models by positing a level of analysis entirely separate from the neurological or biological, on the one hand, and the sociological or cultural, on the other hand (Nuñez & Freeman, 1999). This view reduced the level of cognitive analysis on the individual mind as a passive input–output device that processed information, and it represented reasoning as the logical manipulation of arbitrary symbols (Nuñez & Freeman, 1999). On this basis, traditional linear approaches flourished describing adult cognitive development as a linearlike, simple, fixed progression (Thelen & Smith, 1994). In this view, acquisition of cognitive skills follows a simple ascending progression, with no room for diversion or variance. Moreover, each step is fixed depending on the previous stage or step following a linear progression with monotonic changes (Figure 8.3).

In stark contrast, a weblike metaphor expresses models that account for and describe the variability and tendencies of human cognitive performance over time (Figure 8.4). Deterministic or linear models, on the contrary, focus on descriptions of cognitive trends, freezing purposeful behavior in time in an effort to predict future performance. The cognitive approaches and tools used today have substantially added to the understanding of cognitive developmental changes and variations in adults, but all of them share, to some extent, a linear meta-metaphor. The following are the three primary competing explanations for present cognitive approaches: (a) horizontal décalage, (b) competence versus performance, and (c) cognitive transfer or generalization.

FIGURE 8.3. Linear progression of adult development.

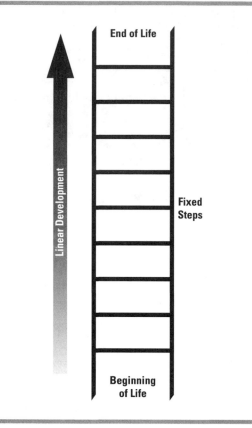

Note. © 2004 Ivelisse Lazzarini. Used with permission.

Horizontal décalage proposes general stability or synchrony across domains, explaining asynchrony or variability as objects' resistance to people's activities (Piaget, 1983). *Competence-versus-performance* approaches contrast between performances demonstrated in activities and lower level performances that arise through processes intervening between competence and activity, frequently hindering the achievement of full competence (Chomsky, 1965; Flavell & Wohlwill, 1969; Overton & Newman, 1982). Last, *cognitive transfer* specifies that the mechanism of knowledge and skill learned in Task A is modified for use in Task B through transferring or generalizing them (Mayer & Wittrock, 1996). Although the linear metaphor helps researchers understand some aspects of complex developmental phenomena by sketching general developmental trends, it does so at the expense of downplaying, neglecting, and even misrepresenting the self-organizing variability and emergent richness of adult cognitive development.

FIGURE 8.4. Cognitive web.

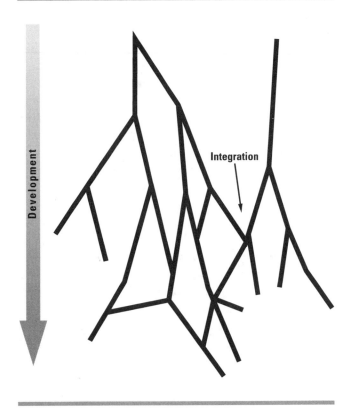

Note. © 2004 Ivelisse Lazzarini. Used with permission.

A weblike metaphor, on the other hand, captures the central concepts of nonlinear dynamical systems—that is, self-organization, asymmetry, and emergent order—by describing the variability found in human behavior. Human beings organize their activities and occupations in specific contexts. Developing and adapting to an ever-changing world demands that social, emotional, and physical aspects of the self are situated to fit the situations at hand. Hence, expressing and describing adult cognition as nonlinear demands serious and rigorous consideration of these concepts. Adult cognition explained from a weblike perspective captures the interconnected complexity of skills in diverse contexts.

Each web contains separate strands for different patterns of brain activity, sometimes converging through coordination and sometimes diverging through differentiation, but always organized in the context of the present state of the limbic system, expressing a desired state that is structured into a goal-directed action and with an awareness of its sensory consequences (Freeman, 2000, 2002). As a result, all previous experiences are contained and operating in a dynamic global web of the forebrain, the primary function of which is to facilitate the shaping of patterns of brain activity (Freeman, 2000; Lazzarini, 2004).

The developmental web metaphor differs conceptually from linear approaches in several important ways:

- An individual's variation in occupation or activities occupies the center stage, as opposed to individual differences being treated as a category error or as noise. Variation is reflected by the individual patterns of assimilation, adaptation, and development, as opposed to conforming to typologies defined by group norms. It helps capture the overt manifestations of individuals' covert neural dynamic processes, including those that are traditionally viewed as static outcomes, such as functional skill and ability (Kelso, 1999; Miller & Coyle, 1999; Yan & Fischer, 2002).
- Variability is a pervasive and ubiquitous concept in human behavior (Yan & Fischer, 2002).
- Nonlinear dynamics help investigate the complexity of growth and variation (Basar, 1990, 1998; Kelso, 1999; Thelen & Smith, 1994).
- An individual's variability in cognitive performance, as opposed to group performance, is the subject of study.
- At any given time, multiple cognitive levels exist in each individual as opposed to a single level (Miller & Coyle, 1999; Yan & Fischer, 2002).
- Interdependence of the pattern of brain activity is explicitly inherent in the dynamics of cognitive performance as opposed to isolated behaviors of causal effects (Ward, 2002).
- Multiple directions, such as forward and backward transition, as opposed to linear forward progression, are observed (Yan & Fischer, 2002).

Thus, the weblike approach to cognition can facilitate a better understanding of what, where, when, how, and why adult cognitive performance rises or falls in complex spatiotemporal situations.

CONSIDERATIONS FOR OLDER ADULTS AND AGING

The hallmark of adult cognition is the multiple levels and stages of performance embedded in the flexibility of patterns of brain activity generated from the prior sensory consequences of actions (Freeman, 2000; Juarrero, 2002; Kelso, 1999; Lazzarini, 2004). Moreover, adult cognitive function continues to increase beyond Piaget's formal operations stage of development (Inhelder & Piaget, 1955/1958; Piaget, 1972, 1983), which is at the heart of most cognitive approaches. In the absence of most cognitive disabilities, the length of some strands in the web continue to expand into development, representing a continuing increase in adults' optimal cognitive skills and a wide range of variation in the level of skill that adults can use in a domain (Mareschal & Thomas, 2001).

Along with the increase in overall complexity of adults' cognitive development, both developmental research (Thelen & Smith, 1994, 1998) and everyday observations indicate that adults show multiple levels of cognitive development, not performance at one fixed level (van Geert, 1991; Yan & Fischer, 2002). Throughout everyday clinical interventions, adults are observed using simple skills when the situation requires habitual actions, and from time to time they are observed making unpredictable, surprising, erratic decisions when dealing with complex tasks without sufficient contextual support. As I mentioned earlier, cognitive performance varies with prior experience, contextual support, and shared action with other people. Hence, of importance for nonlinear systems is the interdependence of the system, not necessarily the details of the interacting components.

Adult cognition explained from the viewpoint of dynamic developmental webs involves growth combined with decline and acquisition of wisdom along with loss of speed (Fischer & Bullock, 1981; Thelen & Smith, 1998; Valsiner, 1991; van Geert, 1994). All of these concepts are absent in most, if not all, cognitive models. Horn and Cattell's (1967) classic research, for example, shows the interweaving of gain and loss with cognitive aging. Various intellectual skills increase slowly but consistently with age. This fact is demonstrated even by research limited to standardized psychometric tests (Fischer, 1980). Psychometric tests explicate what is known as *crystallized intelligence,* an aggregate of skills that profit from accumulated experiences, such as vocabulary and general knowledge. On the other hand, many skills also decline with age, especially from middle adulthood, and these reflect what is referred to as *fluid intelligence* (Fischer, 1980), which is composed of skills that depend on novel activities and information. Most occupations and activities in which older adults engage involve habits, rituals, and crystallized intelligence that are refined through the years. Schaie's (1996) longitudinal study showed that inductive reasoning increases slightly through middle adulthood, with a gradual decline beginning only in late adulthood.

Conversely, there are obvious small declines in physical strength and speed beginning in middle age (Horn,

1982; Salthouse, Hambrick, & McGuthry, 1998). Illness also is considered an important factor, producing significant declines in skill at any age and becoming more likely in old age. Expressed in a nonlinear way, adult cognition is clearly multidimensional and multidirectional (Baltes, 1987; Berg, 2000; Birren, 1970; Schaie, 1983; Sternberg, 1985). Research that relies on linearlike progression and single aspects of cognition is based on the assumptions and statistical techniques that force nonlinear dynamics into single, monolithic dimensions and preclude consideration of the variability of experiential richness expressed by developmental webs (Gottlieb, Wahlsten, & Lickliter, 1998; Juarrero, 2002; Van Odern, Holden, & Turvey, 2003; Yan & Fischer, 2002).

The standardized tests used in most research involving older adults do not assess the complex skills that develop at the highest levels of abstraction achieved in late years; neither do such tests assess the integration of emotional and cognitive strands that ground the new-found insight. Studies have demonstrated that reductions in mental speed sometimes come from the increased complexity of adult cognitive skills and thinking processes (Baltes & Mayer, 1999; Howe, 1999; Schaie, 1996; Sinnott, 1998; Tennant, 1997). The response time data collected over the years have for the most part concerned attempts to reduce response times to elementary causal components of the mind or brain (Luce, 1986; Van Orden, Moreno, & Holden, 2003). However, experience and wisdom afford older adults a wider range of choices, and at times there are two equally good alternatives from which to select (which places the system in a critical state). This clearly represents increased time lags in adults' ability to make decisions.

With multiple elements interacting with one another over time, a dynamic process of self-organization occurs in which adults actively organize their limited cognitive resources into dynamic skill networks to adapt to their complex life needs (van Geert, 1994). Progress results from a combination of forward and backward movements, with backward movement preparing the way to move forward through the construction of new adaptive skills. Constructing skills in multiple directions helps older adults handle complex tasks effectively and flexibly, ultimately advancing their performance and level of competence (Miller & Coyle; 1999; Nesselroade, 1991; Siegler, 1994, 1996; Siegler & Crowley, 1991; Siegler & Jenkins, 1989). However, older adults' backward transitions of cognitive construction are considered by most as an indicator of failure and malfunction (Fischer & Bidell, 1998; Fischer et al., 1997; Miller & Coyle, 1999). Cognitive limitations can then be conceived as the inability to construct new adaptive skills required for optimal exchange with the environment in the presence of the necessary support and taking into account the variability, flexibility, and self-organization of human performance.

Backward transition seems to be the universal strategy that individuals use when they are trying to construct new skills. This is manifested in explicit problem-solving strategies, such as breaking down a novel activity to its simplest components and starting the task from the beginning (Granott, 1993). In fact, this is precisely the skill used by occupational therapists when facilitating adaptation in people who have experienced trauma or chronic illness. Most occupational therapists have witnessed individuals' ability to slowly but surely improve their performance even in the face of permanent lower levels of abstract thinking and cognitive ability to perform. Although considering it a disability, therapists have intuitively used backward transition to facilitate self-organization. Therefore, through the language and vision of nonlinear dynamics, the fact that individuals regress to a low level of performance to figure out a task they do not have the skills to perform, and gradually build toward high-level skills, has been scientifically validated. Recent studies in adult microdevelopment (Yan & Fischer, 2002) demonstrate that backward transitions are ubiquitous in older adults and play a significant role in older adults' cognition. It is evident that what appear to be unsatisfactory lower levels of performance need to be re-examined and re-evaluated. In summary, backward transition helps adults self-organize and formulate ways of solving complex tasks that initially appear beyond their capabilities.

NUMEROUS RANGES IN ADULT COGNITIVE DEVELOPMENT

The web, which expresses individual variability through the process of self-organization, stresses that many components contribute to any occupation or activity. Consequently, human activities or occupations are nonlinear, because the outcome of an action involves more than the sum of the individual's actions and the environmental mechanism that affords these actions. Each person creates a unique web, while at the same time, control and order parameters or other environmental constraints help generalization across individual webs (Fischer & Silvern, 1985; Yan & Fischer, 2002). *Skill variation* is the primary component incorporated within each web strand (Fischer & Rose, 1994). Skill variation

affords the analysis of short-term cognitive changes that identify the patterns in the dynamic variations in adult performance in a learning situation. Each strand in the cognitive web is arranged by an amalgamation of available developmental ranges, including individual experiences and the contextual support that contributes to its construction (Thelen & Smith, 1998; van der Maas & Molenaar, 1992; van Geert, 1998). For any single strand or domain of action, an individual's cognitive performance may vary along a portion of the strand. Habituation, practice, expertise with a specific domain, contextual support (scaffolding) for complex activity, and shared participation with others all influence the level of performance of an individual's occupation along any given strand (Branco & Valsiner, 1997; Fischer, 1980; Fischer & Granott, 1995; Fogel, 1993; Fogel & Lyra, 1997; Siegler, 1994). Each single strand shows the individual's developmental range of skill and knowledge in regard to that particular task and domain given varying amounts of experience and contextual support (van Geert, 1998).

OPTIMAL AND FUNCTIONAL LEVELS

A core concept in traditional developmental cognitive research is that of a person's highest level of performance, or *upper limit* (Allen, Blue, & Earhart, 1992). According to this view, individuals reach a level of cognitive performance on a given skill, beyond which they cannot surpass. This notion requires major reconsideration, because even in the presence of cognitive disabilities an individual's abilities vary dynamically depending on the experience, habits, and contextual support from others. At present, developmental research makes two distinctions between the types of highest level skill performance that vary with contextual support: (a) *optimal level* and (b) *functional level* (Fischer & Bidell, 1998; Fischer, Hand, & Russell, 1984; Yan & Fischer, 2002).

Neither the functional nor the optimal level of performance holds a single competence domain. Instead, in the absence of assistance or supervision by others, individuals show great variation in skill levels in their everyday performance (Fischer & Bidell, 1998; Fischer et al., 1984; Yan & Fischer, 2002). Research has demonstrated that optimal levels are attained mainly in those occasional circumstances when social and environmental conditions provide strong support for complex performance (Fischer & Rose, 1996; Yan & Fischer, 2002). Circumstances facilitating optimal performance include, but are not limited to, specific instructions; practice; familiar materials; familiar environments; and physical or environmental assistance, which is not present in most situations. Therefore, most individuals demonstrate an unyielding disparity between the functional level under low support and the optimal level facilitated by high support.

Functional levels are usually characterized by slow, gradual, and continuous growth over time, whereas optimal levels depict stagelike spurts and plateaus within an upward trend (Fischer et al., 1997; Kitchener et al., 1993). The two approaches diverge, becoming more dissimilar with age, because they rely on different sets of growth processes (Fischer, Kenny, & Pipp, 1990). The functional level results from the habitual construction of skill in a particular domain over time, whereas the optimal level is attained through strong contextual support for a skill combined with patterns of brain activity and self-organization that reorganize behavior in unceasing growth cycles (Yan & Fischer, 2002). In addition, the disparity between optimal and functional levels increases with age (Kitchener et al., 1993).

Adult cognitive development studies show a larger increase with age in the optimal level for a given skill than in the functional level, and thus the difference increases from early childhood through adulthood (Bullock & Ziegler, 1994; Fischer et al., 1990; Kitchener et al., 1993; Watson & Fischer, 1980). Cognitive development in adulthood takes infinite paths and shapes. Hence, as a dynamic, self-organized process, development is always changing and adapting skills, even in the presence of cognitive limitations.

It takes time for an adult to move from the emergence of an optimal level of performance to consolidation of functional levels of performance. Cognitive scholars, for example, have taken several years of intensive thinking with high self-scaffolding and long-time immersion to move from the prescriptive, disembodied Newtonian theory of cause and effect to the framework of nonlinear dynamics. Forward consolidation is both a challenging cognitive journey and a significant intellectual accomplishment, whether for an extraordinary scholar, an ordinary adult, or a person diagnosed with a cognitive disability.

Why are there such gaps in the timing and performance of cognitive capacities and the development of other skills? *Catastrophe theory* is a type of nonlinear approach that can be used to explain how gradually changing forces lead to abrupt changes in behavior. Models based on catastrophe theory aid in explaining sudden, discontinuous changes of events and global patterns of instabilities. When several influences act together, they can produce a nonlinear pattern with a complex shape that includes powerful discontinuities called *catastrophes* (Guastello, 1995; Zeeman, 1976).

Catastrophe theory describes how a developing pathway can stretch back and fold on itself over time as it progresses, giving a distinctive scalloped shape to the uprising pathway. Thus, catastrophes are sudden, discontinuous changes of events that, when modeled, geometrically depict the shapes of human behavior (Guastello, 1995).

NONLINEAR DYNAMICS, CATASTROPHE THEORY, AND OCCUPATION

The appeal of catastrophe theory to occupational therapy clinical practice is that it can explain the sudden changes in entire dynamical systems—including human activities and occupations—at nearly all system levels, and in particular to cross-level hypotheses about such systems. Most of the models for understanding the dynamics of human activities and occupations within occupational therapy practice are linear. The implication is that there is a direct and simple correlation between therapists and clients with respect to treatment interventions and outcomes, whereby one action (therapy) neutralizes the other action (the client's unwanted behavior). The more the client participates in the activities dictated by occupational therapy protocols, the greater the opportunities to decrease aggressive or unwanted behaviors. At times, however, the interactions between the client and the therapist place them in direct conflict with each other.

Zeeman (1976) used catastrophe theory to reaffirm that aggressive behavior is influenced by two conflicting drives: rage and fear. Zeeman's studies demonstrate how linear and nonlinear dimensions of fear and anger relate to aggressive behavior. For example, if the client feels enraged, then he or she will become aggressive; on the other hand, if the client feels fearful, then he or she will most likely flee. If, however, the person feels both rage and fear, then the two factors are in direct conflict, but they will not cancel each other out, as predicted by simple linear models; neither will this conflict lead to neutral behaviors. This principle exemplifies the shortcomings of such linear and simple models. Likewise, therapists practicing in rehabilitation services who embrace these principles fail to acknowledge the infinite variability and complexity that affect treatment interventions and outcomes. I next present a case study to demonstrate the use of nonlinear dynamics, using catastrophe theory to help readers understand the variability and complexity of client–therapist interactions.

CASE STUDY

This case study was conducted in an inpatient acute psychiatric unit to assist therapists in understanding the client's ability to self-organize and observe the catastrophic jumps leading to changes in behavioral variables.

Mary, a patient diagnosed with schizophrenia, resides in an acute psychiatric unit. She exhibits "florid, positive-symptom schizophrenia." The framework of treatment at the hospital is the standard psychiatric approach. Definitions of *schizophrenia* are very much a matter of interpretation that could present problems with treatment interventions. In this case, Mary's view of her illness differed from that of the mental health professionals in the unit, including the occupational therapy professionals. The discordance between patient–staff views negatively influenced Mary's ability to engage in any kind of activity within the psychiatric unit.

At the time the intervention started, Mary was aggressive, verbally abusive, paranoid, avoiding, and noncompliant. The severity of these behavioral variables was classified as an inability to participate in therapy and therapeutic activities, moderate participation, and full participation. Furthermore, the quality of therapeutic interventions was measured by Mary's ability to describe her state of mind and feelings through a self-selected medium: drawing. Thus, drawing became her primary occupation. The consistency of therapeutic interventions as it relates to space and time, therapist involvement, level of assistance or scaffolding provided, and questions asked were the independent or control variables used in this case study. After the completion of every drawing, Mary was asked two questions: (a) Can you explain your drawing? and (b) What does it mean to you today?

In regard to her first drawing, Mary explained her feelings of isolation and the perceptual incongruence between her internal environment and the external environment. The amount of incongruence or discontinuity related by Mary was treated as the *bifurcation* (sudden-jumps) parameter. The positive aspects of prior occupational or simple activity performance were hypothesized as the *asymmetry* (variability) parameter.

Drawing 1 (Figure 8.5)

- Can you explain your drawing?
  "I would like to take all of the people in my world and put them in this cage so they can see what it is like to

have a mental illness and what it is like to be in a bubble and be a prisoner of your own mind. Sometimes I am in their [*sic*] by myself; because it is safe, I cannot harm anyone, and no one can harm me."

- What does it mean for you today?
  "I think the whole world is after me. My thoughts are very negative, and I do not want to be like this. However, I do want people to understand me and understand how difficult it is to live with this type of illness. It is not easy when you are afraid most of the time and your perceptions are different than from most people. I want to tear this picture up and start over tomorrow. Hopefully then, things will appear different to me."

Drawing 2 (Figure 8.6)

- Can you explain your drawing?
  "I was asked by you to draw my morning routine. As you can see, I do not have a morning routine. My daughter yells at me all of the time to get up, but the medications that I take make it hard for me to get up, so I usually sleep until 2 or 3 in the afternoon. Once I am up, I usually eat something, and if I feel good, I go to the park by my house. Sometimes when I am there I just start running as fast as I can. I do not know where I am going; I just want to run because it makes me feel free."

- What does it mean for you today?
  "When I stop taking my medications, I stay in my room more and more, but sometimes, I simply for-

FIGURE 8.5. Case study drawing 1.

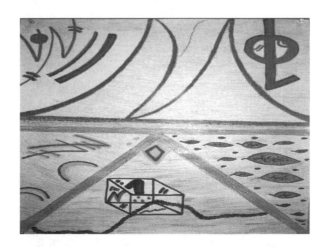

FIGURE 8.6. Case study drawing 2.

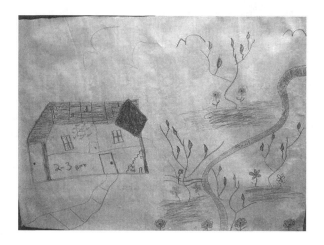

FIGURE 8.7. Case study drawing 3.

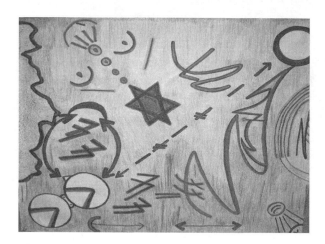

get to take them and I become depressed and the negative voices return, where I do not want to go out. When I get like this my daughter gets very mad at me, and my stress level gets to the point where I want to stay in bed all of the time. The park is meaningful to me. I like watching the animals, flying my kite, and running. However, when things at home get hectic or my stress level is high, I forget to take my medications and then I end up here. I want to learn how to communicate with my daughter and control my stress level so I can continue to spend time at the park."

Drawing 3 (Figure 8.7)

- Can you explain your drawing?
  "I see these symbols in my head all of the times, so I decided to draw them. This is how I see my world some days. When I look in the sky, I often see two suns or two moons. I am not sure what the symbols mean; they just stay with me in my head."
- What does it mean for you today?
  "I am trying to place meaning with the picture I just drew. I do not really know what it means other than these are things that I keep vividly seeing in my mind. I know that I am not ready to go home yet; the voices are still pretty negative and loud. I am trying to control them, and until I can, I need to stay here until I feel better before the doctor send[s] me home. Do you ever see things like this?"

Drawing 4 (Figure 8.8)

- Can you explain your drawing?
  "I am feeling better today, so I drew a rainbow. The sadness is lifting some, but I feel anguish because nobody really understands me. My mood keeps changing, and I feel like crying a whole lot. I am 43 years old, and my daughter will not listen to me. The night before I was admitted here I tried to have a conversation with her about having sex, and she would not listen to me. My daughter does not think I understand these things, and it makes me sad that we fight about this subject often."
- What does it mean for you today?
  "From talking to you, I realize that I need to learn to communicate with my daughter, but it is hard because she is a teenager, and she thinks she knows everything. Because I have a mental illness, my daughter does not think I know any better. My daughter believes that I cannot help myself, so I cannot help her. I have a hard time with this because I have a mental illness [and] my daughter thinks that I do not know any better, and if I cannot help myself, how can I help her?"

Drawing 5 (Figure 8.9)

- Can you explain your drawing?
  "Remember when I told you that when I look in the sky I often see two suns or two moons? Well, this is what it looks like to me. I am feeling much better

FIGURE 8.8. Case study drawing 4.

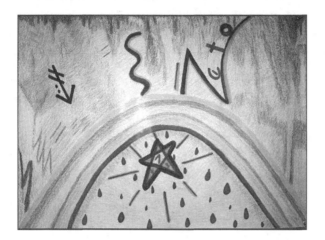

today. I still feel like I am growing inside, so I drew some flowers. Things are beginning to look much clearer, and my stress is pretty much gone."

- What does it mean for you today?
  "I am getting stronger because the staff is helping me in ways that they have not before. My stress is going away because I have been able to communicate through my drawings. The staff this time is interested in what I am doing, and they have not restrained me since I arrived here. I have been able to tell people for the first time my life story and how I view my world. Before I did not know how to articulate what I was feeling or my life story. I am get-

ting better at articulating how I feel when I am sad, feeling crazy, or when I am happy."

Drawing 6 (Figure 8.10)

- Can you explain your drawing?
  "This is how I feel today. Inside I am blooming, and I feel like I am ready to go home."
- What does it mean for you today?
  "I feel strong, and I am ready to go home today. I have learned some new ways to communicate with my family, when and why I should take my medications, and ways to control and cope with my stress. This picture depicts how I feel today. My only hope is that I will be able to continue with my drawings in order to communicate with my family."

REHABILITATION TREATMENT IMPLICATIONS

Mary's drawings demonstrated backward transitions throughout her treatment interventions. She was able to function at higher levels of cognitive capacity while engaged in therapeutic interventions because of the assistance she requested and was offered by the therapists and other staff members. The backward transitions to lower levels of cognitive performance show a remarkable parallel to the asymmetry (irregularities) and gaps mentioned in the development of optimal level in a given domain. In a sense, the cognitive capacities required of Mary under high-support conditions were unstable until she consolidated them through extensive practice and experience in

FIGURE 8.9. Case study drawing 5.

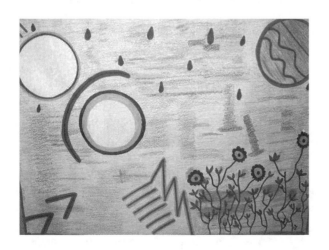

FIGURE 8.10. Case study drawing 6.

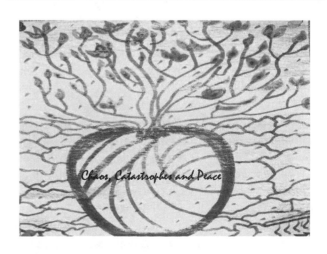

the therapeutic milieu. Consequently, her drawing began to show the self-organizing patterns of brain activity within particular situations. The sudden collapse observed on Mary's critical states—taking medication or not taking medication—versus the sensory consequences of her actions—feeling depressed and trapped in her room—captured something essential to choice and to her ability to self-organize. The state of criticality constrained past behavior while at the same time creating alternative and more flexible choices. Mary was able to create new options for actions that allowed choices of behavior that fit the specific circumstance at a specific time. Her struggle to annihilate habitual activities (which are strong patterns of brain activity) was surpassed by her new understanding of the unwanted sensory consequences of her prior actions.

In Mary's case, the instabilities were eminent in two forms: (a) She demonstrated development of optimal performance when showing sudden jumps and drops, as witnessed in her drawings, and (b) her performance level appeared and disappeared with variation in contextual support (therapist and environmental fitness). When there were changes in the time of treatment and staff support, Mary verbalized her inability to maintain her level of performance. The relationship between the two controls, asymmetry (variation) and the sudden jumps and drops (bifurcations), helped explain why Mary's changes went from uncooperative, nonparticipatory, violent, and verbally abusive to cooperative, able to engage in meaningful participation, and ultimately independent in her occupations. Her drawings delineated and pointed out her personal struggles and incongruent views of the world and, most important, provided a medium for sharing her stories in the most creative and unique way. The freedom to draw served as an important control parameter leading to explosive jumps in performance and ultimately to the changes observed by the staff in the psychiatric unit. Drawing also allowed her to feel in control of what she drew and what she shared with the occupational therapist.

Mary's essential mechanism for the construction of new skills was backward transition to lower levels of occupations (patient/student to mother/teacher) followed by frequent rebuilding of a skill until it was consolidated and finally generalized. This was demonstrated by Mary's drawings and by the reflective written and verbal interactions with therapists. Even when particular skills emerge at one level, such as when Mary realized the need to consistently take her medication to help her daughter's situation, she continued to demonstrate difficulty generalizing the influence of her decision into other aspects of her life. This change was not an imposition or a mere suggestion from the therapists; it was Mary reflecting on the past, struggling with the present, and hypothesizing about the future. Mary required high support at critical states to construct an optimal plan to tackle important issues (e.g., family, disease, medication) as well as extended time to assimilate the meaning of the information exchanged (mostly proposed by her) to annihilate prior self-organized patterns (habits) to ultimately achieve the transformational changes she was expecting to occur.

Backward transition and forward consolidation are important foundations for the dynamic phenomena of adult self-organization and continuous changes. These processes operate within the strands of the developmental web, and they create the wide range of levels of everyday skills. Mary's skills ranged from large drops to basic levels in backward transition to high levels of new skills constructed on these basic actions (e.g., medication, family issues, returning home). The ranges observed went from low levels of habitual actions to functional levels of unaided actions and further up to optimal levels of supported actions. In her case, some of the reasons accounting for this broad variation were her capability to flow from elementary sensorimotor actions to complex abstractions; prior educational level; and the facts that she was contained within a culture that supported her prior occupation and that she had the freedom to choose the particulars of how, when, and where the therapeutic exchange was to occur. Last, her life choices and situations were fully acknowledged, giving her the opportunity to validate her view of the disease process and desired outcomes.

Occupational therapists need to be sensitive to the positive or negative gradual changing forces leading to abrupt changes in clients' behavior that significantly influence rehabilitation interactions. Monitoring gradual changes in the behavioral variables and influencing the control parameters through rehabilitation treatment interventions affords the therapist and client a greater chance to establish a congruent relationship based on shared representational abstractions and not on linear cause-and-effect notions.

The influence and importance of this case study for occupational therapy practice resides in the depth of the meaning of the information exchanged through understanding the skill variability in each strand of the developmental range. It is obvious that, for any single domain of action (e.g., cooperating with treatment, talking about family issues, taking medication, drawing), which equals a single strand on the developmental web, Mary's competence was not fixed at a particular point on the strand but varied along a portion of the strand. Contextual support for the most complex activities, familiarity and practice with specific activities, and joining other therapeutic groups all affected her level of performance along a particular strand. The therapist's understanding of her role—as a facilitator—truly placed the client in the driver's seat, a position of responsibility and accountability. Facilitation of the process of self-organization, in this case, came from the therapist's acknowledgment of and respect for the client's beliefs, their shared professional and occupational cultural values, and the lack of judgment demonstrated by the therapist in her willingness to respect the client's decisions. The case further underscores that, although the energy exchanged was mostly dictated by Mary's ability to participate or not participate in the treatment sessions, it permitted her to self-organize and experience the gradual changes that ultimately led to huge jumps within the functional and optimal levels that finally influenced rehabilitation treatment outcomes in real time and in a positive way.

IMPLICATIONS FOR RESEARCH

Future research should further explore the richness, dynamics, and complexity of adult self-organized cognitive development, building knowledge of the developmental webs and dynamic processes I have described in this chapter. By opening up the scope of research and theory to analysis of the dynamics of the inherent variability and change contained within human actions, researchers can better understand the true richness and complexity of each adult's adaptive, ever-changing construction of knowledge. Discoveries of why, what, and how adult cognition changes can eventually help millions of adults face new challenges from their complex natural, social, and spiritual worlds more successfully and enjoyably.

SUMMARY

Cognition, from its beginning, is the process by which an individual grows, new psychomotor skills emerge, and social engagement is achieved. In other words, it is the process of experiencing and engaging in the complexities of everyday life. Conceived as a nonlinear dynamical process, embodied cognition (the mind as a brain and as a body in the environment in which it exists) arises from bodily interactions with the world and is continually webbed with them (Nuñez, 1999; Thelen, 2003). Cognition depends on the kinds of experiences that come from having a body with particular perceptual and motor capabilities that are inseparably linked and together form

a matrix within which reasoning, memory, emotion, language, activity, and all other aspects of mental life are embedded.

The focus of occupational therapy treatment interventions is on assisting individuals with cognitive deficits to return to productive and meaningful everyday life activities or occupations. The spontaneous meaningfulness of experiences (occupations) is an essential characteristic of mind that everyone counts on in their daily lives. As such, occupation in its broadest sense, and through a nonlinear lens, is the vehicle to facilitate change in daily clinical interventions between occupational therapists and their clients. Hence, taking the concepts of nonlinear dynamics seriously fortifies the scientific quest to account for both ordinary experiences (occupations) and scientific data. Developing cognitive models and tools that could assist in understanding the variability and tendencies of human systems, as opposed to their trends, places occupation at the heart of therapeutic interventions: It becomes the vehicle to facilitate change.

The application of nonlinear dynamics, however, continues to be the missing link in overall therapeutic approaches, including the therapist–patient relationship. Popular therapeutic approaches in mental health are usually paradigmatic, following a linear approach. Although linear explanations have generally framed the clinical problems of motivation and engagement in therapeutic activities, nonlinear dynamics can offer valuable explanations to present traditional views. Nonlinear approaches are useful for understanding unexpected and uncertain rehabilitation outcomes, such as a therapist's inability to establish a positive course of therapeutic interventions based on already established program goals and objectives and the individual's inability to engage in routine established rehabilitation interventions. In this chapter, I have dynamically reframed adult cognitive development, giving particular attention to the complex dynamics behind the variability in adult cognitive development.

Treating adult cognitive development as a static, progressive, unfolding, linear process along a series are approaches to understanding cognition and the mind that retain a substantial dose of residual cognitivism (where mind is viewed in a specific place and time in history) hidden behind attractive possibilities of the ever-developing computer technology. However, a nonlinear dynamical cognitive system emerges when the behavior of each neuron suddenly depends both on what the neighboring neurons are doing and on what went on before (Bressler & Kelso, 2001; Freeman, 2002; Llinas, 2002). By understanding and making a system's current states and behavior systematically dependent on its history and the feedback loops of autocatalysis (self-dynamic properties leading to change), researchers start to incorporate the effects of time onto those states and behavioral (occupational) patterns.

REVIEW QUESTIONS

1. Explain the meaning of the nonlinear dynamical approach to cognition and its significance for assessing adult cognitive impairments.
2. Explain the importance of the concept of self-organization in adult cognitive development as it refers to cognitive impairments.
3. Describe at least two ways in which a nonlinear approach to cognition differs from a linear approach.
4. Give two examples of the importance of understanding cognitive variation and pattern formation in adult cognitive development.
5. How is a weblike approach to cognition different from a ladderlike approach to cognition?
6. What is the hallmark of adult cognitive development?

ACKNOWLEDGMENT

I acknowledge Patrice Stange, CPT, OTR/L, for her contribution to the case study.

REFERENCES

Allen, C. K., Blue, T., & Earhart, C. (1992). *Occupational therapy treatment goals for the physically and cognitively disabled.* Rockville, MD: American Occupational Therapy Association.

Aquinas, T. (1948). *Introduction to Saint Thomas Aquinas* (A. C. Pegis, Ed. & Trans.). New York: Modern Library.

Aquinas, T. (1988). *The philosophy of Thomas Aquinas: Introductory readings* (C. Martin, Ed. & Trans.). New York: Routledge.

Bak, P. (1993). Self-organized criticality and Gaia. In W. B. Stein & F. J. Varela (Eds.), *Thinking about biology* (pp. 255–268). Reading, MA: Addison-Wesley.

Baltes, P. B. (1987). Theoretical propositions of life-span developmental psychology: On the dynamics between growth and decline. *Developmental Psychology, 23,* 611–626.

Baltes, P. B., & Mayer, K. U. (1999). *The Berlin Aging Study: Aging from 70 to 100.* New York: Cambridge University Press.

Basar, E. (1990). *Chaos in brain function.* Berlin: Springer.

Basar, E. (1998). *Brain function and oscillations.* Berlin: Springer-Verlag.

Berg, C. A. (2000). Intellectual development in adulthood. In R. J. Sternberg (Ed.), *Handbook of intelligence* (pp. 117–140). New York: Cambridge University Press.

Berkinblit, M. B., Feldman, A. G., & Fukson, O. I. (1986). Adaptability of innate motor patterns and motor control mechanisms. *Behavioral and Brain Sciences, 9,* 585–638.

Bernstein, N. (1967). *The coordination and regulation of movements.* New York: Pergamon.

Birren, J. E. (1970). Toward an experimental psychology of aging. *American Psychologist, 25,* 124–135.

Branco, A. U., & Valsiner, J. (1997). Changing methodologies: A co-constructivist study of goal orientations in social interactions. *Psychology and Developing Societies, 9,* 35–64.

Bressler, S. (2002). Understanding cognition through large-scale cortical networks. *Current Directions in Psychological Science, 11,* 58–61.

Bressler, S. (2003). Cortical coordination dynamics and the disorganization syndrome in schizophrenia. *Neuropsychopharmacology, 28,* S35–S39.

Bressler, S., & Kelso, S. (2001). Cortical coordination dynamics and cognition. *Trends in Cognitive Science, 11,* 58–61.

Bullock, M., & Ziegler, A. (1994). *Scientific reasoning.* In F. E. Weinert & W. Schneider (Eds.), *The Munich Longitudinal Study on the Genesis of Individual's Competencies (LOGIC).* Munich: Max Planck Institute for Psychological Research.

Chomsky, N. (1965). *Aspects of the theory of syntax.* Cambridge, MA: MIT Press.

Commons, M. L., Trudeau, E. J., Stein, S. A., Richards, F. A., & Krause, S. R. (1998). Hierarchical complexity of tasks shows the existence of developmental stages. *Developmental Review, 18,* 237–278.

Depew, D. J., & Weber, B. H. (1995). *Darwinism evolving: System dynamics and the genealogy of natural selection.* Cambridge, MA: MIT Press.

Diebner, H., Druckrey, T., & Weibel, P. (2001). *Sciences of the interface.* Tübingen, Germany: Genista.

Eoyang, G. (1997). *Coping with chaos: Seven simple tools.* Circle Pines, MN: Lagumo.

Fischer, K. W. (1980). A theory of cognitive development: The control and construction of hierarchies of skills. *Psychological Review, 87,* 477–531.

Fischer, K. W., Ayoub, C. C., Noam, G. G., Singh, I., Maraganore, A., & Raya, P. (1997). Psychopathology as adaptive development along distinctive pathways. *Development and Psychopathology, 9,* 751–781.

Fischer, K. W., & Bidell, T. R. (1998). Dynamic development of psychological structures in action and thought. In R. M. Lerner (Ed.) & W. Damon (Series Ed.), *Handbook of child psychology: Vol. 1. Theoretical models of human development* (5th ed., pp. 467–561). New York: Wiley.

Fischer, K. W., & Bullock, D. (1981). Patterns of data: Sequence, synchrony, and constraint in cognitive development. In K. W. Fischer (Ed.), *Cognitive development: New directions for child development* (pp. 1–20). San Francisco: Jossey-Bass.

Fischer, K. W., & Granott, N. (1995). Beyond one-dimensional change: Parallel, concurrent, socially distributed processes in learning and development. *Human Development, 39,* 302–314.

Fischer, K. W., Hand, H. H., & Russell, S. L. (1984). The development of abstractions in adolescence and adulthood. In M. Commons, F. A. Richards, & C. Armon (Eds.), *Beyond formal operations* (pp. 43–73). New York: Praeger.

Fischer, K. W., Kenny, S. L., & Pipp, S. L. (1990). How cognitive processes and environmental conditions organize discontinuities in the development of abstractions. In C. N. Alexander & E. J. Langer (Eds.), *Higher stages of human development: Perspectives on adult growth* (pp. 162–187). New York: Oxford University Press.

Fischer, K. W., & Rose, S. P. (1994). Dynamic development of coordination of components in brain and behavior: A framework for theory and research. In G. Dawson & K. W. Fischer (Eds.), *Human behavior and the developing brain* (pp. 3–66). New York: Guilford.

Fischer, K. W., & Rose, S. P. (1996). Dynamic growth cycles of brain and cognitive development. In R. Thatcher, G. R. Lyon, J. Rumsey, & N. Krasnegor (Eds.), *Developmental neuroimaging: Mapping the development of brain and behavior* (pp. 263–279). New York: Academic Press.

Fischer, K. W., & Silvern, L. (1985). Stages and individual differences in cognitive development. *Annual Review of Psychology, 36,* 613–648.

Flavell, J. H., & Wohlwill, J. F. (1969). Formal and functional aspects of cognitive development. In D. Elkind & J. H. Flavell (Eds.), *Studies in cognitive development* (pp. 197–217). London: Oxford University Press.

Fogel, A. (1993). *Developing through relationships: Origins of communication, self, and culture.* Chicago: University of Chicago Press.

Fogel, A., & Lyra, M. (1997). Dynamics of development in relationships. In I. Masterpasqua & P. Perna (Eds.), *The psychological meaning of chaos* (pp. 73–94). Washington, DC: American Psychological Association.

Freeman, W. J. (1988a). Strange attractors that govern mammalian brain dynamics as shown by trajectories of electroencephalographic (EEG) potential. *IEEE Transactions on Circuits and Systems, 35,* 781–783.

Freeman, W. J. (1988b). Nonlinear neural dynamics in olfaction as a model for cognition. In E. Basar (Ed.), *Dynamics of sensory and cognitive processing by the brain* (pp. 19–29). Berlin: Springer.

Freeman, W. J. (1990). Nonlinear neural dynamics in olfaction as a model for cognition. In E. Basar (Ed.), *Chaos in brain function* (pp. 63–73). Berlin: Springer.

Freeman, W. J. (1995). *Societies of brains.* Mahwah, NJ: Lawrence Erlbaum.

Freeman, W. J. (1997). Three centuries of category errors in studies of the neural basis of consciousness and intentionality. *Neural Networks, 10,* 1175–1183.

Freeman, W. J. (1999). Consciousness, intentionality, and causality. *Journal of Consciousness Studies, 6,* 143–172.

Freeman, W. J. (2000). Brains create macroscopic order from microscopic disorder by neurodynamics in perception. In P. Arhem, C. Blomberg, & H. Liljenstrom (Eds.), *Disorder versus order in brain function* (pp. 205–219). NJ: World Scientific.

Freeman, W. J. (2001). *Self-organizing brain dynamics by which the goals are constructed that control patterns of muscle actions.* Retrieved March 6, 2004, from http://www.cse.cuhk.edu.hk/~apnna/proceedings/iconip2001/papers/324a/pdf.

Freeman, W. J. (2002). Brains create macroscopic order from microscopic disorder by neurodynamics in perception. In P. Arhem, C. Blomberg, & H. Liljenstrom (Eds.), *Disorder versus order in brain function* (pp. 205–219). Singapore: World Scientific.

Freeman, W. J., & Barrie, J. M. (1994). Chaotic oscillations and the genesis of meaning in cerebral cortex. In G. Buzsaki, R. Llinas, W. Singer, A. Berthoz, & Y. Christen (Eds.), *Temporal coding in the brain* (pp. 13–37). Berlin: Springer.

Gibbs, R. W., & Van Orden, G. C. (2002). Are emotional expressions intentional? A self-organization view. *Consciousness and Emotion, 29,* 530–539.

Goldberg, A. (1996). Nonlinear dynamics for clinicians: Chaos theory, fractals, and complexity at the bedside. *The Lancet, 347,* 1312–1314.

Gottlieb, G., Wahlsten, D., & Lickliter, R. (1998). The significance of biology for human development: A developmental psychobiological systems view. In R. M. Lerner (Ed.) & W. Damon (Series Ed.), *Handbook of child psychology: Vol. 1. Theoretical models of human development* (5th ed., pp. 233–273). New York: Wiley.

Granott, N. (1993). *Microdevelopment of co-construction of knowledge during problem solving: Puzzled minds, weird creatures, and wuggles.* Unpublished doctoral dissertation, Massachusetts Institute of Technology, Cambridge.

Guastello, S. (1995). *Chaos, catastrophe, and human affairs.* Mahwah, NJ: Lawrence Erlbaum.

Haken, H. (2000). A physicist's view of brain functioning: Coherence, chaos, pattern formation, noise. In P. Arhem, C. Blomberg, & H. Liljenstrom (Eds.), *Disorder versus order in brain function* (pp. 135–184). Singapore: World Scientific.

Haken, H. (2002). *Brain dynamics: Synchronization and activity patterns in pulse-coupled neural nets with delays and noise.* New York: Springer.

Haken, H. (2003). Intelligent behavior: A synergetic view. In W. Tschacher & J.-P. Dauwalder (Eds.), *The dynamical systems approach to cognition* (pp. 3–16). Singapore: World Scientific.

Hendriks-Jansen, H. (1996). *Catching ourselves in the act.* Cambridge, MA: MIT Press.

Horn, J. L. (1982). The aging of human abilities. In B. B. Wolman (Ed.), *Handbook of developmental psychology* (pp. 847–870). Englewood Cliffs, NJ: Prentice Hall.

Horn, J. L., & Cattell, R. B. (1967). Age differences in fluid and crystallized intelligence. *Acta Psychologica, 26,* 107–129.

Howe, M. J. A. (1999). *The psychology of high abilities.* New York: New York University Press.

Inhelder, B., & Piaget, J. (1958). *The growth of logical thinking from childhood to adolescence* (A. P. S. Seagrim, Trans.). New York: Basic Books. (Original work published 1955)

Juarrero, A. (2002). *Dynamics in action: Intentional behavior as a complex system.* Cambridge, MA: MIT Press.

Katagiri, F., Lazzarini, I., Singer, F., & Shen-Orr, S. (2003). *Mapping the mind.* Retrieved April 26, 2004, from http://www.necsi.org/education/oneweek/winter03/projectsa.html.

Kay, L. M., Lancaster, L., & Freeman, W. J. (1996). Reafference and attractors in the olfactory system during odor recognition. *International Journal of Neural Systems, 7,* 489–496.

Kelso, S. J. A. (1999). *Dynamic patterns: The self-organization of brain and behavior.* Cambridge, MA: MIT Press.

Kitchener, K. S., Lynch, C. L., Fischer, K. W., & Wood, P. K. (1993). Developmental range of reflective judgment: The effect of contextual support and practice on developmental stage. *Developmental Psychology, 29,* 893–906.

Kugler, P. N., & Turvey, M. T. (1987). *Information, natural law, and the self-assembly of rhythmic movement.* Hillsdale, NJ: Lawrence Erlbaum.

Lazzarini, I. (2004). Neuro-occupation: The nonlinear dynamics of intention, meaning, and perception. *British Journal of Occupational Therapy, 67,* 342–352.

Llinas, R. (2002). *I of the vortex: From neurons to self.* Cambridge, MA: MIT Press.

Luce, R. (1986). *Response times: Their role in inferring elementary mental organization.* New York: Oxford University Press.

Mareschal, D., & Thomas, M. (2001). Self-organization in normal and abnormal cognitive development. In A. F. Kalverboer & A. Gramsbergen (Eds.), *Handbook on brain and behavior in human development* (pp. 743–766). Norwell, MA: Kluwer Academic.

Markman, A. B., & Dietrich, E. (2000). In defense of representation. *Cognitive Psychology, 40,* 138–171.

Mayer, R. E., & Wittrock, M. C. (1996). Problem-solving transfer. In D. C. Berliner & R. C. Calfee (Eds.), *Handbook of educational psychology* (pp. 47–62). New York: Macmillan.

McLaughlin, J., Kennedy, B., & Zemke, R. (1996). Dynamic system theory: An overview. In R. Zemke & F. Clark (Eds.), *Occupational science: The evolving discipline* (pp. 297–308). Philadelphia: F. A. Davis.

Merleau-Ponty, M. (1962). *Phenomenology of perception* (C. Smith, Trans.). New York: Humanities Press. (Original work published 1945)

Miller, P. H., & Coyle, T. R. (1999). Developmental change: Lessons from microgenesis. In E. K. Scholnick, K. Nelson, & P. Miller (Eds.), *Conceptual development: Piaget's legacy* (pp. 209–239): Mahwah, NJ: Lawrence Erlbaum.

Nesselroade, J. R. (1991). Interindividual differences in intraindividual change. In L. M. Collins & J. Horn (Eds.), *Best methods for the analysis of change: Recent advances, unanswered questions, future directions* (pp. 92–105). Washington, DC: American Psychological Association.

Nuñez, R. (1999). Could the future taste purple? Reclaiming mind, body, and cognition. In R. Nuñez & W. Freeman (Eds.), *Reclaiming cognition* (pp. 41–60). Bowling Green, OH: Imprint Academic.

Nuñez, R., & Freeman, W. J. (1999). Restoring to cognition the forgotten primacy of action, intention, and emotion. In R. Nuñez & W. Freeman (Eds.), *Reclaiming cognition* (pp. ix–xix). Bowling Green, OH: Imprint Academic.

Overton, W. F., & Newman, J. L. (1982). Cognitive development: A competence–activation/utilization approach. In T. M. Field, A. Huston, H. C. Quay, L. Troll, & G. E. Finley (Eds.), *Review of human development* (pp. 217–241). New York: Wiley.

Piaget, J. (1930). *The child's conception of physical causality.* New York: Harcourt Brace.

Piaget, J. (1972). Intellectual evolution from adolescence to adulthood. *Human Development, 15,* 1–12.

Piaget, J. (1983). Piaget's theory. In P. H. Mussen (Ed.), *Handbook of child psychology: Vol. 1. History, theory, and methods* (pp. 103–126). New York: Wiley.

Port, R. F., & van Gelder, T. (Eds.). (1995). *Mind as motion: Explorations in the dynamics of cognition.* Cambridge, MA: MIT Press.

Prigogine, I. (1994). *Order out of chaos.* New York: Bantam.

Prigogine, I. (1997). *The end of certainty: Time, chaos, and the new laws of nature.* New York: Free Press.

Prigogine, I., & Stengers, I. (1984). *Order out of chaos: Man's dialogue with nature.* New York: Bantam.

Salthouse, T. A., Hambrick, D. Z., & McGuthry, K. E. (1998). Shared age-related influences on cognitive and noncognitive variables. *Psychology and Aging, 13,* 486–500.

Schaie, K. W. (1983). Consistency and changes in cognitive functioning of the young-old and old-old. In M. Bergerner, U. Lehr, E. Lang, & M. Schmidt-Scherzer (Ed.), *Aging in the eighties and beyond* (pp. 249–257). New York: Springer.

Schaie, K. W. (1996). *Intellectual development in adulthood: The Seattle Longitudinal Study.* New York: Cambridge University Press.

Shaw, R. E. (2001). Processes, acts, and experiences: Three stances on the problem of intentionality. *Ecological Psychology, 13,* 275–314.

Sheer, D. E. (1989). Sensory and cognitive 40-Hz event-related potentials: Behavior correlates, brain function, and clinical application. In E. Basar & T. H. Bullock (Eds.), *Brain dynamics* (pp. 339–374). Berlin: Springer.

Siegler, R. S. (1994). Cognitive variability: A key to understanding cognitive development. *Current Directions in Psychological Science, 3,* 1–5.

Siegler, R. S. (1996). *Emerging minds: The process of change in children's thinking.* New York: Oxford University Press.

Siegler, R. S., & Crowley, K. (1991). The microgenetic method: A direct means for studying cognitive development. *American Psychologist, 46,* 606–620.

Siegler, R. S., & Jenkins, E. (1989). *How children discover new strategies.* Hillsdale, NJ: Lawrence Erlbaum.

Sinnott, J. D. (1998). *The development of logic in adulthood: Postformal thought and its applications.* New York: Plenum.

Skarda, C., & Freeman, W. J. (1987). How brains make chaos in the order to make sense of the world. *Behavioral and Brain Sciences, 10,* 161–173.

Sperry, R. W. (1950). Neural basis of the spontaneous optikinetic response. *Journal of Comparative Physiology, 43,* 482–489.

Sternberg, R. (1985). *Beyond IQ: A triarchic theory of intelligence.* New York: Cambridge University Press.

Szentagothai, J. (1984). Downward causation? *Annual Review of Neuroscience, 1,* 1–11.

Tennant, M. (1997). *Psychology and adult learning* (2nd ed.). New York: Routledge.

Thelen, E. (2003). Grounded in the world: Developmental origins of the embodied mind. In W. Tschacher & J. P. Dauwalder (Eds.), *The dynamical systems approach to cognition* (pp. 17–44). Singapore: World Scientific.

Thelen, E., & Smith, L. B. (1994). *A dynamic approach to the development of cognition and action.* Cambridge, MA: MIT Press.

Thelen, E., & Smith, L. B. (1998). Dynamic systems theories. In R. M. Lerner (Ed.), *Handbook of child psychology: Vol. 1. Theoretical models of human development* (5th ed., pp. 5–34). New York: Wiley.

Tschacher, W., & Dauwalder, J.-P. (2003). *The dynamical systems approach to cognition.* New York: World Scientific.

Tsuda, I. (1991). Chaotic itinerancy as a dynamical basis of hermeneutics in brain and mind. *World Futures, 32,* 167–184.

Tsuda, I. (1996). A new type of self-organization associated with chaotic dynamics in neural networks. *International Journal of Neural Systems, 7,* 451–459.

Ulanowicz, R. E. (1997). *Ecology, the ascendent perspective.* New York: Columbia University Press.

Valsiner, J. (1991). Construction of the mental: From the "cognitive revolution" to the study of development. *Theory and Psychology, 1,* 477–494.

van der Maas, H. L., & Molenaar, P. C. M. (1992). Stagewise cognitive development: An application of catastrophe theory. *Psychological Review, 99,* 395–417.

van Geert, P. (1991). A dynamic systems model of cognitive and language growth. *Psychological Review, 98,* 3–53.

van Geert, P. (1994). *Dynamic systems of development: Change between complexity and chaos.* London: Harvester Wheatsheaf.

van Geert, P. (1998). A dynamic systems model of basic developmental mechanisms: Piaget, Vygotsky, and beyond. *Psychological Review, 105,* 634–677.

Van Orden, G., & Holden, J. G. (2002). Intentional contents and self-control. *Ecological Psychology, 14,* 87–109.

Van Orden, G., Holden, J. G., & Turvey, I. (2003). Self-organization of cognitive performance. *Journal of Experimental Psychology, 132,* 331–350.

Van Orden, G., Moreno, M., & Holden, J. (2003). A proper metaphysics for cognitive performance. *Nonlinear Dynamics, Psychology, and Life Sciences, 7,* 1.

Ward, L. (2002). *Dynamical cognitive science.* Cambridge, MA: MIT Press.

Watson, M. W., & Fischer, K. W. (1980). Development of social roles in elicited and spontaneous behavior during the preschool years. *Developmental Psychology, 16,* 484–494.

Wegner, D. M., & Wheatley, T. (1999). Sources of the experience of will. *American Psychologist, 54,* 480–492.

Wright, J., & Liley, D. T. (1996). Dynamics of the brain at global and microscopic scales: Neural networks and the EEG. *Behavioral and Brain Sciences, 19,* 365–375.

Yan, Z., & Fischer, K. W. (2002). Always under construction: Dynamic variations in adult cognitive development. *Human Development, 45,* 141–160.

Zeeman, C. E. (1976). Catastrophe theory. *Scientific American, 234,* 65–83.

IV

PART

Pediatrics

9

Helene J. Polatajko, PhD, OT Reg. (Ont.), OT(C), FCAOT
Angie Mandich, PhD, OT Reg. (Ont.), OT(C)

Cognitive Orientation to Daily Occupational Performance With Children With Developmental Coordination Disorder

LEARNING OBJECTIVES

By the end of this chapter,
readers will
1. Understand developmental
coordination disorder and its impact
on daily occupational performance
in children
2. Understand the CO-OP approach
and its theoretical foundation
3. Identify the seven key features
of CO-OP
4. Identify the two types of cognitive
strategies used in CO-OP
5. Discuss the evidence supporting
the effectiveness of the CO-OP
approach with children.

This chapter represents a departure from the rest of the chapters in this book in that it treats cognition as a support for successful rehabilitation and does not address cognitive dysfunction. In this chapter, we adopt a very different perspective on cognition and occupation in rehabilitation. Rather than focusing on the remediation of cognitive deficits, we focus on performance and the role of cognition—in particular, the role of cognitive strategies—in supporting performance. The treatment approach we present in this chapter was developed in response to a need for an alternative approach to helping children with motor-based performance problems succeed. The approach emerged as a result of a search for a different paradigm for understanding motor-based performance problems in children like James:

> He decided he wanted to learn how to ride a bike and, yes, this is something he was determined to do for whatever reasons, for comparison reasons with his friends, his sister, whatever. And when I first saw him trying to do it at home and we took off the training wheels and I thought, oh I don't know, "keep trying James." And he came here and I saw him falling over, and he couldn't even get the pedals started and I thought there's just no way. This kid is going to really be disappointed because he's, for whatever reasons, he just isn't, it's not clicking. And even half way through, I still thought, I don't know, he's learning to think about what he's doing and why he's doing it, but is he going to be able to do it? And now it's like he's been riding a bike forever. It's like everything just came together, him thinking about it, and implementing all that stuff. Even the examples, like feet on the pedals are like a Ferris wheel, okay one person gets on and then quickly another person has to get on. And then it just comes. Amazing. He's so proud of that.

> —James's mother
> (Polatajko & Mandich, 2004, p. 47)

James's mother is describing is her son's experience with learning to ride a bike during cognitive orientation to daily occupational performance (CO-OP) treatment. The CO-OP approach, pronounced "COE-ohp," as in the short form of the word *cooperative*, is a treatment approach that was developed specifically for children like James who have a motor-based performance problem called *developmental coordination disorder* (DCD). Children with DCD have a great deal of difficulty learning such everyday skills of childhood as tying shoes, throwing or catching a ball, handling cutlery, running, cutting, writing, or riding a bike. Traditional approaches to the treatment of the motor-based performance problems experienced by these children have been focused on components and have failed to demonstrate significant gains at the performance level (Mandich, Polatajko, Macnab, & Miller, 2001; Pless & Carlsson, 2000; Polatajko & Cantin, in press; Sigmundsson, Pedersen, Whiting, & Ingvaldsen, 1998). As the quote from James's mother indicates, CO-OP is a performance-based approach that results in skill acquisition and performance competence. This approach was described in detail by Polatajko and Mandich (2004).[1] In this chapter, we present an overview of the approach, using excerpts from Polatajko and Mandich's (2004) book. As in other chapters in this volume, the approach, its underlying theories, and main concepts are described, as is the evidence for its use. First, however, we describe DCD. The chapter ends with two case examples showing the use of the CO-OP approach with a school-age child with DCD and with a younger child.

CHILDREN WITH DEVELOPMENTAL COORDINATION DISORDER

DCD has historically been discussed and researched under a variety of terms (Polatajko, 1999). This was due, in part, to the heterogeneity of the disorder and the varying disciplines that were concerned with it. For example, whereas occupational therapists have tended to use terms such as *sensory integrative dysfunction* (Ayres, 1972) and *perceptual–motor dysfunction* (Clark, Mailloux, Parham, & Primeau, 1991), others have used such terms as *developmental dyspraxia* (Dewey, 1995), *clumsy child syndrome* (Gubbay, 1975) or *DAMP* (deficit in attention, motor control, and perception; Gillberg, 1986). In 1994, at an international consensus meeting (Polatajko, Fox, & Missiuna, 1995), a group of 43 experts from 8 countries, representing 11 professions, concluded that the term *developmental coordination disorder,* which is used in the *Diagnostic and Statistical Manual of Mental Disorders* (4th ed.; *DSM–IV;* American Psychiatric Association [APA], 1994) should be adopted.

By definition, DCD is a marked impairment in the development of motor coordination that significantly interferes with academic achievement, activities of daily living, or both; it is not due to a general medical condition, pervasive developmental disorder, or mental retardation and is not consistent with the child's intellectual ability (APA, 1994). DCD can affect gross motor skills, fine motor skills, or both, and is characterized by impairment in the quality of movement (Polatajko & Fox, 1995). Children with DCD form a very heterogeneous group; however, they are generally characterized as having awkward or clumsy movements and as lacking the motor coordination required to execute age-appropriate motor tasks. Although children with DCD learn to perform many of the basic motor skills, they are frequently reported to have a history of delayed milestones and to require much more effort and time to learn motor skills (Polatajko, 1999).

There are, in essence, three schools of thought regarding the performance problems experienced by children with DCD (Polatajko, 1999). One holds that the poor motor skills exhibited by these children simply represent one end of the normal continuum of physical aptitude, arguing that not everyone can be an elite athlete. The second holds that these children simply have a slower rate of motor development and that, in time, the children will outgrow these difficulties. Proponents of this school of thought argue that these children do not require any serious attention because they will grow out of the slow developmental rate on their own. Longitudinal studies, however, have shown that a significant proportion of children with DCD continue to have problems (Losse et al., 1991) even into adulthood, and these children are at increased risk for social, emotional, academic, and psychiatric difficulties and adverse vocational outcomes (Cantell, Smyth, & Ahonen, 1994; Hellgren, Gillberg, Gillberg, & Enerskog, 1993; Rasmussen & Gillberg, 2000). The third school of thought, subscribed to by the APA (see *DSM–IV;* APA, 1994) and the World Health Organization (WHO; see ICD-10 in WHO, 1992),[2] considers these problems to be indicative of a bona fide disorder that requires specific attention.

The motor impairments of children with DCD can result in difficulties in all areas of occupational performance and all domains of participation. In the home, such children may have difficulty with simple self-care activities, such as dressing, especially fastening buttons and snaps and tying their shoes. At school, motor-based academics, especially those that involve handwriting, may present difficulty. At play, motor-based activities such as running, riding a bike, or kicking a soccer ball may be difficult.

Incompetence in the everyday activities of childhood, although not dire in and of itself, can have serious sec-

---

[1]This chapter is based on Polatajko and Mandich (2004) and contains several excerpts from that publication.

[2]The disorder is referred to in the ICD-10 as *specific developmental disorder of motor function* (WHO, 1992).

ondary effects on the lives of children. Observations of school-age children with DCD during organized and free play show that they spend less time in formal and informal team play than do children without this disorder (Smyth & Anderson, 2000). The decreased participation in physical activity and resultant lack of fitness and strength and the vicious cycle of motor activity avoidance is well documented among these children (Rasmussen & Gillberg, 2000; B. Rose, Larkin, & Berger, 1998). Furthermore, parent accounts indicate that it is precisely because of the "minor" nature of the motor impairment that negative consequences result for their children (Mandich, Polatajko, & Rodger, 2003; Segal, Mandich, Polatajko, & Cook, 2002). Parents explain that, because their children fail at the everyday activities of childhood, they are judged by others and by themselves to be less than competent. As a consequence, they frequently withdraw from activities to avoid ridicule and failure, develop low self-esteem and a sense of failure, are teased and bullied by their peers, and experience social isolation and even stigmatization.

The specific nature of DCD is poorly understood; hence, the approaches to treatment have been varied. Treatment approaches have frequently been determined by the theoretical orientation of the professional providing the treatment rather than by the evidence of effectiveness. It was the search for evidence that led to the creation of CO-OP. Because DCD comprises motor impairment that significantly affects a child's ability to perform the everyday activities of childhood, and because little is known about the specific etiology of the disorder, an intervention was sought that would directly address the performance issues faced by these children (Mandich & Polatajko, 2003).

CO-OP APPROACH

CO-OP is "a client-centred, performance-based, problem solving, approach that enables skill acquisition through a process of strategy use and guided discovery" (Polatajko & Mandich, 2004, p. 2). The name was coined to capture the basic elements of CO-OP (see Figure 9.1); the *cognitive orientation* points to the fact that the approach is based on a problem-solving strategy; the *daily occupational performance* indicates that the focus is on the performance, not components; and the short form captures the cooperative relationship that exists between the child and the therapist in a client-centered approach. CO-OP is unique among performance-based approaches because its emphasis is on the role of cognition in the acquisition of motor-based skills.

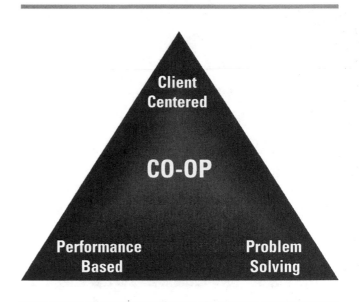

FIGURE 9.1. Fundamental elements of CO-OP.

The primary objective of CO-OP is skill acquisition. Because it is a performance-based approach, it is important that a primary outcome of CO-OP is the acquisition of the specific skills the child wants to, needs to, or is expected to perform. However, CO-OP is designed to meet three additional objectives: (a) cognitive strategy use, (b) generalization, and (c) transfer of learning. Each of these also supports the primary objective: Cognitive strategy use ensures skill acquisition; generalization ensures that the acquired strategies and skills are used outside the therapy setting, without the help of the therapist, in real-world settings; and transfer ensures that the children learn to adapt their skills and strategies to the demands of new skills that they encounter in everyday life.

To meet its objectives, the CO-OP approach draws on the latest research regarding motor performance and the use of strategies to support the mastery of motor-based skills.

Theoretical Foundations of CO-OP

CO-OP was developed within a research context and was designed to be congruent with relevant current theory and evidence-based research. Its foundational theories were drawn from behavioral and cognitive psychology, health human movement science, and occupational therapy (see Figure 9.2), each of which provided ideas on how to approach the problem of helping children with DCD

FIGURE 9.2. Foundations of CO-OP.

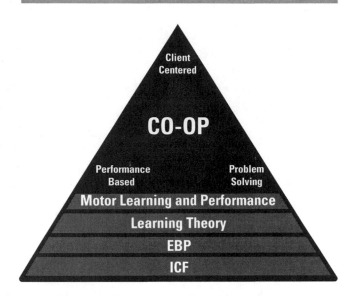

Note. EBP = evidence-based practice; ICF = *International Classification of Functioning, Disability, and Health* (WHO, 2001).

From *Enabling Occupation in Children: The Cognitive Orientation to Daily Occupational Performance (CO-OP) Approach* (p. 18), by H. J. Polatajko and A. Mandich, 2004, Ottawa, Ontario: Canadian Association of Occupational Therapists. Copyright © 2004 by the Canadian Association of Occupational Therapists. Reprinted with permission.

acquire motor skills and become proficient in their performance.

International Classification of Functioning, Disability, and Health

The *International Classification of Functioning, Disability and Health* (*ICF*), created by WHO (2001), presents a new framework for health and disability that acknowledges the interaction of the person and environmental context in producing health or disability. The *ICF* framework identifies three concepts that define health: (a) body function and structure, (b) activity, and (c) participation. Illness or impairments in body function and structure may limit the child's ability to perform activities of daily living and may restrict his or her social participation (WHO, 2001).

In the *ICF*, healthy functioning is nested in the interaction among body function and structure, activity, and participation. Positive health conditions and contextual factors are vital to healthy functioning. Contextual factors are identified as either social or physical environmental factors, such as social attitudes, legal and social structures, geographical structures, or as personal factors, such as gender, age, other health conditions, coping styles, and social background.

As discussed earlier, children with DCD experience difficulty with participation, and this often limits social inclusion and can result in marginalization. The CO-OP approach embraces the views of the *ICF* (WHO, 2001) and is focused on enabling children with DCD to engage in activity and social participation. CO-OP intervention is focused on activity and participation, not on disability and impairment. Thus, in CO-OP the focus is on improving the performance of the child in his or her environment by discovering strategies to eliminate barriers and create facilitators that enable activity and participation.

In summary, the CO-OP approach embraces the *ICF* framework and places emphasis on the interaction between personal and environmental factors to enable successful participation of children with DCD.

Client-Centeredness

An important first step in CO-OP is the identification of the goals for therapy. In CO-OP, the notion of client-chosen goals is considered paramount. CO-OP treatment is centered on the acquisition of skills the child needs to, wants to, or is expected to perform. This focus on client-centeredness is drawn from occupational therapy, which provides the following definition:

> Client-centred practice refers to collaborative approaches aimed at enabling occupation with clients who may be individuals, groups, agencies, governments, corporations, or others. Occupational therapists demonstrate respect for clients, involve clients in decision making, advocate with and for clients in meeting clients' needs, and otherwise recognize clients' experience and knowledge. (Canadian Association of Occupational Therapists [CAOT], 1997, p. 49)

CO-OP is a learning-based intervention requiring active engagement and motivation on the part of the child. A client-centered approach facilitates the identification of skills that have purpose and meaning and that the child is motivated to learn. Client-centeredness is thus a critical feature of CO-OP; the child, the family, and the therapist work together to identify goals and strategies for success.

A Learning Paradigm

CO-OP is embedded in a learning paradigm; it draws on theories of learning found in psychology and human movement science. *Learning* is defined as "an enduring change in behavior or in capacity to behave in a given fashion, which results from practice or other forms of experience" (Shuell, 1986). Learning is influenced by many factors, including occupational, personal, and environmental. CO-OP specifically draws on behavioral and cognitive–behavioral theories of learning.

Cognitive and Behavioral Theories

Behavioral theories focus on the observable relationship among the stimulus, response, and consequence (Martin & Pear, 1996). Behaviorists view learning as a permanent change in the form, duration, or frequency of a behavior. Reinforcement is an integral component of learning. Several techniques have been developed by learning theorists to promote skill acquisition. The CO-OP approach uses reinforcement, modeling, shaping, prompting, fading, and chaining techniques to support skill acquisition.

In contrast to the behavioral theories, cognitive theories view learning as an active mental process of acquiring, remembering, and using knowledge. Cognitive learning theories focus on the role that mental organization of knowledge—including problem solving, reasoning, and thinking—plays in the acquisition and performance of behaviors or skills (Schunk, 2000). Cognitive–behavioral modification is an important part of CO-OP and embraces both cognitive and behavioral theories.

Researchers, such as Meichenbaum (1977), have combined behavioral and cognitive theories in therapy. Fundamental to cognitive–behavioral therapy is the assumption that thinking patterns cause behaviors. In CO-OP treatment, the child is taught to use new thinking patterns that support skill acquisition.

Strategy use, in particular, problem-solving strategy use, is a key component. CO-OP uses the global strategy called *GOAL–PLAN–DO–CHECK,* developed by Meichenbaum (1977, 1991) as a framework to promote skill acquisition. Other domain-specific strategies (DSSs) are developed as well, for example, specific strategies that achieve a specific part of a task (Pressley et al., 1990). Both global strategies and DSSs are used to promote skill acquisition, generalization, and transfer of learning.

Generalization and transfer are important concepts within the learning paradigm. *Generalization of learning* refers to the degree to which a specific skill, learned in a specific context, can be performed in another context. *Transfer of learning* refers to the degree to which learning one skill influences the learning of another skill. Gen-

eralization and transfer allow the child to draw on previous experiences to perform the same or similar skills in a new context.

Motor Learning and Performance Theories

Motor learning is defined as "a set of internal processes that lead to a relatively permanent change in the learner's capacity for skilled motor performance" (D. J. Rose, 1997, p. 144). The process of learning a new skill is not observable and is often inferred by examining the consistent motor performance of the child (Schmidt & Wrisberg, 2000). Motor performance, on the other hand, is observable. Learning a new motor skill also is influenced by many factors, including the child, the task, and the environment in which the task is performed.

Dynamic Systems Theory

Dynamic systems theory emphasizes the relationship between the person and the environment (Thelen, Kelso, & Fogel, 1987; Turvey, 1990). This theory holds that motor behavior is self-organized and arises from a hierarchical, dynamic interaction of multiple subsystems—including the sensory, motor, perceptual, and anatomical systems of the person—and that environmental factors play a key role (Thelen, 1995). Dynamic systems theory takes into account all the factors that influence motor learning and places less emphasis on the central nervous system in determining motor behavior.

Fitts and Posner's (1967) Three-Stage Model of Motor Learning

Fitts and Posner (1967) described a three-stage model of motor learning. In the first stage, called the *cognitive stage,* cognition can be used to guide motor behavior. This first stage is characterized by high error rates in performance. The errors tend to be gross errors; movements are inaccurate and inconsistent, slow and rigid. The child is trying to understand the nature of the task, how to perform the task, and what is required of the task. The child often can be seen talking himself or herself through the movement and may use trial and error as a practice strategy to learn the movement. In the second stage of motor learning, the *associative stage,* the child is able to perform the movement with greater success. During this stage, the child is able to focus attention and perform movements with greater speed and precision. Movements are more relaxed and accurate. The child's error rate is reduced. Repetition and practice are very important during this stage. The final stage of motor learning is the *autonomous stage,* in which the movement is automatic, and the behavior is performed consistently and in a coordinated and smooth movement pattern.

Summary

In summary, the CO-OP approach to motor skill acquisition is based on a learning paradigm, a view that is consistent with contemporary perspectives on motor skill acquisition. CO-OP draws on the dynamic systems perspective, acknowledging that new skills emerge from the interaction of the child, the task, and the environment, but adds to that the acknowledgment of the idea that cognition plays a role in motor learning. Motor learning principles and understanding of the stages of learning allows CO-OP therapists to manipulate the learning environments and design the intervention in ways that support optimal learning and the development of the most advantageous movement strategies.

CO-OP MODEL

The theoretical foundations of CO-OP, in particular the cognitive and motor learning theories, suggest the model underpinning of the CO-OP approach. CO-OP is based on the premise that cognition can act as a mediator between ability and skilled performance (see Figure 9.3). Although this is not a novel premise—there are several examples of such a relationship in this book alone—its application to motor-based performance problems, where there is considered to be an underlying motor deficit, is novel. Traditional views of motor performance in children have been based on developmental models rather than learning paradigms.

FIGURE 9.3. CO-OP model.

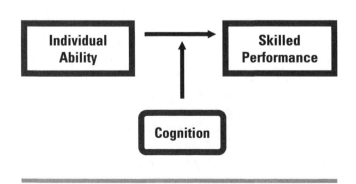

However, the experience of using CO-OP with children with DCD has shown that a learning paradigm, focused on the use of cognitive problem-solving strategies, can be used to successfully to help children with motor deficits acquire motor skills. As can be seen in the case of James, cognitive strategies can bridge the gap between ability—or, in the case of children with DCD, apparent disability—and skilled performance. The data coming out of the use of CO-OP with children with DCD (see Polatajko & Mandich, 2004, for a summary) provide evidence that cognitive strategies act at the interface between the person's ability (or disability) and his or her performance.

The CO-OP model (Figure 9.3) indicates that the relationship between ability and skilled performance can be modified by the use of strategies, that the action within CO-OP is at the interface between ability and skilled performance. The arrows in the model are placed to indicate that strategies are used to mediate the relationship between ability and performance. CO-OP does not target either ability or performance in isolation from each other. Unlike traditional approaches, CO-OP does not focus on changing the ability of the child directly; instead, it uses strategies to augment ability and produce skilled performance. The CO-OP model is consistent with the Canadian Occupational Performance Model (COPM; CAOT, 1997) and several other similar models of performance that consider performance to be the result of the interaction among the person, the task, and the environment. The CO-OP model suggests that cognition, in particular, cognitive strategies, can affect this interaction. The effect can be on the person, the task, the environment, or the interactions among these. The strategies can target the person, the task, the environment, or the interactions among them. As an example, if a child is having difficulty hitting a target with a ball, the child could adopt a strategy that will change his or her physical output ("If I throw higher, I will hit the target"), or the task ("If I use a bigger ball, I will hit the target"), or the environment ("If I throw with the sun behind me, I will see the target better and be able to hit it"), or the interaction ("If I throw higher, with a bigger ball, and with the sun behind me, I will hit the target").

Cognitive Strategies

As the CO-OP model indicates, cognitive strategy use is a hallmark of the approach (Polatajko & Mandich, 2004). Two types of strategies are used: (a) global and (b) domain specific. A global strategy is one that is used to control and coordinate other strategies (Pressley, Borkowski,

& Schneider, 1987). Global strategies are intended to be used for long periods of time in a variety of situations. There are many examples of global or executive strategies in the literature; the one used in CO-OP was developed by Camp, Blom, Herbert, and VanDoorwick (1976) and used by Meichenbaum (1977, 1991). GOAL–PLAN–DO–CHECK is a problem-solving strategy in which the first step is to identify the GOAL. Next, a PLAN for reaching that GOAL is articulated. Then, the PLAN is carried out, which is the DO part of the strategy. Finally, the CHECK part, in which the outcome is evaluated, occurs. If the outcome was successful—that is, the desired GOAL was achieved—then the PLAN is retained; if not, then a new PLAN is devised and again the DO and the CHECK are implemented, and so on and so forth, until the GOAL is achieved (see Figure 9.4).

DSSs are specific to a particular task or part of a task and are intended to be used for only a short time (Pressley et al., 1987). DSSs are not only task specific but also can be child specific; that is, the particular DSS one child uses to perform a particular task may not be the same as that of another child performing the same task. For example, one child may use the DSS "bunny ears" to remind himself to make loops when he is tying his shoes, whereas another may use the strategy "bend and hold" to remind herself of the same thing.

Although CO-OP uses only one global strategy, GOAL–PLAN–DO–CHECK, there are numerous DSSs. Because DSSs are specific to the task and the child, there are potentially as many DSSs as there are children and performance problems. Furthermore, experience with CO-OP has shown that DSSs vary with the specific performance problem the child is experiencing; for example, children with attention deficit disorder appear to require different types of strategies than do children with DCD (Polatajko & Mandich, 2004).

In CO-OP, the DSSs are embedded in the global strategy (see Figure 9.4). DSSs typically emerge when the PLAN is articulated, although they also can emerge when a strategy for accomplishing the CHECK is identified. As described earlier, the global strategy is used in an iterative fashion with frequent modifications of the PLAN, depending on the specific performance issue and the success of the PLAN. Numerous DSSs have been identified during CO-OP sessions with children with DCD. These have been grouped into seven classes, captured by the mnemonic *VG(BATS for 2 Vs;* Polatajko & Mandich, 2004; see Table 9.1). Each of these addresses a different performance problem to support skilled performance (see Table 9.2).

Key Features

As the model suggests, strategy use is the sine qua non of the CO-OP approach (Polatajko & Mandich, 2004). However, strategy use alone does not define the approach. CO-OP has 7 key features that contribute to its definition as a unique approach: (a) client-chosen goals, (b) dynamic performance analysis (DPA), (c) cognitive strategy use, (d) guided discovery, (e) enabling principles, (f) parent–significant other involvement, and (g) intervention structure. Each addresses one or more of the CO-OP objectives (see Figure 9.5), and each is essential to CO-OP's effectiveness. Together, the key features and the factors they subtend (see Figure 9.6) define CO-OP as a client-centered, performance-based, problem-solving approach in which specific strategies, identified through a process of guided discovery, are used to enable skill acquisition.

Client-Chosen Goals

I didn't think that learning to be a goalie was a good goal for therapy. I thought writing was the important thing. Well, I have to tell you that he learned to be a good goalie with you, and then he made the school floor hockey team. They went to the championships and won. He is living his dream!

—Morris's mother
(Mandich et al., 2003, p. 584)

FIGURE 9.4. CO-OP strategy use process.

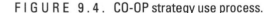

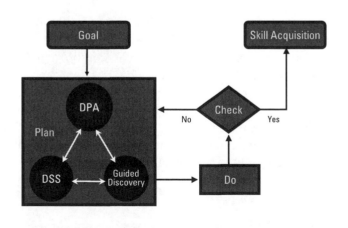

Note: DPA = dynamic performance analysis; DSS = domain-specific strategy. From *Enabling Occupation in Children: The Cognitive Orientation to Daily Occupational Performance (CO-OP) Approach* (p. 73), by H. J. Polatajko and A. Mandich, 2004, Ottawa, Ontario: Canadian Association of Occupational Therapists. Copyright © 2004 by the Canadian Association of Occupational Therapists. Reprinted with permission.

TABLE 9.1. CO-OP Domain-Specific Strategies: VG(BATS For 2 Vs)

Strategy Description	Examples
Verbal Guidance	
Body position: Any verbalization of, attention to, or shifting of the body, whole or in part, relative to the task	"Sit with my back against the chair" "Keep my ankles straight" "Hold the paper with my other hand"
Attention to doing: Any verbalization to cues attending to the doing of the task	"Eyes on the ball" "Listen for the click of the rope" "Where do you need to look?"
Task specification/modification: Any discussions regarding the specifics or modification of the task, or parts of the task, or any modification of the task or any action to change the task, or parts of the task	"Put a mark on the floor so I know where the middle is" "Let's try using pencil grips" "Use paper with lines on it" "Let me do it with you"
Supplementing task knowledge: Any verbalization of task-specific information or how to get task-specific information	"We always start writing at the left" "You make a capital *A* like this" "Let's use these directions to help us make a paper airplane"
Feeling the movement: Any verbalization of attention to the feeling of a particular movement	"Feel the bumps as you make the *B* in the air" "Feel the position of your hand as you hold the scissors"
Verbal motor mnemonic: A name given to the task, component of the task, or body position that evokes a mental image of the required motor performance	"Helper hand" "Ferris wheel" "Bunny ears"
Verbal rote script: A rote pattern of 4–5 clear, concise words that are meaningful to the child to guide a motor sequence	"Dribble, dribble, shoot" "Push, glide; push, glide" "Up, down, and around"

Note. From "Cognitive Strategies and Motor Performance in Children With Developmental Coordination Disorder," by A. Mandich, H. J. Polatajko, C. Missiuna, and L. Miller, 2001, *Physical and Occupational Therapy in Pediatrics, 20*, p. 134. Copyright © 2001 by Haworth Press, Binghamton, NY. Reprinted with permission. Article copies available from The Haworth Document Delivery Service: 1-800-HAWORTH. E-mail address: docdelivery@haworthpress.com.

CO-OP is a client-centered approach with skill acquisition as the primary objective. In CO-OP, the child learns to perform three specific skills, referred to as *GOALS*. In keeping with the concept of client-centeredness, the GOALS are set in collaboration with the child, and great care is taken to ensure that the GOALS are ones that the child wants to, needs to, or is expected to acquire, as they were with Morris. These GOALS are the focal point of the intervention and are the vehicle for addressing the other three objectives of CO-OP. As with Morris, working on child-chosen GOALS ensures that these skills have significance and ecological relevance for the child. This, in turn, ensures that the child will be motivated to learn to perform the skill, to use it beyond the therapy setting, and to apply the new learning to other skills. Furthermore, experience with CO-OP has shown that children frequently choose GOALS that can be viewed as *marker skills*—that is, skills that have a pivotal place in the child's life (as learning to be a goalie was for Morris) and that frequently have *spin-off effects* (Mandich et al., 2003; Segal et al., 2002).

Several techniques (see Figure 9.6) are used in the CO-OP approach to ensure that the three specific skills to be acquired are the GOALs the child wants to, needs to, or is expected to acquire. The child is actively engaged in choosing the GOALs, and all efforts are made to accommodate the child's choices.

Daily Activity Log

The daily activity log is a simple tool used to document the activities carried out in the course of a day. The form of the log structures the recording by listing the times of the day, in half-hour intervals, and providing a

TABLE 9.2. Performance Problems and Their Enabling Strategies

Performance Problems Identified by Dynamic Performance Analysis	Domain-Specific Strategies
Child does not have sufficient task knowledge to even begin to perform the skill or to specify a GOAL, PLAN, or CHECK	• Supplementing task knowledge • Task specification • Body position
Child knows what needs to be done but cannot do it	• Task modification • Body position • Feeling the movement • Attention to doing
Child can do the task but needs support in doing it	• Task modification • Verbal guidance • Verbal self-guidance • Verbal rote script • Verbal mnemonic

Note. From *Enabling Occupation in Children: The Cognitive Orientation to Daily Occupational Performance (CO-OP) Approach* (p. 78), by H. J. Polatajko and A. Mandich, 2004, Ottawa, Ontario: Canadian Association of Occupational Therapists. Copyright © 2004 by the Canadian Association of Occupational Therapists. Reprinted with permission.

place for recording the major activities that were done during that half-hour period. The form can be used as the day progresses to keep track of activities, or it can be used to describe a typical day. In CO-OP, the child is asked to complete the daily activity log, with the as-sistance of his or her parents or significant others, thinking about a typical school day, not a holiday or weekend. The completed daily activity log is used to provide the therapist with information on the child's typical day. The therapist uses the log to help initiate the process of goal setting.

Paediatric Activity Card Sort

The Paediatric Activity Card Sort (PACS; Mandich, Polatajko, Miller, & Baum, 2004) is a picture-based as-sessment used to determine a child's level of occupa-tional engagement. It is composed of 77 cards with color photographs of children between ages 4 and 16 years engaging in typical childhood activities, organized into 4 categories: (a) hobbies, (b) chores, (c) sports, and (d) personal care. The child is asked to sort the pictures into those he or she does do and does not do. The PACS is used to complement the daily activity log in the process of goal setting.

Canadian Occupational Performance Measure

The COPM (Law et. al., 1998) is a client-centered, self-report measure designed to identify treatment goals in the areas of self-care, productivity, and leisure and to mea-sure outcome. The COPM is used in CO-OP to identify

FIGURE 9.5. Key features supporting the CO-OP objectives.

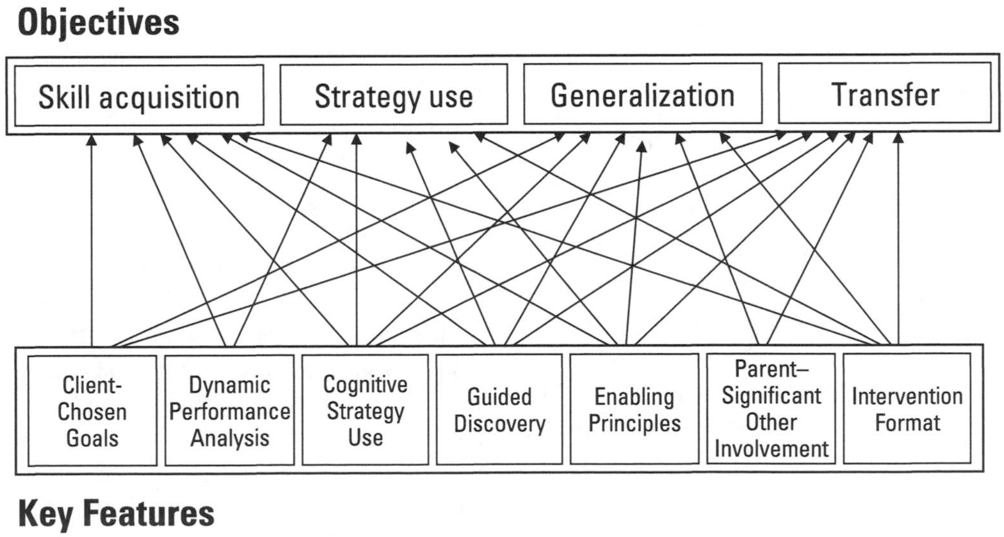

Note: From *Enabling Occupation in Children: The Cognitive Orientation to Daily Occupational Performance (CO-OP) Approach* (p. 53), by H. J. Polatajko and A. Mandich, 2004, Ottawa, Ontario: Canadian Association of Occupational Therapists. Copyright © 2004 by the Canadian Association of Occupational Therapists. Reprinted with permission.

FIGURE 9.6. Key features and factors of the CO-OP.

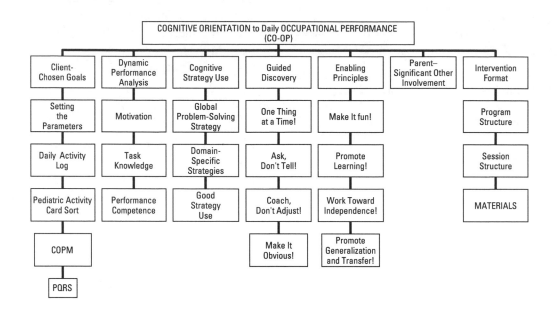

the three client-chosen GOALS that are the focal point of the approach. The therapist uses the information gleaned from the daily activity log and the PACS to initiate the COPM interview and to help guide the questions that are asked to ensure that the child's GOALS are identified. The COPM is administered again at the end of intervention to measure outcome.

Performance Quality Rating Scale

The Performance Quality Rating Scale (PQRS; Henry & Polatajko, 2003; Martini & Polatajko, 1998; Miller, Polatajko, Missiuna, Mandich, & Macnab, 2001) is an observation-based rating scale used to quickly, easily, and repeatedly measure performance and change in performance. Designed as a research tool for use in the development and evaluation of CO-OP, it provides an objective measure of performance to parallel the self-report measure provided by the COPM. The PQRS is used in CO-OP to collect pre- and post-test data.

Dynamic Performance Analysis

Just today, we were having a bowl of chili and you know it was going everywhere around the table practically. Then it occurred to him, "If I hold it, Mommy,

I'm going to hold my bowl. But I can't eat with that hand Mommy." You can tell his mind is going, that he's thinking, you put the spoon in the other hand.

—Mark's mother
(Polatajko & Mandich, 2004, p. 60)

DPA is an observation-based process of identifying performance problems or performance breakdown (Polatajko, Mandich, & Martini, 2000). It was developed specifically for use in CO-OP to support skill acquisition. It is a dynamic, iterative process, embedded in a top-down framework, that is applicable to any performance situation. The DPA process focuses analysis on actual performance, in context, and is carried out while performance is being observed. DPA supports skill acquisition in two ways: (a) identifying performance problems or breakdowns and (b) identifying and testing potential strategies to solve the performance problems. To carry out DPA effectively, the therapist needs to know how to perform the skill in question, what is going wrong with the performance, and potential solutions. The therapist is guided in this process by the DPA decision tree depicted in Figure 9.7.

The DPA decision tree is composed of a series of staged questions and encourages the therapist to consider whether the child has the prerequisite motivation and

FIGURE 9.7. DPA decision tree.

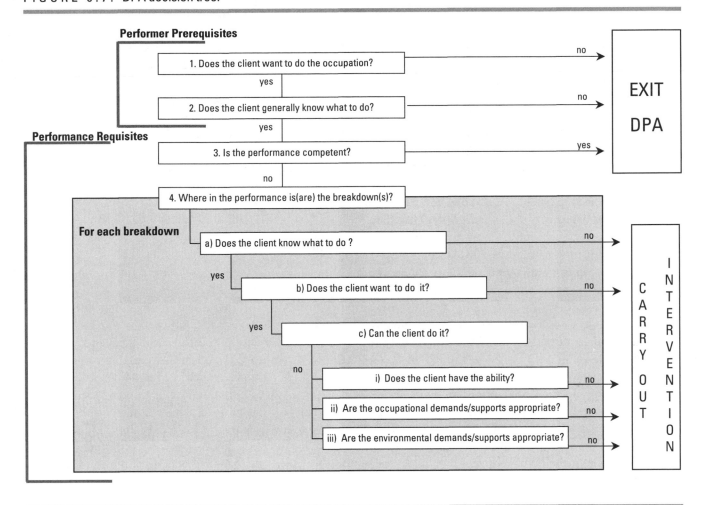

Note: From "Dynamic Performance Analysis: A Framework for Understanding Occupational Performance," by H. J. Polatajko, A. D. Mandich, and R. Martini, 2000, *American Journal of Occupational Therapy, 54,* p. 69. Copyright © 2000 by the American Occupational Therapy Association. Reprinted with permission.

basic task knowledge for performance and whether the performance is competent. If the performance is incompetent, the therapist uses the decision tree to establish the performance problems or to identify the points where the performance breaks down. The therapist uses the DPA process continuously, throughout the intervention, and engages the child in this process. As a result, the child learns to begin to solve performance problems himself or herself, as Mark did in the quote from his mother that opened this section.

Cognitive Strategy Use

You can tell his mind is going, that he's thinking, you put the spoon in the other hand. Then he said, "I can't eat with that hand," then he put the spoon back in his right hand and then it occurred to him, "I'll hold the bowl." Which I still think is kind of, it's slow, but on the other hand, it's quite something that he's pieced all of that together, but it's not natural for him to do that. So that's an interesting thing.

—Mark's mother
(Polatajko & Mandich, 2004, p. 60)

In CO-OP, children learn to think about what to do and how to do it, as Mark did. The children are taught to think their way through a performance problem, to identify a strategy to solve that problem, to implement it, and then to check to see whether it worked. This is done by talking through the performance with the child.

The CO-OP approach uses the global strategy GOAL–PLAN–DO–CHECK to facilitate the process of talking through. The strategy helps the child engage in problem solving a performance issue and monitoring the outcome; in other words, the strategy promotes metacognition. Throughout CO-OP, the therapist and child are engaged in conversation about the GOAL and how it can be performed, the PLAN and how it has been performed, and the CHECK (Batte & Polatajko, 2004).

The global strategy provides the vehicle for discovering the DSSs that are relevant to the particular child and the particular skill. DSSs are used to address specific performance problems as they arise and to support skilled performance. The DPA process is used to identify the need for a DSS and the potential DSSs that will solve the particular performance issue (see Figure 9.4). The DSSs are tailor-made for each child, in each situation. The DSSs one child uses to learn a specific skill may be different from those used by another child to learn the same skill. Similarly, the same child may use several DSSs while learning a skill.

At the outset of CO-OP, the children are specifically taught the global strategy. It is then used throughout the intervention. DSSs, in contrast, are identified and used only if and when they are needed. Therefore, the children are not taught any specific DSSs a priori; instead, they are guided to discover the DSSs that will enable their performance. Experience with CO-OP has shown that guiding the children to discover their own strategies results in much richer, more meaningful strategies than could ever be thought of by a therapist; recall the Ferris wheel strategy used by James.

Guided Discovery

> Remember also that each time one prematurely teaches a child something he could have discovered for himself, that child is kept from inventing it and consequently from understanding it completely. (Piaget, 1970)

Guided discovery is essential to the CO-OP strategy use process (see Figure 9.4). Although it is possible to use strategies without using guided discovery, to do so would rob the child of the ownership and complete understanding that Piaget (1970) said comes with discovery. Guided discovery is an important learning concept. It is rooted in the general principles of learning theory and draws on Meichenbaum's (1977, 1991) scaffolding techniques and the mediational techniques of Feuerstein and colleagues (Feuerstein, Rand, Hoffman, & Miller, 1980; Haywood, 1987, 1988).

In CO-OP, the process of guided discovery is closely entwined with the process of strategy use. It is used in conjunction with the DPA process primarily to elucidate the PLAN and to identify the necessary DSSs (see Figure 9.4). When the child becomes "stuck" in the middle of a performance, the therapist leads the child to discover a PLAN, test it out by DOing it, and CHECKing to see whether it worked. In this way, guided discovery supports not only skill acquisition but also strategy use (see Figure 9.5).

Four key phrases (verbal mnemonics) capture the essence of guided discovery in CO-OP:

1. One thing at a time!
2. Ask, don't tell!
3. Coach, don't adjust!
4. Make it obvious!

One Thing at a Time!

When a child is having difficulty performing a skill, there are typically numerous performance problems. Because CO-OP is embedded in a learning paradigm, and motor-based skills are considered to be learned, not developed, it is important to keep the intervention and the child focused on only one thing at a time. At face value, it seems simple to focus intervention on only one thing at a time; however, the skill lies in knowing on which thing to focus. This comes from knowledge of the child and task and careful use of the DPA process.

Ask, Don't Tell!

When a child discovers the solution to a problem, the likelihood of the child remembering that solution and using it is much greater than when the child is told the solution. An important technique in helping a child discover is to ask just the right question. The art of thoughtful questioning is a Socratic technique, which is known to foster critical thinking, evaluation, and knowledge application. By asking the child questions, attention is drawn to relevant aspects of a performance, and strategy identification is facilitated. The form of the question and the target of the question are informed by knowledge of the child and the task, the DPA process, and the therapist's hypothesis about the solution.

Coach, Don't Adjust!

The physical counterpart to telling a child what to do is to adjust the task or the environment to support his or her performance. Many occupational therapists intuitively, often surreptitiously, adjust heights, weights, angles, noise levels, or levels of difficulty, or they place their finger, hand, or themselves in just the right place to stabilize environments, materials, equipment, and even the child to ensure the child's success. This promotes success in the presence of the therapist, and it ensures that the child is unaware of these enabling strategies and hence likely to fail in the absence of the therapist. In CO-OP, the therapist is required to self-monitor for this type of instinctive behavior; to inhibit it; and to instead bring it to the child's attention by guiding the child to discover the personal, task, or environmental adjustments that will improve performance.

Make It Obvious!

Children with DCD do not readily learn from observation; that is, they do not learn from just watching, as their peers do. They have difficulty knowing what the salient features of a skill to attend to are. Consequently, when working on the PLAN or the CHECK or when the therapist models the DO, the aspect to which the child needs to attend is made obvious; for example, attention is drawn to features of a skill, modeled responses are exaggerated, questions are posed so that the answer is obvious, and coached adjustments are planned to have dramatic outcomes. Furthermore, the relationships between strategy use and outcome are made obvious.

Enabling Principles

He comes out of it excited. He doesn't come out like he's done a lot of work. Like it's a chore. He actually enjoys it, I suppose because he chose the things he's working on, too. It was something that he really wanted to accomplish, and he was quite proud of that. Never had to tell him, we're going to Kid's skills, and he was like aww. No, he was always like okay, today's Kid's skills, good. Do I get to try my bike today, do I get to, what am I doing today? He likes that.

—James's mother
(Polatajko & Mandich, 2004, p. 89)

CO-OP has its foundation in the client-centered philosophy of occupational therapy, which focuses on enabling people to perform the occupations they want to, need to, or are expected to perform. As defined by the CAOT (1997), "Enabling refers to a process of facilitating, guiding, coaching, educating, promoting, listening, reflecting, encouraging, or otherwise collaborating with people so that individuals, groups, agencies, or organizations have the means and opportunity to participate in shaping their own lives" (p. 50).

Central to CO-OP is the idea that the child is a partner in the process. Furthermore, as we have discussed, CO-OP is rooted in a learning paradigm, with the objectives being that the children acquire the specific skills they choose, learn to use strategies, and generalize and transfer both. This suggests a specific set of enabling techniques, one that is consistent with a client-centered philosophy and a learning paradigm, one that ensures motivation for engagement and the willingness to continue when a task becomes challenging.

Four enabling principles (see Figure 9.6) have been identified for use in CO-OP to support skill acquisition, strategy use, generalization, and transfer (see Figure 9.5). The enabling principles are an integral part of the approach and are used throughout the intervention. They are captured in four imperatives:

1. Make it fun!
2. Promote learning!
3. Work toward independence!
4. Promote generalization and transfer!

Make It Fun!

In CO-OP, children like James work on solving performance problems with activities that they want to do but that they have found difficult in the past. This is frequently hard work, so it is important that everything possible is done to engage the child in the process. As James's mother noted, working on the child's chosen GOALs helps in this regard; however, other measures are needed to engage the child. These are captured by the imperative "Make it fun!" which refers to the interaction style of the therapist and a range of props and techniques that are used to make the process fun. Experience with CO-OP suggests that therapists who are playful have the greatest success in engaging the children in strategy use to solve motor performance problems.

Promote Learning!

Because CO-OP is embedded in a learning paradigm, it is important that learning is promoted throughout. The imperative "Promote learning!" is intended to remind the CO-OP therapist to remain cognizant of and use basic learning principles, such as

- Learning progresses through stages.
- Information should be presented in small steps.

- Learners require support, feedback, practice, and review; motivation and contextual factors influence learning.
- Reinforcement, direct teaching, modeling, shaping, prompting, fading, and chaining are important techniques that can be used to promote learning.

Work Toward Independence!

The ultimate goal of CO-OP is that the children are able to perform skills and use strategies on their own—whenever and wherever appropriate. The CO-OP approach is geared toward independence from the very start by working on child-chosen goals, in the way GOAL–PLAN–DO–CHECK is taught, by guiding discovery, and by promoting learning—in particular, by fading the amount of support provided. Early in the therapy, a significant amount of support is provided. As the child becomes more proficient, support is slowly withdrawn, and the child is encouraged to try the skill on his or her own, with fewer and fewer prompts from the therapist. Independence also is fostered through homework, through which the child is required to practice new skills and strategies between sessions and then report to the therapist on how it went.

Promote Generalization and Transfer!

Many of the CO-OP features—for example, focusing on child-chosen skills, guiding discovery, promoting learning, and working toward independence—are designed to promote generalization and transfer.

To support generalization, special care is taken to ensure that the PLANs and DSSs that are created are portable to other situations; for example, if the child identifies marking an *X* on the floor to indicate where in the rope to jump, the therapist might say "That's a great idea; let's see if that works. [Child jumps.] It does! Great! Now, let's talk about how you can use the *X* in the playground, with your friends." Parents and significant others also are included in the planning for generalization.

To support transfer, the therapist creates bridges or links between what the child is learning (i.e., his or her PLANS and DSSs) to other places, situations, or tasks. Both near and far transfers are encouraged. Throughout, attention is explicitly placed on using previous strategies to solve the current problem or on identifying opportunities for future transfer; for example, the therapist might ask the child, "Can you tell me two other letters that use the same shape as *a*"? or "Are there other times when you can use your 'helper hand'? Over the next 2 days I want you to find 5 times when you can use your helper hand." Parents

or significant others also are asked to participate in this process, by helping the child with homework.

Parent–Significant Other Involvement

He's so proud of [learning to ride a bike]. He tells all his friends "and I'm going to get a new bike and I accomplished this," because he knew. He set his own goal: I want to learn how to ride my bike. "Dad, if I learn how to ride my bike, what do I get, what's in this for me? I'd really like a new bike, Dad. I'd really like a bike." So that's what he's getting. He worked towards his goal and he accomplished it and he's happily looking ahead.

—James's mother
(Polatajko & Mandich, 2004, p. 96)

In CO-OP, parents or significant others are called on to be active supporters of the intervention process. The primary role of parents or significant others is to support the child in the acquisition of new skills and to facilitate the generalization and transfer of these skills. They also are asked to provide, within reasonable limits, resources and equipment related to their child's goals; for instance, if the child chooses to learn how to rollerblade, the parents will need to provide the appropriate equipment.

Throughout the intervention, information is shared with the parents or significant others so that they can celebrate successes with the child and support his or her use of newly learned skills and strategies in environments beyond the intervention sessions. Their involvement contributes to all four CO-OP objectives (see Figure 9.5) but is particularly important in promoting generalization and transfer.

To enable parents or significant others to play an active role in helping their child succeed, they are made aware of the essential aspects of the intervention and asked to be involved in specific ways. At the outset, they are oriented to CO-OP, the importance of motivation and task knowledge is explained, and they are asked to work with their child to fill in the daily activity log and to help their child set his or her three skill GOALs. They are asked to attend at least three sessions but are told that they are welcome to observe as many sessions as they wish. By observing, the parents learn the basic principles necessary to help their child develop skills, learn and use cognitive strategies, and transfer and generalize what he or she has learned into everyday life. In discussions, some of the key enabling principles of CO-OP are illuminated. In particular, the importance of guided discovery is emphasized. They, too, are encouraged to remember "One thing at a time!" "Ask, don't tell!" "Coach, don't adjust!" "Make it obvious!" and, most important, "Make it fun!"

The experience of being involved in CO-OP has benefits beyond helping the child acquire the desired skills. By enabling their child to succeed, parents or significant others change their perspective on the child. In the same way that the children learn the relationship between strategy use and outcome and learn to attribute the lack of success to failure of the PLAN rather than to a personal failure, so too can successful strategy use alter parents' perception of themselves and their children. Parents can see that failure can be attributed to an ineffective strategy, as opposed to personal factors. This awareness often results in a new appreciation of the factors that contribute to their child's performance and the realization that there are strategies that can help.

Intervention Format

Delivery of CO-OP follows a particular format (see Figure 9.6). The CO-OP program has an overall structure, as do the individual sessions. Finally, there are specific materials that are used as part of the CO-OP format.

The program structure comprises three distinct phases (see Exhibit 9.1):

1. Phase I, the *Preparation Phase,* is primarily concerned with establishing the GOAL. This phase calls for preparatory work by the child, parent, or significant others and an initial meeting between the child and the therapist. In this phase, the child's chosen goals and

---

EXHIBIT 9.1. Intervention Format: Three Phases of CO-OP

GOAL: Preparation Phase

Prepare to identify client-chosen GOALs	Prior to first meeting: ● Establish contact with parents ● Orient parents to CO-OP ● Ensure parent commitment and involvement ● Provide daily activity log ● Check prerequisites
Identify client-chosen GOALs	At first meeting: ● Review child's completed daily activity log ● Administer PACS ● Administer COPM ● Assess child's baseline performance using the PQRS ● Initiate the DPA process

PLAN and DO: Acquisition Phase

Initiate cognitive strategy use	Session 1: ● Begin to apply enabling principles ● Introduce global strategy: GOAL–PLAN–DO–CHECK ● Have parents or significant others observe
Promote skill acquisition through strategy use	Sessions 2–10: ● Promote the child's use of GOAL–PLAN–DO–CHECK, iteratively, to promote skill acquisition ● Continue the DPA process, iteratively ● Guide discovery of DSSs, iteratively ● Continue to apply enabling principles ● Encourage parents and significant others to observe and promote generalization and transfer of strategies and skills

CHECK: Verification Phase

Verify that the GOALs have been met	Final meeting: ● Readminister COPM and PQRS ● Probe child for generalization and transfer ● Review and reinforce strategy use with parents and significant others

Note. PACS = Paediatric Activity Card Sort; COPM = Canadian Occupational Performance Measure; PQRS = Performance Quality Rating Scale; DPA = dynamic performance analysis.

From *Enabling Occupation in Children: The Cognitive Orientation to Daily Occupational Performance (CO-OP) Approach* (p. 102), by H. J. Polatajko and A. Mandich, 2004, Ottawa, Ontario: Canadian Association of Occupational Therapists. Copyright © 2004 by the Canadian Association of Occupational Therapists. Reprinted with permission.

the baseline level of performance are established. Parent or significant other involvement is initiated.

2. Phase II, the *Acquisition Phase,* is essentially the PLAN and DO phase, in which the work of using strategies to acquire skills is done. This phase is composed of 10 sessions. The first session is devoted to introducing the child to the GOAL–PLAN–DO–CHECK strategy and its use in skill performance. The CO-OP strategy use process (see Figure 9.4) frames the remaining 9 acquisition sessions. Typically, only two GOALs are addressed in the first few sessions. The third GOAL is added when good progress has been made on at least one of the first two GOALs. It is in the acquisition sessions that PLANs are made and DSSs are discovered. The therapist uses the DPA process and guided-discovery techniques throughout these sessions to promote skill acquisition, strategy use, generalization, and transfer (see Figure 9.5). Keeping in mind the enabling principles, the therapist ensures that the experience is fun for the child and that the child learns to become independent in strategy use and skill performance. Each acquisition session is approximately 1 hr in duration and is scheduled to occur once or twice a week. Each session starts with a discussion of the GOAL and PLANs for that session. Next, the homework, if there was any, is reviewed, and then work begins on skill acquisition. Typically, two skills are worked on in any one session; however, depending on the nature of the GOALs and the child's progress with them, only one GOAL, or all three GOALs, could be addressed in any given session. Near the end of each session, the discussion turns to homework. The child usually is sent off with specific things to practice or try outside of the clinic.

3. Phase III, the *Verification Phase,* typically consists of only 1 session, in which CHECK is carried out; the child's progress is reviewed, as are the strategies learned. The child is questioned about the strategies learned and their generalizability and transferability. As well, the COPM and PQRS are readministered to verify that the chosen skills have been acquired. Finally, the child is given a certificate of achievement, one of the CO-OP materials.

Several materials have been developed for use with CO-OP; the first is a puppet that acts as a visual mnemonic for the GOAL–PLAN–DO–CHECK strategy. Others include a strategy log in which the DSSs are recorded; homework sheets, where tasks to be done and their outcome are recorded; strategy supports, such as an alphabet card or a PLAN list; stars or stickers to congratulate the child on his or her work; and whatever equipment is necessary to perform the task.

Although there is a specific CO-OP format and structures for intervention and sessions, it is important to remember that CO-OP is highly individualized; the sessions differ greatly depending on the child or the skill to be learned. CO-OP is tailored to meet the specific needs of a specific child.

CASE EXAMPLES

The case examples on the following pages are adapted from Polatajko and Mandich (2004) and illustrate the application of CO-OP with a school-age child with DCD and with a young child.

EVIDENCE FOR THE CO-OP APPROACH

CO-OP was developed over a period of 10 years through a series of studies conducted by H. J. Polatajko and her colleagues and students. The earlier studies, reported in detail elsewhere (Mandich, 1997; Mandich, Polatajko, Missiuna, & Miller, 2001; Martini & Polatajko, 1998; Polatajko, Mandich, Miller, & Macnab, 2001; Polatajko, Mandich, Missiuna, et al., 2001; Wilcox, 1994; Wilcox & Polatajko, 1993, 1994), elucidated the essential features of CO-OP and provided evidence to support its further development and evaluation. Several additional formal and informal studies were carried out to determine the effectiveness of CO-OP (Polatajko, Mandich, Miller, & Macnab, 2001). The most important of the formal studies was a randomized clinical trial (Miller et al., 2001). Twenty school-age children with DCD were randomly assigned to one of two groups; 10 received CO-OP treatment, while another 10 received the typical treatment approach. The findings indicated that, even with groups as small as 10, the CO-OP treatment was significantly more effective in promoting skill acquisition and skill transfer than the typical treatment approach.

Since the completion of the randomized clinical trial, several other studies have investigated the use of CO-OP in clinical practice. To elucidate the essential differences between CO-OP and the typical treatment approach, Sangster, Beninger, Polatajko, and Mandich (in press) examined the effect of CO-OP on strategy use. They found that, by the end of treatment, the children receiving CO-OP were able to identify significantly more and better strategies than the children

Case Example 9.1. Joseph

Joseph, a 10-year-old boy with DCD, was referred to therapy for assessment and intervention because of difficulties with motor coordination. At the time of the referral, Joseph attended a public school, where he was in fourth grade. Joseph displayed above-average intelligence but was having difficulty meeting the written demands of the classroom environment.

Joseph's mom described him as a clumsy boy who had significant difficult performing such everyday activities as tying his shoes and fastening zippers, snaps, and buttons. Joseph could not play road hockey or rollerblade, the two common neighborhood activities. Joseph's mother felt that he really wanted to join in but was embarrassed about his poor motor skills. Joseph's developmental milestones were within normal limits.

PREPARATION PHASE

Before the first meeting, the therapist did the following:

- Established contact with Joseph's parents,
- Oriented the parents to CO-OP,
- Ensured the parents' commitment and involvement,
- Provided the daily activity log, and
- Checked for child and parent prerequisites.

The therapist carried out an assessment of Joseph's performance skills. The results of standardized testing placed him in the 1st percentile for his age on the Movement Assessment Battery for Children, in the 60th percentile on the Gardner Test of Visual Perceptual Skills (nonmotor), and in the 25th percentile on the Beery Developmental Test of Visual Motor Integration. A parent questionnaire identified functional problems in self-care and school activities.

Using the COPM, the therapist had Joseph choose three GOALs on which to work during CO-OP intervention. These were (a) printing more neatly, (b) learning to throw a baseball, and (c) learning to type on the computer. The therapist observed Joseph's baseline performance of these skills and rated it using the PQRS. Her scores indicated that Joseph's performance was poor. She also used the information she gathered from the observation to carry out the initial DPA. The DPA analysis points of breakdown are given in Table 9.3.

ACQUISITION PHASE

The therapist began the first intervention session by introducing the global strategy. Joseph then used the strategy to teach the therapist how to shuffle cards. Joseph did this well, indicating that he understood the strategy. The therapist then began to work on skill acquisition. With respect to printing, the therapist started by helping Joseph develop a strategy about spacing words and letters. Using exaggeration and experimentation involving comparing and contrasting different positions, the therapist guided Joseph to discover that the words had to be far apart and that, as part of his PLAN, he could use his finger to space his words; the letters, on the other hand, needed to be "close neighbors" but not sitting on top of each other. Later, Joseph developed a PLAN to stop his paper from moving around on the table when he wrote. He developed the verbal mnemonics "helper-hand–doer-hand" to remind him to stabilize the paper. Joseph's PLAN for writing is given in Table 9.4.

Next, the therapist guided Joseph to develop PLANs for baseball and typing. The therapist bridged the helper-hand–doer-hand from writing to basketball and helped Joseph realize that both hands work together and that each has a job to do in performing both skills. Then Joseph worked on typing on the computer. He was able to bridge his body position strategy and his helper-hand–doer-hand strategy to the typing task. Through direct skill teaching, comparison, and verbal guidance, Joseph learned to position his fingers. He called his finger position his "go" position.

(continued)

T A B L E 9 . 3 . Joseph's Breakdown Points

GOAL	Breakdown Points
Cursive writing	His words and letters were too close together. The small and capital letters were all the same size. He had difficulty stabilizing the paper.
Throwing a baseball	He didn't look where he was aiming the ball. He didn't consistently use one hand to throw the ball. He didn't know how to hold the ball.
Typing on the computer	He didn't know how to place his hands on the keys. He looked at the letters when he typed instead of feeling the position of the keys.

Case Example 9.1. Joseph *(Continued)*

TABLE 9.4. Joseph's PLAN for Writing

GOALs	Breakdown Points	Joseph's PLAN
Cursive writing	The small and capital letters were all the same size.	My small letters take up half the space, tall letters take up the full space.
	He had difficulty stabilizing the paper.	I have a helper hand and a doer hand.
	The words and letters were too close together.	Finger spaces between the words; letters need to be neighbors.

As Joseph's skill level improved on each task, the therapist focused Joseph's efforts on how to perform the skill accurately and how to refine the movement patterns. Once Joseph was able to perform the skills, practice was used to solidify the learning. Random practice schedules were used to have Joseph problem-solve new movement patterns. Transfer and generalization were reinforced. The practice environment was varied, and generalization to the home and school settings was established. Joseph created a checklist to help take with him to practice his PLAN and CHECK his own performance. To promote generalization to school, Joseph took a cue card to school and taped it onto the front of his daily planner so he could check his work at school. To promote transfer, the therapist helped Joseph bridge the strategies that Joseph developed to other activities, given in Table 9.5.

Throughout, as the DSSs and PLANs developed, they were all compiled into a strategy summary sheet. The summary sheet was discussed with the parents and taken home to ensure transfer and generalization. Joseph was encouraged to use his strategies at school, at home, and with his peers. The therapist talked with Joseph's teacher to explain the CO-OP approach and to explain the strategies that Joseph had developed. In the final meeting, the therapist repeated the COPM and the PQRS, and both sets of scores revealed significant improvement. Joseph and his parents were very pleased with the results.

TABLE 9.5. Joseph's Strategies to Promote Transfer

DSS Class	Specific Strategy	Bridging of the Strategy
Body position	Helper-hand–doer-hand	Cutting, throwing a football, eating a bowl of soup

Note. DSS = domain-specific strategies.

receiving a typical treatment approach. Batte and Polatajko (2004) examined the role of practice in skill acquisition in CO-OP. They found that, as is typical of cognitive-based approaches, the CO-OP approach was considerably more language-laden than the typical treatment approach. They discovered that in CO-OP a great amount of treatment time was devoted to the discussion of performance, and thus children in the typical treatment approach actually had more practice time than children in the CO-OP approach. Nevertheless, children receiving CO-OP showed significantly greater improvement in performance, indicating that strategy use, not practice, was accountable for the success of the CO-OP approach.

Mandich et al. (2003), as part of a qualitative study, found evidence regarding the impact of CO-OP on the lives of children. During discussion of the impact of DCD on the lives of their children, parents inadvertently offered commentary on the effects of CO-OP and its broad impact on the lives of their children. They indicated that CO-OP not only was effective in having their children reach their goals but also, and more important from their perspective, had far-reaching effects. The children's skills generalized beyond the therapy room to natural settings

Case Example 9.2. Daniel

Daniel was 6 years old when he was referred to therapy by a developmental pediatrician who had diagnosed him with DCD. Daniel attended first grade at a local school. His parents and teacher noted that he was having significant difficulty with fine motor skills. The parents were very frustrated with Daniel's progress and felt that they wanted to intervene early, before significant problems arose. Daniel's parents felt that early intervention would facilitate Daniel's optimal functioning in the classroom. In a developmental regard, Daniel's milestones were all within normal limits; however, he was having significant difficulty printing his letters. He also was having difficulty at mealtime and often spilled his food. He really wanted to use a knife but could not manage to coordinate the movements. He could not tie his shoes or fasten the buttons and zipper on his coat or snowsuit. This often interfered with his ability to go out for recess on time with his friends.

Results of standardized testing on the Movement Assessment Battery for Children placed Daniel in the 5th percentile for his age; on the Gardner Test of Visual Perceptual Skills (nonmotor) he was in the 70th percentile, and on the Beery Developmental Test of Visual Motor Integration he was in the 30th percentile. A parent questionnaire identified functional problems in the areas of self-care and school and leisure activities. Daniel began CO-OP intervention.

The therapist used the COPM with the parents and Daniel, and three goals were identified. The therapist used the DPA decision tree to analyze Daniel's performance and identify these points of performance breakdown (Table 9.6).

As described in recent studies with younger children (Mandich, Polatajko, & Miller, 2001; Taylor & Mandich, 2003, 2004), the CO-OP process was modified to ensure success by administering the COPM to both the parents and to Daniel, reducing the time on task to about 15 min per task, using a variety of modalities with frequent changes in activities

(e.g., pencils, paints, markers for writing), increasing the repetition and reinforcement of the strategies, and incorporating playfulness as a key strategy

Daniel chose to start by working on tying his shoes. The therapist modeled how to tie a shoelace and verbalized the steps. She described the steps in the process to Daniel and then encouraged him to try. She broke the skill into steps. Starting with crossing the laces and making the first knot, the therapist prompted Daniel to describe each step, ensuring that she did not talk while Daniel was concentrating on performing the task. Daniel could make the loops but could not find the hole into which to insert the loop to tie the laces. He developed a strategy of "look for the circle."

The second GOAL Daniel worked on was printing. Daniel often rushed through his work. He developed a strategy—"slow down"—to help him not rush through his work. The therapist began by working on letter formation. Daniel learned to write a *v* by making a check mark; he leaned how to make an *x* by making a "leaning tower." Through questioning, comparison, and exaggeration, Daniel came to realize that not all letters are the same size. Daniel held the pencil with an awkward grasp, so the therapist targeted correcting his pencil grasp. After several sessions, Daniel was able to increase his success with printing and was then willing to work on his pencil grasp. The therapist tried a variety of pencil grips to keep his fingers in the correct position. The therapist used questioning to help Daniel come up with a strategy for an appropriate finger position and pencil grasp. He called it his "takeoff" position.

Daniel also discovered strategies for rollerblading, including "push left, push right" to help him develop the proper rollerblading movement. He learned to keep his ankles straight by using the verbal mnemonic "tall ankles." As DSSs and

(continued)

TABLE 9.6. Daniel's Breakdown Points

GOAL	Breakdown Points
Tying his shoes	He does not know how to put the loops through the hole. He does not know how to tie the final knot.
Rollerblading	He did not know how to hold his ankles in position. He did not focus on where he was going. He could not roll on the blades; he walked instead.
Printing	He takes his time. His letters are too large. He did not know how to form some of his letters. He does not hold his pencil with a functional grasp. He sits on the edge of the chair.

Case Example 9.2. Daniel *(Continued)*

TABLE 9.7. Daniel's PLANs

DSS Class	Specific Strategy	Bridging of the Strategy
Body position	Takeoff position	Computer, eating at the table, doing homework at the desk
Attention to task	Make an *X* Glue my loop to the shoe	Tying his hockey skates and soccer shoes
Body position	Tall ankles	Skating
Task specification–modification	Use of a pencil grip	Provided a grip for school and home

Note. DSS = domain-specific strategies.

PLANs were developed and reinforced, a strategy summary sheet was created for Daniel, which he took home to support generalization. He was encouraged to use his strategies at school. The PLANs and strategies that he developed, as well as the situations to which the strategies were bridged, are given in Table 9.7.

Daniel's parents were informed of the strategies and encouraged to have Daniel use them at home and in school. At the final meeting, the therapist repeated the COPM and the PQRS, and both sets of scores revealed significant improvement. Daniel and his parents were very pleased with the results.

and transfer to other skills, and CO-OP also made the children generally more open to new learning and more willing to participate. As one parent put it,

There is no doubt about it, that for Roger, bike riding has been a lifeline, a lifeline into the social community, and a lifeline so far as his self-esteem it has definitely grown. It sort of was a rite of passage, a real marker for him. It has built his confidence to do other things and to keep trying. (Mandich et al., 2003, p. 588)

In addition to the above-mentioned studies, two studies have investigated the use of CO-OP with preschoolers. The use of CO-OP with a group of 4 children, ages 5 and 6 years, who had been identified by educational resource personnel as experiencing fine motor problems, was evaluated by Mandich, Polatajko, and Miller (2001). Although it is typical in the CO-OP approach for children to identify their own goals, in this case the parents identified the treatment goal. All the children participated willingly in the intervention and made significant gains. The results of independent ratings of the children's handwriting samples and COPM scores indicated that all 4 children improved their printing skills over the 10 sessions.

Taylor and Mandich (2003, 2004) used a single-case experimental design study to examine the effects of CO-OP with four children ages 5 to 7 years. In this study, the children were seen individually and chose their goals in collaboration with their parents. The findings indicated that the children were able to learn and use strategies and achieve their goals; however, slight modifications had to be made to the CO-OP approach for use with these younger children. Sessions had to be more varied, shorter, and more repetitious. Child, parent, and therapist ratings of performance at post-test demonstrated that CO-OP was effective; that children as young as 5 years could acquire, generalize, and transfer the skills using cognitive strategies; and, most importantly, they could acquire, generalize, and transfer strategy use into the home.

Taken together, the findings from these studies provide evidence for the use of the CO-OP approach in improving the performance of children with motor-based problems. Research is ongoing to examine the use of CO-OP with other populations, including children with acquired brain injury, Asperger syndrome, attention deficit disorders, and cerebral palsy. The evidence to date is that CO-OP is effective in helping children with performance problems learn to use strategies to help them perform the skills they choose and to generalize and transfer these skills.

REVIEW QUESTIONS

1. What do the letters in *CO-OP* stand for?
2. What are the characteristics and performance difficulties of children with developmental coordination disorder?
3. What are the main foundational concepts, theories, models, and philosophies underpinning CO-OP?
4. What is the role of cognition in the CO-OP approach?
5. What is the role of the parents or significant others in CO-OP?
6. What is the evidence supporting the use of the CO-OP approach?

REFERENCES

American Psychiatric Association. (1994). *Diagnostic and statistical manual of mental disorders* (4th ed.). Washington, DC: Author.

Ayres, A. J. (1972). *Sensory integration and learning disorders.* Los Angeles: Western Psychological Services.

Batte, M., & Polatajko, H. (2004). *CO-OP vs. practice for children with developmental coordination disorder: A question of strategy.* Manuscript submitted for publication.

Camp, B., Blom, G., Herbert, F., & VanDoorwick, W. (1976). *Think aloud: A program for developing self-control in young aggressive boys.* Unpublished manuscript, University of Colorado School of Medicine, Boulder.

Canadian Association of Occupational Therapists. (1997). *Enabling occupation: An occupational therapy perspective.* Ottawa, Ontario: Author.

Cantell, M. H., Smyth, M. M., & Ahonen, T. P. (1994). Clumsiness in adolescence: Educational, motor, and social outcomes of motor delays detected at 5 years. *Adapted Physical Activity Quarterly, 11,* 115–129.

Clark, R., Mailloux, Z., Parham, L. D., & Primeau, L. A. (1991). Occupational therapy provision of children with learning disabilities and/or mild to moderate perceptual and motor deficits. *American Journal of Occupational Therapy, 45,* 1069–1074.

Dewey, D. (1995). What is developmental dyspraxia? *Brain and Cognition, 29,* 254–274.

Feuerstein, R., Rand, Y., Hoffman, M., & Miller, R. (1980). *Instrumental enrichment: An intervention program for cognitive modifiability.* Baltimore: University Park Press.

Fitts, P. M., & Posner, M. I. (1967). *Human performance.* Belmont, CA: Brooks/Cole.

Gillberg, C. (1986). Attention deficit disorder: Diagnosis, prevalence, management and outcome. *Pediatrician, 13,* 108–118.

Gubbay, S. S. (1975). *The clumsy child: A study of developmental apraxia and agnosic ataxia.* Philadelphia: Saunders.

Haywood, H. C. (1987). A mediational teaching style. *The Thinking Teacher, 4*(1), 1–6.

Haywood, H. C. (1988). Bridging: A special technique of mediation. *The Thinking Teacher, 4*(4), 4–5.

Hellgren, L., Gillberg, C., Gillberg, I. C., & Enerskog, I. (1993). Children with deficits in attention, motor control, and perception (DAMP) almost grown up: General health at 16 years. *Developmental Medicine and Child Neurology, 35,* 881–892.

Henry, L., & Polatajko, H. J. (2003, May). *Exploring the interrater reliability of the Performance Quality Rating Scale.* Paper presented at the meeting of the Canadian Association of Occupational Therapists, Winnipeg, Manitoba.

Law, M., Baptiste, S., Carswell, A., McColl, M. A., Polatajko, H., & Pollock, N. (1998). *Canadian Occupational Performance Measure* (3rd ed.). Toronto, Ontario: Canadian Association of Occupational Therapists.

Losse, A., Henderson, S. E., Elliman, D., Hall, D., Knight, E., & Jongmans, M. (1991). Clumsiness in children—Do they grow out of it? A 10-year follow-up study. *Developmental Medicine and Child Neurology, 33,* 55–68.

Mandich, A. (1997). *Cognitive strategies and motor performance in children with developmental coordination disorder.* Unpublished master's thesis, University of Western Ontario, Waterloo, Ontario, Canada.

Mandich, A., & Polatajko, H. (2003). Developmental coordination disorder: Mechanisms measurement management. *Human Movement Science, 22,* 406–411.

Mandich, A., Polatajko, H. J., Macnab, J. J., & Miller, L. T. (2001). Treatment of children with developmental coordination disorder: What is the evidence? *Physical and Occupational Therapy in Pediatrics, 20,* 51–68.

Mandich, A., Polatajko, H. J., & Miller, L. (2001, May). *Can a cognitive approach be used with preschoolers?* Paper presented at the meeting of the Canadian Association of Occupational Therapists, Calgary, Alberta.

Mandich, A., Polatajko, H. J., Miller, L., & Baum, C., (2004). *The Paediatric Activity Card Sort.* Ottawa, Ontario: Canadian Association of Occupational Therapists.

Mandich, A., Polatajko, H. J., Missiuna, C., & Miller, L. (2001). Cognitive strategies and motor performance in children with developmental coordination disorder. *Physical and Occupational Therapy in Pediatrics, 20,* 125–144.

Mandich, A., Polatajko, H., & Rodger, S. (2003). Rites of passage: Understanding participation of children with developmental coordination disorder. *Human Movement Science, 22,* 583–595.

Martin, G., & Pear, J. (1996). *Behavior modification: What it is and how to do it* (5th ed.). Upper Saddle River, NJ: Prentice Hall.

Martini, R., & Polatajko, H. J. (1998). Verbal self-guidance as a treatment approach for children with developmental coordination disorder: A systematic replication study. *Occupational Therapy Journal of Research, 18,* 157–181.

Meichenbaum, D. (1977). *Cognitive–behavior modification: An integrative approach.* New York: Plenum.

Meichenbaum, D. (1991). *Cognitive–behavior modification.* Presented at the Child and Parent Research Institute, London, Ontario, Canada.

Miller, L. T., Polatajko, H. J., Missiuna, C., Mandich, A. D., & Macnab, J. J. (2001). A pilot trial of a cognitive treatment for children with developmental coordination disorder. *Human Movement Science, 20,* 183–210.

Piaget, J. (1970). Piaget's theory. In P. H. Mussen (Ed.), *Carmichael's manual of child psychology: Vol. 1* (3rd ed., pp. 703–732). New York: Wiley.

Pless, M., & Carlsson, M. (2000). Effects of motor skill intervention on developmental coordination disorder: A meta-analysis. *Adapted Physical Activity Quarterly, 17,* 381–401.

Polatajko, H. J. (1999). Developmental coordination disorder (DCD): Alias the clumsy child syndrome. In K. Whitmore, H. Hart, & G. Willems (Eds.), *A neurodevelopmental approach to specific learning disorders* (pp. 119–133). London: MacKeith.

Polatajko, H. J., & Cantin, N. (in press). A review of current approaches. In R. H. Guetz (Ed.), *Developmental coordination disorder.* Marseille, France: Solal Editeurs.

Polatajko, H. J., & Fox, A. M. (1995). *Final report on the International Consensus Meeting: Children and clumsiness: A disability in search of definition.* London, Ontario, Canada.

Polatajko, H. J., Fox, A. M., & Missiuna, C. (1995). An international consensus on children with developmental coordination disorder. *Canadian Journal of Occupational Therapy, 62,* 3–6.

Polatajko, H. J., & Mandich, A. (2004). *Enabling occupation in children: The cognitive orientation to daily occupational performance (CO-OP) approach.* Ottawa, Ontario: Canadian Association of Occupational Therapists.

Polatajko, H. J., Mandich, A. D., & Martini, R. (2000). Dynamic performance analysis: A framework for understanding occupational performance. *American Journal of Occupational Therapy, 54,* 65–72.

Polatajko, H. J., Mandich, A. D., Miller, L., & Macnab, J. (2001). Cognitive orientation to daily occupational performance: Part II—The evidence. *Physical and Occupational Therapy in Pediatrics, 20,* 83–106.

Polatajko, H. J., Mandich, A. D., Missiuna, C., Miller, L., Macnab, J., Malloy-Miller, T., et al. (2001). Cognitive orientation to daily occupational performance (CO-OP): Part III—The protocol in brief. *Physical and Occupational Therapy in Pediatrics, 20,* 107–124.

Pressley, M., Borkowski, J. G., & Schneider, W. (1987). Cognitive strategies: Good strategy users coordinate metacognition and knowledge. In R. Vasta (Ed.), *Annals of Child Development* (Vol. 4, pp. 89–129). Greenwich, CT: JAI Press.

Pressley, M., Woloshyn, V., Lysynchuk, L. M., Martin, V., Wood, E., & Willoughby, T. (1990). A primer of research on cognitive strategy instruction: The important issues and how to address them. *Educational Psychology Review, 2,* 1–58.

Rasmussen, P., & Gillberg, C. (2000). Natural outcome of ADHD with developmental coordination disorder at age 22 years: A controlled, longitudinal, community-based study. *Journal of the American Academy of Child and Adolescent Psychiatry, 11,* 1424–1431.

Rose, B., Larkin, D., & Berger, B. (1998). The importance of motor coordination for children's motivational orientations in sport. *Adapted Physical Activity Quarterly, 15,* 316–327.

Rose, D. J. (1997). *A multilevel approach to the study of motor control and learning.* Newton, MA: Allyn & Bacon.

Sangster, C. A., Beninger, C., Polatajko, H. J., & Mandich, A. (in press). An exploration of cognitive strategy generation in children with developmental coordination disorder and the impact of a cognitive approach to therapy. *Canadian Journal of Occupational Therapy.*

Schmidt, R. A., & Wrisberg, C. A. (2000). *Motor learning and performance: A problem-based learning approach* (2nd ed.). Champaign, IL: Human Kinetics.

Schunk, D. H. (2000). *Learning theories: An educational perspective* (3rd ed.). Columbus, OH: Merrill.

Segal, R., Mandich, A., Polatajko, H., & Cook, J. V. (2002). Stigma and its management: A framework for understanding social isolation of children with developmental coordination disorder. *American Journal of Occupational Therapy, 56,* 422–428.

Shuell, T. J. (1986). Cognitive conceptions of learning. *Review of Educational Research, 56,* 411–436.

Sigmundsson, H., Pedersen, A. V., Whiting, H. T., & Ingvaldsen, R. P. (1998). We can cure your child's clumsiness! A review of intervention methods. *Scandinavian Journal of Rehabilitation Medicine, 30,* 101–106.

Smyth, M. M., & Anderson, H. I. (2000). Coping with clumsiness in the school playground: Social and physical play in children with coordination impairments. *British Journal of Developmental Psychology, 18,* 389–413.

Taylor, S., & Mandich, A. (2003). *A cognitive intervention for younger children with developmental coordination disorder.* Paper presented at the Occupational Therapy Conference on Evidence Based Practice, London, Ontario, Canada.

Taylor, S., & Mandich, A. (2004). *A cognitive intervention for younger children with developmental coordination disorder.* Manuscript submitted for publication.

Thelen, E. (1995). Motor development: A new synthesis. *American Psychologist, 50,* 79–95.

Thelen, E., Kelso, J. A., & Fogel, A. (1987). Self-organizing systems and infant motor development. *Developmental Review, 7,* 39–65.

Turvey, M. T. (1990). Coordination. *American Psychologist, 45,* 938–953.

Wilcox, A. (1994). *Children with mild motor problems: Exploring a client-centred, cognitive approach in OT intervention.* Unpublished master's thesis, University of Western Ontario, London, Ontario.

Wilcox, A., & Polatajko, H. (1993). Verbal self-guidance as a treatment technique for children with developmental coordination disorder. *Canadian Journal of Occupational Therapy,* (Suppl.), 20.

Wilcox, A., & Polatajko, H. J. (1994). The impact of verbal self-guidance on children with developmental coordination disorder. *11th International Congress of the World Federation of Occupational Therapists Congress Summaries, 3,* 1518–1519.

World Health Organization. (1992). *International statistical classification of diseases and related health problems* (1989 rev.). Geneva, Switzerland: Author.

World Health Organization. (2001). *International classification of functioning, disability and health.* Geneva, Switzerland: Author.

10

Naomi Josman, PhD, OTR

The Dynamic Interactional Model for Children and Adolescents

Children with a variety of developmental or acquired disabilities present a host of functional limitations. People who have sustained traumatic brain injury (TBI) have, in the past, been evaluated and treated with a focus on the recovery of sensory and motor abilities, the underlying assumption being that their developing nervous system would undergo a renewal of weakened cognitive functions. Occupational therapy interventions thus have focused on the areas of sensory and motor abilities and have given less attention to the cognitive functions (Coster, 1998; Cronin, 2001). More recent studies, however, have provided evidence that cognitive therapy provided to children with TBI is efficacious and highly essential.

I begin this chapter by presenting an overview of the theoretical background related to neuropsychological disabilities that are affected in children with brain injury, namely, memory, executive function, and awareness deficits and their critical implications for performing daily functions.

Thereafter, I discuss the dynamic interactional model as adapted for children who have sustained brain injury, with special reference to evaluation and treatment methods for intervention and the implications for the present study with relevant instruments. I then present two case studies to illustrate the intervention. I conclude the chapter with a description of four research studies that used dynamic interactional assessment (DIA) instruments; I detail recommendations for adopting this model for children and propose further research on

the utility and efficacy of the dynamic interactional model for the evaluation, treatment, and rehabilitation of children.

THEORETICAL BACKGROUND

For a variety of reasons, occupational therapists who work with children have only recently begun to explore the use of cognitive approaches for intervention with their clients. Although cognitive approaches have long been used in education and psychology, the stages of problem solving and the relevant techniques used in mediating a child's occupational performance still constitute a novelty to most occupational therapists (Missiuna, Malloy-Miller, & Mandich, 1998).

The pathology and sequelae of pediatric TBI differ from those of the adult TBI population. In childhood TBI, cognitive impairment and secondary delays often are overlooked in the referral intervention process (Cronin, 2001), while the motor components constitute the dominant focus of rehabilitation. Research indicates that even children with mild or moderate TBI without motor impairments demonstrate reduced functional performance. In addition, children with severe brain injury often have long-term cognitive disabilities that might impair school classroom performance (Kinsella et al., 1997). Moreover, problems manifested in preserving sequences of ideas, generalizing, categorizing, or integrating information to main principles are considered critical components that can hinder a child's successful integration into the school class (Josman, Berney, & Jarus, 2000b).

Occupational therapy interventions in acute-stage head trauma recovery include positioning, range of motion, and sensory stimulation (Scott & Dow, 1995; Winkler, 1995). In intermediate care, interventions broaden, including improving motor control and training in activities of daily living, cognitive–perceptual remediation, and community re-entry skills (Cronin, 2001). Although cognitive disability can greatly limit recovery, because voluntary control and independent function rely on cognition (Balskey & Jennings, 1999), cognitive intervention is not a main focus of occupational therapy intervention.

For years, models and approaches in pediatric occupational therapy have focused on sensory integration, perceptual–motor, and neurodevelopmental approaches and overlooked the cognitive aspect and approaches (Kramer & Hinojosa, 1999).

In this chapter, I propose adopting the dynamic interactional model for evaluating and treating children with brain injuries and those with handwriting problems related to learning disabilities. The dynamic interactional model was initially developed by Toglia (1992) for use with adults with brain injuries. Although the effects of head trauma in adults have been extensively researched, head trauma in children has only recently become a topic of research, and a formidable one at that (Dalby & Obrzut, 1991).

A meta-cognitive approach, in conjunction with a perceptual–motor approach, has recently been recommended for intervention to remediate children's handwriting problems (Josman, Sachein, & Sachs, 2004). This study looked at a variety of components that influence handwriting, including self-awareness of performance. It focused on intervention and the efficacy of different approaches, as opposed to most previous studies, which have focused primarily on understanding the basis of handwriting difficulties as well as evaluation and assessment of handwriting.

Handwriting difficulty, or *dysgraphia,* is a disturbance or difficulty in producing written language and is related to the mechanics of writing (Hamstra-Bletz & Blote, 1993). It also has been referred to as a specific learning disability (Brown, Chedwick, Shaffer, Rutter, & Traub, 1981). Dysgraphia is a common complaint among children and adults with learning disabilities, and it may appear accompanied or unaccompanied by other academic difficulties (Cratty, 1994; Johnson, 1995; Rosenblum, Parush, & Weiss, 2003; Waber & Bernstein, 1994).

Neuropsychological Disabilities

Some degree of disability usually persists among children with severe TBI, despite therapeutic intervention (Ylvisaker & DeBonis, 2000). Cognitive deficits are among the main problems that characterize children who have experienced TBI. The most common persistent cognitive deficit areas in children with TBI are attention, concentration, judgment, and impulse control (Anderson, Fenwick, Manly, & Robertson, 1998). Functional limitations associated with these cognitive deficits are related more to meta-cognitive executive functions, for example, poor initiation of tasks and poor task orientation and organization (Ylvisaker, 1998). Difficulties with memory and decreased information-processing speed often are lingering changes following TBI (Porr, 1999). Chadwick, Rutter, Shaffer, and Shrout (1981) observed that, even though children's IQ scores were not decreased, school performance was erratic, attention span was problematic, they were slow to process information, and they had difficulties in problem solving. These deficits are not exclusively manifested at acute stages of the injury but occur even years after completion of the rehabilitation process. Research has shown that young children who have sustained different degrees of TBI might recover from their motor disabilities but might be unable to overcome their cognitive disabilities (Costeff, Groswasswer, & Goldstein, 1990).

Memory

The ability to learn and remember new information is crucial to children's academic performance (Donders, 1992). Deficits in memory are among the most significant and pervasive neuropsychological sequelae of TBI in children (Dalby & Obrzut, 1991; Telzrow, 1987). Goldstein, Levin, Boake, and Lohrey (1990) described the disruption of the specific processes associated with memory impairment: semantic processing and speed of processing, as opposed to traditional quantitative distinctions that usually are documented. Several studies of memory functions in children with TBI were conducted by Levin et al. (1988), focusing on retrieval of newly learned words and on visual recognition. Bassett and Slater (1990) reported that adolescents with TBI demonstrated deficits in immediate and delayed recall of both verbal and visual information. Donders (1992) investigated immediate and delayed recall of a story and of a complex geometric figure in children with TBI and found that performance of participants with mild or moderate TBI tended to be superior to that of participants with severe TBI only for recall of the complex geometric figure. Donders and Woodward (2003) explored the possibility that gender has a moderating effect on memory after pediatric TBI. They studied 70 children with

TBI and 70 demographically matched control participants. The results showed that boys with TBI performed worse than girls with TBI and worse than their control group. However, gender differences were largely attenuated when speed of information processing was used as a covariate. The authors concluded that the effect of TBI on children's memory appears to be moderated by gender and may be mediated by speed of information processing. Farmer et al. (2002) examined the memory functioning of 25 children who had sustained TBI and who had prior learning problems with two control groups: (a) 48 children with TBI who had not had prior learning problems and (b) 23 healthy children. The children with TBI and prior learning problems displayed significantly worse memory abilities than both the control participants and the children with TBI and no prior learning problems. They differed significantly from the other two groups on measures of general memory, verbal memory, sound–symbol learning, and attention. The results suggest that children with premorbid learning problems who have sustained TBI have less cognitive reserve and a lower threshold for the expression of cognitive impairments in areas that reflect preexisting learning and language problems, compared with children without premorbid learning problems.

Executive Functions

Normal development of executive functions begins in infancy and continues throughout adolescence and into the young adult years (Welsh & Pennington, 1988). Furthermore, developments in the executive domains interact dynamically with other aspects of development and are modifiable with experience and training (Bjorklund, 1990; Tranel, Anderson, & Benson, 1995; Welsh & Pennington, 1988).

Mark Ylvisaker, one of the leading theorists in child cognitive functioning, has devoted much contemporary research to the study of executive functions; therefore, in the following paragraphs I cite his literature most often.

The frontal lobes and closely associated limbic regions of the brain have long been known to be most vulnerable in closed-head injury, the most common cause of TBI (Adams, Graham, Scott, Parker, & Doyle, 1980; Levin, Goldstein, Williams, & Eisenberg, 1991; Mendelsohn et al., 1992; Ylvisaker & DeBonis, 2000). Although several factors contribute to this vulnerability, the "bony prominence on the cribriform plate at the base of the frontal lobes" and the "frontal–temporal dissociation secondary to rotational inertial forces inside the skull" account for many of the injuries (Sohlberg, Mateer, & Stuss, 1993).

These neuropsychological vulnerabilities help explain the recurrent finding whereby impairments in executive function constitute the most debilitating disorder after TBI, thus causing the greatest hindrance to academic and social success (Ylvisaker & Freeney, 1995).

The executive system has traditionally been understood to include those mental functions involved in formulating goals, planning how to achieve them, and the carrying out of plans and strategically revising those plans in response to feedback (Lezak, 1982; Luria, 1966). The concept of executive functions is broader than, but closely related to, that of meta-cognitive functions (Ylvisaker & DeBonis, 2000). This is particularly the case when the latter term is broadened to include not only static knowledge of the operation of one's cognitive functions but also a disposition to use such knowledge to succeed when tasks pose difficulties (Flavell, Miller, & Miller, 1993).

The TBI rehabilitation literature has increasingly been dominated by discussions of executive system impairment, although there is no agreement as of yet about intervention strategies (Ylvisaker & DeBonis, 2000).

The assessment of executive function in children poses several formidable theoretical and practical challenges (Anderson, Anderson, Northam, Jacobs, & Mikiewicz, 2002). The majority of clinical measures of executive function have, until recent times, been designed primarily for an adult population. Numerous measures were thus rendered irrelevant for children and limited in their support of normative data. Furthermore, few measures facilitated the due identification and specification of the executive component, despite acknowledgments of the importance of such an approach. Two new instruments have recently been developed especially for children: (a) the Behavior Rating Inventory of Executive Function (Gioia, Isquith, Guy, & Kenworthy, 2000) and (b) the Behavioral Assessment of the Dysexecutive Syndrome in Children (Emslie, Wilson, Burden, Nimmon-Smith, & Wilson, 2003). Extensive research efforts to validate these two instruments with various children populations have been conducted (Anderson et al., 2002; Mahone, Cirono, et al., 2002; Mahone, Hagelthorn, et al., 2002; Mangeot, Armstrong, Colvin, Yeates, & Taylor, 2002; Vriezen & Pigott, 2002).

Awareness

Self-awareness of one's strengths and weaknesses is a critical component of executive functioning (Ylvisaker & DeBonis, 2000). This awareness pertains to any domain of functioning and is needed if one is to deal effectively with problems encountered in daily life. In addition, an understanding of the levels of difficulty in performing specific tasks is associated with self-awareness. Sherer et al. (1998) found that reasonably accurate self-awareness of strengths and weaknesses was strongly related to a return to daily occupations, such as work or vocationally oriented education.

Self-awareness alone does not, however, guarantee success in negotiating and completing tasks; instead, success appears to be contingent on additional executive functions being performed (Ylvisaker & DeBonis, 2000). Butler (1999), in a review of the concept of metacognition and its relation to learning disabilities, delineated the components of *meta-cognitive knowledge* and *meta-cognitive process*. Butler focused on meta-cognition as a framework for understanding effective strategy use in learning and for understanding why students with learning disabilities may fail to coordinate use of knowledge. (For more information about theories and mechanisms related to higher cognitive level functions, e.g., executive functions and awareness, see Chapter 1 of the present volume.)

MAIN CONCEPTS OF THE DYNAMIC INTERACTIONAL MODEL

Toglia's model (Toglia, 1992, 1998, see also Chapter 2 of the present volume) uses a broad definition of *cognition* that encompasses information-processing skills, learning, and generalization. Moreover, cognition is not merely divided into distinct entities; instead, cognitive abilities and deficiencies are analyzed according to underlying processes, strategies, and potential for learning. Awareness is a major component already acknowledged by rehabilitation professionals. Toglia and Kirk (2000) offered a comprehensive model of awareness to guide the development of assessment tools and interventions. In essence, cognition is viewed as an ongoing product of the dynamic interaction among the individual, the task, and the environment. Clinical application of this model provides essential information about individuals' potential for change and helps to answer the following questions: How promptly do individuals learn new material? How well do they retain it? How do they go about organizing new information? How do they proceed with decisions in response to environmental demands? How orderly and comprehensive are their problem-solving strategies?

The dynamic interactional model addresses learning potentials, analyzes individual processing strategies and style, and provides important guidelines for intervention. Implementing this elaborate method with children who have sustained brain injuries or learning disabilities may significantly advance researchers' understanding of the disorders and enhance their capacity for effective therapeutic intervention. (For an in-depth understanding of the dynamic interactional model, see Chapter 2, this volume.)

EVALUATION PROCESS AND INSTRUMENTS

The objectives of evaluating children with TBI are to identify and quantify cognitive deficits to make diagnoses, set intervention goals, build an intervention plan, monitor progress, and supervise family members and teachers (Toglia, 1989).

DIA is a recommended evaluation method for this population. In the next sections I describe assessment tools that have been adapted for use with children. The tools are basically the same as the descriptions given by Toglia in each test manual; however, the wording in the instructions and the cues were changed to suit children's level of understanding.

Toglia Category Assessment

Toglia (1994) designed the Toglia Category Assessment (TCA) to evaluate categorization abilities and the ability to switch conceptual sets among adults who had sustained brain injuries. Functional objects are used in this test. The respondent is asked three types of awareness questions before and after completing the test to determine awareness of his or her abilities: (a) two general awareness questions (the first requires a yes–no answer; the second requires choosing one of three possible answers), (b) two prediction questions asked before test administration, and (c) two estimation questions asked after test completion. The second and third types of questions require answers rated on a scale that ranges from 1 *(easy)* to 4 *(very difficult)*.

The second phase of the test requires the respondent to sort 18 plastic utensils according to three criteria: (a) size, (b) color, and (c) utensil type. After the respondent has sorted the utensils according to simple directions, he or she is then required to sort them in a different way. Cues (graded according to a standardized prompting schedule) are provided by the examiner for individuals who are unable to perform a correct categorization; these cues are dependent on the respondent's error pattern. The examiner determines the relationship between the respondent's performance prediction and estimate and his or her actual TCA score. Performance scores range from 1 *(unable to sort after reduction of amount of items)* to 11 *(sorting independently)*. A total score summing the three scores (for color, type, and size) is given (range, 1–33). In addition, the kind of sorting that was performed first, second, and last is recorded. Also included are scores for general awareness, self-prediction, and self-estimation, which can be related to the actual performance score on the TCA. The test is generally completed in approximately 25 min.

Deductive Reasoning Test

The Deductive Reasoning Test (DR) is administered after the TCA and involves a game requiring the respondent to ask questions regarding an item from the utensil set. The respondent is asked to determine which item from the set the evaluator is thinking about, by asking questions requiring only a "yes" or "no" answer. The respondent is told not to ask a specific, concrete question such as "Is it the green small fork?" and is advised to ask a minimum of questions. The DR, like the TCA, is administered in a dynamic–interactive mode, and cues are provided on a graded schedule. Scores range from 1 *(unable to determine the chosen item)* to 7 *(determines the chosen item by asking five or fewer questions)*. Each cue that is provided lowers the respondent's score. There are three trials in this test, and the final score is a sum of the scores obtained in the three trials. If a score of 7 is obtained twice, testing is discontinued, and the final score is 21. As in the TCA, awareness questions are divided into general awareness, prediction, and estimation questions (asked prior to and after testing).

Contextual Memory Test

The Contextual Memory Test (CMT; Toglia, 1993) measures aspects of memory and meta-memory. Two picture cards, each with 20 objects related to a theme (a restaurant theme or a morning theme) comprise this test. The respondent is shown one of the cards for 90 s and is then asked to name the objects seen, a test of immediate recall. After a 15-min interval, he or she is asked once again to name the objects he or she saw, a test of delayed recall. Forty cards from the same theme are used to evaluate recognition. Twenty cards are identical to the original, and the other 20 cards are similar, but not identical, to the original pictures.

General awareness is tested before and after the memory test. These questions include eight general awareness questions, two questions about self-prediction of memory capacity, and two self-estimation questions following testing. Scores are obtained for performance of immediate and delayed recall and for recognition of items as identical to the originals shown. Self-awareness scores include those for general awareness (range, 7–29), self-prediction (range,

0–20), and self-estimation (range, 0–20). Scores for recall are determined by the number of items remembered, with immediate and delayed recall scored separately (range, 0–20). Scores for recognition are determined by subtracting the number of false-positives from the number of correct answers. *False-positives* are items that the respondent identified incorrectly as having seen earlier on the test card. *True-positives* are items correctly recognized. Eight of the pictures have words on them, because words may improve memory performance. The strategy used by the respondent for remembering is explored as well.

Reliability and validity data for the TCA, DR, and CMT are presented in the section "Evidence-Based Research Supporting the Model." (Data for adults are presented in Chapter 2 of this book.)

Dynamic Occupational Therapy Cognitive Assessment

Recently, the Loewenstein Occupational Therapy Cognitive Assessment (Itzkovitch, Elazar, Averbuch, & Katz, 2000) was adapted for use with pediatric populations, and a dynamic system of cues was added based on the TCA with Toglia's permission. This new evaluation tool, the Dynamic Occupational Therapy Cognitive Assessment for Children (Katz, Parush, & Traub Bar-Ilan, in press), is appropriate for use within the dynamic interactional model. The battery includes 22 subtests in five areas: (a) orientation, (b) spatial perception, (c) praxis, (d) visuomotor construction, and (e) thinking operations. Scores on each subtest range from 1 *(low)* to 5 *(maximal performance)*. Area total scores are summed over the appropriate subtests. The test includes a baseline score, a mediation score (on a five-level cueing system), and a post-test score. Further description and instructions, as well as data on typical children ages 6 through 12 years (the target age range), is provided in the kit manual (Katz et al., in press). In comparing the performance of children with TBI and children with learning disabilities to typical children, significant differences were found on all subtests between each client group and typical children in Israel (Katz & Parush, 2001; Katz, Traub, & Parus, 2003), providing construct validity. All children groups showed improvement with the dynamic/mediation process, enabling evaluation of their potential (Katz et al., in press).

INTERVENTION PRINCIPLES

According to the dynamic interactional model, the role of the occupational therapist working with children with TBI is to evaluate, set intervention goals, provide appropriate intervention, perform ongoing re-evaluations, alter the course of intervention when appropriate, and produce comprehensive reports. Intervention principles include

- Dynamically develop a course of intervention, according to the child's progress.
- Observe and analyze strategies the child uses to process and organize information, and offer more efficient strategies (Ylvisaker & DeBonis, 2000).
- Consider the child's motivational level and personality characteristics.
- Commence intervention at the level of performance problems or when the child can successfully complete the task at hand, relying on up to three cues.
- Use intervention activities appropriate for the child's capabilities and interests.
- Increase task complexity only after observation of generalization at all levels of transfer.
- Use a uniform underlying strategy or conceptual characteristics in all intervention tasks (however, the task's surface characteristics gradually change as intervention moves from near transfer to intermediate and far transfer; Toglia, 1991).

- Relay definitions of the goals of each intervention activity to the child clearly and in concrete terms that he or she can understand.
- Use a spectrum of functional tasks in intervention, including gross motor, tabletop, functional, and computer. Avoid using one type of activity exclusively to ensure that the learned skills may still be accessible in relation to the specific context in which it was embedded (Toglia, 1991).
- Incorporate meta-cognitive training to promote awareness and self-monitoring skills in intervention sessions and in a variety of situations.
- Use both group and individual activities to help the child adapt to different environments.

Below I describe the intervention process through two case examples: Dana and David (discussed later in the chapter).

Evaluation

A battery of DIA assessments, including the CMT and TCA, was chosen to identify deficits and conditions that maximize performance.

Case Example 10.1. Dana

Dana was 15 years old and in the eighth grade. She was hospitalized in the pediatric intensive care unit after she was found unconscious at the foot of a building from which she had fallen after inhaling gas. The emergency team that arrived at the scene rated Dana 3 on the Glasgow Coma Scale. Her pupils responded to light, and her brain CT showed many skull fractures. She had epidural bleeding, a leakage of cerebrospinal fluid from her nose, a hematoma in her eye, fractured ribs, and a pulmonary contusion. She underwent craniotomia and hematoma drainage.

Dana was diagnosed with a diffuse axonal injury, with closed frontal and temporal skull fractures. While still in intensive care, Dana regained consciousness, and she began to speak, to walk with support, to partially control her bladder and bowel, and to eat and drink. She was transferred 1 week later to the pediatric ward, where her mother and other relatives spent most of their waking hours with her.

Dana began rehabilitation 2 weeks after her injury. She was able to walk without support; however, she needed constant supervision because of a tendency to lose her balance. She needed help transferring from sitting to standing. Dana's limbs were weakened, especially on her right (her dominant) side. Sensation remained intact.

In terms of activities of daily living, Dana needed supervision and slight help in drinking and cutting food and in dressing, washing, and bathroom needs. She presented a flat affect, with no facial mimicry, which was related, as a neurological diagnosis, to her extra-aperimedial, which was treated with medication.

Cognitively, Dana exhibited impulsivity in task performance; she did not express her desires or initiation. She had trouble scanning to organize visual information and had trouble creating categories and recalling by any memory channel. However, Dana was able, with verbal mediation and reminders,

to apply a strategy given to her by her therapist. In terms of awareness, Dana was partially oriented; however, she was somewhat confused. She had trouble telling her age and her telephone number, and she claimed she was left-handed while spontaneously reaching out with her right hand. However, Dana was oriented to time and knew where she was. She frequently said "I don't know" as an initial response to questions she was asked.

Dana's attention span was very short—a few moments—and she needed reminders and help with focusing to complete a task. Dana was unable to write at all. She had a tremor, and her motor control of a line was poor. She had difficulty copying basic shapes. Dana's reading was slow and not continuous. She recognized familiar words; however, she made mistakes in adding similar-sounding words. Dana also tired quickly.

This case example was provided by Sharon Zlotnik, an occupational therapist.

Awareness

Dana had little awareness of her abilities. When asked the awareness question of the CMT prior to the memory test, she claimed that she was unaware of any memory difficulties and chose a random answer to each question. After being given some options, she predicted that she would remember 11 (one of the options) out of 20 items to be presented to her.

Memory Abilities

In fact, Dana was able to recall only 9 of 20 items on the immediate-recall test and 7 on the delayed-recall test. After the test, she claimed that her memory was not as good as it had been prior to her injury, and she was able to estimate accurately that she had recalled 9 items on the immediate-recall test and 7 on the delayed-recall test. It should be noted that the average immediate-recall score for healthy adolescents is 12 items and for the delayed-recall test is 11 items.

Categorization

When showing the utensils of the TCA to Dana, she immediately responded, "This is easy, there are three colors here." When asked to sort them into groups, she left utensils out and only after being given a cue from the therapist was she able to sort all utensils into three groups of different colors. In her second sort, she started to classify according to the type of utensil but went back to sorting by color. The therapist provided two different cues, and only after being given those cues was Dana able to classify all utensils into three groups according to type. On the third sorting, Dana had difficulty seeing the option of classifying according to the size of utensils. She needed three cues before she was able to sort the utensils into two groups of large and small utensils. During the assessment sessions, Dana was responsive to cueing and was able to retain information and apply it to other assessment tasks that appeared different, as well as to improve the efficiency of her cognitive operations. After the testing, Dana was aware of her difficulties with the different classifications.

Summary of Evaluation Findings

Both Dana's memory abilities and her abilities to sort items were low for her age group and in the average range of adolescents with TBI. Dana's awareness of her difficulties was inappropriate before task performance but accurate following the performance, which suggests good chances for treatment outcomes. Functionally, Dana needed some practice to be able to perform activities of daily living independently (e.g., dressing, physical organization in the bathroom and while bathing, combing her hair), with minimal supervision. A spontaneous improvement was anticipated, especially in her posture and locomotive ability. Because of her problem in initiation, she needed opportunities in which she could choose among options and encouragement in simple decision making. In the areas of learning and academic functioning, Dana needed graphomotor practice in preparation for writing, combined with cognitive and meta-cognitive training in using strategies for attention, memory, information processing, and information organization.

Intervention

The goals of intervention were

1. Improving attentional functions, so that Dana could perform a continuous activity throughout the session, with no need for reminders
2. Encouraging Dana's ability to initiate, so that she could choose a game or activity and ways in which to perform the tasks, by herself, from several options
3. Improving her cognitive skills of strategy use to plan, remember, organize information, and reach conclusions; Dana should be able to initiate, plan, organize, and perform an activity in a continuous manner, according to stages
4. Improving Dana's writing and typing functions, so that she will be able to copy and produce a full paragraph from a text appropriate for her age, in legible handwriting and in typing, without mistakes
5. Improving meta-cognitive abilities, so that Dana could correctly estimate the level of difficulty of tasks and so that she could say which strategies she should use in order to complete a task and to check herself and correct mistakes while performing the task.

Intervention Plan

The intervention plan designed for Dana included

1. Combining fine motor and graphomotor activities, to prepare her for writing
2. Cognitive and meta-cognitive training in performing tasks that demand continuous and focused attention, visual memory, auditory memory, organization of visual information while copying, arrangement according to a logical sequence, reaching conclusions, and reasoning; for 2 weeks, Dana practiced on computer activities,

worksheets, and movement games (e.g., she learned how to discover the goal of a given game, looking for clues and using strategies for identifying what she had learned in a variety of situations and play activities).

Dana practiced giving instructions by reversing roles with the therapist to perform a brief task, such as giving game instructions. Dana also gave her mother an explanation as to the sequence of activities necessary to turn on and work the computer and how to enter the game file. The meta-cognitive intervention included feedback on performance and improvement of awareness and ability to check herself as well as demanding identification of the necessary strategies for completing the task.

Early in the intervention, Dana was asked about her interest areas and leisure activities, and it was discovered that she liked to design and sew Barbie doll clothes. Because her situation allowed for focusing on functional tasks, this interest area was used as a basis for global and multiple-staged activity. Using the activity of designing and sewing, Dana could practice using strategies that involved executive functions of initiation, planning, performing, and checking her performance. At the beginning of the process, Dana needed close monitoring and much help in formulating an idea before the actual task performance.

After she was given material and sewing tools, Dana immediately got to work cutting, without checking to see whether she was acting efficiently. She was surprised and disappointed to discover that nothing came of her efforts and chose to stop the activity altogether. Even after it was suggested to Dana that she should work in stages and plan them together with the therapist, she refused and asked to take the material and sewing tools to her room and to work alone.

At this stage, Dana went on her first vacation home from the hospital. When she returned, she was asked, using guided questions, to focus on her difficulties and abilities over the weekend as she saw them, as part of intervention of self-awareness. Dana spoke about her difficulty in remembering weakness and pain. In this way, intervention goals were refocused and a new "intervention contract" was made in which Dana became an active participant, carrying responsibility for the intervention.

It also was decided to combine sewing clothes with writing directions, which Dana would dictate to the therapist, so that other clients could enjoy them in the future. This matter stirred up much motivation and a feeling of purpose in Dana. It was agreed that Dana would type the instructions independently later, in the form of a PowerPoint pre-

sentation in her name. Dana needed a great deal of mediation to focus on the instructions she was giving and to organize them in a logical sequence. Throughout the process she needed demonstration by the therapist of how to carry out the instructions, to be able to identify to what degree they were precise and logical.

Conclusion of Intervention

Dana's intervention included 18 sessions; it was terminated before the end of the project, because she was transferred to another rehabilitation facility. By the end of the intervention, there was a significant improvement in Dana's ability to move around independently and in her self-care skills, to the point where she no longer needed assistance. Her handwriting improved greatly and was legible; however, there were still some mistakes, which Dana could identify and correct while writing. There was a significant improvement in her ability to write a sentence from memory and in memorizing instructions for an unfamiliar activity. An improvement was seen as well in her ability to stick with an activity. At this stage, Dana still showed difficulty in her ability to describe, provide details, and to direct precisely. Her use of short sentences and telegraphic communication was still evident and not in keeping with her cognitive ability to reach conclusions and be aware of her difficulties.

EVIDENCE-BASED RESEARCH SUPPORTING THE MODEL

Using the assessment tools developed in the DIA, I report on four studies in this section: (a) a study designed to establish construct-related validity of the TCA and the DR with typically developed children (Josman & Jarus, 2001), (b) a study in which the TCA was administered to children with and without brain injuries (Josman, Berney, & Jarus, 2000a), (c) a study in which the CMT was administered to children with and without brain injuries (Josman et al., 2000a), and (d) a study that introduced a meta-cognitive component to handwriting intervention in children (Josman, Sachein, & Sachs, 2004).

Josman and Jarus's (2001, 2003) study was designed to establish validity and reliability for the TCA and DR for use with children. The aim of this research was to establish construct-related validity for these tests, which were originally developed by Toglia (1994) for the assessment of adults experiencing brain injury. This study represents the first step in validating and adapting the two tests for typically developing children.

The study population consisted of 235 typically developing children, ages 5 through 11, including 112 boys (47.7%) and 123 girls (52.3%). For all children, written parental permission was given for inclusion in the study. The sample was divided into six age groups of varying sizes, the smallest being the group of 5-year-olds ($n = 22$) and the largest the group of 6-year-olds ($n = 71$). The number of boys and girls in each age group differed; however, no significant differences in test scores between boys and girls were found in the t-test analysis. Both the TCA and the DR were administered to all participants.

The results indicated statistically significant differences in the mean performance of children in various age groups, both on the TCA and the DR assessments, but did not show differences among all the age groups. A significant main effect of age was observed in regard to the performance of children, $F(5, 229) = 11.23, p < .001$. Performance of the three older age groups (8- to 11-year-olds) was more accurate than performance of the youngest age group (5-year-olds), and the two older age groups (9- to 11-year-olds) performed more accurately than the 6- and 7-year-olds.

The results indicated a significant main effect of the parameter of categorization, $F(2, 458) = 28.04, p < .001$. Children performed more accurate categorization according to color ($M = 9.39, SD = 2.6$) and type ($M = 9.51, SD = 2.49$) than according to size ($M = 7.88, SD = 3.09$).

Children could not predict their ability in both tests, but most of them were able to estimate their ability following the actual performance of the TCA. Children's predictive ability is based on their capacity to focus on and recall situations similar to that in which they are now being asked to perform and, on the basis of that knowledge, to predict how they will succeed on the test about to be tackled. The ability to estimate, on the other hand, is based on the activity just completed. Thus, it is feasible to hypothesize that estimation ability would be somewhat easier for children insofar as their awareness is enhanced once an activity is performed.

Josman and Jarus (2001, 2003) concluded that the findings of this study provide evidence to support the suitability of the TCA and the DR for use with children. They recommended that both tools be further studied so as to amplify their validity.

Josman et al. (2000a) investigated categorization skills in children following severe brain injury using the TCA. They also explored the capacity to switch conceptual sets, as well as the ability of the TCA to differentiate both between children with brain injuries and typically developing children and between age groups.

The study population was composed of 30 children with severe brain injury, ages 8 through 14 years, and a control group of 30 typically developing children, matched for age and gender. The children in the former group were tested at least 10 months after the onset of their injury. The TCA was administered individually to each child. The results showed that children performed more accurately on categorization according to color ($M = 9.78, SD = 2.19$) and type ($M = 10.17, SD = 1.29$) than according to size ($M = 8.31, SD = 2.71$). Age influenced performance ($p < .05$); the older subgroup (11–14.5 years) performed more accurately ($M = 9.84, SD = 1.82$) than the younger subgroup (8.5–10.11 years; $M = 9.0, SD = 2.31$). Diagnosis group also influenced performance, with typically developing children performing significantly better ($M = 10.08, SD = 1.48$) than children with brain injuries ($M = 8.76, SD = 2.65$), $F(1, 56) = 11.30, p < .001$.

The findings of this study show that typically developing children perform significantly better than do children with brain injuries. The TCA significantly differentiated between children with brain injury and those who are typically developing on all TCA scores at $p < .0001$. In addition, the TCA significantly differentiated between the younger and the older subgroups. This study supports the use of the TCA in assessing children with brain injuries. The discriminant validity of the TCA, which is part of construct validity, was supported by its ability to differentiate among the research groups and ages. Interrater reliability, internal consistency, and concurrent validity already have been established for the TCA (Josman, 1999).

Josman et al. (2000b) studied the performance of children with and without TBI on the CMT, which measures aspects of memory and meta-memory in children. The authors also examined the ability of the CMT to differentiate between children with and without TBI. The same sample as in the previous study (i.e., Josman et al., 2000a) was studied. Thirty children with severe brain injury (ages 8–14 years) and 30 typically developing children (matched for age and gender) participated. The participants were divided according to age into two groups: (a) children (8.5–10.11 years) and (b) adolescents (11–14.5 years). All of the children with brain injury were tested at least 10 months after their injury had been incurred. All participants were evaluated individually.

The results revealed that typically developing children performed better than children with brain injury on the immediate- ($M = 12.23, SD = 1.85$) and delayed-recall tests ($M = 11.06, SD = 1.89$), with no between-groups difference on the recognition test. However, the children with brain injuries improved more from the immediate- and delayed-memory tests to the recognition test than did the typically developing children.

The correlations between general awareness and memory performance components were low for both groups ($r = .20$ for the research group and $r = .26$ for the comparison group). This means that children and young adolescents have difficulties answering general questions about their memory abilities, a fact that needs to be further investigated.

Comparisons among the prediction of the number of items to be remembered, the actual number of items remembered in the immediate-recall test, and estimations of the number of items remembered revealed an overestimation by the research group. As a group, the children with brain injuries predicted that they would remember an average of 11 out of 20 items but actually remembered an average of only 9 items. They correctly estimated they had remembered 9. The opposite picture was obtained for the comparison group, who underestimated their memory performance. The children predicted they would remember a mean of 11 items, actually remembered a mean of 12 items, and estimated that they had remembered a mean of 11.8 items. A chi-square analysis revealed a significant difference between the groups ($p = .01$). No differences were found between age groups.

The study results show that typically developing children perform better on tests of immediate and delayed recall than do children with brain injuries, although there was no difference on the test of recognition. These results support the discriminant validity of the CMT for children with and without brain injury.

Although these three studies relate to assessment instruments developed for the dynamic interactional model, the next study looked at the effectiveness of intervention.

Cognitive approaches are applicable to pediatric populations other than children with brain injuries. Josman et al. (2004) investigated the contribution of a meta-cognitive approach, integrated with a traditional perceptual–motor approach, for children with handwriting problems. A single-case study examined the influence of both approaches, meta-cognitive and perceptual–motor, in intervention for handwriting problems in 4 boys (2 in the second grade and 2 in the third grade). The study's design allowed for the systematic measurement of individual changes in each child's handwriting. Assessment tools used in this study included the HHE (Erez & Parush, 1999), the Purdue Pegboard Test (Tiffin, 1960), and awareness questions developed for this study based on the

CMT (Toglia, 1993). The case example of David outlines the process with 1 child in the study.

The results showed that all children improved in fine motor skills and in handwriting skills over the course of intervention, most significantly after the combined PMI and meta-cognitive intervention. The results also indicated that efficient performance on the Purdue Pegboard Test did not necessarily correlate with efficient handwriting, as examined by the HHE, and vice versa. The differences between the results of the Purdue after each type of intervention indicated that all 4 children improved after the two types of intervention on dominant-hand scores; however, the average improvement was greater after the combined intervention than after the PMI.

Analysis of the nondominant-hand scores for all 4 children after each type of intervention revealed similar results. They all improved in their performance in the two types of interventions; however, the combined intervention produced a greater mean improvement.

Three of the children (other than 1 who showed no change after the PMI) improved in their performance with two hands together on the two types of intervention. However, the combined intervention yielded greater improvement than the PMI. The general score on the Purdue for the 4 children on the two types of intervention indicated that there was greater mean improvement after the combined intervention than after the PMI (other than 1 child who had identical levels of mean improvement).

The scores on the HHE were determined according to five categories: (a) number of letters written in 1 min, (b) total time taken to write a text, (c) number of erasures and corrections, (d) number of unidentifiable letters, and (e) spatial organization on the page. Measurements were taken after each of three phases (prior to intervention, after the first type of intervention, and after the second type of intervention).

The number of letters copied in 1 min improved after each of the three phases for all of the children, more after the combined intervention than after the motor intervention. The child who began with the highest number of letters copied improved more in this area than did the other children.

All four children improved their copying speed after each of the three phases; for all children, this was greater after the combined intervention. The child whose writing speed was slowest before intervention remained the slowest after completing intervention. However, he, like the other children, copied the text more quickly on comple-

Case Example 10.2. David

David is an 8-year, 3-month-old boy in the third grade, and he has one older brother. At the end of first grade, his teacher identified handwriting difficulties that were manifested by poor organization, poor pencil grasp, and slow writing speed. The school psychologist referred David to occupational therapy. David's language abilities were age appropriate, and he performed at an average level relative to his classmates. A single-case study design was used to examine the contribution of a meta-cognitive approach, integrated with a traditional perceptual–motor approach, in handwriting rehabilitation. The design was comprised of a baseline (A), intervention (B), assessment (A), intervention (C), and assessment (A) (an A,B,A,C,A design; Ottenbacher, 1986).

David was assessed (baseline A) in occupational therapy using the Hebrew Handwriting Evaluation (HHE; Erez & Parush, 1999); the Purdue Pegboard Test (Tiffin, 1960); and awareness questions developed specifically for handwriting difficulties, which were based on those included in the CMT (Toglia, 1993). In addition, David was asked to write his first and last names, as well as his home address, at the beginning of every second session. This handwriting task was analyzed according to two criteria in the HHE, unrecognizable letters and spatial arrangement, and proved a useful indicator of change within the intervention process.

After the evaluation, David received perceptual–motor intervention (PMI; intervention B) for 2 1/2 months (10 sessions). During the first 3 sessions, the emphasis was placed on improving basic fine motor skills of the hands and fingers, including in-hand manipulation; using Theraplast, plasticine, and Play Doh; placing different-sized stickers, stringing beads, building with blocks, and so on. In Sessions 4 and 5, David was given motor training on a higher level, which included coloring large and small areas, cutting, and pasting. Intervention tools included worksheets, different coloring tools, and scissors. In Sessions 6 and 7, David was given complex fine motor training, which included copying and building models with different types of

pegs, buttons, and so on. The three final sessions (8–10) comprised specific work on pencil grip, pressure control, quality of the line drawn, using work sheets, mazes, copying using carbon paper, and so on.

During this time, David's handwriting problems, work strategies, and the importance of the various activities to handwriting were not discussed. The directions for the various activities and tasks over the course of intervention were focused and specific to what needs to be done here and now (e.g., "I would like you to try to copy the model in front of you. Take care to work using your first three fingers, and try to be precise in copying."). If David asked a question such as "Why must I do this?" a general answer was given ("To improve things that are hard for you at home and in school"). David was not an active partner in planning the intervention or in choosing the tools used.

At this point, David was reassessed (assessment A) using the initial assessment tools, after which he received an intervention that combined PMI and meta-cognitive approaches (intervention C) for 2½ additional months (10 sessions). This intervention focused on raising his awareness of his handwriting problems, cooperative selection of correct work strategies, and discussing the importance of the various activities for improving these problems.

The interventions were graded such that each 7 to 14 days, a slightly more challenging task was given, each according to David's progress and abilities. In addition, the various strategies were memorized and practiced over the course of the intervention.

During the first session, the main difficulties that David encountered at home and in school were discussed. The discussion consisted of dialogue and the use of directed questions (on the part of the therapist), such as, Do you like to do homework? What about homework is hard for you? Do you write long answers? If not, why? Do you copy everything that your teacher writes on the blackboard? Do you have enough time to answer all the questions on tests? The therapist made it clear to David

that the subject of handwriting would be central to their cooperative work in the coming sessions. Session 2 consisted of cooperative thinking about what is needed for writing and why David was having handwriting problems. For example, he was asked what is difficult for him about writing, and he answered that he tires quickly and his hand hurts. The reasons for these symptoms were discussed, for example, weak wrist and fingers, regulating strong pressure on the pencil, improper pencil grip, and so on.

During Sessions 3 and 4, the main points of the discussions of the previous sessions were repeated. The therapist chose an activity, and before and during the activity she discussed with David, on a general level, its importance for writing. In Sessions 5 and 6, the discussion about handwriting was more specific, and David chose the activity on his own, with little help from the therapist. During the activity, the therapist reflected the strategy used to work on the problem to David and encouraged him to repeat what she said ("What did we say this works on?"). Session 7 consisted of repeating all that had been said previously. David chose the activity independently and reflected how he was working on his problem with mild cues from the therapist, such as "Why did we say it's best to work mainly with the first three fingers?" and performed a self-examination and self-questioning vis-à-vis the quality of his task performance.

During the last three sessions (8–10), David independently named everything he had learned up to that point. He chose the activity independently and explained which work strategy he was using, its importance to handwriting, and how it is similar to other strategies that had been chosen in the past. During task completion, David performed a self-examination and asked himself questions about the quality of his performance (with slight help from the therapist).

David was reassessed (assessment A) once more on termination of the intervention. David's Purdue scores showed improvement in each hand alone and in both hands together throughout the intervention period. There was greater improvement for

(continued)

Case Example 10.2.   David (Continued)

each hand alone at the end of the combined PMI and meta-cognitive intervention. Improvement for performance of two hands together was identical after both types of intervention; however, overall, David improved much more after the combined intervention than after the PMI alone (B). David's HHE scores showed improvement in the number of letters he wrote in 1 min after each type of intervention, but more so after the combined intervention (C), with a smaller change in overall length of time. There was an increase in the number of erasures and rewritten letters after the PMI; however, there was a decrease after

the combined intervention. There were slightly fewer unidentifiable letters, and there was an improvement in David's general organizational score, more so after the combined intervention than after the PMI. David showed greater improvement after the combined intervention on four measures (number of letters, overall time, unidentifiable letters, and organization on the page). He showed a greater improvement on one measure—number of erasures and rewritten letters—after the PMI.

Analysis of the awareness questions revealed that David felt that he had a slight

handwriting problem before the intervention, which demonstrates a certain level of awareness; however, objectively, he had severe handwriting problems at this stage. After completing the intervention program, David felt he no longer had a handwriting problem and, objectively, he had improved greatly and had at this stage only a slight handwriting problem. In other words, David's general level of awareness was higher after completing intervention than prior to its commencement (Josman et al., 2004).

This case example was provided by Sharon Zlotnik, an occupational therapist.

tion of intervention than prior to the intervention. The combined intervention yielded a greater decrease in writing time than the PMI did.

The number of erasures and corrections after each of the two intervention phases was not uniform for the 4 children: One child's number of erasures and corrections increased after the second phase and then decreased after the third phase (regardless of type of intervention); another child showed an increase at the end of intervention, relative to his starting point; and 2 children improved the number of erasures and corrections they made after intervention was terminated, relative to their starting points. The differences in the five test scores for the 4 children after the two types of intervention reveal that the results were consistent, relative to the number of erasures and corrections of each of the participants. They each showed an increased number of erasures and corrections between the first and second types of intervention and a decrease after the second type of intervention. There was an average rise of 1 erasure/correction after the combined intervention and an average decrease of 0.75 erasures after the motor intervention. This result also can be explained by an increase in awareness on the part of the child: Once the child is more aware of his handwriting mistakes, he corrects them.

Two of the children demonstrated a decrease in the number of unrecognizable letters after the first phase (combined intervention); however, after the second phase (motor intervention), this rose. The other children showed a decrease in the number of unrecognizable letters after both phases, more so after the combined phase.

There was a greater decrease in the number of unidentifiable letters after the combined intervention than after the PMI, for all children. All children improved in their spatial organization ability over the course of the intervention, more so after the combined intervention than after the PMI.

The awareness questionnaire included three parts: (a) 7 general questions about the child's handwriting functioning in school, (b) 9 predictive questions about his ability to copy a text, and (c) 10 questions estimating his performance when copying a text. The first question, "Do you prefer to read or to write?" yielded nonuniform results throughout the intervention, relative to the children's initial answers. The second question, "Do you like to write?" showed a positive change for 3 of the children throughout the intervention, relative to their initial answers (this change occurred after the PMI).

The next 5 questions related to the time required to copy from the blackboard and to take a test, fatigue, effort while writing, and legibility. The answers of each of the 4 children were summarized after each intervention phase. Scores ranged from 5 to 25 points. Children with lower scores felt that their handwriting problem was milder. The results for the 4 children were not uniform, and they cannot be related to the type of intervention received.

To analyze the predictive questions, 4 main questions were chosen and matched to the performance norms of the HHE (for second and third graders). This was done to compare the children's level of awareness vis-à-vis their actual performance. One global score was attained, ranging from 4 *(good handwriting ability)* to 16 *(poor handwriting ability)*. Three categories were determined: 4–8 *(mild handwriting problem)*, 9–12 *(moderate handwriting problem)*, and 13–16 *(severe handwriting problem)*.

No uniform correlation was found between level of the children's awareness and type of intervention (combined or motor) received. It must be noted that all 4 children never predicted or estimated themselves worse than their actual performance; instead, their predictions were better than their performance.

All 4 children were asked to write their name and address at the beginning of each intervention session, for additional measurement of their handwriting and to more closely monitor their handwriting. All of the children improved in the components measured (number of unidentifiable letters and spatial organization on the page) throughout the intervention; however, the greatest improvement took place after the combined intervention.

Several analyses were performed to examine the correlation between improvement on the Purdue and improvement on the HHE, for each of the 4 children. An efficient performance on the Purdue did not necessarily correlate with an efficient performance on the HHE, and vice versa. This lack of consistency was found in other measures, such as performance on both hands together, organization, legibility, and number of erasures.

The results of this study, which focused on improvement in the handwriting of children with handwriting problems using a meta-cognitive intervention, led to the conclusion that there is a place for this type of intervention in addition to PMI approaches. This study used a single-case design. Because the results cannot be generalized to a wider population, and the generalization can be made only when speaking of an exact replication of the population, the results need to be replicated using this method (i.e., single-case design) on additional groups of children. In addition, other accepted methods should be used on a larger sample of children.

SUMMARY AND DIRECTIONS FOR FUTURE RESEARCH

In this chapter, I have endorsed adopting the dynamic interactional approach for evaluating and treating children with TBI. Toglia (1992) originally developed this approach for use with adults who had incurred brain injury, and in this chapter I have shown that this approach, including assessment tools and intervention procedures, can successfully be applied to children with brain injuries as well as to children with handwriting difficulties.

Few standardized tests of cognitive functions exist for children with brain injuries. The tools that have been adapted for use with this population need to be tested on larger samples, to increase the strength of the data and to establish norms for different age groups and disabled population. Through this process, the evidence base of using Toglia's assessment tools within children will be supported.

I also reported on an intervention program for handwriting difficulties with the dynamic interactional model of cognitive rehabilitation; this was accompanied by research using single-case study design. This study should be repeated with other therapists and with more children, and then a large group comparison study should be conducted to support the use of dynamic interactional intervention and to add to the evidence base of this approach.

REVIEW QUESTIONS

1. What kinds of cognitive problems do children who have sustained brain injuries experience?
2. What kinds of questions does a clinical application of the dynamic interactional model help answer?
3. What kinds of information can be gleaned by implementing the dynamic interactional model and assessment tools?
4. Which of the assessment tools have been adapted and tested for use with a population of children with brain injuries? What do they examine, and what outcomes resulted from studies of these tools?

ACKNOWLEDGMENT

Thanks to occupational therapist Sharon Zlotnik for providing the case examples.

REFERENCES

Adams, J. H., Graham, D. I., Scott, G., Parker, L. S., & Doyle, D. (1980). Brain damage in fatal non-missile head injury. *Journal of Clinical Pathology, 33,* 1132–1145.

Anderson, V. A., Anderson, P., Northam, E., Jacobs, R., & Mikiewicz, O. (2002). Relationships between cognitive and behavioral measures of executive function in children with brain disease. *Child Neuropsychology, 8,* 231–240.

Anderson, V., Fenwick, T., Manly, T., & Robertson, I. (1998). Attentional skills following traumatic brain injury in childhood: A compotential analysis. *Brain Injury, 12,* 937–949.

Balskey, J., & Jennings, M. (1999). Traumatic brain injury. In S. Campbell (Ed.), *Decision making in pediatric neurologic physical therapy* (pp. 84–140). New York: Churchill Livingstone.

Basset, S. S., & Slater, E. J. (1990). Neuropsychological function in adolescents sustaining mild closed head injury. *Journal of Pediatric Psychology, 15,* 225–236.

Bjorklund, D. F. (1990). *Children strategies: Contemporary views of cognitive development.* Hillsdale, NJ: Lawrence Erlbaum.

Brown, G., Chedwick, O., Shaffer, D., Rutter, M., & Traub, M. (1981). A prospective study of children with head injury III: Psychiatric sequalae. *Psychological Medicine, 11,* 63–78.

Butler, D. L. (1999). Metacognition and learning disabilities. In B. Y. L. Wong (Ed.), *Learning about learning disabilities* (pp. 277–307). New York: Academic Press.

Chadwick, O., Rutter, M., Shaffer, D., & Shrout, P. (1981). A prospective study of children with head injury: Specific cognitive deficits. *Journal of Clinical Neuropsychology, 3,* 101–120.

Costeff, H., Groswasswer, Z., & Goldstein, R. (1990). Long term follow-up with severe closed head trauma. *Journal of Neurosurgery, 73,* 684–687.

Coster, W. (1998). Occupational-centered assessment of children. *American Journal of Occupational Therapy, 52,* 337–344.

Cratty, B. J. (1994). *Clumsy child syndromes, descriptions, evaluation and remediation.* Longhorne, PA: Harwood Academic.

Cronin, A. F. (2001). Traumatic brain injury in children: Issues in community function. *American Journal of Occupational Therapy, 55,* 377–384.

Dalby, P. R., & Obrzut, J. E. (1991). Epidemiologic characteristics and sequelae of closed-head-injured children and adolescents: A review. *Developmental Neuropsychology, 7,* 35–68.

Donders, J. (1992). Memory functioning after traumatic brain injury in children. *Brain Injury, 7,* 429–437.

Donders, J., & Woodward, H. R. (2003). Gender as moderator of memory after traumatic brain injury in children. *Journal of Head Trauma Rehabilitation, 18,* 106–115.

Emslie, H., Wilson, F. C., Burden, V., Nimmon-Smith, I., & Wilson, B. A. (2003). *Behavioral Assessment of the Dysexecutive Syndrome in Children (BADS-C).* St. Edmunds, England: Thames Valley Test Company.

Erez, N., & Parush, S. (1999). *The Hebrew Handwriting Evaluation* (2nd ed.). Jerusalem: School of Occupational Therapy, Faculty of Medicine, Hebrew University of Jerusalem.

Farmer, J. E., Kanne, S. M., Haut, J. S., Williams, J., Johnstone, B., & Krik, K. (2002). Memory functioning following traumatic brain injury in children with premorbid learning problems. *Developmental Neuropsychology, 22,* 455–469.

Flavell, J. H., Miller, P. H., & Miller, S. A. (1993). *Cognitive development* (3rd ed.). Englewood Cliffs, NJ: Prentice Hall.

Gioia, G. A., Isquith, P. K., Guy, S. C., & Kenworthy, L. (2000). Behavior Rating Inventory of Executive Function. *Child Neuropsychology, 6,* 235–238.

Goldstein, F. C., Levin, H. S., Boake, C., & Lohrey, J. H. (1990). Facilitation of memory performance through induced semantic processing in survivors of severe closed-head injury. *Journal of Clinical and Experimental Neuropsychology, 12,* 286–300.

Hamstra-Bletz, L., & Blote, A. (1993). A longitudinal study on dysgraphic handwriting in primary school. *Journal of Learning Disability, 26,* 689–699.

Itzkovitch, M., Elazar, B., Averbuch, S., & Katz, N. (2000). *Loewenstein Occupational Therapy Cognitive Assessment (LOTCA) battery manual.* Pequannock, NJ: Maddak.

Johnson, D. J. (1995). An overview of learning disabilities: Psychoeducational perspectives. *Journal of Child Neurology, 10,* S2–S5.

Josman, N. (1999). Reliability and validity of the Toglia Category Assessment (TCA). *Canadian Journal of Occupational Therapy, 66,* 33–42.

Josman, N., Berney, T., & Jarus, T. (2000a). Evaluating categorization skills in children following severe brain injury. *Occupational Therapy Journal of Research, 20,* 241–255.

Josman, N., Berney, T., & Jarus, T. (2000b). Performance of children with and without traumatic brain injury on the Contextual Memory Test (CMT). *Physical and Occupational Therapy in Pediatrics, 19,* 39–51.

Josman, N., & Jarus, T. (2001). Construct-related validity of the Toglia Category Assessment and the Deductive Reasoning Test with children who are typically developing. *American Journal of Occupational Therapy, 55,* 524–530.

Josman, N., & Jarus, T. (2003). Construct-related validity of the Toglia Category Assessment and the Deductive Reasoning Test with children who are typically developing. In C. B. Royeen (Ed.), *Pediatric issues in occupational therapy* (pp. 108–117). Bethesda, MD: American Occupational Therapy Association.

Josman, N., Sachein, A., & Sachs, D. (2004). *Introducing metacognitive component to handwriting intervention in children: A single case study design research.* Manuscript submitted for publication.

Katz, N., & Parush, S. (2001). *LOTCA for children: Comparison of children with learning disabilities and controls.* Paper presented at the American Occupational Therapy Association Conference, Philadelphia.

Katz, N., Parush, S., & Traub Bar-Ilan, R. (in press). *Dynamic Occupational Therapy Cognitive Assessment for children (DOTCA–Ch).* Pequannock, NJ: Maddak.

Katz, N., Traub, R., & Parus, S. (2003). *Dynamic Occupational Therapy Cognitive Assessment for children (DOTCA–Ch): Performance of brain-injured children.* Paper presented at the 2nd Congress of the International Society of Physical Rehabilitation Medicine, Prague.

Kinsella, G. J., Pirior, M., Sawyer, M., Ong, B., Murtagh, D., Eisenmajer, R., et al. (1997). Predictors and indicators of academic outcome in children 2 years following traumatic brain injury. *Journal of the International Neuropsychological Society, 3,* 608–616.

Kramer, P., & Hinojosa, J. (1999). *Frames of reference for pediatric occupational therapy* (2nd ed.). Baltimore: Lippincott Williams & Wilkins.

Levin, H. S., Goldstein, F. C., Williams, D. H., & Eisenberg, H. M. (1991). The contribution of frontal lobe lesion to the neurobehavioral outcome of closed-head injury. In H. S. Levin, H. M. Eisenberg, & A. I. Benton (Eds.), *Frontal-lobe function and disfunction* (pp. 318–338). New York: Oxford University Press.

Levin, H. S., High, W. M., Ewing-Cobbs, L., Fletcher, J. M., Eisenberg, H. M., Miner, M. E., & Goldstein, F. C. (1988). Memory functioning during the first year after closed-head injuries in children and adolescents. *Neurosurgery, 22,* 1043–1052.

Lezak, M. D. (1982). The problem of assessing executive functions. *International Journal of Psychology, 17,* 281–297.

Luria, A. R. (1966). *Higher cortical function in man.* New York: Basic Books.

Mahone, E. M., Cirino, P. T., Cutting, L. E., Cerrone, P. M., Hagelthorn, K. M., Hiemenz, J. R., et al. (2002). Validity of the Behavior Rating Inventory of Executive Function in children with ADHD and/or Tourette syndrome. *Archives of Clinical Neuropsychology, 17,* 643–662.

Mahone, E. M., Hagelthorn, K. M., Cutting, J., Schuerholz, L. J., Pelletier, S. F., Rawlins, C., et al. (2002). Effects of IQ on executive function measures in children with ADHD. *Child Neuropsychology, 8,* 52–65.

Mangeot, S., Armstrong, K., Colvin, A. N., Yeates, K. O., & Taylor, H. G. (2002). Long-term executive function deficits in children with traumatic brain injury: Assessment using the Behavior Rating Inventory of Executive Function (BRIEF). *Child Neuropsychology, 8,* 271–284.

Mendelsohn, D., Levin, H. S., Bruce, D., Lilly, M. A., Harward, H., Culhane, K., et al. (1992). Late MRI after head injury in children: Relationship to clinical features and outcome. *Child's Nervous System, 8,* 445–452.

Missiuna, C., Malloy-Miller, T., & Mandich, A. (1998). Mediational techniques: Origins and application to occupational therapy in pediatrics. *Canadian Journal of Occupational Therapy, 65,* 202–209.

Ottenbacher, K. J. (1986). *Evaluating clinical change: Strategies for occupational and physical therapists.* Baltimore: William & Wilkins.

Porr, S. (1999). Children with traumatic brain injury. In S. Porr & E. Rainville (Eds.), *Pediatric therapy: A system approach* (pp. 525–544). Philadelphia: F. A. Davis.

Rosenblum, S., Parush, S., & Weiss, P. L. (2003). Computerized temporal handwriting characteristics of proficient and poor handwriters. *American Journal of Occupational Therapy, 57,* 129–138.

Scott, A., & Dow, P. (1995). Traumatic brain injury. In C. Trombley (Ed.), *Occupational therapy for physical dysfunction* (4th ed., pp. 705–733). Baltimore: Williams & Wilkins.

Sherer, M., Bergloff, P., Levin, E., High, W. H., Oden, K. E., & Nick, T. G. (1998). Impaired awareness and employment outcome after traumatic brain injury. *Journal of Head Trauma Rehabilitation, 13,* 52–61.

Sohlberg, M. M., Mateer, C. A., & Stuss, D. T. (1993). Contemporary approaches to the management of executive control dysfunction. *Journal of Head Trauma Rehabilitation, 8,* 45–58.

Telzrow, C. F. (1987). Management of academic and educational problems in head injury. *Journal of Learning Disabilities, 20,* 536–545.

Tiffin, J. (1960). *The Purdue Pegboard Test manual.* Lafayette, IN: Lafayette Instrument.

Toglia, J. P. (1989). Approaches to cognitive assessment of the brain-injured adult: Traditional methods and dynamic investigation. *Occupational Therapy Practice, 1,* 36–57.

Toglia, J. (1991). Generalization of treatment: A multicontext approach to cognitive perceptual impairment in adults with brain injury. *American Journal of Occupational Therapy, 45,* 505–516.

Toglia, J. P. (1992). A dynamic interactional approach to cognitive rehabilitation. In N. Katz (Ed.), *Cognitive rehabilitation: Models for intervention in occupational therapy* (pp. 104–143). Boston: Andover Medical.

Toglia, J. P. (1993). *Contextual Memory Test manual.* Tucson, AZ: Therapy SkillBuilders.

Toglia, J. P. (1994). *Dynamic assessment of categorization: TCA—The Toglia Category Assessment.* Pequannock, NJ: Maddak.

Toglia, J. P. (1998). A dynamic interactional model to cognitive rehabilitation. In N. Katz (Ed.), *Cognition and occupation in rehabilitation* (pp. 5–50). Bethesda, MD: American Occupational Therapy Association.

Toglia, J., & Kirk, U. (2000). Understanding awareness deficits following brain injury. *NeuroRehabilitation, 15,* 57–70.

Tranel, D., Anderson, S. W., & Benson, A. (1995). Development of the concept of "executive function" and its relations to the frontal lobes. In F. Boller & J. Grafman (Eds.), *Handbook of neuropsychology* (pp. 125–148). Amsterdam: Elsevier.

Vriezen, E. R., & Pigott, S. E. (2002). The relationship between parental report on the BRIEF and performance-based measures of executive function in children with moderate to severe traumatic brain injury. *Child Neuropsychology, 8,* 296–303.

Waber, D. P., & Bernstein, J. H. (1994). Repetitive graphomotor output in learning disabled and nonlearning disabled children: The Repeated Patterns Test. *Developmental Neuropsychology, 10,* 51–65.

Welsh, M. C., & Pennington, B. F. (1988). Assessing frontal-lobe functioning in children: Views from developmental psychology. *Developmental Neuropsychology, 4,* 199–230.

Winkler, P. (1995). Head injury. In D. Umphred (Ed.), *Neurological rehabilitation* (3rd ed., pp. 421–453). St. Louis, MO: Mosby.

Ylvisaker, M. (1998). *Traumatic brain injury rehabilitation* (2nd ed.). Boston: Butterworth-Heinemann.

Ylvisaker, M., & DeBonis, D. (2000). Executive function impairment in adolescence: TBI and ADHD. *Topics in Language Disorders, 20,* 29–57.

Ylvisaker, M., & Freeney, T. (1995). Traumatic brain injury in adolescence: Assessment and reintegration. *Seminars in Speech and Language, 16,* 32–44.

11

Sharon A. Cermak, EdD, OTR/L, FAOTA

Cognitive Rehabilitation of Children With Attention-Deficit/Hyperactivity Disorder

LEARNING OBJECTIVES

By the end of this chapter, readers will
1. Understand the characteristics of ADHD and their impact on participation
2. Identify methods and instruments for the assessment of ADHD
3. Understand and appreciate the importance of executive function in children with ADHD
4. Understand current intervention research with children with ADHD
5. Explain the application of the cognitive–mediational and dynamic interaction model with children with ADHD.

Attention-deficit/hyperactivity disorder (ADHD) is a neurological condition that includes difficulty with attention and hyperactivity–impulsivity. Children with ADHD typically exhibit behavior that has been classified into two main categories: (a) poor sustained attention and (b) hyperactivity–impulsivity. There are three subtypes of the disorder (American Psychiatric Association [APA], 1994, 2000): (a) predominantly inattentive, (b) predominantly hyperactive–impulsive, and (c) combined types. The combined type is the most prevalent.

ADHD commonly occurs in conjunction with other conditions; the current literature indicates that approximately 40% to 60% of children with ADHD have at least one co-existing disability (Barkley, 1998; Jensen, Martin, & Cantwell, 1997; Jensen et al., 2001). Although any disability can coexist with ADHD, certain disorders are more common than others. Almost one-third of all children with ADHD have learning disabilities (National Institute of Mental Health [NIMH], 1999), including difficulty in reading, math, written communication, or some combination of these (Anderson, Williams, McGee, & Silva, 1987; Cantwell & Baker, 1991; Dykman, Akerman, & Raney, 1994; Jensen et al., 2001; Zentall, 1993). Additional problems common in children with ADHD include anxiety, depression, and oppositional–defiant disorder. Occupational therapists have noted that a high percentage of children with ADHD also show disorders of sensory integration (Dunn & Bennett, 2002; Mangeot et al., 2001; Mulligan,

1996; Parush et al., 1997; Tseng, Henderson, Chow, & Yao, 2004; Yochman, Parush, & Ornoy, 2004).

In the United States, an estimated 3% to 5% of the student population has ADHD (APA, 1994, 2000), a figure that comprises an estimated 1.46 million to 2.46 million children. Boys are five to nine times more likely than girls to be diagnosed. The disorder is found in all cultures, although prevalence figures differ. The prevalence of ADHD has dramatically increased in recent years (Robison, Sclar, Skaer, & Galin, 2004). Robison, Skaer, Sclar, and Galin (2002) reported that the rate of U.S. office-based physicians visits documenting a diagnosis of ADHD increased from 19.4 per 1,000 U.S. population ages 5 through 18 in 1990 to 59 per 1,000 in 1998. One-third to one-half of all referrals to child mental health facilities are for children with ADHD (Popper, 1988).

PRIMARY CHARACTERISTICS OF ADHD

In the following sections I describe the primary characteristics of ADHD, and the specific criteria for diagnosis of ADHD are listed in the *Diagnostic and Statistical Manual of Mental Disorders* (APA, 2000).

Inattention

Problems in attention may be conceptualized into three aspects: (a) sustained, (b) divided, and (c) alternating (Resnick, 2000). *Sustained attention* is the ability to maintain focus over time. *Divided attention* refers to attending to two competing but relevant stimuli, such as simultaneously driving and listening to the radio. The third aspect of attention is *shifting attention.* For example, if a person hears an ambulance siren while driving, instead of continuing to divide his or her attention between the highway and the radio, he or she fully shifts attention to the road, searching for the ambulance. Individuals with ADHD may continuously be shifting or alternating attention when sustained attention is needed. Individuals with ADHD often do not pay close attention to details; they may make careless mistakes in work, schoolwork, or other activities. Children have difficulty maintaining attention on tasks or play activities. They may not seem to listen, even when spoken to directly. They are easily distracted; often forgetful in daily activities; and often lose things, such as their pens or pencils needed for tasks and activities.

Impulsivity

Children with ADHD often have a low level of frustration tolerance and cannot delay gratification. They may act impulsively and in the moment without thinking. They may make important decisions without adequate information about or reflection on the consequences of their actions. They may have difficulty waiting their turn and with inhibiting emotional reactions to others, such as blurting out answers, interrupting others, or saying tactless things. They often cannot seem to stop behaviors, such as touching things or people. Situations and games that require sharing, cooperation, and restraint with peers are particularly difficult. They may have difficulty exercising impulse control while driving and may get tickets for speeding. They may be able to explain in great deal detail what they should have done and may be the first to point out when another child has not followed the rules. ADHD is a matter not of not knowing what to do but of not being able to inhibit oneself (Selikowitz, 1995). Children with ADHD often take risks and may be accident prone; for example, they may run out from between cars without looking. Accidental poisoning and burning are more common in this group of children (Selikowitz, 1995).

Hyperactivity

Symptoms of hyperactive or restless behavior include fidgeting, excessive speed, difficulty remaining seated in school, and a subjective sense of restlessness. Children with ADHD are often described as constantly "on the go" and may act as if they are "driven by a motor" (Barkley, 1998; Centers for Disease Control and Prevention, 2004).

THEORIES OF ADHD

Many researchers believe that the cause of ADHD is genetic or biological, although they acknowledge that the child's environment affects behavior. Current views of ADHD relate to the dopaminergic systems, frontal and prefrontal lobe function, cerebellum, and multisystem views (Biederman & Faraone, 2002; Roth & Saykin, 2004).

ADHD has traditionally been viewed as a problem related to attention. Barkley (1996, 1997a, 1997b, 1998) has proposed an integrated model of ADHD in which the primary deficit relates to difficulty inhibiting responses. Barkley posited that behavioral disinhibition, the central deficit in ADHD, adversely affects four executive functions: (a) prolongation or working memory; (b) self-regulation of affect, motivation, and arousal; (c) internalization of speech; and (d) reconstitution or analysis and synthesis (see Table 11.1).

The following six assumptions underlie this theoretical model of ADHD:

1. Behavioral inhibition begins earlier in development than the other four executive controls.
2. These executive controls emerge at different developmental stages.
3. The impairments in the four executive functions associated with ADHD arise from the primary behavioral inhibition deficit; if and when this primary deficit is altered, other functions improve.
4. Behavioral inhibition deficits result from genetic and developmental factors.
5. Secondary deficits in self-regulation create further primary deficits in behavioral disinhibition because self-regulation enhances restraint or inhibition.
6. The model does not explain the occurrence of ADHD without hyperactivity.

COGNITIVE IMPAIRMENTS: DEFICITS IN EXECUTIVE FUNCTIONS

There is a strong relationship between executive function and ADHD, and many studies of children with ADHD demonstrate symptoms of executive function difficulties. Castellanos (cited in Spodak, 1999) described executive functioning as "the ability to delay responses and sustain or shift attention so that an individual can set priorities

TABLE 11.1. Executive Functions Affected by Disinhibition in a Model Proposed by Barkley (1996)

Executive Function	Description
Prolongation or working memory	Working memory involves the ability to hold a mental image while preparing for and acting on information. Prolongation or working memory is dependent on the ability to inhibit, which allows the development of mental representations.
Self-regulation of affect	The ability to delay or control emotions allows children to engage in self-directed behaviors that modify not only the behavior itself but also the emotional reactions elicited. Lack of inhibition in children with ADHD results in greater emotional reactivity, less objectivity, decreased social perspective-taking, and decreased motivation to facilitate goal-directed behaviors.
Internalization of speech	Language is used to control one's own behavior as well as to control the behavior of others. Development of language contributes to executive-control functions, with speech serving as a control for behavioral inhibition. The development of language from public speech to private subvocalization is associated with an increase in control over one's behavior. Both language and knowledge of rules of acceptable behavior increasingly control behaviors and are related to the capacity for self-control and the ability to plan and direct behavior toward the goal. In children with ADHD, internalization of speech is less mature and more public, resulting in excessive talking, less reflection, less organization, and less rule-oriented behavior, and it is less influential in controlling children's behaviors.
Reconstitution	Reconstitution is the ability to analyze and synthesize information and enables the generation of new ideas and creativity or new combinations of ideas and problem solving. This develops from the processes of internal speech, mental prolongation, and behavioral inhibition. Fluency affects this process, and as tasks become more goal-directed, speech becomes rapid, efficient, and even creative, informing the internal total message that produces the action. Children with ADHD may have difficulty with problem solving because of their challenges generating multiple plans of actions or alternatives.
Motor control and fluency	Behavioral inhibition and other executive functions influence the ability to inhibit behaviors irrelevant to the task, to execute and persist in goal-directed motor responses, to complete novel or complex motor responses, to re-engage once interrupted, and to control one's behaviors through mentally represented stimuli. Fine and gross motor skills depend on inhibition in neural zones adjacent to those being activated (mirror and overflow movements). The prefrontal areas are involved with more complex motor planning and execution. Children with ADHD often show difficultly with fine and gross motor coordination and with planning and executing motor responses, particularly when lengthy, complex, goal-directed behaviors are required.

Note. ADHD = attention-deficit/hyperactivity disorder.

and respond to various environmental stimuli" and "attention with regard to the future." Denckla (cited in Spodak, 1999) used the acronym ISIS (*i*nitiate, *s*hift, *i*nhibit, and *s*ustain) to stand for core executive function deficits that relate to the ability to plan, organize, and develop strategies or rules.

Executive functions include processes of flexibility, planning, inhibition, and self-monitoring. This includes interference control processes, organization, and goal-oriented preparedness to act. Executive functions involve the regulation, inhibition, and maintenance of behavioral responses as well as problem-solving organization and reasoning (Berlin, Bohlin, Nyberg, & Janols, 2004; Teeter, 1998; Teeter & Semrud-Clikeman, 1997). Children with ADHD fail to sustain goal-directed behaviors and have difficulty shifting from one mental set to another. Although executive-control deficits are common in children with ADHD, they are not unique to this population and have been implicated in other childhood disorders

that share similar behavioral features, including disinhibition and self-control problems (see, e.g., Chapter 10, this volume).

EFFECT OF ADHD ON FUNCTIONAL PERFORMANCE

The effect of ADHD on functional performance can be profound and widespread, affecting every developmental domain, including cognitive, academic, social, emotional, and behavioral. Executive-control deficits, or the inability to regulate and to inhibit one's behavioral responses, can result in impulsivity, carelessness, poor planning and problem solving, and disorganization. Children with ADHD are often not aware of the consequences of their behavior. This interferes with future learning because children do not adequately profit from their experiences in predictable patterns. Barkley (1997a) referred to this as a deficit in *rule-governed behaviors,* or the inability to learn the relationship between behavior and its antecedents and consequences.

School Function

The core symptoms of ADHD make meeting the daily challenges of school difficult. Difficulty sustaining attention to tasks may result in the child missing important details and assignments and having difficulty organizing assignments. Hyperactivity may be expressed by the child disrupting the class verbally or physically. Impulsivity may be characterized by the child responding to questions without fully formulating the best answers and attending only to activities that are entertaining or novel (U.S. Department of Education, Office of Special Education and Rehabilitative Services, Office of Special Education Programs [hereafter *U.S. Department of Education*], 2003). Classroom performance may be characterized by low rates of on-task behavior, low rates of academic task completion, and low rates of positive exchanges with teachers (Wells et al., 2000). These behavior patterns contribute to high rates of academic underachievement, placement in special education services, grade retention, and school dropout. These negative school outcomes occur even if the child does not have specific learning disabilities (Wells et al., 2000). Barkley (1996) suggested that difficultly in executive functions—particularly working memory, internalized speech, and verbal fluency—affect the acquisition of math, spelling, reading comprehension, and oral/written report skills.

Self-Care

Little research exists on the extent to which children and adolescents with ADHD adequately care for their physical and mental health. One aspect of self-care that has been explored involves the extent to which adolescents use substances such as alcohol or drugs. An indication that adolescents with ADHD may have problems with this area of personal care comes from findings that adolescents with ADHD are more likely to qualify for substance dependence and abuse disorders. In one study of young adults with ADHD, Murphy, Barkley, and Bush (2001) found that 11% of the ADHD group felt that they were alcoholic, compared to 3% of the control group. However, 29% of the ADHD group had been told by others that they drank too much, compared with just 2% of the control group. Moreover, 10% of the ADHD group had been treated for alcohol problems, compared with 2% of the control group. Similar results were found for illegal drug use.

Occupational Functioning

Studies of adult outcomes of children with hyperactivity have indicated significantly greater problems in the workplace, significantly lower occupational status, and greater probability of being self-employed by their 30s than was evident in control groups (Mannuzza, Klein, Bessler, Malloy, & LaPadula, 1993; Weiss & Hechtman, 1993). Murphy and Barkley (1996) found that adults with ADHD reported having been fired more often from their places of employment than had control adults (53% vs. 31%). The adults with ADHD also had changed jobs significantly more often than the control group adults during the same period of time.

An area of occupational functioning in teens and adults with ADHD that has been receiving great attention is motor vehicle driving. Teens and young adults with ADHD have been found to have significantly higher risk for motor vehicle accidents, citations (especially speeding), and license revocations and suspensions than do controls (Barkley, Guevremont, Anastopoulos, DuPaul, & Shelton, 1993; Barkley, Murphy, & Kwasnick, 1996; Cox, Merkel, Kovatchev, & Seward, 2000; Nada-Raja et al., 1997; Woodward, Fergusson, & Horwood, 2000).

In a study of driving risks and behavior, Barkley et al. (1996) found that young adults with ADHD were more likely to have been involved in crashes that resulted in bodily injuries. The adults with ADHD had more driving violations on their official records, including speeding tickets, or were more likely to have had their licenses suspended or revoked (48% vs. 9%), and they experienced suspensions more often. No differences were found between the groups in driving knowledge, so knowledge per se did not account for the differences. However, when tested on a computer-driving simulator, the young adults displayed more uneven steering of the vehicle and had more scrapes and crashes while operating the simulated vehicle than did individuals in the control group.

Barkley, Murphy, DuPaul, and Bush (2002) examined multiple levels of driving performance and evaluated adverse outcomes in a large sample of 105 young adults with ADHD. This included basic cognitive functions necessary for driving, driving knowledge and rapid decision making, driving performance (on a simulator), actual driving behavior (self- and other ratings), and history of adverse driving events (self- and Department of Motor Vehicles reports). The authors found increased adverse outcomes, including accidents, license suspensions, citations, and speeding, among the participants with ADHD. Moreover, the young adults with ADHD had difficulties in cognitive abilities that are prerequisites for safe driving, including motor coordination, reaction time, motor inhibition, and sustained attention.

Parent–Child Relationships

Research has indicated that parents of children with ADHD display more negative reactions and fewer positive reactions, as well as more commanding directive behavior, than parents of children without ADHD (Wells et al., 2000). Family life is characterized by increased parenting stress and decreased parental feelings of self-competence (Fischer, 1990; Mash & Johnson, 1990), as well as increased rates of maternal depression and marital conflict (Wells et al., 2000).

Social Functions and Peer Relationships

Children with ADHD do not self-monitor readily and thus may have a difficult time reading others' responses and changing their behavior accordingly. They are often rejected by peers because of their active, demanding, and intrusive behaviors and particularly when aggressiveness is present. Their off-task, disruptive behavior and their noncompliance in the classroom also can result in peer problems. Children receive more negative attention from teachers and are described as irritating, annoying, domineering, and rigid in social situations (Whalen & Henker, 1985). Children with ADHD often have difficultly participating in clubs and sports and engaging in other extracurricular activities (Barkley, 1998; Fletcher, 1999).

ASSESSMENT

Assessments for children and adolescents with ADHD can focus on the symptoms of ADHD (attention, impulsivity, and hyperactivity), on cognitive functions, or on functional and occupational problems. Similarly, they can look at the symptoms of comorbidities, such as conduct disorder, anxiety, or learning disabilities. The form of the assessment can be variable and may include parent/child/teacher rating scales or assessments of the child's performance or interactions, or it can be observationally based. This review focuses on rating scales and methods for direct observation of symptoms of ADHD as well as measures of cognitive performance known to present problems in children and adolescents with ADHD. Some assessments are appropriate for use by occupational therapists; others are in the domain of neuropsychology but are important for therapists to know so they can interpret

findings from other disciplines. Because a primary purpose of an occupational therapy evaluation is to identify the client's current occupational performance and, on the basis of the client's values, interests, and priorities, to examine how the client's current performance compares with what he or she needs and wants to do (American Occupational Therapy Association [AOTA], 2002; Law et al., 1994), occupational therapists may want to begin with an assessment such as the Canadian Occupational Performance Measure (Law et al., 1994) or the Perceived Efficacy and Goal Setting System (Missiuna, Pollack, & Law, 2004) with children, their parents, or both, and teachers. This is particularly important because many of the instruments of ADHD focus on the impairment level.

Rating Scales

Rating scales address not only the presence of ADHD symptoms but also their severity. Rating scales can also assess functional impairment in many domains. Rating scales can be completed by parents and teachers or by self-report for older children; they are cost-effective methods for gathering information from multiple informants across different settings. They can summarize information across longer time intervals than that afforded by observation. Many parent- and teacher-completed rating scales as well as child self-report rating scales are available to assess ADHD and functional impairments. A review of these ratings scales was described by Anastopoulos and Shelton (2001) and is provided in Tables 11.2 and 11.3.

ADHD Symptoms

Broad-based rating scales that include but are not limited to ADHD include the Behavior Assessment System for Children–2nd Edition (BASC–2; Reynolds & Kamphaus, 2004a), Conners' Rating Scales–Revised (Conners, 1997); the Achenbach System of Empirically Based Assessments (Achenbach, 2003), and the Eyberg Behavior Inventories (Eyberg & Pincus, 1999). Assessments that are more specific to ADHD include the ADHD Rating Scale–IV (DuPaul, Power, McGoey, Ikeda, & Anastopoulos, 1998), the Attention Deficit Disorders Evaluation Scales (home and school versions; McCarney, 1989), and the Adolescent Behavior Checklist (Adams, Kelley, & McCarthy, 1997). These assessments and their psychometric properties were reviewed by Anastopoulos and Shelton (2001).

T A B L E 1 1 . 2 . Rating Scales for Assessing ADHD

	Assessment Measure	Authors	Parallel Forms	Age Range	Psychometric Properties
Broad-Band Measure	Behavior Assessment System for Children– 2nd Edition	Reynolds & Kamphaus (2004a, 200b)	Parent Teacher Self-report	2–21	R/V: Excellent Norms: National
	Conners' Rating Scales– Revised	Conners (1997)	Parent Teacher Self-report	3–17	R/V: Excellent Norms: National
	Achenbach System of Empirically Based Assessment	Achenbach (2003)	Parent Teacher Self-report	1.5–30	R/V: Excellent Norms: National
	Devereux Scales of Mental Disorder	Naglieri et al. (1994)	Parent Teacher Self-report	5–18	R/V: Excellent Norms: National
	Child Symptom Inventory–4	Gadow & Sprafkin (1998)	Parent Teacher	5–12	R/V: Excellent Norms: Limited
Narrow-Band Measure	Attention-Deficit/Hyperactivity Disorder Rating Scale–IV	DuPaul et al. (1998)	Parent Teacher Self-report	5–18	R/V: Excellent Norms: National
	Attention Deficit Disorder Evaluation Scales	McCarney (1989)	Parent Teacher Self-report	3–65	R/V: Excellent Norms: National
	Adolescent Behavior Checklist	Adams et al. (1997)	Self-report	11–17	R/V: Satisfactory Norms: National
	Child Attention Problem Rating Scale	Edelbrock (1991)	Parent Teacher	6–16	R/V: Excellent Norms: National
	SNAP	Atkins & Pelhorn (1991); Waschchbusch et al. (1998)	Parent Teacher	5–17	R/V: Satisfactory Norms: Limited
	Barkley Home and School Situations Questionnaires	Barkley & Murphy (1998)	Parent Teacher	4–18	R/V: Satisfactory Norms: Limited

Note. ADHD = attention-deficit/hyperactivity disorder; R/V = reliability/validity.
Adapted from *Assessing Attention-Deficit/Hyperactivity Disorder* (p. 107), by A. D. Anastopoulos and T. L. Shelton, 2001, New York: Kluwer Academic/Plenum. Copyright © 2001 Kluwer Academic/Plenum. Reprinted with permission of Springer Science and Business Media.

Functional Impairment

Rating scales and interviews can address various domains of psychosocial functioning as well as adaptive functioning. Anastopoulos and Shelton (2001) described a series of rating scales that can be used for assessing functional impairment in children with ADHD (see Table 11.3). Most of these make evaluations at the impairment level. Other examples, which are more familiar to occupational therapists and assess participation, include the School Function Assessment (Coster, 1998; Mancini, Coster, Trombly, & Heeren, 2000) and the Vineland Adaptive Behavior Scale (Sparrow, Balla, & Cicchetti, 1984). In a study that used the Vineland Adaptive Behavior Scales to examine the adaptive-skill dysfunction of children with attention deficit disorder (ADD) and ADHD, Stein, Szumowski, Blondis, and Roizen (1995) found that adaptive functioning was well below average and that the level of adaptive functioning relative to IQ was significantly lower for the ADD and ADHD groups than for a group diagnosed with mental retardation/pervasive developmental disorder in the areas of socialization, communication, and daily living. The authors concluded that the deficits in adaptive functioning that characterized children with ADHD and ADD may help explain the poor long-term prognosis of ADHD, and they suggested that increased attention should be paid to the assessment and treatment of adaptive functioning in these individuals. Cohn and Cermak (1998) emphasized the importance of including the family perspective in assessment and treatment planning and reviewed a series of instruments that are appropriate for use with families of children with ADHD. Some of these measures are also described in Table 11.3.

Observational Systems

Direct observational assessments can yield information that may be unavailable in other assessment modalities. Such information also can be invaluable in treatment planning. Several school-based systems have been developed recently.

TABLE 11.3. Rating Scales for Assessing Functional Impairment

Rating Scale	Authors	Area of Functioning Assessed	Psychometric Properties
Academic Performance Rating Scale	DuPaul et al. (1991)	Academic success and academic productivity via teacher report	Satisfactory
Social Skills Rating System	Gresham & Elliot (1990)	Social skills via parent, teacher, and self-report	Very good
Parenting Scale	Arnold et al. (1993)	Dysfunctional parental disciplinary practices	Satisfactory
Parenting Practices Scale	Strayhorn & Weidman (1988)	Parenting style	Satisfactory
Parenting Stress Index	Abidin (1995)	Source and degree of stress in parent–child system	Excellent
Parenting Sense of Competence Scale	Johnston & Mash (1989)	Perceived competence or efficacy and overall satisfaction in parenting role	Satisfactory
Symptom Checklist–90–Revised	Derogatis (1994)	Global and specific types of psychological distress and psychopathology in parents	Very good
Beck Depression Inventory–II	Beck et al. (1996)	Frequency and severity of depression symptoms in parents	Excellent
Beck Anxiety Inventory	Beck (1993)	Frequency and severity of anxiety symptoms in parents	Satisfactory
Adult AD/HD Rating Scale–IV	Barkley & Murphy (1998)	Frequency and severity of AD/HD symptoms in parents	Satisfactory
Lock–Wallace Marital Adjustment Scale, Marital Satisfaction Inventory–Revised, Dyadic Adjustment Scale	Locke & Wallace (1959), Snyder (1997), Spanier (1989)	Overall marital satisfaction	Satisfactory
Parenting Alliance Inventory	Abidin & Brunner (1995)	Degree to which parents work together in parenting roles	Excellent

Note. AD/HD = attention-deficit/hyperactivity disorder.
Adapted from *Assessing Attention-Deficit/Hyperactivity Disorder* (p. 108), by A. D. Anastopoulos & T. L. Shelton, 2001, New York: Kluwer Academic/Plenum. Copyright © 2001 Kluwer Academic/Plenum. Reprinted with permission of Springer Science and Business Media.

Direct Observation Form and Profile

The Direct Observation Form and Profile, for children ages 5 to 14 is part of the Achenbach System of Empirically Based Assessment (Achenbach, 2003). It provides information from direct observation of the child's behavior in group or classroom settings. It includes 96 items scored on a 4-step rating scale. There is a section for scoring on-task behavior at 1-min intervals as well as a section for the observer to write a narrative description of the child's behavior over a 10-min period. It is recommended that the child be observed on three or more occasions to obtain a representative sample of his or her behavior. The form should be completed for the target child and for two other children in the classroom. On-task, externalizing, internalizing, and total problem scores are averaged for up to six observation sessions. The computer-scored profile includes six additional scales: Withdrawn–Inattentive, Nervous–Excessive, Depressed, Hyperactive, Attention-Demanding, and Aggressive.

Behavior Assessment System for Children–2, Student Observational System

The Behavioral Assessment System for Children–2, Student Observational System (BASC–2; Reynolds, & Kamphaus, 2004a) allows coding of directly observed adaptive and maladaptive classroom behaviors. After a 15-min observation period, the observer completes a frequency checklist of 65 behaviors in 13 categories: 4 adaptive and 9 maladaptive. In another part of the observation, the examiner records behaviors during 30 3-s observations across a 15-min total observation period. The BASC Portable Observation Program (Reynolds & Kamphaus, 2004b) is a computer program in which the therapist records information directly onto a PDA or laptop. It includes the BASC Student Observation System.

Behavioral Observation of Students in Schools

The Behavioral Observation of Students in Schools (Shapiro, 2003) is a type of observation system for children in grades pre-K through 12 that allows narrative, continuous, or anecdotal behavior recording. It is designed for direct observation of classroom on-task behavior skills. It measures two categories of engaged (on-task) behavior: (a) active engaged time and (b) passive engaged time. It also measures three categories of nonengaged (off-task) behavior with verbal, motor, or passive responses. It includes event/frequency count recording, in which instances of the specific behavior are observed and recorded in terms of the number of times the behavior occurs and the duration or amount of time that the behavior lasts. A scatter plot shows the number of times over a period of time. It also includes interval recording, in which observation is divided into brief segments, and recording can reflect the moment of time, the whole time interval, or any time during the interval. It allows for the observation of the target student and the peer group and can provide data on teacher-directed instruction. When intervals are the unit being used, the target student may be observed at 15-s intervals, with the peer group and teacher-directed instruction at every 5th interval.

Assessments of Cognitive Function: Performance Measures of Attention

Although these assessments are typically administered by a neuropsychologist, some are appropriate for use by an occupational therapist with specialized training.

Vigilance and Sustained Attention: Continuous Performance Tests

A frequently used instrument for assessing sustained attention is the *continuous performance test* (CPT). There are several assessments that share certain characteristics. One version involves having the child watch for a particular target throughout the entire test. The child responds each time he or she observes the designated target. In a more difficult version, the child responds to the particular target only when it is immediately preceded by different symbol. CPTs require that the child respond to the appropriate targets and also not respond to the inappropriate targets.

Conners' Continuous Performance Test

One example of a CPT is Conners' Continuous Performance Test (Conners, 1994). This computer-assisted procedure assesses attention and impulsivity and can be used in both research and clinical settings. In the standard administration, the child or adolescent responds to any letter except for the letter X for 14 min. (This is a re-

verse of the previously described CPT versions.) The chance of impulsive target errors is maximized in this version because the child or adolescent is continuously responding. In this sense, Conners' CPT places an emphasis on response inhibition, consistent with Barkley's (1998) theoretical conceptualizations of ADHD. There are six trial blocks with each having three sub-blocks containing 20 trials. The interval between stimuli is 1 s, 2 s, or 4 s. The standard administration can be changed to the traditional version by varying the target letters, presentation time, inter-stimulus response time, number of blocks, and number of trials and target per block. The computer program generates information regarding the total number of stimuli; the number of correct responses; omission errors; commission errors; and various reaction times expressed as raw scores, *T* scores, and percentiles.

Test of Variables of Attention

Another example of a CPT is the Test of Variables of Attention (TOVA/TOVA–A; Greenberg & Waldman, 1993; Leark, Dupuy, Greenberg, Corman, & Kindeschi, 1996) for ages 4 to 80 years. The test is standardized and norm referenced on more than 2,000 individuals. The TOVA is the visual version, and the TOVA–A is the auditory version. The tests are designed to measure attentional and impulse control processes in four areas: (a) inattention or omissions, (b) impulse control or commissions, (c) response time, and (d) response time variability. Software records an individual's response and reaction times and calculates raw scores and percentages. Data are reported in standard scores and are presented in quarters, halves, and totals for the 21 min of the test. A printable report shows information in narrative and graphic form. A discriminant function ADHD score is provided.

Test of Everyday Attention

The Test of Everyday Attention for Children (TEA–Ch; Manly, Robertson, Anderson, & Nimmo-Smith, 1999) is a norm-referenced standardized assessment that uses gamelike tests to assess different aspects of attention in children and adolescents ages 6 to 16 years. The materials in the TEA–Ch relate to everyday situations for ecological validity. Nine subtests measure different aspects of attention, including focused (selective) attention (which reflects the ability to resist distraction, to sort through information, and to discriminate elements that are important to the task at hand), sustained attention (which reflects the ability to keep one's mind on a job), attentional control/switching (the ability to divide attention between two tasks, to switch attention smoothly from one thing to another), and the ability to inhibit motor and verbal responses (see Table 11.4 for a description of the subtests). The full assessment takes 1 hr; a shorter screening uses the first four subtests. Two parallel forms allow for retesting.

Measures of Executive Function

Areas of executive function found to be impaired in children with ADHD include self-regulation, inhibition, attention, and planning. I now describe two neuropsychological assessments to illustrate this: (a) the Behavior Rating Inventory of Executive Function (Gioia, Isquith, Guy, & Kenworthy, 2000), which includes several aspects of executive function, and (b) Stroop tests, which assess a particular aspect of executive function (see Chapter 1 of this volume for a more thorough review of assessments of executive function).

Behavior Rating Inventory of Executive Function

The Behavior Rating Inventory of Executive Function (Gioia et al., 2000) is a questionnaire for parents and teachers of children ages 5 to 18 years, designed to assess executive-function behaviors in the home and school environments. It is intended for use with various populations,

TABLE 11.4. Subtests of the Test of Everyday Attention in Children (Manly et al., 1997)

Subtest	Type of Attention Assessed	Description
Sky Search	Selective/ focused attention	A brief, timed subtest. Children have to find as many "target" spaceships as possible on a sheet filled with very similar distracter spaceships. In the second part of the task there are no distracters. Subtracting Part 2 from Part 1 gives a measure of a child's ability to make this selection that is relatively free from the influence of motor slowness.
Score!	Sustained attention	Children have to keep a count of the number of "scoring" sounds they hear on a tape, as if they were keeping the score on a computer game. Because this seems so simple and because of the long gaps between the sounds, the task does very little to "grab" the child's attention. It is therefore a good test of the child's ability to self-sustain attention.
Creature Counting	Attentional control/ switching	Children repeatedly switch between the two relatively simple activities of counting upward and counting downward. They are asked to count aliens in their burrow, with occasional arrows telling them to change the direction in which they are counting. Time and accuracy are scored.
Sky Search DT	Sustained–divided attention	Having previously completed the Sky Search subtest and the Score! subtest, children are asked to combine the two tasks of finding the spaceships and keeping a count of scoring sounds. Some children, who may have completed each aspect of the task well, show a substantial decrement in performance under dual task conditions.
Map Mission	Selective/ focused attention	Children search a map to find as many target symbols as they can in 1 min.
Score DT	Sustained attention	This subtest combines the sustained-attention task of counting the scoring sounds with another listening task. As they count, children also have to listen for an animal name that occurs at some stage during a spoken news report. Because attending to the meaning of speech is relatively easy, children are advised to devote most of their attention to the counting. The subtest measures the capacity to perform strategic attentional allocation over time.
Walk, Don't Walk	Sustained attention/ response inhibition	Children are asked to take one step along a paper path, using a pen, after each tone they hear on the tape. Unpredictably, one tone ends differently from the rest, meaning the next step should not be taken. To perform this task, children must sustain their attention on what they are doing and not engage in a task-driven, automatic style of responding.
Opposite Worlds	Attentional control/ switching	In the Same World, children follow a path naming the digits 1 and 2 that are scattered along it. In the Opposite World, they do the same task except they have to say "one" when they see a 2 and "two" when they see a 1. Speed on the cognitive reversal task is assessed.
Code Transmission	Sustained attention	Children must sustain attention on a monotonous series of spoken numbers—the "code transmission"—listening for two 5 s in a row. When this happens they are asked to say the number that came immediately before the 5 s ended. Over the 12 min of the test the 40-item code number builds up.

Note. DT = dual task.

including individuals with learning disabilities, brain injuries, developmental disorders, and attentional disorders. The parent and teacher forms each contain 86 items within 8 clinical scales that measure different aspects of executive functioning: (a) Inhibit, (b) Shift, (c) Emotional Control, (d) Initiate, (e) Working Memory, (f) Plan/Organize, (g) Organization of Materials, and (h) Monitor. The clinical scales, described in Table 11.5, form an overall score, the Global Executive Composite, as well as two indexes: (a) Behavioral Regulation and (b) Metacognition. The Working Memory and Inhibit scales are considered clinically useful in differentiating the diagnostic subtypes of ADHD.

Stroop Tests

Stroop tests typically require the respondent to rapidly read a series of words of names of colors, many of which are printed in different colors, although there are many variations of this test. Stroop tests are popular neuropsychological tests and are based on the finding that it takes markedly longer to read printed color names when the print ink is in a color different from the word color (e.g., when the word *blue* is printed in red ink; Lezak,

2004). This task requires the ability to attend to only one visual feature while blocking out the processing of the other (e.g., maintaining focused attention and warding off distractions). It is particularly challenging for children with ADHD who are distracted by the competing features. Numerous variations of this test are available with different numbers of items, stimulus formats, and levels of complexity (see Lezak, 2004, for a review). Scoring is based on time required to complete the test, number of errors, or a combination of these. In a meta-analysis of the sensitivity and specificity of the Stroop Color and Word tests, Homack and Riccio (2004) found that children with ADHD consistently performed more poorly than control children, but the Stroop tests did not consistently differentiate children with ADHD from other clinical groups such as children with learning disabilities.

LINKING ASSESSMENT, FUNCTION, PARTICIPATION, AND INTERVENTION

In considering assessment, two aspects must be considered: (a) the core symptoms of ADHD (attention, hyperactivity, and impulsivity) that interfere with the child's ability to function and participate and (b) the child's skill level or occupational performance. It is important to consider how the symptoms of ADHD (and other comorbid disorders, e.g., learning disabilities) affect the individual's ability to participate. The relation between these two aspects is indirect. Much of the literature on executive-function deficits in children with ADHD is based on neuropsychological testing conducted in laboratory environments (Lawrence et al., 2002, 2004). Researchers assume that the core symptoms of ADHD influence function, and one assumes that, if one improves the core symptoms of ADHD, one will improve the individuals' ability to participate. However, this is not always true. An example is based on a study conducted by Pelham et al. (1990), which examined the effect of medication on ADHD symptoms and skill level in a children's baseball game. ADHD symptoms were measured by the child's attention during the task (e.g., during probes, were the children attending to their position? Could they answer key questions? Were their bodies in the "ready" position?). Skill was measured by whether the children hit the ball better. The results indicated that, although children attended better, their skill was not improved. Similarly, in a meta-analysis of research of cognitive and behavioral treatment of impulsivity in children, Baer and Nietzel (1991) found that interventions were successful in slowing children's response times, but this did not necessarily lead to sizable changes in accu-

TABLE 11.5. Scales of the Behavior Rating Inventory of Executive Function Parent and Teacher Forms (Gioia et al., 2000)

Clinical Scale[a]	Description
Inhibit	Control one's impulses; appropriately stop own behavior at the proper time.
Shift	Move freely from one situation, activity, or aspect of a problem to another as the situation demands; transition; solve problem flexibly.
Emotional Control	Modulate emotional responses.
Initiate	Begin a task or activity; generate ideas independently.
Working Memory	Hold information in mind to complete a task; stay with an activity.
Plan/Organize	Anticipate future events; set goals; develop appropriate steps ahead of time to carry out an associated task or action; carry out tasks in a systematic manner; understand and communicate main ideas or key concepts.
Organization of Materials	Keep work space, play areas, and materials in an orderly manner.
Monitor	Check work; assess performance during or after finishing a task to ensure attainment of goal; keep track of the effect of own behavior on others.

[a]The number of items on each scale ranges from 6 to 12.

racy. Thus, in working with individuals with ADHD, one needs to consider both symptoms and skill and their relation to participation.

INTERVENTION: EVIDENCE BASE FOR PRACTICE

ADHD is a condition that has a primary neurological basis, with secondary psychological features. It often exists with coexisting disorders, which must be addressed as well if the treatment for ADHD is to be effective. There is a need to work individuals with ADHD on multiple levels simultaneously. Approaches to intervention may include medication, psychotherapy, treatment of secondary psychological issues, and treatment of comorbid conditions. Use of cognitive rehabilitation models may be used to treat the cognitive problems of individuals with ADHD. Goals may include improving cognitive function, developing internal and external compensatory strategies, and restructuring physical and social environment to maximize function. In this section I examine evidence for the most commonly used and accepted interventions that have been supported by research.

Psychopharmacological Treatment

Psychopharmacological treatment is one of the most common forms of treatment for children with ADHD (Robison et al., 2004). This may include the use of psychostimulants, antidepressants, anti-anxiety medications, antipsychotics, and mood stabilizers (NIMH, 2000). Stimulants are the most common and include methylphenidate (Ritalin), dextroamphetamine, and Cylert. In January 2003, the Food and Drug Administration approved a new type of nonstimulant medication for the treatment of children and adults with ADHD, atomoxetine, also known as Stratera (U.S. Department of Education, 2003).

In a review of the National Ambulatory Medical Care Survey records of children ages 5 to 18 years from 1995 to 1999, Robison et al. (2004) found that, of approximately 14 million total office visits for the diagnosis of ADHD, 42% used medication alone, and 32% used medication plus other approaches, resulting in a total of approximately 74% of physicians who prescribed stimulant medication. (N.B.: The National Ambulatory Medical Care Survey is an ongoing annual survey of U.S. office-based physicians conducted by the National Center for Health Statistics of the Centers for Disease Control and Prevention.)

Stimulants predominate in clinical use and have been found to be effective in 75% to 90% of children with ADHD (Goldman, Genel, Bezman, & Slanetz, 1998; U.S. Department of Education, 2003; U.S. Department of Health and Human Services, 1999). Medications have been well researched for children with ADHD. A review of literature from 1975 to 1997 found more than 170 studies, involving more than 6,000 school-age children, that had examined the effectiveness of medication (Goldman et al., 1998). The largest controlled trial of intervention for children with ADHD recently found stimulant medication to be highly effective in reducing core ADHD symptoms (MTA Cooperative Group, 1999a; this study is discussed in more detail later in this chapter).

Although common, medications are still the most controversial forms of treatment for children with ADHD. Even when effective, stimulant medications do not normalize the entire range of behavior problems, and children continue to manifest higher levels of behavior problems than their peers (U.S. Department of Health and Human Services, 1999). Because of this and the controversy surrounding medication, various other approaches also have been used with children with ADHD.

Multimodal Cognitive and Behavioral Approaches

When working with individuals with ADHD, a combination of medication and other approaches (multimodal approaches) often are used. These approaches may include psychoeducation, behavior therapy, environmental changes, and psychotherapy. The focus of the remaining section deals with studies that include cognitive–behavioral intervention.

Baer and Nietzel (1991) completed a meta-analysis of 36 outcome studies that used cognitive treatment or behavioral treatment, or both, including self-statement modification (self-instructional techniques), reinforcement contingencies, modeling, strategy training, problem-solving training, and numerous intervention combinations to reduce impulsivity in samples that included but were not limited to children with ADHD. The results indicated that, relative to untreated or placebo controls, cognitive or behavioral intervention or both was associated with improvements of one-third to three-quarters of a standard deviation.

In a meta-analysis of studies conducted between 1966 and 1995, DuPaul and Eckert (1997) reviewed 63 studies that looked at outcomes of school-based interventions for children with ADHD. Interventions were categorized as academic, contingency management, or cognitive–behavioral. Dependent variables were classified into one of three categories: (a) academic measures (e.g., norm-referenced achievement tests), (b) behavioral measures (e.g., child rating scales), and (c) clinic-based measures (e.g., reaction intensity or vigilance tasks). Contingency management strategies and academic interventions were more effective for behavior change than were cognitive–behavioral interventions; on the other hand, cognitive–behavioral interventions were more effective for academic outcomes (although this finding was not supported in an earlier qualitative review by Abikoff, 1991).

Multimodal Treatment Study of Children With ADHD: A Randomized Controlled Trial

A recent study conducted by the National Institute of Mental Health—the Multimodal Treatment Study of Children With ADHD (MTA)—is the longest and most comprehensive study of the intervention for children with ADHD (MTA Cooperative Group, 1999a, 1999b). It is important for occupational therapists to be aware of this study, because it will be cited by individuals in other disciplines as the most current and comprehensive randomized clinical trial of treatment for children with ADHD. Details of the intervention protocol are provided so therapists can compare this to alternate or supplemental approaches that they may recommend. In the MTA study, 579 children with ADHD between ages 7 and 10 years were followed at six sites nationwide and in Canada. All children had primary diagnoses of ADHD, combined type, based on *Diagnostic and Statistical Manual of Mental Disorders* (APA, 1994) criteria. In addition, the following comorbidities were present: aggressive-spectrum disorders such as conduct disorder or oppositional defiant disorder (54%), anxiety disorders (33%), and affective disorders (3.8%; MTA Cooperative Group, 1999b). Four interventions were compared: (a) medication alone under carefully controlled conditions; (b) psychosocial/behavioral interventions alone; (c) a combination of medication and psychosocial/behavioral interventions; and (d) community care, which frequently included medication prescribed by the child's own physician. Children were randomly assigned to one of these conditions.

Because this study is considered the most comprehensive investigation of intervention for children with ADHD, and the psychosocial/behavioral intervention effects are of particular interest to occupational therapists, I spend time describing this intervention and its rationale. I heretofore refer to this as *psychosocial treatment,* with the recognition that it includes a strong behavioral component.

Psychosocial (Cognitive–Behavioral) 3 Treatment Strategies in the MTA Study

The intervention was designed on the basis of a review of the literature of the most effective interventions for "improving the symptoms, comorbidities, and functional impairments associated with ADHD" (Wells et al., 2000, p. 500). Treatment was an intensive 14-month program combining direct contingency management and clinical behavior therapy. It consisted of three major integrated components: (a) a parent training component; (b) a school intervention component; and (c) a child treatment component, which included an intensive summer treatment program. Intervention was integrated across settings with similarities of specific treatment procedures such as point systems and token economies across school, home, and summer settings.

Parent Training

Parent training consisted of 27 group sessions and 8 individual sessions. Group sessions were based on social learning theory and consisted of behavior management skills, including setting up a daily report card with target behaviors; attending to, rewarding, and positively reinforcing prosocial child behaviors; giving effective directions and rules; and using time-out and response cost as a consequence for negative child behaviors. Parents also learned to implement a home token economy system. Additionally, training included techniques for stress, anger, and mood management; strategies for assisting their children with peer interactions and friendships; skills for supporting their child's academic homework performance; and skills for interacting with their child's school. Methods included didactic presentation, modeling, role playing, and group discussion. Individual sessions were designed to review and support the parent training skills taught in group sessions and problem solve individual needs.

School Intervention

There were two main components for the school intervention: (a) a teacher consultation program and (b) a paraprofessional program. In the teacher consultation program, therapist–consultants met with teachers twice monthly at the beginning and monthly later in the program. The first goal was to establish a daily report card that would be coupled with a home-based reward system implemented by parents as part of the parent training program. During a preliminary assessment, the teacher helped choose priorities for consultation so that, by the end of consultation, the teacher would have skills in classroom rules and enforcement procedures, contingent attention and ignoring, clear commands and soft reprimands, individualizing instructional materials, modifying class structure, school-based reinforcement, classroom token economies, group-based contingencies, response cost, and time-out.

The paraprofessional program, an educational intervention based on behavior modification techniques (including frequent prompting and reinforcement), focused on classroom concerns such as staying on task, interacting with others, completing work, and shifting activities. Paraprofessionals were trained and participated in three phases. First, during the spring of the 1st school year of the program, paraprofessionals received extensive training in skills to assess and implement behavioral intervention. They participated in supervised field experience in the children's classrooms, observing children and practicing data collection of interactions and target behaviors, and they worked as classroom aides. The paraprofessionals were camp counselors and teachers' aides during the summer treatment program. After this, the paraprofessionals participated in a program in the fall of the children's 2nd school year. Each paraprofessional was assigned two children and spent the morning in one child's classroom and the afternoon in the other. The paraprofessionals provided direct intervention for the target child, kept data on the target child's progress, implemented the changes to the child's daily report card that were decided on by the teacher and the therapist–consultant, and served as instructional aides to the teachers for all children in the classrooms.

The paraprofessional program used two major behavior modification interventions. The first system was the daily report card. A set of 4 to 6 target behaviors was identified for each child based on a set of 10 behaviors: (a) getting started, (b) interacting with others, (c) following rules about being quiet, (d) following rules about remaining seated, (e) attending to assigned work, (f) performing assigned work, (g) stopping and preparing for the next period, (h) following directions, (i) following classroom rules, and (j) an individualized category. At the end of specified time intervals that were individualized by the child's teacher and teacher–consultant, the paraprofessional awarded a token to the child if the child met the daily report card criteria during that interval. The paraprofessional's use of appropriate behavioral interventions in the classroom served as a model for teachers to use effective strategies. The time interval was increased gradually to shape the child's behavior and enable delay of reward and transition to teacher mainte-

nance of the program. The second system was a merit badge system in which target behaviors related to social skills such as cooperation and communication were reinforced by awarding merit badge points. Parents also awarded merit badge points.

Child-Based Treatment

The 8-week Summer Treatment Program met daily on weekdays from 8:00 a.m. to 5:00 p.m. Children participated in age-matched groups of 12 with two classroom staff members and five paraprofessional counselors for each group. The group stayed together for all activities, and children received intensive experience in functioning as a group. Three hours were spent in classroom sessions; the rest of the day was spent on recreation and therapeutic group activities. Interventions targeted improving children's peer relationships, interactions with adults, academic performance, and self-efficacy. Components of the program and strategies used are described in Table 11.6.

Overarching Principles and Guidelines

The MTA program was comprehensive and designed to address ADHD symptoms as well as comorbidities and functional impairments. It was based on the theoretical conceptions of the nature and course of ADHD as

> a chronic disease with symptoms, co-morbidities, and impairments that multiply, intensify, and persist into adolescence and even adulthood, and the treatment of which may require intensive intervention in multiple areas of functioning, in multiple settings over years rather than weeks or months. (Wells et al., 2000, p. 500)

On the basis of previous research, it was recognized that (a) psychosocial intervention is setting specific and is not maintained when once treatment is withdrawn, and (b) generalization must be specifically programmed. This is similar to Toglia's emphasis on the need for a multicontext approach to intervention (see Chapter 2, this volume). Three forms of generalization were built into the MTA program: (a) across settings, including school (including classroom, lunchroom, recess), home, and social situations; (b) across symptom domains; (c) and across time (maintenance of treatment effects). Specific strategies and techniques such as the daily report card, points, tokens, and response cost were used to monitor and reinforce similar target behaviors across home and school settings to promote generalization.

TABLE 11.6. Components and Strategies Used in the Multimodel Treatment Study of Children With ADHD Summer Program (MTA Cooperative Group, 1999a, 1999b)

Component	Description
Point systems	Points earned or lost were exchanged for privileges, social honors, and home-based rewards.
Positive reinforcement, Appropriate commands	Use of praise and public recognition. Directions were brief, explicit, and phrased to minimize noncompliance.
Time-out	Discipline provided for prohibited behaviors such as aggression, intentional destruction of property, and repeated noncompliance.
Peer intervention	Social skills training with modeling, coaching, role playing, and practice, with feedback and reinforcement to facilitate learning. Included daily sessions in which children worked cooperatively in small groups to achieve a goal; inclusion of a peer buddy program.
Sports skills training	Included because children with ADHD often do not know and/or follow game rules and often have poor motor skills. Poor performance in these areas contributes to social rejection and low self-esteem. One period each day was devoted to skill development, and two periods each day were devoted to playing age-appropriate games and sports.
Daily report card	Included target behaviors for each child derived for both academic and recreational group settings. Integrated with parent daily report card.
Classrooms	3 hr daily in the classroom, with 1 hr in each: academics; computer-assisted instruction in reading, math, and written language; and art class for less structured activity. Use of response cost system, points for assignment completion and accuracy.
Individualized programs	Functional analysis or problem behaviors with individualized program as needed.

Note. ADHD = attention-deficit/hyperactivity disorder.

Results of the MTA Study

Outcome variables of the MTA study included primary ADHD symptoms rated by parents and teachers; aggressive and oppositional behavior rated by parents, teachers, and classroom observers; internalizing symptoms, including anxiety and sadness rated by parents, teachers, and children; social skills rated by parents, teachers, and children; parent–child relationships rated by parents; and academic achievement assessed by standardized achievement tests (MTA Cooperative Group, 1999a, 1999b). Children in all four groups showed reductions in levels of symptoms over time in most areas. However, some interventions were more effective than others. Combined treatment and medication alone were superior to the behavioral/psychosocial treatment alone for both parent and teacher ratings of primary ADHD symptoms. Combined treatment and medication management intervention did not differ significantly on any of the domains. However, when rank ordering was considered on different outcomes, children in the combined treatment group did best on 12 of 19 outcome measures, whereas those in the medication management group were best on only 4 measures.

In addition, when the individual outcome measures were combined into composite measures, or when children's outcomes were grouped into excellent responses versus less dramatic response categories, children receiving combined treatment did significantly, but modestly (in terms of effect size), better. When combined treatment was compared with psychosocial/behavioral treatment alone, combined treatment was superior on parent and teacher ratings of primary ADHD symptoms, on parent ratings of aggressive/oppositional behavior, on parent ratings of children's internalizing symptoms, and on standardized reading assessments. Thus, the results indicated that adding medication to the psychosocial treatment of a child yielded substantial benefits. Of the four interventions investigated, the combined treatment and the medication-alone treatment worked significantly better than psychosocial/behavioral therapy alone or community care alone at reducing the symptoms of ADHD.

The study also found that a lower medication dosage was effective in the combined treatment, whereas higher doses were used to achieve similar results in the medication-alone treatment. This is an important finding for parents who may be reluctant to use medication and may want the minimal dosage possible.

Considerations for Occupational Therapy

The results of the MTA trial indicated that medication, when coupled with cognitive–behavioral intervention, was effective in improving function in children with ADHD. An important factor to remember when considering these results is that the treatments investigated in this study were limited to those that had the greatest empirical support at the time the study was designed: medication and psychosocial/behavioral treatment. This study does not provide any information about the effectiveness of other types of treatment for ADHD, such as dietary intervention, biofeedback, or sensory integration. Moreover, participants in this study were all diagnosed with the combined ADHD type; thus, this study does not provide information about the inattentive type. The study only included children ages 7 to 10 years; thus, the results may not be applicable to younger children or older children with ADHD. Finally, motor skills were not examined in this sample, even though it has been reported that 50% of children with ADHD also have significant motor impairment/ or meet criteria for developmental coordination disorder, or both (Gillberg, 2003). This is particularly important for occupational therapists, because it is this population that is likely to be referred.

OCCUPATIONAL THERAPY APPLICATION

The goal of occupational therapy intervention, regardless of the theoretical model, frame of reference, or techniques used, is "improved client performance" (AOTA, 2002, p. 614). Although the literature on ADHD is replete with descriptions of children's impairment in basic and higher order cognitive function, including executive function, there is little written in the occupational therapy literature regarding cognitive approaches to intervention with children with ADHD or intervention for the cognitive impairments experienced by children with ADHD. Some investigators have examined the comorbidity of ADHD and disorders of sensory modulation (e.g., Dunn & Bennett, 2002; Mangeot et al., 2001; Mulligan, 1996) and have proposed that occupational therapy using sensory integration principles may enhance attention and on-task behaviors (Kimball, 2002; Schilling, Washington, Billingsley, & Deitz, 2003; VandenBerg, 2001). Other investigators have identified the comorbidity of ADHD and developmental coordination disorder (e.g., Gillberg, 2003; Tseng et al., 2004) and have focused on remediation of motor planning and handwriting difficulties. Shaffer et al. (2001) examined the effects of a specific intervention, the Interactive Metronome, on selected aspects of motor and cognitive skills in boys with ADHD. Finally, although there is extensive literature outside of occupational therapy on the use of behavioral principles and behavior modification for children with ADHD, there is little research within occupational therapy. A recent publication by Watling and Schwartz (2004) emphasized the importance of understanding and implementing positive reinforcement as an intervention strategy for children with disabilities, although this was not specific to children with ADHD.

DYNAMIC INTERACTIONAL MODEL OF COGNITION

Current research indicates that a combined approach using medication and psychosocial/cognitive–behavioral therapy is an appropriate intervention for children with ADHD. Principles from Toglia's dynamic interactional model of cognition (see Chapter 2, this volume) can be applied and integrated with use of a cognitive–behavioral approach when working with children and adolescents with ADHD. These approaches are not mutually exclusive, and application of principles of the dynamic interactional model can enhance intervention strategies.

Although the dynamic interactional model of cognition has not been applied to children with ADHD, several studies with children with ADHD have used cognitive–mediational approaches (e.g., Goldstein & Goldstein, 1990), on which this approach is based. Furthermore, dynamic interaction has been applied to children and adults with head injury (see Chapter 10, this volume) who share with children with ADHD symptoms of impulsivity, difficulty with attention, and other executive-function disorders.

As discussed in Chapter 2, "Cognition is an ongoing product of the dynamic interaction among the individual, the task, and the environment" (pp. 29–30). As such, cognitive function can be enhanced by modifications in any of the components. In the following sections, I discuss each component (person, task, environment) and its influence on function of children with ADHD.

There are no published dynamic interactional assessments designed to assess attention or impulsivity in children with ADHD. The Contextual Memory Test (Toglia, 1993), although designed for adults, can be used with older children with ADHD to assess memory, an area found to be impaired in some children with ADHD (see Chapters 2 and 10, this volume, for a description of this test and its application). Moreover, existing tests can be adapted to incorporate aspects of dynamic interaction, including awareness and self-evaluation. I discuss this in the next section.

Disorders of awareness are characteristic of individuals with brain injuries but have not been empirically documented in the ADHD population. However, there are abundant clinical descriptions of children with ADHD who have limited awareness of their feelings and problems and tend to overestimate their potential for success (Barkley, 1997a; Fletcher, 1999). The behavior of the children with ADHD often is characterized by impulsivity and inadequate online monitoring of their performance.

In dynamic interactional assessment the individuals are asked to predict their performance, perform the task, and evaluate their performance. Assessment uses cues and task alterations to identify the person's potential for change. Intervention may focus on "changing the person's strategies and self-awareness; modifying external factors such as the activity demands and environment; or simultaneously addressing the person, activity, and environment to facilitate performance" (Toglia, Chapter 2, p. 29). The following are the underlying assumptions of a dynamic interactional approach.

- Occupational performance requires the ability to recognize one's strengths and limitations, use efficient processing strategies, and monitor one's performance.
- Performance can be facilitated by changing the demands of the activity or task, the environment, the person's use of strategies and self-awareness, or a combination of these.
- External cues and modifications of the environment or the activity (task) can support and enhance occupational performance. This can be done without changes in the individual's strategy use and self-awareness when another person is responsible for the modifications, or it can be done by the individual through strategies and self-awareness.

On the basis of the above assumptions, it is important in an assessment to identify not only an individual's performance level but also his or her ability to recognize his or her strengths and limitations, to use efficient processing strategies, and to monitor his or her own performance. It also is important to determine whether performance can be facilitated by changing the task or activity demands, restructuring the environment, or enhancing the individual's use of strategies and self-awareness. Most standardized assessments of attentional abilities, such as CPTs, do not include dynamic interactional components. However, aspects of dynamic interactional assessment can be integrated into any assessment.

An example of a recent test that includes both a static and dynamic components is the Dynamic Occupational Therapy Cognitive Assessment for Children (Katz, Parush, & Traub Bar-Ilan, in press). This assessment, although not specifically designed for children with ADHD, provides a standardized administration, followed by a cueing protocol to examine the child's potential for learning. A task, such as a CPT, can be modified to allow for a dynamic component. However, adapting the test in this manner may invalidate its use as a norm-referenced test. Thus, it is critical for the therapist to identify, in advance, the purpose of testing (see Chapter 2, this volume). If the primary purpose of the assessment is to identify whether the child has attentional problems and how severe these problems are relative to one's peers, then use of a CPT in its standardized format as a norm-referenced test is appropriate. If the therapist wants information on the child's awareness of his or her attentional difficulties and wants information on the child's potential for learning through cueing or task modification procedures, or both, then the test can be adapted using a dynamic interactional framework.

Dynamic assessment, as used within Toglia's dynamic interactional model of cognition, includes three components: (a) investigation of self-perception and awareness prior to task performance, (b) facilitating change in performance, and (c) investigating self-perception of performance and strategy use after the task (see Chapter 2, this volume). Consider, for example, a CPT test in which the child is required to watch a series of letters on a computer screen for 15 min and press a key every time the letter X appears. In a dynamic approach, one might say to the child

> I am going to have you watch a computer screen for 15 minutes. There will be different letters on the screen. I am going to ask you to push a key on the computer every time the X appears on the screen. Do you think you will have any difficulty with this task?

If the child responds "yes," the examiner would then ask the child to rate the difficulty (a little, medium, a lot) and might ask when (beginning of task, after 2–3 min, after 5 min) and what kind of difficulty the child thinks he or she would have.

After the child has completed this task, the examiner asks

> Do you think this task was harder or easier than you thought it would be? Do you think you missed any Xs? How many do you think you missed? Do you think you pushed the key at the wrong time and chose other letters that weren't Xs?

The examiner also might question the child about the strategies the child used. For example, if the child says that the task was boring and it was hard to pay attention, the examiner might ask what the child did to help himself or herself continue paying attention. One child might say that he bounced in the chair. Another might say that she tapped her foot. Both of these children are indicating that they used movement to help keep themselves alert. They have given the therapist information about their awareness and the strategies they use and have provided cues for intervention.

It also is important for the therapist to observe the child while the child performs the test. Did the child recognize when he or she made an error? This is often easy to spot by children's verbal or nonverbal responses as they perform a task. This provides the therapist with information about children's online awareness and their ability to monitor their performance while they are completing the task. Self-awareness is critical to judgment, safety, and independent performance across all areas of occupation. It is also important for children to understand why they are having difficulty. A child who is aware that he or she is constantly not meeting standards, but does not understand why, may experience severe anxiety.

Dynamic assessment methods examine change in performance with cues, mediation, feedback, or task changes to provide an estimate of the child's learning potential. Thus, after the standard administration of the task, the therapist may try several variations with cueing. For example, the therapist may now ask the child to push the key when he sees the letter *A* on the computer screen. For some letter *A*s the therapist will modify the stimulus and make the *A* boldface or in color. In this manner, the therapist will be able to determine whether enhancing the salience of the stimulus improves performance.

Another strategy that has been used in intervention studies is to provide an external cue, such as an auditory beep, periodically. The child may be asked to push the key when the beep sounds and continue with the task. In this manner, the therapist can determine whether a simple alerting device, provided periodically, enhances general attention and performance. An alternative modification may be to give the child a "movement break" (such as chair push-ups) every 5 min to observe whether movement enhances ability to sustain performance.

Other methods for evaluating children's or adolescents' awareness include a comparison of the child's rating of his or her performance with that of a parent or guardian, a teacher, or both. This method involves examining the discrepancy in ratings and has been commonly used in assessing awareness in individuals with head injuries (see Chapters 1, 2, and 10, this volume).

To an increasing extent, the literature is indicating that performance is enhanced when an activity is meaningful to the child and his or her family. This is particularly true for children with ADHD. Strategy use can be enhanced in tasks that are relevant for children. Moreover, engagement in familiar and meaningful occupations may be more effective in facilitating the emergence of awareness (see Chapters 2 and 9, this volume). Self-monitoring skills are most likely to emerge in activities that are the "just-right challenge" so that the child or adolescent can integrate the experience (Ayres, 1979; see also Chapter 2, the present volume). An individual who does not understand the purpose or relevance of the activity will be less likely to pay attention and more likely to lose interest.

INTERVENTION: THE PERSON, TASK, ENVIRONMENT

Treatment for a child with ADHD may focus on changing the child or adolescent's strategies and self-awareness; modifying external factors, such as the task or activity demands or the physical and social environment; or simultaneously addressing the person, activity, and environment to facilitate performance.

As Toglia emphasizes in the dynamic interactional model of cognition (see Chapter 2), occupational performance provides feedback that influences an individual's self-perceptions about his or her abilities and performance, often resulting in an individual changing or modifying his or her processing strategies. However, many children with ADHD do not appear to be aware of their difficulty or modify their performance in response to the feedback they receive, either because they do not accurately interpret the feedback or because they are unable to inhibit their actions and change course. Because of this, their judgment may be impaired, and they are at significant risk for safety. Thus, online monitoring is a significant challenge for individuals with ADHD. Feedback also may be provided by another person or by an external source, including use of a contingent reward system as described in detail in the MTA studies (MTA Cooperative Group, 1999a, 199b; Wells et al., 2000).

(Re)Structuring the Physical and Social Environments

The type of environment that a child with ADHD is in can affect his or her ability to process information and adapt to task demands. For example, an adult who gives multiple instructions to a child with attentional problems will elicit a different response than an adult who enhances information processing by presenting information in a straightforward, simple way. Mediation by a more skilled partner, such as an adult who presents the information in a clear, structured manner, can help the child attend to information that is relevant and can help him or her extract meaning, make connections, and deepen experiences. Vygotsky (1978) described the importance of a more knowledgeable partner who can move the child from his or her current performance to a higher level. Vygotsky referred to the difference between what a child can accomplish on his own and what he or she can accomplish with a more skilled partner as the *zone of proximal development*. Social restructuring may include educating family members, teachers, and significant others about the individual cognitive challenges and ways to facilitate performance by supporting information processing and adapting the task or environment.

Features of the physical environment, such as the extent of visual and auditory distractions and the arrangement and organization of materials, affect a child's ability to perform a task. For example, a child may be asked to do his homework. In one instance, the television may be on, the telephone intermittently ringing, and the work space cluttered with toys; in the other instance, he has a quiet work space with the materials he needs to complete his homework such as his textbook, pens, pencils, and papers. Physical restructuring may involve modifying aspects of the individual's physical environment to minimize ADHD challenges. This might mean organizing and uncluttering the child's work space or using a ball instead of a chair so that he can get movement input as he works.

According to Hallowell and Ratey (1995), structure allows an individual with ADHD to use his or her abilities rather than dissipating them. Structure includes tools such as lists, reminders, notepads, appointment books, filing systems, Rolodexes, bulletin boards, schedules, receipts, in- and outboxes, answering machines, computer systems, alarm clocks, and alarm watches. *Structure* refers to the set of external controls that one sets up to compensate for the unreliable or ineffective internal controls (p. 221). Improving cognitive functioning also can be supported through improved sleep patterns, regular exercise, improved nutrition, and reduced stress (Goldstein & Ellison, 2002).

The Task

The task itself also can be modified. It can be simplified, or the complexity can be increased. Key features can be highlighted, increasing their salience. Time to complete the task can be increased or decreased. Tasks can be divided into short steps with time between. Each of the changes has the potential to influence an individual's performance.

The Person

Processing strategies are ways that information is processed across domains. These strategies include "orga-

nized approaches, methods, or tactics, that operate to select and guide the efficient processing of information" (see Chapter 2, p. 33, this volume). An example of a processing strategy that people use to handle large amounts of information is *grouping*. When a person is trying to remember a telephone number, he or she usually mentally groups the numbers into units of 3 (area code), 3 (first three digits), and 4 (last four digits). In this way, one has three groups of information to recall instead of 10 discrete bits of information. Left-to-right scanning is another processing strategy used by most people when searching for information in a page of written material.

Cognitive dysfunction may be conceptualized in terms of deficiencies in processing strategies and self-monitoring skills. Children with ADHD often display inefficient strategy use; they do not initiate and use self-regulatory or monitoring behaviors such as anticipating, monitoring, checking, and revising solutions (Barkley, 1998, 2004). Difficulties in a wide range of attention, memory, visual-processing and problem-solving tasks may reflect the same underlying behavior or inefficient strategy use. For example, a tendency to focus on or be distracted by irrelevant details may interfere with a child's performance on a memory task or a problem-solving task. Time use is a major problem for many individuals with ADHD. A child or adolescent may have difficulty deciding how to prioritize steps, or he or she may spend excessive time on less important details. Several studies have identified that children with ADHD exhibit more self-talk than their peers (Goldstein & Goldstein, 1990; Lawrence et al., 2002), although the self-talk is less mature (Goldstein & Goldstein, 1990).

Teaching compensatory strategies is highly useful in working with individuals with ADHD and should appropriately be a major function of therapy. Goldstein and Ellison (2002) referred to such strategies under the umbrella of "learning how to take charge of ADHD" (p. 110). Helping the individual develop compensatory strategies such as making lists, writing down reminders, and using date planners to record homework assignments and activities are all important strategies.

FOCUS OF COGNITIVE REHABILITATION

Difficulty with impulse control will lead individuals with ADHD to act spontaneously, without thinking ahead or considering the consequences of their actions. Their search for thrills and novelty may stem from excessive attraction to immediate reward. They also may have difficultly inhibiting the impulse to avoid aversive tasks and situations.

Their decision-making processes may be impulse driven, and they may make important choices too rapidly and without careful consideration or planning. Important components of therapy should aim to teach self-regulation such as stop and think, consider the consequences of an action, and generate appropriate alternatives (Barkley, 1997a, 1997b). Interventions that focus on the development of self-control skills and reflective problem-solving strategies as methods to regulate an individual's behavior (DuPaul & Eckert, 1997) are important for children with ADHD.

Core deficits in attention are likely to cause individuals with ADHD to act without consideration of small details or planning and be easily distracted by irrelevant stimuli. Intervention should focus on helping children examine information in a systematic manner, prioritize information, formulate a plan of action, maintain goal-directed behavior, and persist with activity over time. Intervention may involve asking questions about a task, answering these questions in the form of cognitive rehearsal, providing self-instruction that guides the task, or providing self-management intervention.

Individuals with ADHD may be unaware of the impact of their behavior on others, with cognitive deficits causing them to miss the cues in social situations. Inattention and distractibility may be perceived by others as an inability to listen or as the lack of interest. Impulsivity may be interpreted as rudeness if an individual makes untimely and inappropriate interruptions to conversations. Failure to follow instructions, mood swings, and unpredictable temperament may be perceived by others as unacceptable behavior, and individuals may become ostracized socially. Individuals with ADHD may possess inadequate or underdeveloped social skills. They may have difficultly modifying their social behavior in accordance with situational demands. For individuals with ADHD, therapy may focus on strategies involving micro-level skills such as maintaining eye contact, using an appropriate voice volume, and maintaining body position, as well as macro-level skills such as giving compliments and constructive feedback, turn-taking, and listening skills. Individuals may need to be taught to pay attention to social cues, enabling them to recognize and engage in more appropriate social behavior.

In all instances, it is important to help children learn to self-regulate and to reflect on their thinking and the contextual feedback from their behavior. Awareness of performance can be enhanced through predicting one's performance and evaluating and comparing actual performance with one's prediction. Consistent with occupational therapy philosophy, interventions need to be context

sensitive, and everyday routines, including parent–child, teacher–child, and peer interactions, are the ideal context in which to provide strategy training. A list of strategies to consider when working with children with ADHD is provided in Exhibit 11.1.

CASE STUDY: MICHAEL

"Michael has been a difficult child from the time I can remember," said Michael's mother:

> He hardly slept as an infant. He walked earlier than my daughter, and from the moment he took his first steps at 8 months, he has been on the go. When he was a toddler, he had to be watched all the time. He's like a walking disaster. He takes risks all the time; he's broken his arm twice and has numerous scars. He acts without stopping to think of the consequences, and he never seems to learn from his mistakes. He starts things but doesn't finish them. Even getting dressed in the morning is a problem. He will put on a few things and then get distracted by something in his room, such as a toy. I constantly have to call upstairs and remind him to get ready. Michael seems to be driven by a motor and constantly on the go. By the time nighttime comes, I'm exhausted watching him. Even sleep is difficult. We can't get him to go to bed, and when he does go, we can't get him to stay in bed.

When asked about school, Michael's mother replied,

> School is a disaster for Michael. His teacher complains that he is unable to sit still and do his work; he calls out in class, he's noisy, and he disrupts the other children. In preschool, his teacher complained that he had difficultly sitting down during circle time and staying on his mattress during naptime. He needed a teacher's assistant to sit with him so he would not disrupt the other children. When in kindergarten, his teacher complained that, when other children were in the block-building area, he would go over to their blocks and, for no apparent reason, knock them over.

Michael's mother also talked about homework being a major conflict at home. She stated that he had to read for 20 min each night and had to complete one or two worksheets. She stated that it usually took an hour or 2 to get 20 min of reading because Michael was constantly up and down. He would start, get up for a drink, and then go to the television. She would call him back, he would work

EXHIBIT 11.1. Examples of Processing Strategies and Behaviors Relevant for Children With ADHD

Attention
- Detects subtle changes in task conditions.
- Initiates exploration or search of the environment.
- Searches for information in a planned, systematic manner.
- Inhibits automatic responses.
- Maintains goal-directed behavior.
- Is unhindered by internal or external distractions peripheral to the task.
- Sustains focus of attention on task.
- Persists with the repetitive activity over time.
- Paces and monitors speed of response.
- Reduces stimuli/identifies irrelevant information (e.g., cross out, sort, remove what is unnecessary).
- Identifies relevant information (highlights, distinguishes critical details spontaneously, compares stimuli and chooses important facts).
- Pays attention to detail.
- Simultaneously attends to overall stimulants as well as details.
- Keeps track of rules, facts, and pieces of information (external vs. internal methods).
- Allocates resources by placing greater effort and concentration on more critical aspect of the task.
- Easily disengages focus of attention when necessary.
- Follows changes in task, stimuli, or rules without error, withdrawal, or resistance.
- Verbalizes each step of a task to focus attention.
- Persists and maintains consistency of performance.
- Attends to relevant details, highlights or lists critical information.

Problem Solving
- Predicts the consequences of an obstacle or action.
- Analyzes the condition of the problem.
- Recognizes when information is incomplete and actively searches for needed information.
- Prioritizes information.
- Distinguishes critical facts, assumptions, and irrelevant information.
- When stuck, re-examines the problem in a different way, reorganizes information differently, asks questions for clarification, talks out loud through each step, or brainstorms.
- Formulates a plan or sequence of action.
- Shifts to alternate strategies, plans when needed.
- Persists with the task in searching for a solution.
- Spontaneously checks work.
- Detects errors.

Impulsivity
- Considers alternatives before making a choice.
- Waits for question to be completed before answering.
- Waits for directions to be completed before starting task.
- Waits for one's turn.
- Paces speed of response.
- Visualizes the steps before performing them.
- Formulates and adheres to a plan or sequence of action.
- Checks own work.
- Attends to relevant details, highlights or lists critical information.
- Organizes items prior to beginning a task.
- Makes and uses a list to stay on task.

Note. ADHD = attention-deficit/hyperactivity disorder. The information in this table is based on Toglia (see Chapter 2, this volume).

for another minute or two, and then he would leave for the computer. Michael's mother said that homework was a constant source of conflict and caused nightly arguments.

When Michael's teacher was interviewed, she stated,

Michael is smart, but his work doesn't show it. His schoolwork is rarely completed. When the students in class are independently working on assignments, Michael looks out the window, watches the other children, opens and closes his desk, and gets out of his seat constantly. His work is always very messy; his writing is all over the page. When he copies his math homework problems from the board, he makes numerous mistakes, because he doesn't pay attention to the numbers or their alignment. When Michael does math problems, he doesn't pay attention to the plus and minus signs. If he starts adding, he continues adding, even when the problems call for subtraction.

The teacher added that lack of attention to detail is characteristic of Michael's performance in many areas.

Interviews with Michael's teacher indicated that her concerns were with his inability to stay on task and his frequent "sloppy errors." She also was concerned about his illegible handwriting and found it difficult to grade his assignments. When an occupational therapist examined Michael's handwriting papers, it appeared that part of the reason for his messy work was that Michael was not attending to the lines on the page and wrote all over the page. Michael stated that he wanted to do better in school and wanted to be on the honor roll.

Michael had been diagnosed with ADHD and was using medication. Reports by a neuropsychologist indicated that, on a CPT, Michael made many errors of omission (missed the Xs) and commission (pressed the key on incorrect letters). This indicated that he had difficulty sustaining attention, and it showed impulsivity. The occupational therapist concluded, on the basis of Michael's CPT performance and coupled with his teacher's reports, that Michael had difficulty paying attention to detail, as indicated by his not attending to the lines when writing, not attending to the plus and minus signs when doing math problems, and not checking his work as when copying from the blackboard.

The therapist wanted to know if Michael was aware of his performance and so repeated the CPT using a different target stimulus. As described in the "Assessment" section, the therapist first asked Michael to predict how he would do. Michael stated that he thought the task would be easy and that he would get everything correct. In fact, he again made many errors. However, he was not aware of this and felt that he had done well.

The occupational therapist also wanted to look at the effects of task and environmental supports on Michael's task performance. She examined the effect of external cueing on performance on the CPT task. She put half the *A*s in boldface type and left half in a regular typeface. This form of cueing increased accuracy by 20% for the highlighted stimuli.

In math, instead of giving Michael a worksheet with addition and subtraction problems mixed together, as was typically done in class, the therapist gave him one page with addition problems and put a large plus (+) sign with the word *ADD* at the top of the page. She gave him a second sheet with all subtraction problems and put a large minus (−) sign with the word *SUBTRACT* at the top of the page. Michael's accuracy went from 60%–70% to 85%–90% with this change. Thus, the therapist concluded that the problem was not that Michael did not know how to accurately do the operations but rather that he was not attending to the details of the sign and therefore was missing many problems.

Although one solution would be to always structure Michaels' work in this manner, the teacher felt that Michael would not learn to work in a contextually relevant manner needed for school. The next thing the therapist tried was using the page of mixed addition and subtraction but color coding the plus and minus signs so that all plus signs were green and all minus signs were red. Use of a strategy such as this required the teacher to mark the signs. Increasing the salience of the plus and minus signs seemed to facilitate performance, although not to the same extent as presenting addition and subtraction problems separately.

The next strategy transferred responsibility to Michael instead of the teacher. The therapist asked Michael to circle the plus or minus sign before starting each problem. This helped for a few problems, but Michael seemed to be more focused on circling the mathematical symbol than on paying attention to what the symbol was. Thus, the next strategy the therapist tried was asking Michael before each problem to trace the sign in green if it was an

addition problem and trace the sign in red if it was a subtraction problem and to say to himself "add" or "subtract." This seemed to force him to attend to the sign and resulted in enhanced performance. This is an example of a situation-specific strategy that was effective for his math work but that would not automatically generalize to other situations that also required attention to detail.

The occupational therapist also considered the difficulty that Michael was having copying math homework from the board. An example of an external strategy would be to have another child copy the problems for Michael. Another method would be to teach Michael to use graph paper to align the numbers. An example of an internal strategy would be to teach Michael the strategy of checking the accuracy of his copying after each problem. When Michael was cued to slow his copying and check its accuracy after each item, copying was improved. The strategy of "stop and check" is an example of a general strategy that can be applied across multiple tasks for which attention to detail is important. Obviously, some approaches, such as using graph paper and checking work, can be combined.

Another concern that Michael's teacher expressed was Michael's difficulty staying seated and on task during independent seatwork. Michael's teacher reported that he often looked out the window and watched the other children. Review of his seating placement indicated that he was seated in the aisle next to the window at the rear of the class. We suggested that his teacher move his seat to the front row, in the middle. This is an example of an environmental manipulation that influenced performance. Michael's teacher reported that Michael attended better. She was not sure whether this was because he was less distracted because he was farther from the window and couldn't see all the children or because she provided more cues to him and monitored him more closely because he was closer to her. Michael still had difficulty staying on task, so a behavioral approach was implemented in conjunction with strategy training (see below).

The occupational therapist wanted to work with Michael's mother on her goal to have Michael stay on task with his homework and reduce the number of times she needed to remind him to sit down and continue working. The objective was to have Michael remain seated and work on homework for 20 min. The strategy was to stay focused on the task. The therapist implemented an external strategy that involved the use of a vibratory cue. Michael wore a watch with a built-in vibrator programmed to go off randomly every 30 to 90 s. Michael was asked to record whether he was on task doing his assignment each time the vibrator went off. If he was seated at the table and on task, he was asked to put a chip into a container (contingent reinforcement). If he was off task, he was asked to take a chip out of the container (response cost). (N.B.: Earphones with a tape programmed to make an audible beep also could be used instead of a vibrating watch, and a page with spaces in which to make a check mark could be used instead of chips.)

Use of dynamic interactional assessment was incorporated as follows: Before starting the task, the procedure was described to Michael. He was told that he was going to be asked to do homework for 20 min. He was asked if he thought it would be difficult for him and to rate the level of difficulty from *a little* to *a lot*. He was then told that during this 20 min he would have the opportunity to earn up to 20 chips for being on task and sticking to his homework. He was asked how many chips he thought he would be able to earn. The protocol was then implemented. After this, Michael was asked if he thought that the task was easier or harder than he expected. He was asked to compare the number of chips he had thought he would earn with the number of chips he actually earned. He was asked about strategies he used to stay on task. If his performance was less than he predicted, he was asked why he had difficulty and what strategies he could use next time so he could earn more chips. The plan was to grade the vibration cues by gradually spacing out the cues so that at the end of 3 months they were to occur 5 to 7 min apart. The next step was to fade the self-recording procedure (use of chips) so that self-directed tracking could be accomplished.

To promote generalization, these strategies were practiced in different contexts (home and school). Another strategy that was targeted was "pay attention to detail," because this was an issue in multiple contexts. Different activities were selected that involved attending to detail. See Exhibit 11.1 for examples of strategies that may be used to enhance attention and decrease impulsivity.

SUMMARY

In this chapter, I reviewed the major characteristics of ADHD and discussed their impact on the children and adolescents' function in the areas of school function, self-care, work, and parent and peer relationships. Traditional assessments, including rating scales, observational systems, performance measures, and measures of executive function, were reviewed. The need to link assessment with the child's function and participation when planning intervention was emphasized. Current evidence for intervention with children with ADHD was reviewed,

with emphasis on the MTA study, the most comprehensive intervention study with children with ADHD that reported that medication combined with a cognitive–behavioral approach was more effective than either treatment alone or than standard community-based care. The relevance of these findings for occupational therapy was discussed. I proposed that principles of the dynamic interactional model of cognition described by Toglia (see Chapter 2, this volume) can be applied and integrated with use of a cognitive–behavioral approach to intervention. I reviewed and illustrated application of dynamic interactional questioning to more traditional ADHD assessments. I also applied, through a case study, consideration of the person–task–environment in intervention to a child with ADHD.

REVIEW QUESTIONS

1. Describe the three main characteristics of ADHD, and give examples of behaviors of each.
2. According to Barkley's model of ADHD, what is the primary deficit, and how does this affect executive functions?
3. Discuss the impact of ADHD on school, work, play and leisure, and activities of daily living.
4. What are the differences among rating scales, observational systems, and measures of performance to assess ADHD? Give an example of each.
5. What are *executive functions?* Give an example of a test used with children with ADHD.
6. Medication is a commonly used intervention for children with ADHD. Discuss research on its effectiveness.
7. Describe the national NIMH-funded multimodal treatment study. What were the primary results? Why is it important for therapists to be aware of this study?
8. How can principles of the dynamic interactional model of cognition be applied to children with ADHD? Give an example in terms of how a traditional test can be adapted to assess awareness.
9. Give an example of intervention to improve attention to task and task performance targeting the task, the environment, and the person.

REFERENCES

Abidin, R. R. (1995). *Parenting Stress Index* (3rd ed.). Lutz, FL: Psychological Assessment Resources.

Abidin, R. R., & Brunner, J. F. (1995). Development of a parenting alliance inventory. *Journal of Clinical Child Psychology, 24,* 31–40.

Abikoff, H. (1991). Cognitive training in ADHD children: Less to it than meets the eye. *Journal of Learning Disabilities, 24,* 205–209.

Achenbach, T. M. (2003). *Achenbach System of Empirically Based Assessment* (ASEBA). San Antonio, TX: Harcourt Assessment.

Adams, C. D., Kelley, M. L., & McCarthy, M. (1997). The Adolescent Behavior Checklist (ABC): Development and initial psychometric properties of a self-report measure for adolescents with ADHD. *Journal of Clinical Child Psychology, 26,* 77–86.

American Occupational Therapy Association. (2002). Occupational therapy practice framework: Domain and process. *American Journal of Occupational Therapy, 56,* 609–639.

American Psychiatric Association. (1994). *Diagnostic and statistical manual of mental disorders* (4th ed.). Washington, DC: Author.

American Psychiatric Association. (2000). *Diagnostic and statistical manual of mental disorders* (4th ed., text rev.). Washington, DC: Author.

Anastopoulos, A. D., & Shelton, T. L. (2001). *Assessing attention-deficit/hyperactivity disorder.* New York: Kluwer Academic.

Anderson, J. C., Williams, S., McGee, R., & Silva, P. A. (1987). *DSM–III* disorders in preadolescent children. *Archives of General Psychiatry, 44,* 69–76.

Arnold, D. S., O'Leary, S. G., Wolff, L. S., & Acker, M. M. (1993). The Parenting Scale: A measure of dysfunctional parenting in discipline situations. *Psychological Assessment, 5,* 137–144.

Arnold, L. E., Abikoff, H. B., Cantwell, D. P., Conners, C. K., Elliott, G. R., Greenhill, L. L., et al. (1997). NIMH Collaborative Multimodal Treatment Study of Children with ADHD (MTA): Design, methodology, and protocol evolution. *Journal of Attention Disorders, 2,* 141–158.

Atkins, M. S., & Pelham, W. E. (1991). School-based assessment of attention deficit-hyperactivity disorder. *Journal of Learning Disabilities, 24,* 197–204, 255.

Ayres, A. J. (1979). *Sensory integration and the child.* Los Angeles: Western Psychological Services.

Baer, R. A., & Nietzel, M. T. (1991). Cognitive and behavioral treatment of impulsivity in children: A meta-analytic review of the outcome literature. *Journal of Clinical Child Psychology, 20,* 400–412.

Barkley, R. A. (1990a). *Attention-deficit hyperactivity disorder: A handbook for diagnosis and treatment.* New York: Guilford Press.

Barkley, R. A. (1990b). A critique of current diagnostic criteria for attention deficit hyperactivity disorder: Clinical and research implications. *Journal of Developmental and Behavioral Pediatrics, 11,* 343–352.

Barkley, R. A. (1996). Attention-deficit/hyperactivity disorder: Diagnostic, developmental and conceptual issues. In M. J. Breen & C. R. Fiedler (Eds.), *Behavioral approach to assessment of youth with emotional/behavioral disorders: A handbook for school-based practitioners* (pp. 413–449). Austin, TX: Pro-Ed.

Barkley, R. A. (1997a). *ADHD and the nature of self-control.* New York: Guilford Press.

Barkley, R. A. (1997b). Behavioral inhibition, sustained attention, and executive functions: Constructing a unifying theory of ADHD. *Psychological Bulletin, 121,* 65–94.

Barkley, R. A. (1998). *Attention-deficit hyperactivity disorder: A handbook for diagnosis and treatment* (2nd ed.). New York: Guilford Press.

Barkley, R. A. (2004). Attention-deficit/hyperactivity disorder and self-regulation: Taking an evolutionary perspective on executive functioning. In R. F. Baumeister & K. D. Vohs (Eds.), *Handbook of self-regulation* (pp. 301–232). New York: Guilford Press.

Barkley, R. A., Guevremont, D. C., Anastopoulos, A. D., DuPaul, G. J., & Shelton, T. L. (1993). Driving-related risks and outcomes of attention deficit hyperactivity disorder in adolescence and young adults: A 3–5 year follow-up survey. *Pediatrics, 92,* 212–218.

Barkley, R. A., & Murphy, K. R. (1998). *Attention-deficit hyperactivity disorder: A clinical workbook* (2nd ed.). New York: Guilford Press.

Barkley, R. A., Murphy, K. R., DuPaul, G. J., & Bush, T. (2002). Driving in young adults with attention deficit hyperactivity disorder: Knowledge, performance, adverse outcomes, and the role of executive functioning. *Journal of the International Neuropsychological Society, 8,* 655–672.

Barkley, R. A., Murphy, K. R., & Kwasnik, D. (1996). Motor vehicle driving competencies and risks in teens and young adults with attention deficit hyperactivity disorder. *Pediatrics, 98,* 1089–1095.

Beck, A. T. (1993). *Beck Anxiety Inventory.* San Antonio, TX: Harcourt Assessments.

Beck, A. T., Steer, R. A., & Brown, G. K. (1996). *Beck Depression Inventory II.* San Antonio, TX: Harcourt Assessments.

Berlin, L., Bohlin, G., Nyberg, L., & Janols, L. O. (2004). How well do measures of inhibition and other executive functions discriminate between children with ADHD and controls? *Child Neuropsychology, 10,* 1–13.

Biederman, J., & Faraone, S. V. (2002). Current concepts on the neurobiology of attention-deficit/hyperactivity disorder. *Journal of Attention Disorders, 6*(Suppl. 1), S7–S16.

Cantwell, D. P., & Baker, L. (1991). *Psychiatric and developmental disorders in children with communication disorder.* Washington, DC: American Psychiatric Association.

Centers for Disease Control and Prevention. (2004, February 4). *ADHD attention-deficit/hyperactivity disorder.* Retrieved August 16, 2004, from http://www.cdc.gov/ncbddd/adhd/symptom.htm.

Cohn, E., & Cermak, S. A. (1998). Including the family perspective in sensory integration outcomes research. *American Journal of Occupational Therapy, 52,* 540–546.

Conners, C. K. (1994). *Conners' Continuous Performance Test, users manual.* Toronto, Ontario: Multi-Health Systems.

Conners, C. K. (1997). *Conners' Rating Scales–Revised, users manual.* North Tonawanda, NY: Multi-Health Systems.

Coster, W. J. (1998). Occupation-centered assessment of children. *American Journal of Occupational Therapy, 52,* 337–344.

Cox, D. J., Merkel, L., Kovatchev, B., & Seward, R. (2000). The effect of stimulant medication on driving performance of young adults with ADHD: A preliminary double-blind placebo-controlled trial. *Journal of Nervous and Mental Disease, 18,* 230–234.

Derogatis, L. R. (1994). *Symptom Checklist–90-R.* Minneapolis, MN: Pearson Assessments.

Dunn, W., & Bennett, D. (2002). Patterns of sensory processing in children with attention deficit hyperactivity disorder. *OTJR—Occupation, Participation, and Health, 22,* 4–15.

DuPaul, G. J., & Eckert, T. L. (1997). The effects of school-based interventions for attention-deficit hyperactivity disorder: A meta-analysis. *School Psychology Review, 26,* 5–27.

DuPaul, G. J., Power, T. J., Anastopoulos, A. D., & Reid, R. (1998). *Attention-Deficit/Hyperactivity Disorder Rating Scale IV: Checklists, norms, and clinical interpretation.* New York: Guilford Press.

DuPaul, G. J., Power, T. J., McGoey, K. E., Ikeda, M. J., & Anastopoulos, A. D. (1998). Reliability and validity of parent and teacher ratings of attention-deficit/hyperactivity disorder symptoms. *Journal of Psychoeducational Assessment, 16,* 55–68.

DuPaul, G. J., Rapport, M. D., & Perriello, L. M. (1991). Teacher ratings of academic skills: The development of the Academic Performance Rating Scale. *School Psychology Review, 20,* 284–300.

Dykman, R. A., Akerman, P. T., & Raney, T. J. (1994). *Assessment and characteristics of children with attention deficit disorder.* Report prepared for the Office of Special Education Programs, Office of Special Education and Rehabilitative Services, U.S. Department of Education.

Edelbrock, C. S. (1991). Child Attention Problem Rating Scale. In R. A. Barkley (Ed.), *Attention-deficit hyperactivity disorder: A clinical workbook* (pp. 49–50). New York: Guilford.

Eyberg, S., & Pincus, D. (1999). *Eyberg Child Behavior Inventory and Sutter–Eyberg Student Behavior Inventory–Revised.* Odessa, FL: Psychological Assessment Resources.

Fischer, M. (1990). Parenting stress and the child with attention deficit hyperactivity disorder. *Journal of Clinical Child Psychology, 19,* 337–346.

Fletcher, J. (1999). *Marching to a different tune: Diary about an ADHD boy.* London: Taylor & Francis.

Gadow, K. D., & Sprafkin, J. (1998). *Child Symptom Inventory–4* (CSI–4). Stony Brook, NY: Checkmate Plus.

Gillberg, C. (2003). Deficits in attention, motor control, and perception: A brief review. *Archives of Diseases of Childhood, 88,* 904–910.

Gioia, G. A., Isquith, P. K., Guy, S. C., & Kenworthy, L. (2000). *Behavior Rating Inventory of Executive Function.* Odessa, FL: Psychological Assessment Resources.

Goldman, L. S., Genel, M., Bezman, R. J., & Slanetz, P. J. (1998). Diagnosis and treatment of attention-deficit/hyperactivity disorder in children and adolescents. *Journal of the American Medical Association, 279,* 1100–1107.

Goldstein, S., & Ellison, A. J. (2002). *Clinicians' guide to adult ADHD: Assessment and intervention (Practical resources for the mental health professional).* New York: Elsevier.

Goldstein, S., & Goldstein, M. (1990). *Managing attention disorders in children.* New York: Wiley.

Greenberg, L. M., & Waldman, I. D. (1993). Developmental normative data on the Test of Variables of Attention (TOVA). *Journal of Child Psychology and Psychiatry and Allied Disciplines, 34,* 1019–1030.

Gresham, F. M., & Elliot, S. N. (1990). *Social Skills Rating System* (SSRS). Circle Pines, MN: AGS.

Hallowell, E. M., & Ratey, J. J. (1995). *Driven to distraction: Recognizing and coping with attention deficit disorder from childhood through adulthood.* New York: Touchstone.

Homack, S., & Riccio, C. A. (2004). A meta-analysis of the sensitivity and specificity of the Stroop Color and Word Test with children. *Archives of Clinical Neuropsychology, 19,* 725–743.

Jensen, P. S., Hinshaw, S. P., Kraemer, H. C., Lenora, N., Newcorn, J. H., Abikoff, H. B., et al. (2001). ADHD comorbidity findings from the MTA Study: Comparing comorbid subgroups. *Journal of the American Academy of Child and Adolescent Psychiatry, 40,* 147–158.

Jensen, P. S., Martin, D., & Cantwell, D. P. (1997). Comorbidity in ADHD: Implications for research practice, and *DSM–IV. Journal of the American Academy of Child and Adolescent Psychiatry, 36,* 1065–1079.

Johnston, C. (2002). The impact of attention deficit hyperactivity disorder on social and vocational functioning in adults. In P. S. Jensen & J. R. Cooper (Eds.), *Attention deficit hyperactivity disorder: State of the science, best practices* (pp. 1–21). Kingston, NJ: Civic Research Institute.

Johnston, C., & Mash, E. (1989). A measure of parenting satisfaction and efficacy. *Journal of Clinical Child Psychology, 18,* 167–175.

Katz, N., Parush, S., & Traub Bar-Ilan, R. (in press). *Dynamic Occupational Therapy Cognitive Assessment for Children (DOTCA–Ch).* Pequannock, NJ: Maddak.

Kimball, J. G. (2002). Developmental coordination disorder from a sensory integration perspective. In S. A. Cermak & D. Larkin (Eds.), *Developmental coordination disorder* (pp. 210–220). Albany, NY: Delmar Thomson.

Law, M., Baptiste, S., Carswell, A., McColl, M. A., Polatajko, H., & Pollock, N. (1994). *Canadian Occupational Performance Measure* (2nd ed.). Toronto, Ontario: Canadian Association of Occupational Therapists.

Law, M., Baptiste, S., Carswell, A., McColl, M. A., Polatajko, H., & Pollock, N. (1994). Pilot testing of the Canadian Occupational Performance Measure: Clinical implications and measurement issues. *Canadian Journal of Occupational Therapy, 61,* 191–197.

Lawrence, V., Houghton, S., Douglas, G., Durkin, K., Whiting, K., & Tannock, R. (2004). A comparison of children's performance during neuropsychological and real-world activities. *Journal of Attention Disorders, 7,* 137–149.

Lawrence, V., Houghton, S., Tannock, R., Douglas, G., Durkin, K., & Whiting, K. (2002). ADHD outside the laboratory: Boys' executive function performance on tasks in videogame play and on a visit to the zoo. *Journal of Abnormal Child Psychology, 30,* 447–462.

Leark, R. A., Dupuy, T. R., Greenberg, L. M., Corman, C. L., & Kindechi, C. (1996). *Test of variables of attention: Professional manual.* Los Alamitos, CA: Universal Attention Disorders.

Lezak, M. D. (2004). *Neuropsychological assessment* (4th ed.). New York: Oxford University Press.

Locke, H. J., & Wallace, K. M. (1959). Short marital adjustment and prediction tests: Their reliability and validity. *Marriage and Family Living, 21,* 251–255.

Mancini, M., Coster, W. J., Trombly, C. A., & Heeren, T. C. (2000). Predicting elementary school participation in children with disabilities. *Archives of Physical Medicine and Rehabilitation, 81,* 339–347.

Mangeot, S. D., Miller, L. J., McIntosh, D. N., McGrath-Clarke, J., Simon, J., Hagerman, R. J., et al. (2001). Sensory modulation dysfunction in children with attention-deficit/hyperactivity disorder. *Developmental Medicine and Child Neurology, 43,* 399–406.

Manly, T., Robertson, I. H., Anderson, V., & Nimmo-Smith, I. (1999). *Test of Everyday Attention for Children (TEA–Ch).* London: Thames Valley Test Company.

Mannuzza, S., Klein, R. G., Bessler, A., Malloy, P., & LaPadula, M. (1993). Adult outcome of hyperactive boys: Educational achievement, occupational rank, and psychiatric status. *Archives of General Psychology, 50,* 565–576.

Mash, E. J., & Johnston, C. (1990). Determinants of parenting stress: Illustrations from families of hyperactive children and families of physically abused children. *Journal of Clinical Child Psychology, 19,* 313–328.

McCarney, S. B. (1989). *Attention Deficit Disorders Evaluation Scales (ADDES).* Columbia, MO: Hawthorne Educational Services.

Missiuna, C., Pollack, N., & Law, M. (2004). *Perceived Efficacy and Goal Setting System.* Toronto, Ontario: Psychological Corporation.

MTA Cooperative Group. (1999a). A 14-month randomized clinical trial of treatment strategies for attention-deficit/hyperactivity disorder (ADHD). *Archives of General Psychiatry, 56,* 1073–1086.

MTA Cooperative Group. (1999b). Moderators and mediators of treatment response for children with attention-deficit/hyperactivity disorder. *Archives of General Psychiatry, 56,* 1088–1096.

Mulligan, S. (1996). An analysis of score patterns of children with attention disorders on the Sensory Integration and Praxis Tests. *American Journal of Occupational Therapy, 50,* 647–654.

Murphy, K. R., & Barkley, R. A. (1996). Attention deficit hyperactivity disorder in adults: Comorbidities and adaptive impairments. *Comprehensive Psychiatry, 37,* 393–401.

Murphy, K. R., Barkley, R. A., & Bush, T. (2001). Executive functioning and olfactory identification in young adults with attention-deficit hyperactivity disorder. *Neuropsychology, 15,* 211–220.

Nada-Raja, S., Langley, J. D., McGee, R., Williams, S. M., Begg, D. J., & Reeder, K. I. (1997). Inattentive and hyperactive behaviors and driving offenses in adolescence. *Journal of the American Academy of Child and Adolescent Psychiatry, 36,* 515–522.

Naglieri, J. A., LeBuffe, P. A., & Pfieffer, S. I. (1994). *Devereux Scales of Mental Disorder* (DSMD). San Antonio, TX: Harcourt Assessment.

National Institute of Mental Health. (1999). *Questions and answers: NIMH Multimodal Treatment Study of Children With ADHD.* Bethesda, MD: Author.

National Institute of Mental Health. (2000). *NIMH research on treatment for attention deficit hyperactivity disorder (ADHD): The Multimodal Treatment Study—Questions and answers.* Retrieved March 5, 2004, from http://www.nimh.nih.gov/events/mtaqa.cfm

Parush, S., Sohmer, H., Steinberg, A., & Kaitz, M. (1997). Somatosensory functioning in children with attention deficit hyperactivity disorder. *Developmental Medicine and Child Neurology, 39,* 464–468.

Pelham, W. E., Harper, G. W., McBurnett, K., Milich, R., Murphy, D. A., Clinton, J., et al. (1990). Methylphenidate and baseball playing in ADHD children—Who's on 1st? *Journal of Consulting and Clinical Psychology, 58,* 130–133.

Popper, C. W. (1988). Disorders usually first evident in infancy, childhood, or adolescence. In J. A. Talbott, R. E. Hales, & S. C. Yudofsky (Eds.), *Textbook of psychiatry* (pp. 649–735). Washington, DC: American Psychiatric Association.

Resnick, R. J. (2000). *The hidden disorder: A clinician's guide to attention deficit hyperactivity disorder in adults.* Washington, DC: American Psychological Association.

Reynolds, C. R., & Kamphaus, R. W. (2004a). *Behavior Assessment System for Children–2 (BASC–2).* Circle Pines, MN: American Guidance Service.

Reynolds, C. R., & Kamphaus, R. W. (2004b). *Behavior Assessment System for Children Portable Observation Program* [Computer software]. Circle Pines, MN: American Guidance Service.

Robison, L. M., Sclar, D. A., Skaer, T. L., & Galin, R. S. (2004). Treatment modalities among US children diagnosed with attention-deficit hyperactivity disorder: 1995–1999. *International Clinical Psychopharmacology, 19,* 17–22.

Robison, L. M., Skaer, T. L., Sclar, D. A., & Galin, R. S. (2002). Is attention deficit hyperactivity disorder increasing among girls in the US? Trends in diagnosis and the prescribing of stimulants. *CNS Drugs, 18,* 129–137.

Roth, R. M., & Saykin, A. J. (2004). Executive dysfunction in attention-deficit/hyperactivity disorder: Cognitive and neuroimaging findings. *Psychiatric Clinics of North America, 27,* 83–96.

Schilling, D. L., Washington, K., Billingsley, F. F., & Deitz, J. (2003). Classroom seating for children with attention deficit hyperactivity disorder: Therapy balls versus chairs. *American Journal of Occupational Therapy, 57,* 534–541.

Selikowitz, M. (1995). *All about ADD: Understanding attention deficit disorder.* New York: Oxford University Press.

Shaffer, R. J., Jacokes, L. E., Cassily, J. F., Greenspan, S. I., Tuchman, R. F., & Stemmer, P. J., Jr. (2001). Effect of interactive metronome training on children with ADHD. *American Journal of Occupational Therapy, 55,* 155–162.

Shapiro, E. S. (2003). *Behavioral Obsservation of Students in Schools (BOSS).* San Antonio, TX: Harcourt Assessment.

Snyder, D. K. (1997). *Marital Satisfaction Inventory–Revised.* Los Angeles: Western Psychological Services.

Spanier, G. (1989). *Dyadic Adjustment Scale.* North Tonawanda, NY: MHS.

Sparrow, S. S., Balla, D. A., & Cicchetti, D. V. (1984). *Vineland Adaptive Behavior Scales (VABS).* Circle Pines, MN: American Guidance Service.

Spodak, R. (1999). *Executive functioning—What is it and how does it affect learning?* Retrieved March 5, 2004, from http://www.washingtonparent.com/articles/9906/executive-functioning.htm.

Stein, M. A., Szumowski, E., Blondis, T. A., & Roizen, N. J. (1995). Adaptive skills dysfunction in ADD and ADHD children. *Journal of Child Psychology and Psychiatry and Allied Disciplines, 36,* 663–670.

Strayhorn, J. M., & Weidman, C. S. (1988). A parent practices scale and its relation to parent and child mental health. *Journal of the American Academy of Child and Adolescent Psychiatry, 27,* 613–618.

Teeter, P. A. (1998). *Interventions for ADHD: Treatment in developmental context.* New York: Guilford Press.

Teeter, P. A., & Semrud-Clikeman, M. (1997). *Child neuropsychology: Assessment and intervention for neurodevelopmental disorders.* Newton, MA: Allyn & Bacon.

Toglia, J. P. (1993). *Contextual Memory Test.* San Antonio, TX: Psychological Corporation.

Tseng, M. H., Henderson, A., Chow, S. M., & Yao, G. (2004). Relationship between motor proficiency, attention, impulse, and activity in children with ADHD. *Developmental Medicine and Child Neurology, 46,* 381–388.

U.S. Department of Education, Office of Special Education and Rehabilitative Services, Office of Special Education Programs. (2003). *Identifying and treating attention deficit hyperactivity disorder: A resource for school and home.* Washington, DC: Author.

U.S. Department of Health and Human Services. (1999). *Mental health: A report of the Surgeon General.* Washington, DC: Author.

VandenBerg, N. L. (2001). The use of a weighted vest to increase on-task behavior in children with attention difficulties. *American Journal of Occupational Therapy, 55,* 621–628.

Vygotsky, L. S. (1978). *Mind in society: The development of higher psychological processes.* Cambridge, MA: Harvard University Press.

Waschbusch, D. A., Willoughby, M. T., & Pelham, W. E. (1998). Criterion validity and the utility of reactive and proactive aggression: Comparisons to attention deficit hyperactivity disorder, oppositional defiant disorder, conduct disorder, and other measures of functioning. *Journal of Clinical Child Psychology, 27,* 396–405.

Watling, R., & Schwartz, I. S. (2004). Understanding and implementing positive reinforcement as an intervention strategy for children with disabilities. *American Journal of Occupational Therapy, 58,* 113–116.

Weiss, G., & Hechtman, L. T. (1993). *Hyperactive children grown up.* New York: Guilford Press.

Wells, K. C., Pelham, W. E., Kotkin, R. A., Hoza, B., Abikoff, H. B., Abramowitz, A., et al. (2000). Psychosocial treatment strategies in the MTA study: Rationale, methods, and critical issues in design and implementation. *Journal of Abnormal Child Psychology, 28,* 483–505.

Woodward, L. J., Fergusson, D. M., & Horwood, J. (2000). Driving outcomes of young people with attentional difficulties in adolescence. *Journal of the American Academy of Child and Adolescent Psychiatry, 39,* 627–634.

Yochman, A., Parush, S., & Ornoy, A. (2004). Responses of preschool children with and without ADHD to sensory events in daily life. *American Journal of Occupational Therapy, 58,* 294–302.

Zentall, S. S. (1993). Research on the educational implications of attention deficit hyperactivity disorder. *Exceptional Children, 60,* 143–153.

PART

Healthy Elderly People and Elderly People With Dementia

12

Linda L. Levy, MA, OTR/L, FAOTA

Cognitive Aging in Perspective

Information Processing, Cognition, and Memory

LEARNING OBJECTIVES

By the end of this chapter,
readers will
1. Name and define the three
information-processing stages of
cognition
2. Identify the components of short-
term memory
3. Explain the concept of working
memory
4. Name three forms of long-term
memory and describe how each is
developed
5. Discuss the differences between
explicit and implicit memory.

In this chapter I synthesize neuroscientific and cognitive information-processing concepts as they apply to cognitive theoretical models in occupational therapy practice. I begin with an overall definition of the broad construct known as *cognition,* including its multiple component processes and functions. I go on to explore the information-processing model of cognition as it is evolving in the cognitive psychology and neuroscience literature. I detail this model because it provides an indispensable conceptual framework for the examination of cognition, component processes of cognition, and the sources of the cognitive difficulties that emerge in the event of cognitive impairment that are addressed in the succeeding chapters of this book.

COGNITION

Cognition is a difficult concept for students to grasp because it is so often taken for granted. The better it works, the less conscious of it one is. Hence, cognition is something people tend not to think much about—unless they are confronted with some kind of impairment. So, just what is cognition?

Cognition is usually defined simply as the acquisition of knowledge, yet both the acquisition and the use of knowledge involve a number of complex mental processes. Neisser (1967) broadened the definition of cognition to include "all the processes by which sensory input is transformed, reduced, elaborated, stored, recovered, and used" (p. 4). This definition contains several important implications

for understanding the term (Reed, 2000). The reference to *sensory input* implies that all cognition begins with contact with the external environment. The reference to *transformation* of sensory input implies that one's representation of the world is not necessarily identical to the actual nature of the world, that is, that people actively construct their representations of the world. *Reduction* refers to the information that may reach one's cognitive receptors but is eventually lost (forgotten). *Elaboration* is an essential process that occurs when one adds to sensory input, in light of previous experiences. The *storage* and *recovery* of information are what are typically referred to as *memory;* the distinction between the two implies that storage of information does not necessarily mean that one will recover that information. The last part of Neisser's definition is perhaps the most important. After information has been perceived, stored, and recovered, it must be put to use—for example, to make decisions, to solve problems, to reason; to formulate goals; to meet psychological needs; and to engage in instrumental activities of daily living (IADLs), activities of daily living (ADLs), and in all occupational behaviors.

Hence, cognition can be characterized as a number of mental components. Together, these form a complex system of interdependent mental processes. These components can be grouped into three major categories: (a) mental power (endurance), (b) specific cognitive abilities, and (c) executive functions.

The first category, *mental power* (stamina, or endurance), refers to the basic energy that supports all mental operations. More specifically, it refers to the capacity to maintain a state of wakefulness wherein the individual is ready and able to respond to events in the environment (Posner & DiGirolama, 2000; Tootell & Hadjikhani, 2000), as well as the amount of cognitive work that can be performed per unit of time. Hence, this category of cognitive function makes reference to issues such as arousal level (coma would be an example of not having enough power, or endurance, or both), alertness (vs. persistent fatigue), attention and concentration span, and the number of lines of thought a person can manage simultaneously (task-switching efficiency). Mental energies (alertness) and efficiency (speed) are significant issues to be considered in any kind of neurocognitive disorder; these powers are also worsened by sleep deprivation, illness (acute or chronic), dehydration, and stress.

The second category, *specific mental abilities,* refers to abilities that are identified as the cognitive substrates of performance. They include

- The ability to maintain attention and focus on meaningful and relevant information when multiple stimuli are presented at the same time (attention)
- The ability to learn and retain information (memory)
- The ability to perform calculations and solve problems
- The ability to accurately recognize objects (visual perception)
- The ability to determine where visual objects are (visual spatial processing)
- The ability to understand and use language.

Note that, although people with neurocognitive disorders may have extensive brain injury and demonstrate numerous behavioral changes, they may score within normal ranges on neuropsychological tests that assess these components in isolation. Their functional deficits tend not to be measured within conventional neuropsychological testing.

Executive abilities refers to perhaps the largest, and most complex, array of cognitive functions. They are linked to intentionality, purposefulness, and complex decision making (Lezak, 1995; Luria, 1966) and are crucial for all higher order purposive behavior—including identifying the objective, projecting the goal, forming plans to reach it, organizing the means by which such plans can be carried out, and judging the consequences to see that all is accomplished as intended. Executive functions reach significant development only in humans and are the last functions in the brain to fully mature (i.e., in late adolescence). In essence, they serve as a type of supraordinate system coordinating all of the other processes of the brain.

They release the person from fixed repertoires and reactions (i.e., a *re*active approach to the environment) and allow for the mental representation of alternatives, imagination, and freedom (i.e., a *pro*active approach to the environment; Fernandez-Duque, Baird, & Posner, 2000; Goldberg, 2001). All aspects of executive functions regulate mental activities that allow for self-control. These are also the functions that allow individuals to meet social, vocational, occupational, IADL, ADL, and internal psychological (emotional) needs.

As I show in the discussion that follows, executive functions rely on working memory processes for their operation (Carpenter, Just, & Reichle, 2000), processes that are particularly vulnerable to damage in neurocognitive disorders. As a result, executive functions are among the first to break down in the event of neurocognitive disease. At mild levels of impairment, the consequences become apparent in difficulties related to overall occupational performance in general, and the ability to carry out IADLs in particular (e.g., planning and preparing meals, shopping for personal items, managing finances, using the telephone, doing heavy and light housework, and managing one's medications). At more severe levels of impairment limitations in executive functions become evident in the more basic ADLs as well (e.g., dressing, bathing, toileting, grooming, eating, transfers, and ambulation; Schwartz, 1995; Schwartz, Mayer, Fitzpatrick-DeSalme, & Montgomery, 1993).

In the following section I examine the cognitive information-processing model to provide a framework for conceptualizing the components and functions of cognition and for furthering readers' understanding the processes that are especially vulnerable to impairment in the event of neurocognitive disorders. Understanding what occurs at each of the stages is particularly important when individuals experience difficulties in occupational performance; practitioners can then identify which stage is the primary source of the difficulty and design interventions within the context of personally relevant everyday academic, vocational, social, leisure, and self-care occupations to address them.

INFORMATION PROCESSING, COGNITION, AND MEMORY

The cognitive information-processing model has been the major perspective in cognitive research for more than 30 years. It serves as the predominant conceptual framework in the cognitive neuroscience and cognitive psychology literature and determines how most students of cognition currently think and talk about the workings of cognition (Tulving, 2000). One of the primary objectives of the information-processing model is to identify the major information-processing stages involved in the acquisition, storage, retrieval, and use of information, as well as what happens during these stages at both psychological and neurological levels. It was first represented in Atkinson and Shiffrin's (1968) model of memory and has more recently been honed and refined in the neural-network, parallel distributed processing (or *connectionist*) models of cognition (Giles, Horne, & Lin, 1995; Levine, Long, & Parks, 1998; McClelland, McNaughton, & O'Reilly, 1995). The information-processing model has generated broad-based behavioral and neuroscientific support.

The model proposes that cognition involves the processing (i.e., preservation, transformation, and transfer) of information through three functionally distinct stages

identified in Figure 12.1: (a) sensory–perceptual memory, (b) short-term memory, and (c) long-term memory. Short-term memory is further divided into *primary memory* and *working* (or "scratch-pad") *memory,* and long-term memory is conceptualized as *explicit* (i.e., episodic and semantic) and *implicit* (automatic) memory (i.e. procedural, perceptual priming, and conditioned memories). According to this model, information is first processed through sensory–perceptual memory to reach short-term memory and is then processed through short-term memory in order to enter long-term memory. Thoroughly processed information becomes part of long-term memory and can be reactivated at any time to return to either short-term working memory or to sensory–perceptual memory. Hence, the model identifies a two-way flow of information required to help us make sense of the world around us we constantly use information that we gather through our senses

FIGURE 12.1. Cognitive information-processing model.

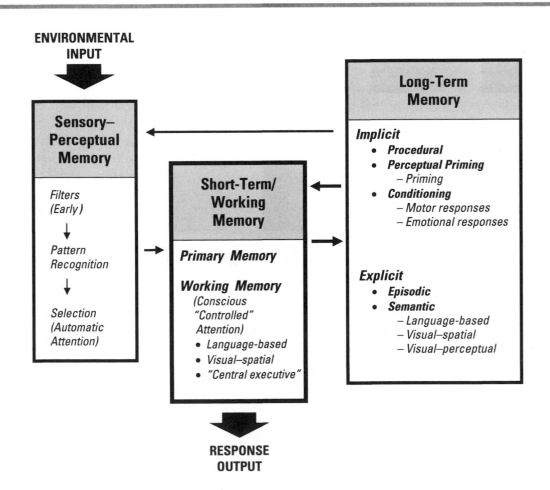

(often referred to as *bottom-up processing*) and information that we have stored in our imaginations (often called *top-down processing*) in a dynamic process, as we construct meaning about our environments and our relations to it. However, information not processed and passed to the next stage is lost, or forgotten.

The handling of information at each memory stage has been likened to the information processing of a computer. Like a computer, the mind takes in information, performs operations on it to change its form and content, stores the information, retrieves it when needed, and generates responses to it. Similarly, each of the three stages involves transforming information into a memory trace that can be stored (*encoding*), holding or maintaining the to-be-remembered information for immediate or later use (*storage*), and accessing the information when needed (*retrieval*). There is evidence that memory can fail at any of these stages. "Forgetting" may be due to failure to encode (i.e., inattention), destruction (i.e., displacement or decay) of the memory trace, or failure to retrieve (i.e., occasions when the memory is stored but cannot be brought to mind). I address each of these contingencies later in this chapter.

Note that, in information-processing models, *learning* is very difficult to differentiate from *memory*. Learning involves the acquisition of new information; memory involves the retention and retrieval of that information. Clearly, there can be no memory if learning has not occurred first, and learning has no meaning without memory. Hence, in information-processing models learning is considered within the acquisition or *encoding* stage of memory—or, more simply, as whatever the individual has encoded through experience.

Figure 12.1 is a schematic representation of a typical information-processing model of memory, synthesizing the ideas of several theorists. To better understand the model, I examine each component in further detail. This will provide the background necessary for identifying the specific components that are most frequently affected by aging, as well as those that remain strong. It will also serve as the basis for examination of how compensatory strategies can be introduced to improve cognitive competency and to optimize occupational performance and participation.

SENSORY–PERCEPTUAL MEMORY

Sensory–perceptual memory is the initial phase of intake of sensory information. Stimuli from the environment (sights, sounds, touches, smells, tastes) and internal sensations constantly bombard our sensory receptors. Sensory–perceptual information is registered automatically and lasts for perhaps a few hundred milliseconds to 4 or 5 s after the physical stimulus is withdrawn. This phase allows us to hold information long enough for additional analysis and filtering by perceptual and attentional processing.

Encoding

Sensory–perceptual memories are sense specific. The information is encoded as nearly an exact replica of the original stimulus (e.g., as fleeting visual images or sound patterns) and is stored according to the sensory modality that is activated (i.e., there are separate stores for visual, auditory, tactile, olfactory, gustatory, and proprioceptive information; Poon, 1985). The visual sensory–perceptual memory store is called *iconic memory,* because it stores information as a visual image (an icon); it lasts for approximately 0.3 s. The auditory sensory–perceptual memory store is called *echoic memory,* because sounds linger in it; it stores information for 3 to 5 s. Tactile sensory–perceptual memory (e.g., the feel of a passing breeze) lasts between 1 and 2 s. Because it is sensory information, this information remains primitive and unanalyzed.

Storage

Sensory–perceptual memory initially has a massive storage capacity; it can store virtually all information that has activated our sensory receptors. However, sensory information that activates our sense receptors is far greater than what our brains can fully process. Hence, the sensory–perceptual memory store filters down the vast amounts of information through the intertwined mechanisms of *perception* and *attention*. Ultimately, only the most relevant information (i.e., information that is selected as worth remembering) is perceived, attended to, and transferred for further memory processing. The vast majority of sensory information disappears quickly (*decays*) and is forgotten.

Retrieval

Information in sensory–perceptual memory is retrieved and retained by perception and attention. *Perception* involves the capacity to process relevant sensory stimuli while filtering out the rest. The perceptual filters that assist in this process are based on complex factors, including prior knowledge, experience, motivation, expectations, and predispositions. Hence, the sensory stimuli that are perceived are, in large part, those that make contact with neural connections (association networks) that are known (i.e., information that has already been stored).

Ultimately, perception organizes the selected sensory information into meaningful patterns based on prior experiences and memories (Gibson, 1969; Treisman & Gelade, 1980). For example, we generally interpret ambiguous clusters of visual stimuli as though they represent objects (e.g., a chair or a cup) in the real world. Accordingly, we are able to construct three-dimensional objects out of two-dimensional visual images, and we are able to identify complete objects while ignoring complex background distractions (i.e., *figure–ground discrimination,* the most elemental form of perceptual organization). We also organize sensory information, such as light, color, spatial position, and depth perception, into physiologically "hardwired," or species-specific, patterns. We also know that, in addition to clusters of stimuli that activate familiar patterns, those that are particularly intense (in terms of amount of sensory activation) or novel (i.e., exceptionally unfamiliar) are also likely to be attended to and perceived (Hampson, Pons, Stanford, & Deadwyler, 2004).

As indicated, information in sensory–perceptual memory is also retained by attention. Like perception, attention is complex (Posner & DiGirolama, 2000; Stuss, Binns, Murphy, & Alexander, 2002; Tootell & Hadjikhani, 2000). It has been described as a looplike process involving complex interactions among the prefrontal cortex, ventral brain stem, and posterior cortex (Goldberg, 2001; Johnson, 2004). In essence, attention acts as an additional filter that determines which perceptual patterns will be recognized (and carry potential for being remembered) and which will be filtered out (blocked; Broadbent, 1958; Deutsch & Deutsch, 1963; Treisman & Gelade, 1980). It consists of at least three distinct processes, including

1. A system that helps us maintain a general state of readiness to respond
2. A system that sets our threshold for responding to an external stimulus
3. A system that helps us selectively attend to appropriate stimuli and inhibit responses to competing stimuli.

In the sensory–perceptual memory stage, attention is automatic, unconscious, and "effortless." (Conscious—a.k.a. *controlled*—attention is addressed in the next stage.) Here, attention continually monitors the vast array of percepts that reach our sensory and perceptual receptors and selects only those that are of greatest relevance; at the same time, it inhibits responses to irrelevant, or distracting, information. The *cocktail party effect* is an illustra-

tion of this phenomenon (Wood & Cowan, 1995): While focused on a conversation with one person in a crowded and noisy room, our auditory systems are continually scanning the environment, filtering out irrelevant information and alert to other relevant information—particularly emotionally toned words, or the mention of one's own name. (And, as will be seen, this shift in attention disrupts processing of the original conversation.) This selective component of automatic attention is developed through extensive, consistent practice and experience with the environment (Gibson, 1969).

Note also that both perception and attention are activated in light of previous memories (e.g., prior knowledge, expectations, and experience), particularly those with affective significance (Davidson, 2000; Hamann, 2001; LeDoux, 2000). As well, even when unconscious (i.e., in coma or dreaming states), the brain both attends to and perceives relevant stimuli. In reality, however, both processes are so inextricably intertwined that they cannot truly be separated.

In sum, sensory–perceptual memory is the essential first stage toward the acquisition and consolidation of memories for longer term storage. This stage filters down vast amounts of sensory information and permits sensory and perceptual information that has been selected to "linger" for further processing, although we are largely unaware of the information that has been selected, and the memories retained are little more than fleeting images or sound bites. Sensory–perceptual impressions remain to be sorted through and organized in the next processing system, the short-term memory store.

SHORT-TERM/WORKING MEMORY

Once perceived; attended to (here, automatically, *unconsciously,* or effortlessly); and transformed into transitory patterns of images, sounds, or other types of sensory codes, the information is transferred to the short-term memory store. Short-term memory consists of those pieces of information to which the mind can *consciously* attend and process at any one time. In essence, it represents conscious awareness. This ability has long been recognized as the primary indicator of one's cognitive abilities (Jacobs, 1887; James, 1890). Short-term memory is also referred to as *active memory* (Anderson, 1983, 1993; Anderson & Lebiere, 1998). This is because the content of short-term memory is *activated information,* that is, what a person is thinking about and processing at the moment, and because we must keep information active in short-term memory or it will be lost.

Two sources of activated information are processed in short-term memory. One source is incoming impressions being attended to that one has just transferred from sensory–perceptual memory. The other source is more complex. It includes relevant information being retrieved from associated networks in already-established memory stores to help us to interpret and understand incoming information, unrelated ideas of which we are aware and "just happen to be thinking about" at the time, or both. Thus, short-term memory is used to process information from both sensory–perceptual memory and long-term memory stores. It is a system that involves a combination of storage (i.e., keeping things in mind) and processing (i.e., providing a work space for reflection and thought). This capability is reflected in its component memory systems: *primary memory* and *working memory* (Baddeley, 1992).

Primary memory was the first component of short-term memory to be recognized. It reflects the amount of recently experienced information to which one can attend, while filtering out and disregarding the numerous distractions that might otherwise interfere, and can then recall immediately. Note that in this component there are no additional processing requirements. It is roughly synonymous with the quantitative aspect of attention commonly known as *attention span* (or, more accurately, *memory span*). The digit span test found on most mental status tests is a measure of primary memory. In digit span, the longest string of digits an individual can immediately remember without making an error reflects one's short-term memory capacity and, hence, one's attention (or memory) span.

As I discuss more fully later, conscious (or *controlled*) attention is a limited cognitive resource. We can reliably pay attention to only a few items (e.g., approximately seven digits) while filtering out the numerous distractions that undermine that attention. Because it is possible to pay attention to only a limited amount of information at any one time, attentional resources are strained whenever individuals engage in activities that require attending to multiple tasks (i.e., multitasking), or in tasks that necessitate divided attention. Researchers now recognize that we can attend effectively to only one line of thought processing at a time, whether a string of digits, a world event, or conversation on the telephone. Although it may seem as though we are attending to several lines of thought simultaneously, we are actually dealing with them sequentially (Rubinstein, Meyer, & Evans, 2001); as a result, what has been termed *multitasking*, or *divided attention*, is actually *task switching*. In addition, researchers have found that when we seek to undertake two activities at once (e.g.,

talking on a cell phone while driving, conversing at a cocktail party and hearing one's name mentioned across the room, reading this chapter while watching a television program), each activity receives less than 50% of the neuronal energies (measured in the form of oxygen on functional magnetic resonance imaging) that might otherwise be available. When we switch back and forth between the two activities, there is also a 20%–30% decrease in the activation required to complete the two separate problems (Justa et al., 2001). Hence, shifting attention between lines of thought significantly reduces the cognitive resources (e.g., controlled attention, concentration, and the quantity of relevant activated information) that might otherwise be devoted to each task.

Working memory entails not only holding information in mind (i.e., it relies on attentional processes) but also "working on" or processing the information to find its underlying meaning and to prepare it for long-term storage (Anderson, 1993, 1995; Anderson & Lebiere, 1998; Baddeley, 1992, 1996b; Miyake & Shah, 1999). More than merely storage system (as would be reflected in the term *short-term memory*), working memory is conceived as more like a process, or pattern, of activation; as such, it serves as the more contemporary term for short-term memory. This memory component is at work when you are trying to understand this concept as you are reading it, while simultaneously keeping in mind background information provided in previous sentences, calling up relevant prior knowledge to increase your understanding and inhibiting irrelevant distractions in the surrounding environment.

Working memory capacity is a critical factor in determining the ability to focus one's conscious attention; to concentrate; to override automatic reactions when they are unwarranted; to move from concrete data to abstract concepts; to understand language; to set goals and to adjust behavior in relation to external circumstances; to engage in planning; to solve problems; and to engage in decision making, reasoning, creativity, judgment and in the service of all other higher order executive functions (including the ability to carry out IADLs; Carpenter et al., 2000).

In this effort, working memory coordinates all of the other cognitive substrates of performance (i.e., perception, attention, language, and implicit and explicit memory) and allows us to formulate goals and objectives (a mental image of where we are headed) and to devise plans to attain those goals. This, in turn, entails a complex process of overriding fixed repertoires and automatic reactions to the problem at hand, deciding what type of information is useful to the preconceived goal (a.k.a. controlled attention or *executive control*), and then selecting this information from the huge totality of knowledge available in implicit and explicit long-term stores. All of these search-and-retrieval activities require vast and intricate neural computations and connections, which are guided and coordinated by the frontal and prefrontal lobes (Bunge, Ochsner, Desmond, Glover, & Gabrieli, 2001; Goldberg, 2001). Note that, in large part, it is the exceptional richness of these connections and the fact that they are also the last nerve pathways in the brain to fully mature that makes the frontal lobes particularly vulnerable to damage by dementia, traumatic brain injury, schizophrenia, and a host of other neurocognitive and dementia-associated diseases. As a consequence, working-memory processes and associated executive functions are among the first to be eroded in neurocognitive disease.

Researchers now understand that working memory uses distinct subsystems (Anderson, 1993; Anderson & Lebiere, 1998; Baddeley, 1992, 1996a; Baddeley & Hitch, 1974; Baddeley & Logie, 1999; Miyake, Friedman, Rettinger, Shah, & Hegerty, 2001; Shallice, 1988). These include at least two storage subsystems, used to temporarily store different kinds of information prior to further processing and to allow for divided attention (i.e., *task switching*) while processing information and the *central executive system* (a.k.a. the *supervisory attentional system* and the *executive control system*), which serves an essential oversight function to coordinate and manage the various tasks needed.

The first subsystem is known as the *phonological loop.* It temporarily stores and processes retrieved (or activated) language-based information, for example, vocabulary, speech-based information, and reading-based information. For instance, when we bring to mind the name of England's prime minister, that information is temporarily activated from long-term memory to this subsystem. The second subsystem is known as the *visuospatial sketchpad.* It temporarily stores and processes retrieved (or activated) visuospatial information, for example, nonverbal information, information about positions of objects, information required to orient one's self in space, geometric information, or mental images (e.g., images of one's mother's face, the configuration of one's living room, or positions of players on a football field). To date, more is known about the phonological (language-based) system than about the visuospatial system in working memory. However, researchers know that these components have different capacities, such that one's capacity for language may well be quite different than one's capacity for visual images, and there is likely a separate system for numbers. In addition, there is evidence from positron emission tomography that the phonological and visuospatial systems are mediated by different brain structures (Awh et al., 1996; Smith & Jonides, 1997); verbal storage requirements activate left frontal hemisphere activity, and spatial information storage requirements activate right frontal hemisphere activity, consistent with the brain's tendency toward hemispheric specialization.

The most important, and perhaps least understood, subsystem of working memory is the *central executive,* which is conceptualized as the oversight system that selects and regulates information flow within working memory, retrieves relevant information for temporary storage and subsequent processing, and allocates limited energy resources to each of the working-memory subsystems. Hence, it orchestrates the selection, initiation, planning, monitoring, and termination of all processing routines (e.g., encoding, storing, and retrieving). In addition, it plays the key role in troubleshooting, or recognizing the need to override (i.e., inhibiting) automatic patterns of thought and action when these processes appear to be unwarranted by external circumstances (I discuss "automatic" levels of processing more fully later).

As would be expected, working-memory assessments require individuals to maintain attention to target memory items while performing an additional processing task. One such assessment is the *alphabet span test,* in which the individual is asked to repeat a series of words after arranging them in alphabetical order. Another is the *backward digit span test,* in which the individual is asked to repeat a list of digits in reverse order. Spelling a word such as *world* backward and subtracting from 100 sequentially by 7s are also assessments of working memory.

Problems with working memory are most visibly reflected in problems with comprehension of sentences in general, in decision making in ambiguous situations, in complex problem solving, and in difficulties with IADLs. In large part, these difficulties are due to the inability to focus on and keep track of all the clauses and relevant information that one ordinarily manages to coordinate in one's mind, while inhibiting automatic responses and irrelevant information (distractions). Working-memory assessments are also highly related to performance on intellectual aptitude and achievement tests (Engle, Kane, & Tuholski, 1999; Kyllonen, 1996; Kyllonen & Cristal, 1990; Mukunda & Hall, 1992). Indeed, it is likely that working-memory capacity best measures the construct of intelligence.

Encoding

Information in short-term (working) memory is encoded in one of three forms: (a) visuospatial images (including visual imagery and nonverbal information), (b) sounds of words that are similar to the fleeting impressions transferred from sensory memory, or (c) in semantic codes, based on meaning through association to information activated from long-term memory stores (e.g., chunking and elaboration, which I discuss later in this chapter). Nevertheless, most information in short-term/working memory is encoded semantically, as words. This includes our "inner voices" as we call on prior knowledge to help us think through the steps of a problem to ourselves.

Storage

Short-term (working) memory has a relatively small storage capacity. On average, short-term memory is limited to seven (plus or minus two) items, or bits, of information that can be held in conscious awareness, or attention, at any one time (Miller, 1956). This capacity is evident in our ability to retain a phone number long enough to dial it (N.B. A *bit* is any unit of meaningful new information, e.g., a number, date, word, sight, sound, or idea.) The limit does not involve underlying memory processes that eventually become automatic, such as dialing the phone number, as I discuss more fully later. Short-term/working-memory storage limitations have also been conceptualized in terms of the length of time that information can remain active, that is, the amount of verbal material that can be articulated within 1 or 2 s (Baddeley, 1992). As a result, our short-term memory span holds fewer words when the words take longer to say (e.g., *bird, kid, vat, foot, pen, tree,* and *brick,* vs. *unintentional, chrysanthemum, imaginary, simultaneous, possibility, application,* and *disinfectant*). Slow speakers are therefore penalized.

Both capacity and time limitations impose significant constraints on cognitive processing because, in essence, we are able to keep only seven items active at once. (The actual number is debated, and there are reasons to believe it may be less, perhaps around three or four [Cowan, 2000]. However, for the present purposes, the exact limitation is not as important as the fact that there are space and time limits on the maximum amount that can be attended to, and that it is surprisingly small.) Nonetheless, this limitation is considered critical for reflection, deliberation, and thought. It narrows down the information in conscious awareness to manageable limits, while comprehension occurs.

It is also important to recognize that capacity limitations are significantly constrained by anxiety, and although mild degrees of stress may enhance arousal and controlled attention (Luu, Tucker, & Derryberry, 1998), higher degrees of stress (i.e., chronic stress), anxiety, and depression significantly disrupt working-memory functioning. This is because chronically stressed, anxious, and depressed individuals are besieged by extraneous intrusive and worrisome thoughts that divide attention and pre-empt limited working-memory resources (Ashcraft, 2002; Ashcraft & Kirk, 2001; Eysenck, 1997; Eysenck & Calvo, 1992; Hasher & Zacks, 1979; Luu et al., 1998). As a result, they may become too inattentive and unfocused to process external information into working memory. For these reasons, stress management strategies such as deep breathing, muscle relaxation, and exercise are important cognitive strategies, because they help to clear the mind of extraneous thoughts and thereby enhance one's working-memory capacity.

It should also be recognized that short-term (working) memory capacity is strongly linked to *information-processing speed;* that is, differences in the speed with which one is able to process information have significant effects on the capacity of short-term (working) memory (recall time limitations) and, consequently, its function (Fry & Hale, 1996; Salthouse, 1996). Information-processing speed can be informally assessed by determining how quickly an individual responds to questions and task demands. Declines in information-processing speed and associated capacity limitations significantly affect individuals with neurocognitive disorders. These issues are detailed in subsequent chapters.

The limited capacity in short-term (working) memory is the number of bits of information rather than the size of each bit. As a result, limitations can be somewhat circumvented by an encoding strategy known as *chunking,* the ability to group together a number of elements into larger, more meaningful units, thereby increasing the amount of information in each bit. For example, the numbers 106874153 can be thought of as a series of nine different numbers (difficult for most of us to remember), or as the three chunks 106–87–4153 (manageable for most of us to remember), as with Social Security numbers (here, elements that are close in time and space are combined). Moreover, a short-term working memory of seven chunked words can become a memory of seven sentences, or even (with practice) a memory of seven paragraphs. Hence, chunking is used to organize concrete information (e.g., shopping lists, telephone numbers, credit card numbers) as well as complex abstract ideas. Even experts in their fields encode their knowledge bases in huge chunks (Chase & Ericsson, 1982; Patel & Groen, 1986). Miller, Galanter, and Pribram (1960) described the efficacy of this recoding process in short-term/working memory in this manner: "To use a rather farfetched analogy, it is as if we had to carry all our money in a purse that could contain only seven coins. It doesn't matter to the purse, however, whether these coins are pennies or silver dollars" (p. 132).

As will be seen, there are countless ways to chunk similar information into recognizable units, from the use of visual patterns (e.g., a shape), auditory patterns (e.g., a rhyme), or idiosyncratic features (e.g., similarities to numbers in one's birth date or to an important historical date). In any case, chunking makes use of knowledge already stored in long-term memory to recode new information into larger, more meaningful units. This strategy not only reduces the number of items in short-term working memory but also increases the amount of information that can be transferred to long-term memory. It is an essential age- (and/or diagnosis-) irrelevant strategy for enhancing cognitive processing.

Retrieval

As in sensory–perceptual memory, the duration of information that can be retrieved in short-term (working) memory is very short, lasting from 1 to 2 s up to about 30 s. Once we are distracted by incoming sights, sounds, or thoughts, our most recent short-term working memories are lost and "forgotten." As indicated, information in short-term memory must be kept activated to be retained and eventually retrieved. Activation levels are high as long as we are focusing attention on selected information. However, if we do not continue to focus attention, the activation level weakens (decays) over time and finally drops so low that the information cannot be reactivated (Anderson, 1993). Hence, failing to pay conscious attention to selected information is the most significant way in which information is lost from the short-term memory store. Information is also lost through the displacement of old information by new information. This is because, as indicated, only about seven chunks of information can be simultaneously maintained at a level of activation that permits them to be attended to and recalled and, once an additional item is added, the activation given to the new item is taken away from the items that were presented earlier (Anderson, 1983, 1993). Short-term working memory thereby updates itself by dropping items to make room for more.

An important principle should be emphasized here. Short-term working memory depends on consciously "controlled" attention. Because we are limited in what we can consciously attend to, our short-term memory contains only what has been selected. This means that most of the information to which we are exposed either will never enter short-term memory or will enter so briefly that it will not be processed for later retrieval. Accordingly, what are often perceived as "memory lapses" are actually a consequence of attention mechanisms specifically designed to filter out information not currently being paid attention to (in this case, potential distractions), and "forgetfulness" through this kind of "inattention" is actually not forgetting (as would occur in retrieval failure) but rather the fact that the desired information was never registered in the first place. When we experience difficulty remembering the names of people to whom we were introduced, or where we placed the keys, or where in the parking lot we parked the car, it is likely that we were not paying sufficient attention to this information in the first place (or, put another way, we were excluding the information from the main path of our thoughts at the time).

The impact on eventual retrieval of paying conscious attention is substantial. In one revealing study, Gordon (2003) asked two groups of students to read paragraphs. One group was told that they would be tested on the material; the second group was not. Those who had been told that they would be tested remembered more than 90% of what they had read, whereas those who had not been told remembered less than 10%. (Note that the latter group would have demonstrated *incidental* rather than *intentional* learning, as was distinguished by Hasher and Zacks, [1979].) Hence, perhaps the single most important strategy to offset what we all experience as "forgetting" is developing the habit of consciously paying attention to the process of registering information that we want to retain while making deliberate attempts to resist distractions.

Activation in short-term working memory can be maintained to retain information longer than 1 to 30 s through the use of *rehearsal strategies* (Craik & Lockhart, 1972). These further capitalize on our ability to pay conscious and focused attention to information that we want to retain. *Maintenance rehearsal* involves repeating the information subvocally to ourselves (or to others; that's why salespeople use our names in just about every sentence). As long as the verbal information is repeated, it can be maintained in short-term memory indefinitely. Although this kind of rehearsal is considered a shallow form of mental processing that is less easily transferred and retrieved later (a.k.a. *rote learning* or *rote memory*), it is particularly useful for retaining concrete information that one plans to use temporarily and then forget, such as a phone number. As will be seen, it also serves an essential role in maintaining information long enough for deeper and more effective (i.e., elaborative) processing for transfer.

Elaborative rehearsal involves the capacity of working memory to actively organize the information for transfer out of short-term/working memory by connecting it with other information already stored. This kind of rehearsal transforms information into a form that can be more easily retrieved, because it encodes the information in terms of its meaning relative to already-acquired information. (As I discuss later, long-term memory most effectively files information in terms of its meaning.) For example, if I meet someone whose name is the same as my daughter's, I don't have to repeat the name to keep it in memory (as would be the case if I were using rote memory); I just have to make the association with an already-established memory. This association also allows me to quickly shift the information out of limited short-term/working memory stores, and it serves as an easily accessed cue when I seek to retrieve the information from long-term memory stores again. Hence, elaborative rehearsal focuses on the *meaning* of information to be learned and its relationship to information that is already stored. This association not only allows new information to shift out of short-term memory and into long-term memory but also provides the necessary cues for retrieval when needed at a later time. Note that chunking, described earlier, is another form of elaborative rehearsal. Chunking establishes associations between different items and recodes them into larger, more meaningful units (chunks) relative to one's previous memories.

Regardless, elaborative rehearsal (i.e., associating the information with previous memories) produces deeper, more meaningful, more readily transferred, and more easily retrievable memories than merely rehearsing verbal information repeatedly (i.e., absent association with previous memories; Craik & Tulving, 1975). Again, although rote memorization is useful for keeping information in short-term/working memory, it is not an efficient way to move information to long-term memory for eventual retrieval.

Neuroscientists have found that there are additional processes that determine retention and transfer of information from sensory–perceptual memory through working memory (Anderson & Phelps, 2001; Davidson, 2000; Erk, 2003; Kempermann, 2002; LeDoux, 2000; McClelland et al., 1995; Parkin, 1997; Rolls, 2000; Zeineh, Engel, Thompson, & Bookheimer, 2003). The hippocam-

pus (and related entorhinal, perirhinal and parahippocampal cortical structures, including the amygdala—referred to collectively as the *medial temporal lobe*), deep in the center of the brain, initiates short-term/working-memory processing. Researchers now know that the decision to store or discard incoming sensory–perceptual information is handled by the hippocampus and that the process can also occur relatively automatically. It does not appear to necessitate as much conscious attention and deliberate thought (as in maintenance or elaborative rehearsal) as was previously believed.

In essence, neuroscientists view the hippocampus as a switching station for the formation of new explicit memories. As sensory neurons in the cortex receive and filter vast amounts of sensory information through sensory–perceptual mechanisms, they relay it to the hippocampus. If the hippocampus responds (activates), the neurons start the process of forming a durable network of new synaptic connections to each another that will evolve into cortical long-term memories. (Note that memories are not stored in the neurons or synapses themselves; instead, they are stored in the pattern of connections between neurons.) However, without the activation of the hippocampus to initiate the process of forming new connections, the information will likely be lost.

Hippocampal activation appears to hinge on two related questions. First, does the information have any emotional significance? The name of a potential date is likely to generate more activation from the hippocampus than the name of Warren Harding's secretary of agriculture. The second question is whether the information is associated with information already stored in long-term memory (i.e., whether it activates neural connections that are known). If one has already devoted neural circuitry in long-term memory to American political history, then the name of Harding's agricultural secretary may actually activate some response, and if the hippocampus designates the name as sufficiently meaningful for transfer to long-term storage, then it will connect easily to the related bits of information already linked together in the cortex in long-term memory.

Hence, emotional significance and meaning are fundamental to the activation of the hippocampus. In addition, emotion appears to be an essential precursor for activation of the entire information-processing system (the hippocampal complex includes the amygdala, the brain region most strongly related to emotional memories). In essence, emotions are the means by which the individual unconsciously appraises the meaning and survival value of information as either worth thinking about or not.

Hence, emotional significance helps us maintain a readiness to respond (i.e., the initial attentional process) and has a selective effect on the information we notice to encode (Davidson, 2000; Hamann, 2001; LeDoux, 2000). It is the source of intrinsic motivation essential to all behavior. When hippocampal activation occurs automatically (e.g., memories of one's first love, or where one was on the morning of September 11, 2001), durable memories are formed without effort. Nevertheless, the hippocampus can also be prodded into activation by information with less inherent (unconscious) emotional significance that one nonetheless *consciously* considers to be significant, interesting, or meaningful (or, perhaps information that one knows might appear on a future test). This activation occurs through the effortful (controlled or intentional) process of paying attention to selected information discussed earlier. Here, paying attention involves not only deciding that the information is interesting, significant, or meaningful but also focusing all one's senses on the information (i.e., tuning in with all senses) and filtering out distractions (i.e., not letting one's mind wander to extraneous stimuli). Once again, perhaps the most important strategy for enhancing memory function is to increase one's interest (emotional connection) and conscious attention to desired information—or, as expressed in these terms, to make a strong impression on one's hippocampus.

More than 100 years ago, William James (1890) anticipated these contemporary understandings of short-term/working memory. In *Principles of Psychology,* he wrote (emphasis mine),

> Everyone knows what attention is. It is the taking possession by the mind, in clear and vivid form, of one or a few stimuli from many alternatives. Millions of items of the outward order are present to my senses which never properly enter into my experience. Why? *Because they have no interest for me. My experience is what I agree to attend to.* Only those items which I notice shape my mind—without selective interest, experience is an utter chaos. *Interest alone* gives accent and emphasis, light and shade, background and foreground—intelligible perspective, in a word. (pp. 403–404)

In effect, we use the network that we have already acquired from our past to capture new information that forms new memories. As a result, what we already know determines to a great extent what we will learn, remember, and forget.

LONG-TERM MEMORY

Long-term memory is the permanent, apparently limitless, component of the information-processing system. It refers to any information that is no longer in short-term working memory or conscious awareness but has been stored for potential future recall. Long-term memories eventually come to be consolidated in the neocortex and cortex surrounding the hippocampus, particularly in the regions where sensory information is interpreted (McClelland et al., 1995; Rolls, 2000; Squire & Alvarez, 1998), and although relatively "new" long-term memory representations are fragile, sensitive to disruption, and stored temporarily in the hippocampus, these memories eventually undergo a series of processes (e.g., glutamate release, protein synthesis, neural growth and rearrangement) that render them more stable and no longer dependent on hippocampal regions for their endurance (Frankland, O'Brien, Ohno, Kirkwood, & Silva, 2001; Haist, Gore, & Mao, 2001; Kelleher, Govindarajan, Jung, Kang, & Tonegawa, 2004; Kempermann, 2002; McClelland et al., 1995; Rolls, 2000). (N.B.: Implicit memories evolve within different areas of the brain. I address these shortly.) Hence, long-term memory includes the store of information that was transferred as recently as minutes ago (e.g., a point made earlier in this chapter) as well as very remote long-term memories. One can appreciate this capability by trying to recall some early childhood memories.

Our ability to recall early memories at will demonstrates the ease with which information can move from long-term memory back into short-term/working memory. Similarly, as we seek to problem-solve or learn any new information, we transfer relevant prior knowledge to working memory to help us resolve the problem or to understand and use the new information.

Encoding

Information in long-term memory can be encoded verbally (i.e., through sequences of words), visually (i.e., through images representing spatial configurations), or acoustically (i.e., through sounds), as well as through tastes and smells. These items of information are organized for eventual retrieval either by time, place, and affective state (*episodic memory*) or by meaningful relations (*semantic memory*). (Episodic and semantic memory are discussed more fully in the next section.) There is considerable evidence that we recall visual experiences much more reliably than verbal ones. For example, we are able to remember faces more easily than names. One explanation is that we tend to store visual images as both words and images, whereas we store words only as words (Clark & Paivio, 1991). Another explanation is that a larger portion of one's brain is devoted to visual functions than to any other function (e.g., the occipital lobe comprises approximately 40% of the brain). Regardless, constructing visual images of material to be memorized (e.g., figures, organizational charts) can significantly enhance memory for verbal material.

Nevertheless, the dominant mode for encoding items of information in long-term memory is in semantic codes, that is, in terms of the items' meanings. When we hear a sentence, we tend to remember a meaningful interpretation of that sentence (i.e., in a sequence of words) rather than the exact words of the sentence itself. Similarly, when we remember a picture or image, we tend to remember a meaningful interpretation of the picture rather than the exact specifics of the visual image. Hence, we tend to remember an abstracted gist of our experiences more than the precise details of the sensory input.

Storage Systems

Long-term memory is divided into *explicit* or *implicit* stores. There are two explicit memory stores, identified as *episodic* and *semantic,* and at least three kinds of implicit memory stores, identified as *procedural, perceptual priming,* and *conditioning* stores (Schacter & Tulving, 1994; Squire, 1994; Tulving, 2000; see Figure 12.2). *Explicit memory* involves the conscious recollection of information, whereas *implicit memory* refers to information that can be accessed automatically, unconsciously, or "effortlessly."

Episodic memory is the explicit store that involves memory of personally relevant facts and events. It includes the ability to remember individual pieces of factual information (e.g., faces, names, bits of conversation heard 10 min ago, names of past presidents) and the ability to remember events tied to a particular place and time. Such events can range from the significant (e.g., birthdays, graduations, weddings) to the mundane (remembering

FIGURE 12.2. Long-term-memory stores.

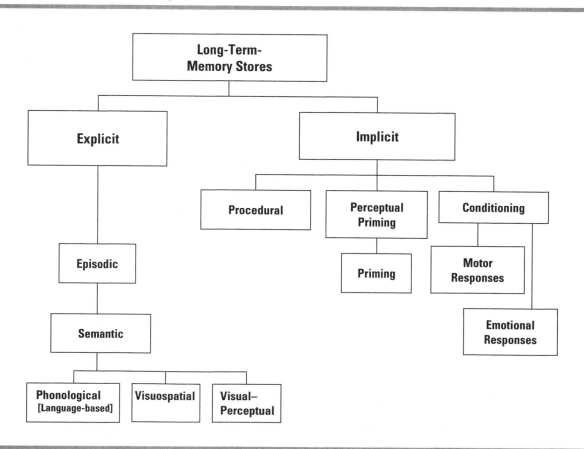

where one put one's keys, what one wore yesterday, or what one had for breakfast).

Episodic memory is considered as *recent* or *remote* for events related to the past or as *prospective* for events that are to take place in the future. Recent episodic memory is reflected in the ability to remember a therapist's name for periods of 5 or 10 min in the face of distraction and orientation to time and place—items that must be learned daily. This capacity is particularly significant because it reflects the individual's potential for new learning. Remote episodic memory is reflected in one's memory of personal wedding dates, current events from the past, or lists of past presidents. Prospective episodic memory involves remembering to take action in the future, for example, as in remembering to take one's medication, to get to an appointment, to purchase some item after work, or to return a phone call.

Recent episodic facts and events are the least durable of all types of memory (Smith, Petersen, Ivsnik, Malec, & Tangalos, 1996). When older adults (or their younger counterparts under stress) complain that they are experiencing "short-term memory loss," they are actually referring to recent episodic memory loss. This memory loss is particularly significant for those pieces of information with minimal emotional significance (i.e., birthdays and special events are retained). It is also significant for pieces of information that are unrelated to facts that one already knows (e.g., names of new acquaintances, dates of past or future appointments, items or tasks on a list, locations of recently placed objects, names and dosage of current medications). As indicated, information that is related to one's existing body of knowledge is relatively easy to assimilate and remember, whereas information that is unrelated to other facts that one already knows is more easily forgotten.

Recent episodic memory is typically assessed using a word list or story-retelling learning task with both immediate and delayed recall. It is also assessed by tests such as the ability to remember a therapist's name for periods of 5 or 10 min in the face of distraction and orientation to time and place (items that must be learned daily). Tests for recent episodic memory are particularly significant because they assess new learning potential. Remote episodic memory is assessed by tests for memories such as personal wedding dates, events from the past, or lists of past presidents.

Retrieval from episodic memory is significantly enhanced by the ability to recall contextual information about the originating experience, particularly time and place. For instance, investigators found early on that words learned underwater were best recalled underwater, whereas words learned on land were best recalled on land (Godden & Baddeley, 1975). In addition to external contextual information, retrieval from episodic memory is related to internal contextual cues. One's internal state during the encoding of the original experience can vary, whether one is happy or sad, calm or anxious, sober or intoxicated, and so on. Individuals demonstrate better recall when their internal state at test matches their state at learning. Here, the feelings evoked by the particular state serve as cues for retrieving information encoded while in that state (Eich, 1980; Lewis & Critchley, 2003). Note that, as a result, depressed individuals tend to remember (and focus on) mostly negative and unhappy (depressing) experiences.

However, the most effective strategies for improving memory, by which is most often meant improving recent episodic memory, are based on learning strategies that elaborate new information by associating it with a pre-existing body of knowledge. These *mnemonic* strategies are introduced in the next section; however, as discussed next, they transform episodic memories into semantic memory stores that are far more resistant to decay.

Semantic memory is the explicit store that builds on episodic memory. It involves one's knowledge and beliefs about facts and concepts, without reference to how, when, or in what state they were originally learned. What we understand—whether the ability to speak one or more languages, to prepare a holiday meal, to produce a successful harvest, or to write a chapter on cognition—is clearly based on memory for facts. However, semantic memory is much more complex than the mere accumulation of facts and events. It involves a synthesis of facts into an associated memory network that provides means for insight, knowledge, judgment and, perhaps, even wisdom. Semantic memories are also organized conceptually, by principles more complex than the time, place, and affective state wherein they originated. In addition, whereas episodic memories are retrieved by contextual cues, semantic memories are retrieved conceptually, by elaborated associational concepts and meanings related to an already-accumulated knowledge base.

Semantic memory is more durable than episodic memory, because semantic knowledge is made up of so many tightly associated facts that it is unlikely that they will all be forgotten at the same time. In effect, information is so tightly woven together that none of it can easily slip through the cracks. The remembered facts provide the associational cues for those that might otherwise be forgotten.

There are several types of semantic memory, including

- Phonological (i.e., language-based knowledge)
- Visuospatial (e.g., perception of the spatial layout of one's environment, perception of the position of objects in space, geometric knowledge, information encoded as visual images, imaginative thought)
- Visual–perceptual (e.g., face recognition, comprehension of nonverbal communication, object identification).

Measures of semantic memory are typically language based. One common assessment is a verbal fluency task, wherein individuals are given 1 min to produce items from a given category (e.g., animals or vegetables); here, individuals must retrieve knowledge of concepts to complete the task. Within intelligence tests (e.g., the Wechsler Adult Intelligence Scale, the Scholastic Aptitude Test), semantic assessments are incorporated in the general information subtests (answering questions such as "What was Mark Twain's real name?") or the vocabulary test sections. Semantic measures are often considered *crystallized intelligence* on most intelligence tests.

Procedural memory is the implicit store that is the most basic and extensive type of memory. It is believed to reside in the cerebellum, basal ganglia, and associated structures and has been likened to the bedrock upon which all of one's short- and long-term memories rest. It is also the most durable form of memory. Even with severe cognitive impairment, many of these basal memories persist.

Procedural memory involves the amalgam of motor, perceptual, and cognitive skills associated with the acquisition of movement- or skill-based information (e.g., skills, rules, and plans; Anderson, 1983, 1993; Squire, 1987; Tulving, 1985, 2000). Whereas explicit memory comprises the facts that we know, procedural memory comprises the skills we know how to perform. Producing the correct overt response to an environmental cue evidences this type of memory. Hence, it provides us with knowledge about "how" to throw a ball or ride a bicycle rather than knowledge "about" balls and bicycles, as provided by semantic (explicit) memory. Additionally, although procedural skills are in large part founded on episodic or semantic memories, with repetition and practice they eventually become *proceduralized;* that is, once acquired, they evolve into memories that are processed automatically, without conscious effort, when we are confronted with that stimulus again.

An example is shifting gears in a standard transmission car. At first, one has to consciously think about every step, but with time and practice the procedure becomes more and more automatic: One can even drive while attention is focused elsewhere, as on conversation with a passenger (i.e., when driving conditions are not demanding; otherwise, conscious attention and working memory override these automatic reactions and quickly take over). Similarly, athletes (e.g., divers, gymnasts, swimmers) and musicians (e.g., pianists, flutists, violinists) must turn their complex movements into automatic procedural memories through relentless repetition. Procedural memory forms the basis for high-proficiency skills that generally all people share, such as speaking a native language, reciting the alphabet, reading (albeit not for comprehension), basic mathematical skills (multiplication, long division), and interacting with other people (e.g., social skills; Anderson, 1983, 1993). Similarly, it serves as the basis for idiosyncratic skills that one may acquire, such as playing chess, tennis, or a musical instrument, or proficiency in carpentry, typing, or computer programming. It is also the foundation for routine functional skills, such as driving, getting dressed, putting together a jigsaw puzzle, brushing one's teeth, tying one's shoes, or peeling a potato.

As indicated, actions and skills that were once consciously monitored and controlled and that once required deliberate recollection, through repeated doing, gradually become automatic and are shifted from the cortex to deeper structures in the brain. In this way, procedural memories become independent of their originating (explicit) memory processes and evolve into a more efficient, faster, and more durable form of cognitive functioning. They bypass the need to devote a great deal of attention to the task and to consciously retrieve relevant information. Hence, they significantly reduce demand on the limited capacity of short-term/working memory and thus free that system to focus on more problematic aspects of tasks. At the same time, they enable us to deal adaptively with our environment in a variety of skill-based situations automatically, with a minimum of cognitive effort. And although, as discussed previously, we are capable of attending to only one conscious line of thought processing at a time (given the limitations of short-term memory resources), we can maintain a number of procedural processes simultaneously, at an unconscious "automatic-pilot" level. Neuroscientists estimate that 90% of information processing is based on this implicit, automatic-pilot processing system and that it serves as the basis for most of the information processing that occurs in the brain (Bargh & Barndollar, 1996; Goldberg, 2001; Johnson, 2004; Montague & Berns, 2002). Researchers now recognize that the vast majority of mental processes are automatic;

by contrast, effortful and consciously controlled cognitive operations represent only a minor portion of mental life.

It is unfortunate that procedural memory has yet to be included in assessments of mental status. To date, mental status tests are designed to tap episodic and semantic memory processes alone. The problem is that mental status instruments are generally used to predict rehabilitation potential in the cognitively disabled. As I have argued elsewhere (Levy, 1998a), this poses a significant problem for occupational therapy practitioners, because procedural memories are a pivotal source of cognitive capacity that is capitalized on in rehabilitation for individuals with any kind of cognitive disabilities. (Note that the Cognitive Performance Test, described in Chapter 14, provides occupational therapists with an invaluable tool to assess procedural, as well as semantic, episodic, and working memory, for individuals with dementias.)

As indicated, procedural memories are categorized as implicit in contrast to explicit. This means that they share characteristics with other memories that process information automatically, effortlessly, and without conscious awareness (Schacter & Tulving, 1994; Squire, 1994; Tulving, 2000). We tend to be aware of the products of these kinds of memories rather than the processes themselves. Other examples of implicit memories include those evidenced in *perceptual priming* and *priming*. (N.B. Incidental learning, mentioned earlier, is another form of implicit memory.)

Perceptual priming involves a process by which prior exposure to a stimulus activates association networks that prime later perceptual processing of that stimulus, without conscious awareness that the stimulus had been perceived earlier. *Priming* is a similar process wherein prior exposure to a stimulus makes a memory more available, unconsciously. For example, when people are asked to identify words that are flashed quickly on a screen, they are able to recognize that *doctor* is a word more quickly after prior exposure to the word *nurse* rather than the word *sandwich*. The word *nurse* then has served to prime the second word, *doctor*. Similarly, people may be asked to complete a word beginning with the letters "BRE." If they have heard the words *bread* or *breakfast* in casual conversation prior to the test, they are more likely to complete the completion cue quickly, and with those particular words, rather than the numerous alternatives; again, this occurs without having had conscious awareness of having prior exposure to the words that primed the response. Note that priming processes are closely related to our perceptual representation systems, whose function is to facilitate perceptual identification of objects based on

prior memories. They also reflect learning within our perceptual systems wherein information is primed unconsciously (a.k.a. *subliminal learning*).

Finally, implicit memories include those memories acquired through *conditioning*. These are memories that are formed more or less automatically through the processes of classical and operant conditioning, and they include both motor and emotional responses (Watson & Rayner, 1920). Recall that, in contrast, episodic and semantic memory systems are considered "explicit"; that is, they require conscious recollection, awareness, and effort for their operation. With explicit memories, there is awareness that a given piece of information was encountered before.

There are indications that the implicit-memory system developed before the explicit system both in the evolution of the species and in the development of the individual (Goldberg, 2001; Sherry & Schacter, 1987). As a result, this system is more resistant to neurological injury or aging processes. In addition, there is evidence that implicit-memory tasks call on different areas of the brain than do explicit ones. In particular, it appears that the hippocampus (and related cortical structures), as well as the frontal lobes of the cerebral cortex, are critical for explicit-memory processes but not for implicit ones. Implicit memories appear to reside in the motor cortex, basal ganglia, and cerebellum, bypassing the hippocampus (Esiri, Lee, & Trojanowski, 2004; McClelland et al., 1995; Moscovitch & Winocur, 1992; Rolls, 2000; Squire, 1994).

Storage

Episodic, semantic, and procedural memories must be stored in a systematic way. Unlike short-term/working memory, in which a few pieces of information can be stored and retrieved efficiently, long-term memory requires that millions of pieces of information be stored in an organized manner. Long-term memory is estimated to contain up to a quadrillion (10^{15}) bits of information! Memory retrieval is not a random process. As indicated earlier, the way that new information is initially processed in short-term/working memory determines how it is stored for effective recall later. An important requirement is that new information is associated with information already stored in long-term memory, as we construct our own understandings of the material in short-term/working memory. *Elaboration, organization, context,* and *repetition* significantly influence this process.

Elaboration, introduced earlier, is the addition of new meaning to information through its connection with existing knowledge, wherein episodic (rote) information is transformed into semantic memory and, as I have discussed, the process of finding connections can be automatic or conscious. We draw on existing knowledge to build an understanding of new information and, perhaps, to enhance or change that knowledge in the process. New information is stored by associating it with other relevant information that is already stored. Material that is elaborated when first processed in short-term/working memory will be more efficiently recalled later. This is because elaboration builds extra associations to existing knowledge stored in long-term memory and establishes the kinds of cues that will be necessary for retrieval at a later time. Again, the more deeply (elaborately) we associate a piece of information with other pieces in long-term memory, the more retrieval cues we will have to find the information that we are seeking, and the more extensive the retrieval cues, the stronger our memory (Craik & Tulving, 1975).

Practitioners should note that that elaborated memories can be directly contrasted to *rote memories* (or *rote learning*), terms that are often misunderstood. *Rote memories* are those that are learned in isolation from meaningful association, with extensive repetition and practice (e.g., numbering systems, months of the year, multiplication tables, a Shakespearean sonnet); hence, the information to be remembered is not linked to existing memories, but the words are linked to themselves. It is fairly limited and requires many repetitions for formation sufficient for later recall. Anyone who has had the experience of memorizing a poem can attest to the difficulty in learning the poem, and if one line in the stanza is not recalled, recall of the rest fails. Note also all the material that you have tried to learn this way and the little that you are able to remember after 6 months. To reiterate, rote learning (a form of maintenance rehearsal) is learning through repetition rather than through understanding. It is not an efficient way to organize information for transfer and eventual retrieval from long-term memory stores (Craik & Tulving, 1975).

Organization is a second storage strategy. As indicated earlier, organization of material in long-term memory is dependent on how we have previously organized information for coding and transfer from working memory. It is clear that information that is well organized, grouped into categories, or chunked when encoded and elaborated in short-term/working memory is more effectively stored than unrelated pieces of information, particularly if the information is complex or extensive. Additionally, we are capable of storing and retrieving a massive amount of

information if we organize it effectively. Placing a concept in some organizing structure or classification category provides a guide or framework to direct us back to individual pieces of information when needed. For example, lists of names or concepts are far easier to recall when we encode the information into categories (i.e., classes and subclasses) and then retrieve them on a category-by-category basis; in addition, hierarchical organization appears to be preferable (Bower, Clark, Winzenz, & Lesgold, 1969; McClelland et al., 1995; Nelson, 1995). Note that Figures 12.1 and 12.2 organize information about memory systems into categories and diagrams (visual images) to assist in recalling the information later, and the organizational structure of this chapter (outlines, headings, and other kinds of textual cues) are intended to indicate major and minor ideas and to reveal relationships among concepts; nevertheless, memory processing seems to benefit most when the organization is done by the person who needs to remember the material (i.e., in light of one's own idiosyncratic memory stores).

Context is the third element that affects storage and eventual retrieval, particularly for episodic memory. (Recall that semantic information is retrieved conceptually rather than contextually.) This is because the contextual cues available when an event is encoded are learned with the event, and this information provides some of the most powerful retrieval cues. As a result, recall is significantly enhanced when the internal and external context present during the encoding of memory is also present during later attempts at retrieving it (a.k.a. the *encoding specificity principle*). Hence, an important retrieval strategy for episodic information is to re-create, as much as possible, the objective and subjective contextual situation that was experienced initially. For example, if one's neuroscience class always meets in a particular room, recall of the material provided will be better when one is in that room, because the context of the room serves as a cue for retrieving the lecture material. Also, it helps to picture the setting, time of day, affective state, and companions who were with us, to retrieve the information—perhaps a name—that we are seeking. In a similar manner, one's ability to retrieve the names of first-grade classmates would be significantly enhanced were one to again walk through the hallways of that elementary school.

Repetition also has a powerful effect on storage. Neuroscientists have found that the brain stores memories by altering connections between individual neurons. These connections are always in flux. If a particular memory is not used often, then the neuronal connections between the nerve cells weaken, and eventually the memory fades through lack of regular use. However, if one activates the memory repeatedly, the pattern of connections strengthens (Haist et al., 2001; Lopez, 2000), similar to the way a well-worn path in a dense forest becomes easier to follow. Hence, we can significantly enhance processes of information retrieval by rehearsing, using, and practicing what it is that we want to remember. Note also that thoughtful practice serves as an additional form of elaboration (i.e., a source of new associations), because each time the material is repeated, we have an opportunity to expand on it. In addition, repetition both strengthens learning and speeds retrieval time.

Retrieval

For stored information to be useful, it must be retrievable, that is, accessible on demand. As indicated, the retrieval process relies on information that has already been stored by association with other relevant information into an association network. These associations serve as the essential links and cues for activation of the network and retrieval of that information, and so retrieval from long-term memory depends primarily on effective retrieval cues.

Despite the massive size of the associational network (i.e., a quadrillion bits of information stored in the vast web of neurons in the cerebral cortex), only one small area is activated at any one time. Recall that, although information that we are consciously thinking about is based in short-term/working memory, we are always retrieving information from long-term memory to help us "work on" that information. This information is retrieved and transferred to short-term/working memory through what is known as *spread of activation* (Anderson, 1983, 1993; Herrmann, Ruppin, & Usher, 1993; McClelland et al., 1995). When a particular thought or image is active—that is, when we hear a word or are thinking about it (in working memory)—other closely associated information (i.e., neuronal connections) become activated as well. Spread of activation in evidenced in thoughts that come to mind when we are in the middle of a conversation. Regardless, retrieval from long-term memory is based on the spread of activation from one bit of information to related bits in the association network. This, in turn, depends on the extent to which the information is elaborated, organized, embedded in context, and has been activated repeatedly.

Previously stored information can be retrieved in two ways: (a) recall or (b) recognition. *Recall* is what most of us think of as memory. It involves the ability to retrieve a particular piece of information by means of working memory's ability to mount an internal process of search and retrieval for cues to the information from long-term memory stores. This process occurs without the assistance of any externally provided associational cues. Note that when we say "I can't remember," we usually mean "I can't recall."

In contrast, *recognition* is a form of retrieval that is reflected in our ability to "match" information presented to us with previously learned information. Information in storage is matched with an externally provided associational cue, and the associational cue activates the relevant stored memories with which they are linked. Hence, with recognition the cue is processed directly into the long-term store, in large part bypassing the need for working memory to mount a complicated retrieval process from long-term stores. Instead, the associational cue triggers more elemental processes of attention and requires the individual to make a yes or no decision concerning whether the information had been seen or heard (i.e., recognized) before. As a result, recognition memory tasks significantly reduce the demands of the memory task. Recall is clearly a far more demanding test of retrieval than recognition, as we have all discovered from experience with essay versus multiple-choice examinations.

The implication here is that individuals process information more effectively when relevant information in long-term memory has been preactivated. In addition, information stored in long-term memory that is seemingly forgotten may nonetheless be accessed and "recalled" by recognition, as long as relevant associational cues are provided. Often, retrieval failure is considered the better interpretation of forgetting; people may never truly forget memories but instead just lose access to them. Indeed, some researchers suggest that nothing is ever lost in long-term memory; instead, it is the means of retrieving it that is lost (e.g., the phone number that my family had when I was a child is likely still stored—but at this point, I can no longer retrieve it). Regardless, it probably makes more sense to think of forgetting as resulting in memories becoming less and less available rather than being deleted entirely.

As has been observed (Levy, 1996, 1998b), recognition memory is an area of reserved cognitive capacity that is elemental to the cognitive disability model for cognitive rehabilitation. Occupational therapy practitioners using this model capitalize on this spared retrieval capacity by providing the just-right kinds of physical, psychological, and social environmental cues. These external cues activate relevant networks of stored memories necessary for the retrieval of productive behavioral responses to enable the individual to function to the best of his or her capacities despite significant cognitive impairment.

Regardless, findings such as these from the information-processing literature are applied in a number of occupational theoretical models to a consideration of how best to optimize the fit between individuals with cognitive impairments and their home, work, or leisure environments (contexts). I expand on these rehabilitative strategies in subsequent chapters of this book.

CONCLUSION

In this chapter I have provided an overview of the basic definitions and functions of cognition, along with the fundamental mechanisms of the cognitive information-processing model as it is emerging in the cognitive neuroscience and cognitive psychology literature and a brief review of applications of concepts emerging from this work. Cognition can be conceptualized not as a unitary construct but rather as a complex amalgam of different component systems. As a result, there are many means of acquiring and forgetting information, including recall versus recognition, episodic versus semantic, explicit versus procedural, working versus sensory–perceptual, and implicit versus explicit. Occupational therapy practitioners who understand cognitive information-processing concepts will be prepared to integrate the cognitive rehabilitation concepts introduced in subsequent chapters of this book, in which I discuss optimal rehabilitative strategies to maximize functional abilities, occupational performance, and quality of life for people experiencing the devastating impairments presented by neurocognitive disease.

REVIEW QUESTIONS

1. What must people do to remember?
2. How many types of memory are there?
3. Why do people forget?
4. Are there limits on memory capacity?
5. What is happening with memory when we experience "tip-of-the-tongue" phenomena?

REFERENCES

Anderson, A., & Phelps, E. (2001). Lesions of the human amygdala impair enhanced perception of emotionally salient events. *Nature, 411,* 305–309.

Anderson, J. R. (1983). *The architecture of cognition.* Cambridge, MA: Harvard University Press.

Anderson, J. R. (1993). *Rules of the mind.* Hillsdale, NJ: Erlbaum.

Anderson, J. R. (1995). *Learning and memory: An integrated approach.* New York: Wiley.

Anderson, J. R., & Lebiere, C. (1998). *The atomic components of thought.* Mahwah, NJ: Erlbaum.

Ashcraft, M. (2002). Math anxiety: Personal, educational, and cognitive consequences. *Current Directions in Psychological Science, 11,* 181–185.

Ashcraft, M., & Kirk, E. (2001). The relationships among working memory, math anxiety, and performance. *Journal of Experimental Psychology: Learning, Memory, and Cognition, 130,* 224–237.

Atkinson, R. C., & Shiffrin, R. M. (1968). Human memory: A proposed system and its control processes. In K. Spence & J. Spence (Eds.), *The psychology of learning and motivation* (Vol. 2, pp. 89–195). New York: Academic Press.

Awh, E., Jonides, J., Smith, E., Schumacher, R., Koeppe, R., & Katz, S. (1996). Dissociation of storage and rehearsal in verbal working memory: Evidence from PET. *Psychological Science, 7,* 25–31.

Baddeley, A. (1992). Working memory: The interface between memory and cognition. *Journal of Cognitive Neuroscience, 4,* 281–288.

Baddeley, A. (1996a). Exploring the central executive. *Quarterly Journal of Experimental Psychology: Human Experimental Psychology, 49,* 5–28.

Baddeley, A. (1996b). The fractionation of working memory. *Proceedings of the National Academy of Sciences, 93,* 13468–13472.

Baddeley, A., & Hitch, G. (1974). Working memory. In G. A. Bower (Ed.), *The psychology of learning and motivation* (Vol. 8, pp. 47–89). New York: Academic Press.

Baddeley, A., & Logie, R. (1999). Working memory: The multiple-component model. In A. Miyake & P. Shah (Eds.), *Models of working memory: Mechanisms of active maintenance and executive control* (pp. 521–539). New York: Cambridge University Press.

Bargh, J., & Barndollar, K. (1996). Automaticity in action: The unconscious as repository of chronic goals and motives. In P. Gollwitzer & J. Bargh (Eds.), *The psychology of action: Linking cognition and motivation to behavior* (pp. 457–481). New York: Guilford Press.

Bower, G., Clark, M., Winzenz, D., & Lesgold, A. (1969). Hierarchical retrieval schemes in recall of categorized word lists. *Journal of Verbal Learning and Verbal Behavior, 8,* 323–343.

Broadbent, D. E. (1958). *Perception and communication.* London: Pergamon.

Bunge, S., Ochsner, K., Desmond, J., Glover, G., & Gabrieli, J. (2001). Prefrontal regions involved in keeping information in and out of mind. *Brain, 124,* 2074–2086.

Carpenter, P., Just, M., & Reichle, E. (2000). Working memory and executive function: Evidence from neuroimaging. *Current Opinion in Neurobiology, 10,* 195–199.

Chase, W., & Ericsson, K. (1982). Skill and working memory. In G. H. Bower (Ed.), *The psychology of learning and motivation* (pp. 1–58). New York: Academic Press.

Clark, J., & Paivio, A. (1991). Dual coding and education. *Educational Psychology Review, 3,* 149–210.

Cowan, N. (2000). The magical number 4 in short-term memory: A reconsideration of mental storage capacity. *Behavioral and Brain Sciences, 24,* 87–185.

Craik, F., & Lockhart, R. (1972). Levels of processing: A framework for memory research. *Journal of Verbal Learning and Verbal Behavior, 11,* 671–684.

Craik, F., & Tulving, E. (1975). Depth of processing and the retention of words in episodic memory. *Journal of Experimental Psychology, 104,* 268–294.

Davidson, R. (2000). Cognitive neuroscience needs affective neuroscience (and vice versa). *Brain and Cognition, 42,* 89–92.

Deutsch, J., & Deutsch, D. (1963). Attention: Some theoretical considerations. *Psychological Review, 70,* 80–90.

Eich, J. (1980). The cue dependent nature of state dependent retrieval. *Memory and Cognition, 8,* 157–173.

Engle, R., Kane, M., & Tuholski, S. (1999). Individual differences in working memory capacity and what they tell us about controlled attention, general fluid intelligence, and functions of the prefrontal cortex. In A. Miyake & P. Shah (Eds.), *Models of working memory: Mechanisms of active maintenance and executive control* (pp. 102–134). New York: Cambridge University Press.

Erk, S. (2003). Emotional context modulates subsequent memory effect. *Neuroimage, 18,* 439–447.

Esiri, M., Lee, V., & Trojanowski, J. (2004). *The neuropathology of dementia* (2nd ed.). New York: Cambridge University Press.

Eysenck, M. (1997). *Anxiety and cognition: A unified theory.* Hove, England: Psychology Press.

Eysenck, M., & Calvo, M. (1992). Anxiety and performance: The processing efficiency theory. *Cognition and Emotion, 6,* 409–434.

Fernandez-Duque, D., Baird, J., & Posner, M. (2000). Executive attention and metacognitive regulation. *Consciousness and Cognition, 9,* 288–307.

Frankland, P., O'Brien, C., Ohno, M., Kirkwood, A., & Silva, A. J. (2001). CaMKII-dependent plasticity in the cortex is required for permanent memory. *Nature, 411,* 309–313.

Fry, A., & Hale, S. (1996). Processing speed, working memory, and fluid intelligence: Evidence for a developmental cascade. *Psychological Science, 7,* 237–241.

Gibson, E. (1969). *Principles of perceptual learning and development.* New York: Appleton-Century-Crofts.

Giles, C., Horne, B., & Lin, T. (1995). Learning a class of large finite state machines with a recurrent neural network. *Neural Networks, 8,* 1359–1365.

Godden, D., & Baddeley, A. (1975). Context-dependent memory in two natural environments: On land and under water. *British Journal of Psychology, 66,* 325–331.

Goldberg, E. (2001). *The executive brain: Frontal lobes and the civilized mind.* New York: Oxford University Press.

Gordon, B. (2003). *Intelligent memory.* New York: Viking.

Haist, F., Gore, J., & Mao, H. (2001). Consolidation of human memory over decades revealed by functional magnetic resonance imaging. *Nature Neuroscience, 4,* 1139–1145.

Hamann, S. (2001). Cognitive and neural mechanisms of emotional memory. *Trends in Cognitive Sciences, 5,* 394–400.

Hampson, R., Pons, T., Stanford, T., & Deadwyler, S. (2004). Categorization in the monkey hippocampus: A possible mechanism for encoding information into memory. *Proceedings of the National Academy of Sciences, 101,* 3184–3189.

Hasher, L., & Zacks, R. (1979). Automatic and effortful processes in memory. *Journal of Experimental Psychology: General, 108,* 356–388.

Herrmann, M., Ruppin, E., & Usher, M. (1993). A neural model of the dynamic activation of memory. *Biological Cybernetics, 68,* 455–563.

Jacobs, J. (1887). Experiments on "prehension." *Mind, 12,* 75–79.

James, W. (1890). Attention. In W. James *Principles of Psychology* (Vol. 1, pp. 402–459). New York: Henry Holt.

Johnson, S. (2004). *Mind wide open: Your brain and the neuroscience of everyday life.* New York: Scribner.

Just, M., Carpenter, P., Kellera, T., Emerya, L., Zajaca, H., & Thulborn, K. (2001). Interdependence of nonoverlapping cortical systems in dual cognitive tasks. *NeuroImage, 14,* 417–426.

Kelleher, R., Govindarajan, A., Jung, H.-Y., Kang, H., & Tonegawa, S. (2004). Translational control by MAPK signaling in long-term synaptic plasticity and memory. *Cell, 116,* 467–479.

Kempermann, G. (2002). Why new neurons? Possible functions for adult hippocampal neurogenesis. *Journal of Neuroscience, 22,* 635–638.

Kyllonen, P. (1996). Is working memory capacity Spearman's *g?* In I. Dennis & P. Tapsfield (Eds.), *Human abilities: Their nature and measurement* (pp. 46–76). Mahwah, NJ: Erlbaum.

Kyllonen, P., & Cristal, R. (1990). Reasoning ability is (little more than) working memory capacity. *Intelligence, 14,* 389–433.

LeDoux, J. (2000). Emotion. In M. Gazzaniga (Ed.), *The new cognitive neurosciences* (2nd ed., pp. 1065–1066). Cambridge, MA: MIT Press.

Levine, D., Long, D., & Parks, R. (Eds.). (1998). *Fundamentals of neural network modeling: Neuropsychology and cognitive neuroscience.* Cambridge, MA: MIT Press.

Levy, L. (1996). Cognitive integration and cognitive components. In K. O. Larson, R. Stevens-Ratchford, L. Pedretti, & J. Crabtree (Eds.), *The role of occupational therapy with the elderly (ROTE)* (2nd ed., pp. 573–598). Rockville, MD: American Occupational Therapy Association.

Levy, L. (1998a). Cognitive changes in later life: Rehabilitative implications. In N. Katz (Ed.), *Cognition and occupation in rehabilitation: Cognitive models for intervention in occupational therapy* (pp. 307–322). Bethesda, MD: American Occupational Therapy Association.

Levy, L. (1998b). Cognitive disabilities model in rehabilitation of older adults with dementia. In N. Katz (Ed.), *Cognition and occupation in rehabilitation: Cognitive models for intervention in occupational therapy* (pp. 195–221). Bethesda, MD: American Occupational Therapy Association.

Lewis, P. A., & Critchley, H. D. (2003). Mood-dependent memory. *Trends in Cognitive Sciences, 7,* 431–433.

Lezak, M. (1995). *Neurological assessment.* New York: Oxford University Press.

Lopez, J. (2000). Shaky memories in indelible ink. *Nature Reviews Neuroscience, 1,* 6–7.

Luria, A. (1966). *Higher cortical functions in man* (2nd ed., B. Haigh, Trans.). New York: Basic Books. (Original work published 1962)

Luu, P., Tucker, D., & Derryberry, P. (1998). Anxiety and the motivational basis of working memory. *Cognitive Therapy and Research, 22,* 577–594.

McClelland, J., McNaughton, B., & O'Reilly, R. (1995). Why are there complementary learning systems in the hippocampus and neocortex: Insights from the connectionist models of learning and memory. *Psychological Review, 102,* 419–457.

Miller, G. A. (1956). The magical number seven, plus or minus two: Some limits on our capacity for processing information. *Psychological Review, 63,* 81–97.

Miller, G., Galanter, E., & Pribram, K. (1960). *Plans and the structure of behavior.* New York: Holt, Rinehart & Winston.

Miyake, A., Friedman, N., Rettinger, D., Shah, P., & Hegerty, M. (2001). How are visuospatial working memory, executive functioning, and spatial abilities related? A latent-variable analysis. *Journal of Experimental Psychology, 130,* 621–640.

Miyake, A., & Shah, P. (Eds.). (1999). *Models of working memory: Mechanisms of active maintenance and executive control.* New York: Cambridge University Press.

Montague, P., & Berns, G. (2002). Neural economics and the biological substrates of valuation. *Neuron, 36,* 265–284.

Moscovitch, M., & Winocur, G. (1992). The neuropsychology of memory and aging. In F. Craik & T. Salthouse (Eds.), *The handbook of aging and cognition* (pp. 315–372). Hillsdale, NJ: Erlbaum.

Mukunda, K., & Hall, V. (1992). Does performance on memory for order correlate with performance on standardized measures of ability? A meta-analysis. *Intelligence, 16,* 81–97.

Neisser, U. (1967). *Cognitive psychology.* New York: Appleton-Century-Crofts.

Nelson, C. (1995). The ontogeny of human memory: A cognitive neuroscience perspective. *Developmental Psychology, 31,* 723–738.

Parkin, A. J. (1997). Human memory: Novelty, association, and the brain. *Current Biology, 7,* R768–R769.

Patel, V., & Groen, G. (1986). Knowledge based solution strategies in medical reasoning. *Cognitive Science, 10,* 91.

Poon, L. (1985). Differences in human memory with aging: Nature, causes, and clinical implications. In J. E. Birren & K. Schaie (Eds.), *Handbook of the psychology of aging* (2nd ed., pp. 427–462). New York: Van Nostrand Reinhold.

Posner, M., & DiGirolama, G. (2000). Attention in cognitive neuroscience: An overview. In M. Gazzaniga (Ed.), *The new cognitive neurosciences* (2nd ed., pp. 621–632). Cambridge, MA: MIT Press.

Reed, S. (2000). *Cognition* (5th ed.). Belmont, CA: Wadsworth.

Rolls, E. (2000). Memory systems in the brain. *Annual Review of Psychology, 51,* 599–630.

Rubinstein, J., Meyer, D., & Evans, J. (2001). Executive control of cognitive processes in task switching. *Journal of Experimental Psychology: Human Perception and Performance, 27,* 763–797.

Salthouse, T. (1996). The processing speed theory of adult age differences in cognition. *Psychological Review, 103,* 403–428.

Schacter, D., & Tulving, E. (1994). What are the memory systems of 1994? In D. Schacter & E. Tulving (Eds.), *Memory systems 1994* (pp. 1–5). Cambridge, MA: MIT Press.

Schwartz, M. (1995). Re-examining the role of executive functions in routine action production. In J. Grafman, K. Holyoak, & F. Boller (Eds.), *Annals of the New York Academy of Sciences (Structure and Function of the Human Prefrontal Corte; Vol. 769,* pp. 321–335). New York: New York Academy of Sciences.

Schwartz, M., Mayer, N., Fitzpatrick-DeSalme, E., & Montgomery, M. (1993). Cognitive theory and the study of everyday action disorders after brain damage. *Journal of Head Trauma Rehabilitation, 8,* 59–72.

Shallice, T. (1988). *From neuropsychology to mental structure.* New York: Cambridge University Press.

Sherry, D., & Schacter, D. (1987). The evolution of multiple memory systems. *Psychological Review, 94,* 439–454.

Smith, E., & Jonides, J. (1997). Working memory: A view from neuroimaging. *Cognitive Psychology, 33,* 5–42.

Smith, G., Petersen, R., Ivsnik, R., Malec, J., & Tangalos, E. (1996). Subjective memory complaints, psychological distress, and longitudinal change in objective memory performance. *Psychology and Aging, 11,* 272–279.

Squire, L. (1987). *Memory and brain.* New York: Oxford University Press.

Squire, L. (1994). Declarative and nondeclarative memory: Multiple brain systems supporting learning and memory. In

D. L. Schacter & E. Tulving (Eds.), *Memory systems 1994.* Cambridge, MA: MIT Press.

Squire, L., & Alvarez, P. (1998). Retrograde amnesia and memory consolidation: A neurobiological perspective. In L. R. Squire & S. M. Kosslyn (Eds.), *Findings and current opinion on cognitive neuroscience* (pp. 75–83). Cambridge MA: MIT Press.

Stuss, D., Binns, M., Murphy, K., & Alexander, M. (2002). Dissociations within the anterior attentional system: Effects of task complexity and irrelevant information on reaction time speed and accuracy. *Neuropsychology, 16,* 500–513.

Tootell, R., & Hadjikhani, N. (2000). Attention: Brains at work. *Nature Neuroscience, 3,* 206–208.

Treisman, A., & Gelade, G. (1980). A feature integration theory of attention. *Cognitive Psychology, 12,* 97–136.

Tulving, E. (1985). How many memory systems are there? *American Psychologist, 40,* 385–398.

Tulving, E. (2000). Introduction to memory. In M. Gazzaniga (Ed.), *The new cognitive neurosciences* (2nd ed., pp. 727–732). Cambridge, MA: MIT Press.

Watson, J., & Rayner, R. (1920). Conditioned emotional reactions. *Journal of Experimental Psychology, 3,* 1–14.

Wood, N., & Cowan, N. (1995). The cocktail party phenomenon revisited: Attention and memory in the procedure of Cherry 1953. *Journal of Experimental Psychology: Learning, Memory, and Cognition, 21*(1), 255.

Zeineh, M., Engel, S., Thompson, P., & Bookheimer, S. (2003). Dynamics of the hippocampus during encoding and retrieval of face–name pairs, *Science, 299,* 577–580.

13

Linda L. Levy, MA, OTR/L, FAOTA

Cognitive Aging in Perspective

Implications for Occupational Therapy Practitioners

LEARNING OBJECTIVES

By the end of this chapter, readers will

1. Identify the three information-processing stages of cognition and how each is affected by cognitive aging

2. Identify the memory components that are affected by the aging process and those that remain strong

3. Identify three forms of long-term memory and describe how each is affected by cognitive aging

4. Identify the focus of the cognitive vitality approach to the treatment of cognition

5. Describe the changes that occur in memory and attention with normal aging, including age-associated memory impairment

6. Discuss the effect that normal age-related cognitive change has on occupational performance, instrumental activities of daily living, and activities of daily living

7. Identify compensatory strategies that address the effects of age-related memory decline on the effectiveness of occupational therapy intervention or on day-to-day occupational performance

8. Identify practical methods that can be used with older adults to enhance performance on and satisfaction with daily life activities.

Cognitive vitality is essential for optimal aging. This maxim has been recognized for thousands of years. In the words of Cicero (106–43 BC), "To live is to think" (Cicero, 1923). Over the past decade, the disciplines of cognitive psychology and neuroscience have made enormous strides in our understanding of cognitive aging. As the proportion of older people in the U.S. population grows, it becomes increasingly important to understand age-related changes. For older adults in good physical condition, cognitive decline is the foremost threat to their overall productivity and quality of life. For those whose physical activities are limited, cognitive decline is the major additional threat to quality of life. Understanding how cognitive functioning changes with age offers practitioners new opportunities for designing interventions to minimize the effects of those changes on cognitive functioning to optimize occupational participation and engagement.

In this chapter I review recent findings in cognitive aging related to functional performance in older adults. Note that the focus here is on the changes in cognitive function in individuals who are not experiencing a dementia-causing disease—that is, on "normal" rather than "pathological" aging. (Dementia is discussed in Chapter 14.) I synthesize knowledge on the specific nature of cognitive changes that occur with age in light of information-processing concepts introduced previously (see Chapter 12). Understanding patterns of impaired and preserved cognitive functions provides the requisite groundwork for understanding the impact of these impairments on occupational performance. I also present guiding principles and intervention strategies that practitioners can introduce to assist older adults with the problems in cognitive functioning that they may experience, to maximize occupational performance, functional independence, and quality of life. I conclude the chapter with discussion of diagnostic and assessment issues related to the experience of age-related cognitive decline and an overview of evidence supporting cognitive remediation to improve cognitive skills.

INFORMATION PROCESSING AND OLDER ADULTS

As indicated, most older adults experience detectable changes in cognitive function as they age. Although serious decline that severely interferes with occupational performance and engagement is associated with dementing conditions of aging (e.g., Alzheimer's disease), more moderate degrees of change occur with normal aging (National Research Council, 2003). These changes are likely to be annoying or frustrating to the older adult, although by definition (American Psychiatric Association, 1994; Crook et al., 1986) they are not disabling (i.e., they do not impair the ability to perform basic activities of daily living [ADLs] and instrumental activities of daily living [IADLs]). Hence, the intervention strategies I discuss are meant to help these older adults better understand expected changes and to develop alternative ways to manage the cognitive problems that they experience that interfere with overall occupational performance, productivity, and quality of life. Within the rehabilitation population, however, physical conditions such as hypertension, hyperlipidemia, cardiovascular disease, and diabetes significantly accentuate age-related changes (see Levy, 1996a; Waldstein, 2003, for full discussions). These changes can affect the potential to optimally benefit from occupational therapy rehabilitation; thus, practitioners will need to introduce specific intervention strategies to enable these older adults to compensate for the increased problems they experience, particularly those confronted in the learning and retrieving of newly acquired information.

The human information-processing model has served as the predominant conceptual framework in the cognitive aging psychology literature for more than 30 years (Tulving, 2000). In the following sections I examine each element of the information-processing model (i.e., sensory–perceptual memory, working memory, and long-term memory) addressed in Chapter 12 to identify the patterns of spared and impaired information-processing capacities that can occur as aging progresses, along with associated implications for intervention. (It would also be helpful to review concepts introduced in Chapters 12 and 14 and Table 12.1 before proceeding.) At the outset, it is important to emphasize that declines in these areas represent averages of group performance, such that cognitive decline is by no means inevitable. Many older adults, including some centenarians, appear to avoid cognitive decline even into the 11th decade of life (Schaie, 1988; Silver, Jilinskaia, & Perls, 2001).

SENSORY–PERCEPTUAL MEMORY AND AGING EFFECTS

Recall that the first stage of information processing relies on sensory stimulation by sight, sound, taste, touch, and smell. Because the sensory–perceptual memory store processes this input, it will be significantly affected by sensory impairments. The vision, hearing, taste, smell, vestibular, and proprioceptive difficulties experienced by most older adults restrict information processing by slowing, limiting, blurring, or distorting the sensory information that the individual receives (Baltes & Mayer, 1999; see also Levy, 1996a, for a full discussion). For example, try to imagine reading the newspaper while wearing blurry eyeglasses. How much information would you remember later? Likewise, if you cannot fully hear the name of the person you are meeting for the first time, you can hardly expect to remember it later. To remember something that you read, or to recall someone's name, information must first be clearly and firmly registered in your sensory cortex.

Unfortunately, even when corrections are made for common forms of sensory loss (e.g., hearing aids, eyeglasses), older adults still tend to perform more poorly on perceptual tasks than do younger people, particularly in relation to speed of perceptual processing (Salthouse, 1996). (A typical perceptual-processing speed task measures how many perceptual judgments a person can make in a specified time frame, e.g., identifying single letters or numbers or deciding whether two letter strings are the same). This change in perceptual speed begins in young adulthood and declines in a linear fashion (i.e., the rate of decline is constant) thereafter (Schaie, 1998). As a result, the speed of putting component pieces of sensory–perceptual information into a meaningful whole becomes progressively slower (e.g., recognizing someone's face or comprehending signs while speeding past them on the expressway). In addition, strong correlations have been found between sensorimotor decline (especially visual and auditory acuity) and declines in cognitive functioning (Anstey, Luszcz, & Sanchez, 2001; Lindenberger & Baltes, 1994; National Research Council, 2003; Wahl & Heyl, 2003).

The sensory–perceptual store is also influenced by a variety of physical factors that affect central nervous system functioning, dull one's senses, and reduce one's ability to fully perceive and attend to information in the surroundings. Medications are by far the major offenders here. Especially problematic are the many substances used to treat sleep disorders (sedative–hypnotic agents), as well as antianxiety drugs, tricyclic antidepressants, anti-inflammatories, antihistamines, antidiabetics, antipsychotics, stomach acid suppressants, and anti-Parkinson's agents (Agency for Health Care Policy and Research [AHCPR], 1996).

Other factors that reduce perceptual and attention capacities though their direct biological effects on the brain are pain (both acute and chronic), nutritional deficiencies, persistent use of alcohol or illicit drugs, chronic stress, depression, sleep deprivation, hypertension, hypotension, hyperlipidemia (high cholesterol), hyperglycemia (diabetes), and thyroid problems. These factors are also the most common causes of reversible memory loss (AHCPR, 1996; McDowell, 2001). By some measures, hypertension alone accounts for half the variance in cognitive performance of older adults (Elias, Robbins, Elias, & Streeten, 1998; Madden & Blumenthal, 1998).

Hence, although most changes in cognition and memory represent normal changes of aging, some may be caused by temporary or treatable physical or medical problems. Practitioners need to be alert to these potentially remediable causes of memory loss and, when indicated, to refer older adults to appropriate specialists to address them. Older adults who effectively manage these factors can also reduce the risk of cognitive decline and, perhaps, even Alzheimer's disease in late life (Fillit et al., 2002; Peters, 2001). More specific considerations include the following:

- *Vision and hearing impairment:* Every older adult needs to have routine vision and hearing tests. Common causes of impairments such as cataracts, glaucoma, presbycusis (mild hearing loss), and impacted cerumen (earwax) should be treated with a view to their importance for maintaining cognitive functioning. At the same time, environmental cues should be presented using methods that compensate for the probable sensory–perceptual declines experienced by older adults (e.g., increased intensity, yet glare-free, lighting; magnification and large-print visual cues; use of color contrast; lowered voice pitch; and reduction of background noise).

- *Medication side effects:* Most older adults take multiple medications, a number of which are known to impair cognition. If the start of an older adult's memory problems coincides with the use of a new medication, then it is likely that the two are related. Practitioners need always to consider the cognitive effects of an older adults' medications and to investigate whether alternative medications or lowered dosages are possible.

- *Nutritional deficiencies:* Individuals who have low levels of B vitamins (particularly vitamin B12, B6, thiamine, and folate) are more likely to develop fatigue, depression, memory loss, and dementia (Toole & Jack, 2002; Wang et al., 2001). Any older adult with memory loss should be referred for testing.

- *Alcohol and illicit drug effects:* Heavy drinking damages the brain directly. Although a recent study demonstrated that drinking one to three glasses of alcohol a day reduced the risk of developing dementia, individuals who had more than four drinks a day were 1.5 times more likely to develop dementia (Ruitenberg et al., 2002). Drugs of abuse (e.g., opiates and cocaine) are also associated with poorer cognitive performance (Carlin & O'Malley, 1996). Although drug or alcohol abuse is not curable, it can be successfully managed; referrals for treatment are clearly warranted if drug or alcohol abuse is suspected.

- *Stress:* Animal studies have shown that chronic stress damages the hippocampus and can impair cognitive function (Lee, Ogle, & Sapolsky, 2002; Shors, 2001). Older people are particularly susceptible to this effect. Hence, stress reduction techniques should be among the daily activities of older people. Physical exercise is particularly useful through its release of endorphins, the body's natural antidepressant hormones. There is also recent evidence that exercise improves attention and decision-making capability among older adults (Colcombe et al., 2004).

- *Depression:* Older adults who are experiencing changes in memory, attention, or executive function may actually be experiencing the symptoms of depression, and yet depression in older adults is frequently missed and thereby left untreated. In large part, this is because depressed older adults typically experience more somatic symptoms, such as severe pain (usually headache or backache), abdominal problems, and ill-defined shortness of breath, and they are less likely than younger people with depression to report depressed mood (Levy, 1996b). Hence, practitioners and family members need to be alert to the symptoms of depression (i.e., loss of interest in usual activities, inactivity, apathy) and to encourage the older adult to seek treatment if warranted. Practitioners should note that brief self-report questionnaires can facilitate screening. Both the Geriatric Depression Scale (Yesavage et al., 1983) and the Center for Epidemiological Studies Depression Scale (Radloff, 1977) can be administered in 5 to 10 min and have well-established reliability and validity (AHCPR, 1996).

- *Sleep disorders:* Older people are often plagued by sleep disturbances and a decrease in REM (rapid eye movement sleep, during which dreaming occurs) sleep that can impair the ability to learn new information and to organize previously acquired memories (Siegel, 2001). Chronic sleep deprivation and fatigue can also lead to high blood sugar levels and elevated cortisol levels, both of which damage brain cells in the hippocampus (Spiegel, Leproult, & Van Cauter, 1999). All older adults should be encouraged to implement sleep hygiene strategies (e.g., avoiding daytime napping, passing up caffeine and nicotine after noontime, daytime mild exercise, adopting presleep relaxation rituals, etc.) and to seek treatment, when warranted, for sleep disorders.

- *Management of medical illnesses*
  - *Hypertension.* It is estimated that 42 million Americans have hypertension, but only 10 million have it under control (American Heart Association, 1998). Chronic moderate to high blood pressure reduces the amount of blood flow to cells, which translates into less oxygen, glucose, and nutrients for neurons in the brain. This markedly increases a person's vulnerability to the damage caused by Alzheimer's disease. Hypertension can also cause dementia through the development of ministrokes (vascular dementia) or larger strokes that affect the hippocampus.

    Several studies demonstrate that high blood pressure in midlife leads to poor cognitive function later in life (Launer, Masaki, Petrovitch, Foley, & Havlik, 1995; see also Waldstein, 2003, for a review). It has also been established that risk factors that double or triple the risk for developing a heart attack also increase the risk of memory loss and dementia. Studies have shown that people who take blood pressure and cholesterol-lowering medications regularly cut their risk of developing memory loss to less than half of what it would otherwise be (Forette et al., 1998). In addition, keeping blood pressure controlled (below 120/80 mmHg) prevents stroke and maximizes blood flow to the brain.

  - *Diabetes.* Diabetes is a risk factor for stroke and vascular dementia. It is also a risk factor for cognitive impairment (Arvanitakis, Wilson, Bienias, Evans, & Bennett, 2004; Convit, Wolf, Tarshish, & de Leon, 2003; Gregg, Jaffe, & Cauley, 2000). There is evidence that control of blood sugar can prevent some of the vascular complications of diabetes, so it is likely that appropriate glucose control by diet and medication will lower the likelihood of developing memory problems.

  - *Hyperlipidemia.* High cholesterol is associated with cognitive impairment (Auperin, Berr, & Bonithon-Kopp, 1996); it has also been identified as a risk factor for dementia (Kivipelto et al., 2001). There is evidence that people with high cholesterol levels (more than 250 mg/deciliter) in midlife are 2.2 times more likely to develop dementia in later life, compared with those with normal levels at midlife. High cholesterol is clearly deleterious to cognitive functioning and overall health and should be treated.

SHORT-TERM MEMORY AND AGING EFFECTS

Recall that short-term memory is the "working memory" that enables one to combine information that arrives from the environment with information retrieved from long-term memory.

Minimal age-related differences have been found in primary memory, the storage component of short-term memory. As a result, older adults attend to, perceive, and briefly retain amounts of information within the normal short-term memory span of approximately seven items with little difficulty (Craik & Jennings, 1992). Recall that with primary memory there are no additional processing requirements.

In contrast, age-related differences have been found in working memory, the component that both stores and processes new information to prepare it for long-term storage. Tasks that require one to transform and manipulate complex new information (i.e., complex reasoning and problem solving) become progressively more difficult with age, and the capacity of working memory (i.e., the amount of information that is immediately accessible to assist in processing) is reduced (Park et al., 1996; Salthouse, 1992, 1994). There is much theoretical debate as to why this occurs (Chow & Nesselroade, 2004; Park, 2000; Salthouse, 2004). Currently, deficits are being attributed to declines in attention, speed of processing, or both.

Attention

One body of research holds that age differences in working memory are explained by problems older adults experience with the inhibitory mechanisms of attention (Hasher, Tonev, Lustig, & Zacks, 2001; Hasher & Zacks, 1988; Zacks & Hasher, 1997). Older adults experience increasing difficulty distinguishing between information that is relevant and irrelevant to a particular task; they demonstrate more difficulties filtering out external distractions that interfere with attention, and they are less able to inhibit automatic responses when confronted with novel situations (known as *response inhibition*). This inhibitory deficit increases as the demands and complexity of the task increase (Backman, Small, & Wahlin, 2001; Salthouse, 1992; West, 1999; Zacks & Hasher, 1997). As a result, extraneous sights, sounds, or irrelevant thoughts are more likely to intrude on the already limited (approximately seven-bit) capacity of short-term/working memory, displacing more relevant thoughts. This leaves older adults with less space for other purposes, such as higher-level processing (e.g., elaboration) of information that one wants to remember.

Older adults also experience greater difficulty than younger adults with divided attention (task switching), a decline that may also be related to inhibitory difficulties. Divided-attention deficits are seen in a reduced capacity to process information that comes from two or more sources simultaneously, or while one is seeking to perform two tasks concurrently (Whiting & Smith, 1997); to switch tasks successfully, the brain must marshal the resources required to perform the new task while inhibiting the demands of the previous one. If two sources of information are in direct competition (e.g., two sources of communications at once, an unexpected caller, or an unavoidable interruption), older adults tend to select one source to remember and disregard the other. By contrast, younger adults try to remember both, and although they are likely to remember less of either, they tend not to disregard one source of information completely. As a result, older adults, if they are distracted in some way, find it more difficult to remember what one intended to buy at the store, meant to do "in this room," or even one's initial train of thought in conversation. The memory performance of older adults is clearly optimized when they are focused on one task at a time.

Note also that divided-attention difficulties are accentuated when both tasks involve new information rather than more familiar skills (Rubinstein, Meyer, & Evans, 2001). As indicated earlier, although we are capable of thinking through consciously only one main topic at a time, a number of automatic processes (e.g., procedural) can be maintained at an unconscious level; hence, multitasking becomes easier when parts of the process are routine.

Speed of Processing

Another body of research holds that age differences in working-memory processing are largely explained by processing speed (Birren & Fisher, 1995; Salthouse, 1996, 2000, 2004). As in sensory–perceptual memory, the aging process slows the rate at which information is processed in working memory: Older adults take more time than their younger counterparts to process and accurately retrieve new information. Proponents of this theory argue that slowed speed of processing may be the bottleneck that causes the other deficits in cognitive function. Specifically, slowing of basic-level cognitive processes may impair more complex working-memory functions, such as inhibiting distraction, which later results in slowed or inaccurate retrieval. Slower processing may also reduce the amount of relevant information that can

be activated for higher-level processing of intricate material. Similarly, important cognitive operations, such as association, chunking, elaboration, and rehearsal, may be executed too slowly; as a result, products of early processing may decay or be displaced when needed in later processing. At the same time, slower processing may limit the amount of attentional resources required to effectively divide attention, that is, sufficient to maintain attention to one task (while inhibiting distractions) and to transition smoothly to another.

Note that slowed speed of information processing is related to the overall slowing of neural transmission that occurs with aging. This slowing is also reflected in declines in motor function, including decreased reaction time, dexterity, coordination, grip strength, and a slower gait (see Levy, 1996a, for an overview of age-related neurological changes). The cause for this slowing has been attributed to modest disruptions of connections within the neural network with age; specifically, each neuron loses some of its dendritic branches, the density of synapses diminishes, and the protective covering of axons becomes thinner (Terry & Katzman, 2001). Additionally, although thinning results in slower signal transmission between neurons (particularly in the temporal, frontal, or parietal lobes), it does not result in loss of their function. As a result, older adults retain their abilities to form new memories, although their processing abilities may become slower with age, and although older adults do not seem to mind walking more slowly, or having a weaker grip (acknowledging that no one is the same athlete at 60 as they were at 30), they very much mind the effects of the slowing that occur in information processing. This anxiety is understandable because we intuitively recognize that memory is the neural sum of who we are, have been, and hope to be, and to lose memory is to lose our sense of self. In addition, recent publicity about Alzheimer's disease has greatly heightened anxiety that memory slippage ("senior moments") may be a sign of a more serious problem. As indicated, however, normal changes take place in cognition with age, and it is important reassure older adults that these kinds of changes are not signs of disease and are amenable to intervention.

Intact but Slower Learning

Although the speed of the learning process slows with increasing age, the baseline ability to learn and remember is retained. Hence, although it may take longer for older adults to take in complex new information and retain it, all evidence indicates that, if older adults take the time and make the effort to learn something, they will remember it as accurately as younger adults (Albert, 2002; Arenberg & Robertson-Tchabo, 1977; Gounard & Hulicka, 1977; Hayslip & Kennelly, 1985; Hultsch & Dixon, 1990; Labouvie-Vief, 1976; Ostwald & Williams, 1985; Sharit & Czaja, 1994). Additionally, although older adults may think that they are forgetting information more easily, what is actually happening is that they are not learning it as well in the first place. The problems that they experience are primarily related to attention (i.e., working memory) rather than retention. At the same time, there is evidence that an older adult's learning performance is improved with the kinds of instructions and practice I discuss here (Backman, 1989; Ball et al., 2002; McDougall, 2002).

Life moves at a more rapid pace than it did even 30 years ago. More individuals are on fast tracks and find the need to multitask. Newscasters and interviewees speak more rapidly, as do professionals and other service workers who are overwhelmed by shorter appointments, staff reductions, deadlines, and the bottom line. At the same time, ever-changing technologies require new skills to be mastered and updated regularly. These societal changes place current older adults at a particular disadvantage. It becomes more and more difficult to keep up with the mere tempo and sheer volume of information presented to them. To reiterate, however, once older adults have the opportunity to register the information at their own pace, they learn just as well as younger people. It is likely that contemporary older adults will need to rely to an even greater extent on the self-paced opportunities available through (large-print) reading materials and computer resources to keep up to date and informed.

Implications

Practitioners can do much to assist older adults in compensating for the working memory deficits they experience; by recognizing that many older adults are aware of their memory deficiencies, practitioners can develop useful strategies to help them improve their cognitive functioning. Perhaps the most important intervention occurs through providing older adults with sufficient metacognitive knowledge (i.e., knowledge about the workings of the cognitive system) so that they can implement the keystone strategy conveyed throughout this chapter, that is, making deliberate effort to pay extra attention to information one wishes to learn or retain. Here, *paying extra attention* refers to the ability to heighten one's focus on and interest in information that one considers impor-

tant, such that the information selected is more likely to activate the hippocampus than, perhaps, all the other information that is activating sensory–perceptual processing. *Paying extra attention* also refers to the determination to monitor the distracting elements in the environment and focus on selected information while discarding stray thoughts and disregarding distractions. Teaching this age-irrelevant memory enhancement strategy can do much to mitigate the increased difficulties in working memory that older adults experience (Backman, 1989; Ball et al., 2002; McDougall, 2002; Saczynski, Willis, & Schaie, 2002; Willis & Nesselroade, 1990; Willis & Schaie, 1986). Additional strategies and principles for intervention include the following:

- As might be expected, the foremost consideration in offsetting working memory learning deficits is ensuring that one has the older adult's attention. Attention can be intensified, for example, through the use of bright colors, underlining, highlighting, or some combination of these for written words and changes in lighting, voice level, or pacing for verbal information. Attention is enhanced when information is presented through more than one modality (e.g., verbal, written, and graphic). Hence, auditory and visual information (e.g., handouts, overheads, and videos) should be used together whenever feasible (note that handouts serve also as powerful recall cues). The intent is to use mere emphasis to help direct the older adult's selective attention to new information to be learned.

- Speed of information processing declines. Slow your rate of speech to allow more time for processing, encoding, storage, and retrieval. Similarly, be ever cognizant of the need to allow more exposure time to process new information and to allow more time for visual and verbal elaborations and organization at the time the information is presented. In addition, allow more time for tasks requiring information retrieval.

- As indicated, older adults do best when tasks are self-paced and not timed. Be cognizant of the need to allow individuals to pace their own learning. This often means reducing content in a given time period to offer greater clarity, specificity, and opportunity for depth. Provide self-paced instructional materials to serve as additional memory cues whenever possible.

- Practitioners need to encourage older adults to think aloud (i.e., to talk to oneself) when practicing a new skill. This entails useful repetition and review of new information, and it generates auditory cues that enhance attentional processes. It also ensures that the principles taught are being remembered correctly.

- Related to the above, recognize that repetition alone is a weak way of learning; it is far more effective to rehearse with elaboration. Hence, encourage active verbalization and elaboration of new information. As in the traditional classroom setting, learners should be encouraged to take notes and to paraphrase the information in their own words.

- Recognize that attention may be thought of as a state of activity that is triggered by various kinds of emotional arousal. Hence, only information or skills that are directly relevant and emotionally significant to the individual are likely to be remembered. Precede all teaching with an assessment of the older adult's interest in what will be taught, what is already known, and what the individual thinks he or she needs (or does not need) to know.

- Organize and simplify the teaching environment. Chaos and clutter are underrecognized, albeit significant, memory deterrents. They serve as distractions that clutter (i.e., overload) one's working memory, divide one's attention, and limit processing resources.

- Similar to the above, minimize the number of potential sources of information. Limit all background noise, interruptions, and other distractions that may compete for the older adult's attention. This includes common distractions, such as noise levels in the surrounding environment, talking to the older adult while he or she is attempting a new skill (especially small talk), and inadvertently incorporating nonessential information. Again, one can dramatically improve the person's ability to attend by limiting the amount of information that is registered.

- Provide clearer instructions for organizing a complex task into its basic components. Separate essential from nonessential details and focus on one major concept, comprising no more than three to seven chunks of information, at a time. This further reduces the need for the older adult to divide attention. Note also that recall is enhanced for information that is logically grouped, chunked, categorized, or sequenced when encoded in the first place.

- Recognize that new information or skills are best retained when they build on previous ways of doing things. It is always easier and faster to find an existing connection than to create new ones from scratch. Help the individual find personal associations for new information with previously known information

(i.e., to activate the hippocampus and enhance elaborative rehearsal). Note that older adults have an advantage here because they have so many more experiences to which to relate. Begin with statements such as "Does this look like anything that you have ever done before?" or "What I want you to do is similar to . . . ." to preactivate relevant information in long-term memory and to enhance attention.

- Encourage older adults to find ways to avoid using limited memory resources, for example, by developing the habit of placing one's keys, eyeglasses, or wallet in the same place or parking one's car in the same space when going to places one visits routinely (i.e., grocery store, doctor's office, drycleaners, and pharmacy). This strategy frees working memory of the need to process and remember varying locations daily. The objects will be found in an already-remembered place.

- Encourage older adults to make whatever they need to remember more interesting, more meaningful, more emotionally significant, and more connected to already learned information. Note that this principle serves also as the basis for many of the mnemonic techniques used to encode information that are discussed in the following section. Regardless, information that is perceived to be more interesting, meaningful, or emotionally significant is far more easily learned.

- Encourage older adults to avoid multitasking as much as possible. If one is forced to do many things at once, it is likely that several things will be forgotten. If remembering details is important, recommend doing one thing at a time.

- Encourage older adults to practice active listening (elaboration) to new information that needs to be remembered.

- It is true for all individuals that memory works best when a person is relaxed and can think clearly. Reassure older adults that the more irritated, anxious, or depressed they become, the less they are likely to remember. It is important to slow down and relax when trying to remember information. In addition, stress management resources are essential for everyone.

- Reassure older adults that memory lapses are normal and are not a harbinger of Alzheimer's disease. Our information-processing systems are designed to enable us to attend to and remember only information that is relevant and important to us in the long run, not all the details of everyday life. Hence, we usually remember what we need to and forget what we usually do not need to know.

- Reassure older adults that learning capacity does not necessarily diminish with age; it just takes more dedication and attention, necessitating more practice, rehearsal, and review of the information. In contrast to the adage that "You can't teach an old dog new tricks," you *can*. It just takes longer.
- Reassure older adults that it is not that they have forgotten information; it is more likely that the information was never really stored in the first place. Again, this is a deficit that can be significantly ameliorated by making a point of identifying information that one wants to remember and then paying extra attention.
- No one should ever take for granted that one will remember anything that one has made no deliberate attempt to remember.

LONG-TERM MEMORY AND AGING EFFECTS

Beginning around age 50, age-related deficits occur in the *recent* components of long-term memory's episodic store. *Prospective* and *remote* episodic-memory components are more stable, at least until the late 70s (Schaie, 1998). Similarly, both semantic and procedural long-term memory stores are minimally affected (Schacter, 1996). At the same time, there is evidence that semantic memory (e.g., vocabulary world knowledge and an individual's knowledge stores) can be significantly enhanced with advancing age (Schaie, 1998; Schaie & Willis, 1991). Hence, age-related declines are in large part confined to recent episodic-memory processing, and these are reflected in increased difficulties in remembering and recalling newly learned day-to-day information unrelated to facts already known. They are much less likely to occur either in the higher levels of memory processing, which involve synthesis and integration (e.g., semantic memory knowledge stores), or in the foundational components of memory processing (e.g., procedural, automatic, and other implicit memories). This is likely the reason that a far greater proportion of older adults exhibit the quality known as "wisdom" (i.e., good judgment and advice about important but uncertain matters of life), compared with their young or middle-aged counterparts (Baltes & Graf, 1996; Baltes, Staudinger, & Lindenberger, 1999), and indeed, the most outstanding senators, judges, doctors, and lawyers tend to be older adults who carry with them several decades of knowledge and experience. It is also the reason that older adults maintain intact or even

superior performance on most everyday tasks (see Parks, 2000; Park & Hall-Gutchess, 2000, for reviews). (N.B.: Most tasks of daily living involve complex combinations of implicit cognitive processes triggered by environmental cues.) Researchers have also noted that the greater knowledge and experience associated with increased age probably reduce the need for the type of novel problem solving that declines with age; that is, much of what we typically do may be more dependent on successful access and retrieval of information from the wealth of experiences that we already know rather than our ability to solve truly novel problems or reason with greatly unfamiliar material (Salthouse, 2004).

Age-related differences also occur in the ability to use recall mechanisms to retrieve episodic information (Park et al., 1996); hence, they are at a disadvantage in retrieving information when there are few cues or environmental supports. Typical examples include forgetting where one left the car keys, eyeglasses, scissors, or parked the car; forgetting the name of a person, movie, or book; forgetting why one entered a particular room; forgetting whether one already told someone something; or "blocking" a name, movie, or book title when needed and proceeding to remember it later (the initial cue does not sufficiently activate the target word for retrieval, until later). However, when associative cues are provided (i.e., in recognition tests), older adults perform almost as well as their younger counterparts (Craik & Jennings, 1992).

Recall deficits appear to reflect the decreased ability of working memory to search for and activate relevant episodic memories and thereby to independently generate cues necessary for retrieval. Thus, difficulties in retrieving previously acquired information can be mitigated by teaching the older adult to think of associated information to cue recall of needed new information. It can also be diminished by the provision of environmental recognition cues. An example of the implementation of both principles would be remembering a particular item, going into another room to get it, being unable to remember what the item was, and then returning to the original room where the memory was formed. This return will often result in remembering the item because of exposure to the environmental cue that initiated the memory.

Practitioners should note that recent episodic-memory deficits are particularly salient because rehabilitation protocols so often rely on retrieval of episodic information (e.g., hip replacement precautions, transfer sequences, one-handed ADL strategies, techniques for using long-handled dressing equipment, and sequencing the operating buttons on a microwave or an answering machine).

Yet, as indicated earlier, given sufficient attention and repetition, these episodic skills carry potential to become *proceduralized*; that is, once acquired consciously and practiced to a sufficient level, they become automatic and never completely lost.

Throughout history, a variety of strategies have been devised for compensating for deficits in episodic memory. Known as *mnemonic devices* (from the Greek *mnemon,* meaning "mindful"), these strategies involve learning to make better use of conscious, elaborative, and meaningful associations when information is initially processed, to provide enduring cues for recall later, or to make use of external environmental prompts to assist in generating necessary recognition cues. When older adults are taught to use these strategies, the deficits that they experience in recalling recent episodic memories are reduced. It is important to provide exposure to a variety of strategies, so that older adults can select ones that are consistent with their particular learning styles and preferences as well as those deemed most useful given their specific situations.

One mnemonic strategy, the *method of loci,* dates back to the time of Cicero. Here, the individual creates a visual association between items to be remembered (e.g., a grocery list) and varying locations along a path through a familiar site (e.g., one's apartment complex) where items might be placed. The otherwise-isolated items are automatically linked into a previously well-learned associational chain, no matter how improbable. This strategy was commonly used by Greek and Roman orators to remember long speeches without notes, before materials such as paper and pencils were available. It is considered one of the most powerful and effective mnemonic techniques.

Other mnemonic strategies use words (acronyms), rhymes, or sentences to enhance episodic retention. These strategies are effective because stronger associations exist between letters comprising words, or between words in rhymes or sentences, than between bits of isolated information. For example, we still remember that the notes in the spaces between the lines of the treble clef spell the word *FACE.* We remember the notes on the lines by making an association with the sentence "Every Good Boy Does Fine." In geography, we remembered the Great Lakes because they spell the word *HOMES:* Huron, Ontario, Michigan, Erie, and Superior. To reset our clocks, we remember "Spring forward, fall back." Rhymes have been identified as particularly effective mnemonic techniques because words that rhyme tend to be recalled from our memory banks effortlessly and other words that rhyme with the word that is needed provide cues to recall it (Higbee, 1988). The first stories that we were able to remember were in the form of nursery rhymes. We often use a rhyming technique to remember how many days there are in a month ("Thirty days hath September, ..."); many remember the notes of the scale with the song from *The Sound of Music* that begins, "Doe, a deer, a female deer, ..." (and song lyrics are remembered when other memories fail); we also remember that "In 1492, Columbus sailed the ocean blue." In addition "Righty tighty, lefty loosy" is useful for remembering that screws are turned to the right to make them tighter and to the left to loosen them. Creating rhymes (or songs), sentences, or acronyms for teaching rehabilitative strategies such as hip replacement precautions, tub transfers, dressing sequences, and use of adaptive equipment would likely do much to enhance retention of these newly learned (episodic) strategies and the potential for them to become proceduralized.

Mnemonic strategies also use imagery and visualization to retrieve isolated bits of information. These strategies capitalize on our capacity to remember what we see better than what we hear, even if those images are solely within our "mind's eye" (recall that vision is our strongest memory system). Visual imagery also adds richness to the material to be remembered (it adds more sensory modalities). Note also that use of visualization is the principle underlying the method of loci.

Visualization entails associating episodic information with vivid visual images. For example, suppose I am driving home and think of a phone call I should make when I return home. I might associate the telephone with a very familiar object, such as imagining a telephone hanging on the garage door. When I return home, the sight of the garage door should remind me to make the call. Or, suppose I need to remember to call my sister about my nephew's birthday and to call a mechanic about repairing the car. If I imagine my sister getting my nephew a new car for his birthday, I have associated isolated pieces of information into one more easily recalled visual image, and I have provided two chances to remember something, both visual and verbal. Similarly, to remember where in the parking lot I parked the car, it is helpful to make a conscious effort to look back and form a detailed mental image of the car's location before exiting the lot. Hence, visualization is another mnemonic strategy that can be taught to older adults to offset the episodic-memory difficulties that they experience. Note that the more unusual (and perhaps funny or ridiculous) the image is, the more dramatic the impact will be on one's hippocampus, and the easier it will be to remember. Practitioners need also to encourage older adults to create mental images of the rehabilitation techniques they are teaching through literal demonstration of those techniques. Use of illustrations or videotapes that the older adult can view at a later time also provides useful reinforcement.

The most common mnemonic strategies are those that originate externally. *External memory strategies* are methods for remembering that depend on tangible objects, places, or people. They provide concrete cues to facilitate retrieval of desired episodic information. Commonly used examples include handouts; reminder notes; checklists (i.e., to keep track of task steps); lists for shopping, errands, and telephone messages; daily planners; asking others for reminders; putting everything back where it belongs; and object placement (putting reminder objects in a conspicuous place). Specific external strategies include bookmarks, medication organizers, colored jackets for specific keys, interval timers, watch alarms, and whistling teapots. New products on the market also provide means of compensating for these vulnerabilities; for example, steam irons are now available that shut themselves off after a short period of not being used, and many car models come equipped with headlights that automatically shut off within a few minutes of the ignition key being removed. Currently, a vast commercial enterprise is devoted to the design, manufacture, and sale of technological devices to compensate for episodic-memory deficits. These include computer software packages, pocket-size tape recorders, speed dial features on telephones, and personal digital assistants.

Memory researchers report extensive use of external memory strategies. In fact, writing things down is considered the greatest memory strategy ever devised, and yet researchers have found that older adults tend to perceive the use of techniques such as Post-It notes, making lists, and using handouts as "crutches" as "cheating" (Scogin & Prohaska, 1993). They seem to fear that relying on external aids will only hasten memory decline instead of enhancing memory by reducing memory load. Hence, although practitioners need to encourage older adults to make use of external memory aids to assist in remembering rehabilitative strategies or engagement in important activities in their everyday lives, it may also be important to dispel beliefs that external strategies are inferior methods to offset episodic-memory decrements. It is probable that most people used these aids earlier in their lives, and there is no reason to stop using them as they age.

More specific considerations include the following:

- Although a decline in memory function can be irritating or upsetting for the older adult who experiences it, it is important to reassure him or her that the consequences are minimal for managing daily life activities. Older adults tend to perform well on everyday tasks because the cognitive processes involved are in large part automatic and are driven by external cues in the environment.

- Practitioners need to understand that age-related declines represent a genuine problem for people who remember the high levels of skills that they had in the past and contrast these with present levels of memory functioning.

- It is reassuring for older adults to be informed that memory for knowledge actualization (i.e., semantic knowledge accumulated over a lifetime) does not deteriorate with age. Instead, the changes that do occur are mild, are not disabling, and appear to be restricted to changes in encoding (working memory) and recent episodic retrieval processes. Additionally, as indicated throughout this chapter, these difficulties are amenable to intervention.

- As discussed in the previous section, recall for newly learned information may be enhanced by teaching older adults how to organize the information more efficiently in relation to other well-learned (e.g., semantic) information that is more readily accessible for recall. In addition, teaching these encoding strategies helps to compress more information into a form that is more effectively processed by the limited capacity working memory system.

- One of the simplest ways to remember episodic information (appointments, phone numbers, shopping lists, and important tasks for the day), and to reduce memory load, is to write it down. Using Post-It notes is particularly helpful. Keeping a calendar for appointments and making a list of tasks that need to be done in a given day are ways that even the most accomplished people in the world use to remember important events and tasks (consider the explosion in popularity of personal digital assistants). Note that even the mere act of writing notes and making lists reinforces attention and memory. This kind of organization also brings a sense of control and reduces stress, allowing one's memory to function better.

- Memory pathways weaken when not used over time. As a result, older adults will require more time than younger adults to retrieve early events because they have many more years between the laying down of those events in memory and subsequent recall.

- Although the memory lapses experienced may result in blocking of information (i.e., an episodic-recall delay), it is important to reassure the older adult that nonetheless, these memories are not lost and that, although it may take longer to retrieve the information, the information is typically jogged and remembered later.
- In light of the above, difficulty in recalling specific information reflects a decline in the ability to retrieve information instantaneously. Older adults need to be apprised of the need to devote more time to the process of retrieving the information they seek, bearing in mind that the accumulation of information that they have stored expands greatly with increasing age.
- Once information is in long-term memory, it generally stays there. If one cannot remember something that is in one's long-term memory, it generally represents a retrieval problem. Searching for or providing additional cues or information can often improve retrieval.

DIAGNOSTIC ISSUES

Three types of cognitive decline with aging have been identified: (a) *age-associated memory impairment* (*AAMI*), (b) *mild cognitive impairment* (*MCI*), and (c) *dementia*.

Age-Associated Memory Impairment

AAMI refers to the mild symptoms of cognitive decline that occur as part of the normal aging process that have been discussed throughout this chapter. It can be applied to nearly 90% of the older adult population. Older adults experiencing AAMI complain of memory loss relative to their younger years but generally have normal scores on psychometric testing for their age group (Crook et al., 1986). Hence, impairment may marginally increase with age but does not exceed the normal range of functioning for one's particular age group. AAMI does not impair the ability to perform ADLs. Typical problems that older adults report include the following:

- Thinking is slower.
- Speed of recall is slower.
- Paying attention is more difficult.
- Recalling information is slower following interruptions.
- Organizing information takes more time.
- Remembering names following introductions or in subsequent encounters is more difficult.

- Misplacing objects becomes problematic.
- Remembering multiple items to be purchased or a series of tasks to be done within a specified period of time is more difficult.
- Tasks that require multiple actions become more problematic.
- Being distracted in some way compounds these problems.

These lapses are more likely to occur when the older adult is tired, sick, distracted, or under stress. Under less stressful circumstances, the older adult is usually able to remember the necessary information. Note that older adults who worry about memory loss are unlikely to experience a serious cognitive decline; those with more serious conditions tend not to be aware of their lapses, do not worry about them, or attribute them to other causes. In addition, most data indicate that AAMI does not progress to dementias such as Alzheimer's disease. Moreover, most data indicate that AAMI does not progress to MCI because less than 1% of people with AAMI go on to develop dementia (Fillit et al., 2002).

Mild Cognitive Impairment

MCI refers to memory loss that falls outside normal limits for one's age group (1.5 *SD*s below age-matched control participants; Peterson et al., 1999; Sherwin, 2000). Hence, the memory lapses of MCI are more severe than AAMI, and people retain less information than most people their age (i.e., usually recent memory). This memory impairment is persistent and begins to interfere with more complex daily activities. For example, a person with AAMI might occasionally forget the name of casual acquaintances or an appointment and then remember later. In contrast, a person with MCI might struggle repeatedly to remember names of close colleagues during meetings, need frequent reminders for events and appointments, and may ask the same question a number of times; he or she may also forget information in a paragraph that he or she just read. These kind of memory lapses can begin to interfere with one's professional life. Nevertheless, people with MCI do not have pronounced impairments in daily function (they are essentially independent in routine ADLs) and therefore, by definition, do not have dementia (Peterson et al., 1999). Hence, they are generally able to live independently but may be less active socially and at work. Once the individual loses the ability to take care of typical ADL responsibilities, however, his or her cognitive impairment is no longer considered mild. At least in some individuals, MCI can progress to dementia. Up to 12% of individuals with MCI develop dementia each year, and 50% with MCI will develop dementia within 3 years of diagnosis (Peterson et al., 1999). Symptoms may be present for as long as 7 years before they become severe enough to indicate a diagnosis of dementia. Intervention trials are under way to determine whether treatments for Alzheimer's disease can slow this rate of conversion. Note also that the strategies introduced in this chapter are also useful for people experiencing MCI (Fillit et al., 2002), particularly the approximately 50% who may not go on to develop dementia.

Dementia

Dementia can be broadly defined as a syndrome of progressive global cognitive impairment severe enough to affect daily function. The term is reserved for chronic, progressive, irreversible, global cognitive impairment. This generally occurs within individuals who have little insight into their profound memory losses. A recent study found that individuals with MCI who lack awareness of their functional deficits (i.e., those who reported fewer problems than their spouse or adult child reported) were eight times more likely to subsequently develop dementia than those who reported deficits similar to those reported by informants (Tabert et al., 2002). The differences between AAMI and dementia are substantial (see Table 13.1).

In early dementia, impairments in executive function are most noticeably reflected in IADLs, which are among the most sensitive signs of the disease. The earliest changes seen are in the abilities to manage money and medications, to use the telephone, and to use transportation (Karlawish & Clark, 2003). Later, individuals lose the ability to find their way in their own neighborhoods; to recognize their grandchildren; and eventually to take care of basic needs, such as showering and getting dressed.

Note that the pathological changes associated with Alzheimer's disease differ substantially from normal brain aging (Selkoe, 1999; Small, Tsai, DeLaPaz, Mayeux, & Stern, 2002). Hence, there is no known neuropathogenic relationship between cognitive aging and Alzheimer's disease. Alzheimer's disease is *not* considered an accelerated form of cognitive aging; it is a disease primarily of old persons (Fillit et al., 2002). Rehabilitation for older adults with dementia requires very different strategies. This topic is addressed in Chapter 15.

T A B L E   1 3 . 1 . Age-Associated Memory Impairment vs. Dementia

Age-Associated Memory Impairment	Dementia
Independent in daily living	Becomes dependent on others for activities of daily living
Follows written or spoken instructions	Gradually unable to follow instructions
Forgets, but remembers later	Rarely remembers later
Is able to use memos, lists, and notes	Gradually unable to use notes
Complains of memory loss	May complain of memory problems only if specifically asked; unable to recall instances of memory loss
Is more concerned about forgetfulness than are close family members	Is much less concerned about incidences of memory loss than family members are
Maintains recent memory for important events, affairs, and conversations	Notably declines in memory for recent events and ability to converse
Has occasional word-finding difficulties	Has frequent word-finding difficulties and substitutions
Does not get lost in familiar places; may have to pause momentarily to remember the way	Gets lost in familiar places while walking or driving; may take hours to eventually return home
Able to operate common appliances (although may be unwilling to learn how to operate new ones)	Becomes unable to operate common appliances; unable to learn to operate even simple new ones
Maintains prior level of interpersonal skill	Demonstrates loss of interest in social activities; gradually shows signs of socially inappropriate behaviors
Performs normally on mental status examinations (when education and culture are taken into account)	Performs abnormally on mental status examinations not accounted for by education or cultural factors

Cognitive Screening Instruments

Several mental status tests are available to screen and assess cognitive function in older adults. The most widely used and validated for use in institutional and community settings is the Mini-Mental State Examination (MMSE; Folstein, Folstein, & McHugh, 1975; see Appendix 13.1). The MMSE provides specific age and education norms for older adults (Crum, Anthony, Bassett, & Folstein, 1993); has excellent test–retest reliability (Folstein et al., 1975; Tombaugh & McIntyre, 1992), validity (Folstein et al., 1975; Tombaugh & McIntyre, 1992), and sensitivity (Bachman et al., 1993; Tombaugh & McIntyre, 1992); and is correlated with physiological tests such as CT scans (Colohan, 1989) and tests of cerebral ventricular size (Pearlson & Tune, 1986). It assesses a broad range of cognitive abilities, including attention (i.e., immediate recall of three items), recent episodic memory (i.e., recent recall of three items and responses to questions related to temporal orientation), semantic language (i.e., naming common objects, repeating a linguistically difficult sentence, following a three-step command, and writing a sentence), semantic spatial ability (i.e., copying a two-dimensional figure), and working memory (i.e., performing serial 7s or spelling the word *world* backward).

The MMSE requires no test-specific training, can be administered by a variety of clinicians with general skill and knowledge of test administration, and takes approximately 10 min. To reiterate, however, it is a screening tool, not a diagnostic tool. A score of more than 24 out of a possible 30 points is generally recommended as indicative of normal cognitive functioning, albeit this score must *always* be considered relative to one's age and education and in light of the effects of sensory deficits (e.g., vision and hearing), tremor (Anthony, LeResche, Niaz, Von Korff, & Folstein, 1982), or both; in contrast, a score of less than 24 is generally recommended as indicative of cognitive impairment (Anthony et al., 1982), although "of unknown origin," warranting referral for more comprehensive evaluation. For example, before a diagnosis of dementia would be considered, an older adult's low MMSE score is interpreted within the context of other clinical data, such as informant-based history of cognitive decline; evidence of impairment in salient IADLs; and assessment for depression, sensory impairment, and factors other than dementia (e.g., as have been discussed above) that may account for impaired cognitive performance (AHCPR, 1996).

Functional status/IADL assessment is also important in detecting more severe impairment (Morris et al., 1991; Tabert et al., 2002; Wilder et al., 1994). Specifically, the Functional Activities Questionnaire (FAQ; Pfeffer, Kurosaki, Harrah, Chance, & Filos, 1982) has been identified as the most useful measure to discriminate between older adults either with and without severe cognitive impairment (AHCPR, 1996) and with and without incipient MCI (Tabert et al., 2002). The FAQ is an informant-based measure of functional abilities that provides performance ratings on 10 IADLs. Scores range from 0 to 30. A score of less than 9 out of a possible 30 points is generally recommended as indicative of normal cognitive functioning, whereas people with scores of 9 or greater should be referred to specialists to be screened for the presence of dementia or other physiological conditions that are potential causes of cognitive decline (AHCPR, 1996).

Cognitive screening instruments are primarily focused on the detection of severe cognitive impairment due to dementia; as such, they are neither intended nor sensitive enough to detect the mild cognitive changes associated with normal aging. Hence, older adults who complain of memory impairment who may have either AAMI or MCI generally score normally on screening instruments such as the MMSE (Fillit et al., 2002). If indicated, more extensive psychometric testing by neuropsychologists is required to distinguish between those with AAMI (or, more likely, MCI) and those with early dementia. Neuropsychological assessments particularly sensitive to MCI include those that measure memory (e.g., story recall), aphasia (e.g., verbal fluency), and executive functioning (e.g., trail-making tests).

Cognitive Training Programs

There is growing evidence that relatively brief cognitive training programs can reverse age-related decline in a number of older adults. Findings indicate that specific cognitive functions in older adults—including visual perception, attention, reasoning, and memory storage and retrieval—can be improved by cognitive intervention as well as generalized to independent tests of the cognitive functions of interest (not just on procedures used in training; Ball, Beard, Roenker, Miller, & Griggs, 1988; Ball et al., 2002; Baron & Mattila, 1989; Kramer, Larish, Weber, & Bardell, 1999; McDougall, 2002; Saczynski et al., 2002; Schaie, 1998; Schaie & Willis, 1986; Verhaeghen, Marcoen, & Goossens, 1993; Willis & Nesselroade, 1990; Willis & Schaie, 1986). The largest program was entitled ACTIVE (Advanced Cognitive Training for Independent and Vital Elderly; cf. Ball et al., 2002). This randomized, controlled, multisite intervention study has generated the highest strength of evidence for practice (Class I) and, as such, is described in detail here.

The ACTIVE study examined the effects of cognitive training on more than 1,800 adults aged 65 to 94 experiencing normal aging changes (i.e., free of any probable cognitive impairments). Three groups of older adults received training to improve memory (i.e., episodic memory), reasoning (i.e., working memory), and attention–processing speed, whereas the fourth group received no training. Training sessions took place in small groups twice a week over a 5-week period, and each session lasted from 60 to 75 min. In large part, training focused on helping these older adults develop strategies introduced in this chapter (tutored training) as well as workbook exercises to practice these new strategies. For example, participants in the memory training groups were taught how to remember word lists and sequences of items, text material (newspaper articles), and the main ideas and details of stories by using techniques such as chunking, categorizing, and mnemonics (specifically, visual imagery); participants in the reasoning group learned how to solve problems that follow patterns by organizing information and identifying repetitive patterns to determine what should come next (e.g., learning how to use a schedule for taking medications and for understanding bus routes); and participants in the attention–processing speed training group focused on practicing the ability to identify and locate visual information quickly (a car vs. a truck), and in multiple locations, using a touch-screen computer.

After the intervention, 26% of the memory group, 74% of the reasoning group, and 87% of the attention–processing speed group had made significant improvements in memory, reasoning, and attention–speed of processing, respectively. These improvements were maintained 2 years later. In addition, the magnitude of overall improvement in these cognitive abilities was found to be equivalent to the amount of cognitive decline one would expect over a 7- to 14-year interval among older adults of these ages. These positive outcomes, then, strongly suggest that remediation can help stem the cognitive declines reported in cognitively healthy (without dementia) older adults.

Note that, unlike training young children, where it can be assumed that new skills are being conveyed, older adults have had previous access to the skills being trained. As a result, the improvements cited in these cognitive intervention studies suggest that the plasticity in cognitive function demonstrated is likely due to the activation of already-available cognitive skills that have lost their proficiency or efficiency (i.e., they have become "rusty") through disuse (Heckhausen & Singer, 2001; Schaie, 2004).

Armed with the information provided in this chapter, occupational therapy practitioners are well placed to design and institute cognitive intervention programs such as those just described. Indeed, the promotion of cognitive vitality through primary and secondary prevention programs has been designated a national health priority by the National Institute on Aging and the Centers for Disease Control and Prevention (American Society on Aging, 2003; Fillit et al., 2002). In large part, these programs combine education on how memory works and the specific mechanisms that underlie the changes in memory that occur with normal aging, along with training in compensatory strategies for attending, learning, and recalling new information. To reiterate, older adults who are considered most appropriate for formal memory training programs are those who report age-related memory problems similar to those noted in AAMI and who also score normally (for one's age) on cognitive screening assessments (e.g., the MMSI and FAQ), although those with MCI are also likely to benefit. The overall intent is to promote functional adaptation through education, metacognition, and the use of compensatory strategies to help older adults overcome deficits in occupational performance and quality of life that they may experience.

SUMMARY

Cognitive change is a normal consequence of aging. Changes are selective, however, and primarily occur in specific components of short-term (working) and long-term (episodic) memory. Significant declines, however, are related to brain disease (discussed in Chapter 15).

The key to helping older adults minimize the effects of age-related decline is an understanding of how memory processing works as well as an appreciation of the variety of compensatory strategies that can be introduced to help older adults organize information more effectively for eventual retrieval. Occupational therapy practitioners can initiate either formal or informal cognitive training protocols to teach older adults metacognitive strategies to strengthen their attentional capabilities and to inhibit internal and external distracters that may undermine attention; they can also help older adults choose from the variety of rhyming, imagery, visualization, note-taking and other mnemonic strategies deemed useful for their particular situations. Practitioners need also to recognize that tasks and teaching environments for older adults should routinely be adapted to place fewer demands on limited attentional capacities and thereby to promote encoding and retention of newly learned information. In these ways, occupational therapy practitioners play a critical role in helping older adults minimize day-to-day difficulties experienced in cognitive functioning that may affect occupational performance, productivity, and quality of life; compensate for any adverse effects of age-related memory changes on retention of rehabilitation strategies; and help stem the age-related declines experienced by most older adults.

REVIEW QUESTIONS

1. How is the use of encoding strategies related to memory among older adults?
2. Define *age-associated memory impairment* and give an example of how this might affect an older adult's daily functioning.
3. How might an older adult be instructed to compensate for the effects of age-related cognitive decline?

REFERENCES

Agency for Health Care Policy and Research. (1996, November). *Recognition and initial assessment of Alzheimer's disease and related dementias: Clinical Practice Guideline No. 19* (AHCPR Publication No. 97-0702). Rockville, MD: U.S. Department of Health and Human Services, Public Health Service, Agency for Health Care Policy and Research.

Albert, M. (2002). Memory decline: The boundary between aging and age-related disease. *Annals of Neurology, 51,* 282–284.

American Heart Association. (1998). *1999 heart and stroke statistical update.* Dallas, TX: Author.

American Psychiatric Association. (1994). *Diagnostic and statistical manual of mental disorders* (4th ed.). Washington, DC: Author.

American Society on Aging. (2003). *Strategies for cognitive vitality.* San Francisco: Author.

Anthony, J. C., LeResche, L., Niaz, U., Von Korff, M., & Folstein, M. (1982). Limits of the "Mini-Mental State" as a screening test for dementia and delirium in aging hospital patients. *Psychological Medicine, 12,* 397–408.

Anstey, K., Luszcz, M., & Sanchez, L. (2001). Two year decline in vision but not hearing is associated with memory decline in very old adults in a population based sample. *Journal of Gerontology, 47,* 289–293.

Arenberg, D., & Robertson-Tchabo, E. A. (1977). Learning and aging. In J. E. Birren & K. W. Schaie (Eds.), *Handbook of the psychology of aging* (pp. 421–449). New York: Van Nostrand Reinhold.

Arvanitakis, Z., Wilson, R., Bienias, J., Evans, D., & Bennett, D. (2004). Diabetes mellitus and the risk of Alzheimer disease and decline in cognitive function. *Archives of Neurology, 61,* 661–666.

Auperin, A., Berr, C., & Bonithon-Kopp, C. (1996). Ultrasonic assessment of carotid wall characteristics and cognitive functions in a community sample of 59–71 year olds. *Stroke, 27,* 1290–1295.

Bachman, D. L., Wolf, P. A., Linn, R. T., Knoefel, J. E., Cobb, J. L., Belanger, A. J., et al. (1993). Incidence of dementia and probable Alzheimer's disease in a general population: The Framingham Study. *Neurology, 43,* 515–519.

Backman, L. (1989). Varieties of memory compensation by older adults in episodic remembering. In L. Poon, D. Rubin, & B. Wilson (Eds.), *Everyday cognition in adulthood and late life* (pp. 509–544). New York: Cambridge University Press.

Backman, L., Small, B., & Wahlin, A. (2001). Aging and memory: Cognitive and biological perspectives. In J. E. Birren & K. W. Schaie (Eds.), *Handbook of the psychology of aging* (5th ed., pp. 349–377). San Diego, CA: Academic Press.

Ball, K., Beard, B., Roenker, D., Miller, R., & Griggs, D. (1988). Age and visual search: Expanding the useful field of view. *Journal of the Optical Society of America, 5,* 2210–2219.

Ball, K., Berch, D., Helmers, K., Jobe, J., Leveck, M., Marsiske, M., et al. (2002). Effects of cognitive training interventions with older adults. *Journal of the American Medical Association, 288,* 2271–2281.

Baltes, P., & Graf, P. (1996). Psychological aspects of aging: Factors and frontiers. In D. Magnusson (Ed.), *The lifespan development of individuals: A synthesis* (pp. 427–460). New York: Cambridge University Press.

Baltes, P., & Mayer, K. (Eds.). (1999). *The Berlin Aging Study from 70 to 100.* New York: Cambridge University Press.

Baltes, P., Staudinger, U., & Lindenberger, U. (1999). Wisdom: A metaheuristic to orchestrate mind and virtue toward excellence. *American Psychologist, 55,* 122–135.

Baron, A., & Mattila, W. (1989). Response slowing of older adults: Effects of time contingencies on single and dual tasks performances. *Psychology and Aging, 4,* 66–72.

Birren, J., & Fisher, L. (1995). Aging and speed of behavior: Possible consequences for psychological functioning. *Annual Review of Psychology, 46,* 329–353.

Carlin, A., & O'Malley, S. (1996). Neuropsychological consequences of drug abuse. In I. Grant & K. Adams (Eds.), *Neuropsychological assessment of neuropsychiatric disorders* (2nd ed., pp. 486–503). New York: Oxford University Press.

Chow, S., & Nesselroade, J. (2004). General slowing or decreased inhibition? Mathematical models of age differences in cognitive functioning. *Journal of Gerontology, 59B,* P101–P109.

Cicero. (1923). *On old age* (W. A. Falconer, Trans.). Cambridge, MA: Harvard University Press.

Colcombe, S., Kramer, A., Erickson, K., Scalf, P., McAuley, E., Cohen, N., et al. (2004). Cardiovascular fitness, cortical plasticity, and aging. *Proceedings of the National Academy of Sciences, 101,* 3316–3321.

Colohan, H. (1989). An evaluation of cranial CT scanning in clinical psychiatry. *Israeli Journal of Medical Science, 158,* 178–181.

Convit, A., Wolf, O., Tarshish, C., & de Leon, M. (2003). Reduced glucose tolerance is associated with poor memory performance and hippocampal atrophy among normal elderly. *Proceedings of the National Academy of Sciences, 100,* 2019–2022.

Craik, F. I., & Jennings, J. (1992). Human memory. In F. Craik & T. Salthouse (Eds.), *Handbook of memory disorders* (pp. 51–110). New York: Wiley.

Crook, T., Bartus, R., Ferris, S., Whitehouse, P., Cohen, G., & Gershon, S. (1986). Age associated memory impairment: Proposed diagnostic criteria and measures of clinical change: Report of a National Institute of Mental Health work group. *Developmental Neuropsychology, 2,* 261–276.

Crum, R., Anthony, J., Bassett, S., & Folstein, M. (1993). Population based norms for the Mini-Mental Status Examination by age and educational level. *Journal of the American Medical Association, 269,* 2386–2391.

Elias, M., Robbins, M., Elias, P., & Streeten, D. (1998). A longitudinal study of blood pressure in relation to performance on the Wechsler Adult Intelligence Scale. *Health Psychology, 17,* 486–493.

Fillit, H. M., Butler, R. N., O'Connell, A. W., Albert, M. S., Birren, J. E., Cotman, C. W., et al. (2002). Achieving and maintaining cognitive vitality with aging. *Mayo Clinic Proceedings, 77,* 681–696.

Folstein, M. F., Folstein, S. E., & McHugh, P. R. (1975). Mini-Mental State: A practical method for grading the cognitive state of patients for the clinician. *Journal of Psychiatric Research, 12,* 189–198.

Forette, F., Seux, M. L., Staessen, J. A., Thijs, L., Birkenhager, W. H., Babarskiene, M. R., et al. (1998). Prevention of dementia in randomized double-blind placebo-controlled systolic hypertension in Europe (Syst-Eur) trial. *The Lancet, 352,* 1347–1351.

Gounard, B. R., & Hulicka, I. M. (1977). Maximizing learning efficiency in later adulthood: A cognitive problem-solving approach. *Educational Gerontology, 2,* 417–427.

Gregg, E., Jaffe, K., & Cauley, J. (2000). Is diabetes associated with cognitive impairment and cognitive decline among older women? *Archives of Internal Medicine, 160,* 174–180.

Hasher, L., Tonev, S., Lustig, C., & Zacks, R. (2001). Inhibitory control, environmental support, and self-initiated processing in aging. In M. Naveh-Benjamin, M. Moscovitch, & R. L. Roedinger (Eds.), *Perspectives on human memory and cognitive aging: Essays in honour of Fergus Craik* (pp. 286–297). East Sussex, England: Psychology Press.

Hasher, L., & Zacks, R. (1988). Working memory comprehension and aging: A review and new view. In G. Bower (Ed.), *The psychology of learning and motivation: Advances in research and theory* (Vol. 22, pp. 193–225). New York: Academic Press.

Hayslip, B., Jr., & Kennelly, K. J. (1985). Cognitive and noncognitive factors affecting learning among older adults. In D. B. Lumsden (Ed.), *The older adult as learner* (pp. 73–98). Washington, DC: Hemisphere.

Heckhausen, J., & Singer, T. (2001). Plasticity in human behavior across the life span. In P. Baltes & N. Smelser (Eds.), *International encyclopedia of the social and behavioral sciences* (pp. 11497–11501). St. Louis, MO: Elsevier.

Higbee, K. (1988). *Your memory: How it works and how to improve it* (2nd ed.). New York: Paragon House.

Hultsch, D., & Dixon, R. (1990). Learning and memory and aging. In J. Birren & K. Schaie (Eds.), *Handbook of the psychology of aging* (3rd ed., pp. 259–274). New York: Academic Press.

Karlawish, J., & Clark, C. (2003). Diagnostic evaluation of elderly patients with mild memory problems. *Annals of Internal Medicine, 138,* 411–419.

Kivipelto, M., Helkala, E.-L., Laakso, M. P., Hänninen, T., Hallikainen, M., Alhainen, K., et al. (2001). Midlife vascular risk factors and Alzheimer's disease in later life: Longitudinal population based study. *British Medical Journal, 322,* 1447–1451.

Kramer, A., Larish, J., Weber, T., & Bardell, L. (1999). Training for executive control: Task coordination strategies and aging. In D. Gopher & A. Koriat (Eds.), *Attention and performance XVII* (pp. 617–652). Cambridge, MA: MIT Press.

Labouvie-Vief, G. (1976). Toward optimizing cognitive competence in later life. *Educational Gerontology, 1,* 75–92.

Launer, L., Masaki, K., Petrovitch, H., Foley, D., & Havlik, R. (1995). The association between midlife blood pressure levels and late life cognitive function: The Honolulu–Asia Aging Study. *Journal of the American Medical Association, 274,* 1846–1851.

Lee, A., Ogle, W., & Sapolsky, R. (2002). Stress and depression: Possible links to neuron death in the hippocampus. *Bipolar Disorders, 4,* 117–128.

Levy, L. (1996a). Health and impairment: The performance context. In K. O. Larson, R. Stevens-Ratchford, L. Pedretti, & J. Crabtree (Eds.), *The role of occupational therapy with the elderly (ROTE)* (2nd ed., pp. 169–198). Rockville, MD: American Occupational Therapy Association.

Levy, L. (1996b). Mental disorders in aging adults. In K. O. Larson, R. Stevens-Ratchford, L. Pedretti, & J. Crabtree (Eds.), *The role of occupational therapy with the elderly (ROTE)* (2nd ed., pp. 221–229). Rockville, MD: American Occupational Therapy Association.

Lindenberger, U., & Baltes, P. (1994). Sensory functioning and intelligence in old age: A strong connection. *Psychology and Aging, 9,* 339–355.

Madden, D., & Blumenthal, J. (1998). Interaction of hypertension and age in visual selective attention performance. *Health Psychology, 17,* 76–83.

McDougall, G. (2002). Memory improvement in octogenarians. *Applied Nursing Research, 15,* 2–10.

McDowell, I. (2001). Alzheimer's disease: Insights from epidemiology. *Aging, 13,* 143–162.

Morris, J. C., McKeel, D. W., Storandt, M., Rubin, E., Price, J., Grant, E., et al. (1991). Very mild Alzheimer's disease: Informant-based clinical, psychometric, and pathologic distinction from normal aging. *Neurology, 41,* 469–478.

National Research Council. (2003). Structure of the aging mind. In P. Stern & L. Carstensen (Eds.), *The aging mind: Opportunities for cognitive research* (pp. 37–53). Washington, DC: National Academy Press.

Ostwald, S. K., & Williams, H. Y. (1985). Optimizing learning in the elderly: A model. *Lifelong Learning: An Omnibus of Practice and Research, 9,* 10–15.

Park, D. (2000). The basic mechanisms accounting for age related decline in cognitive function. In D. Park & N. Schwartz (Eds.), *Cognitive aging: A primer* (pp. 3–21). Philadelphia: Psychology Press.

Park, D., & Hall-Gutchess, A. (2000). Cognitive aging in everyday life. In D. Park & N. Schwartz (Eds.), *Cognitive aging: A primer* (pp. 217–232). Philadelphia: Psychology Press.

Park, D., Smith, A., Lautenschlager, G., Earles, J., Frieske, D., Zwahr, M., & Gaines, C. (1996). Mediators of long term memory performance across the lifespan. *Psychology and Aging, 11,* 621–637.

Pearlson, G., & Tune, L. (1986). Cerebral ventricular size and cerebrospinal fluid acetylcholinesterase levels in senile dementia of the Alzheimers type. *Psychiatry Research, 17,* 23–29.

Peters, R. (2001). The prevention of dementia. *Journal of Cardiovascular Risk, 8,* 253–256.

Peterson, R., Smith, G., Waring, S., Ivnik, R., Tangelos, E., & Kokmen, E. (1999). Mild cognitive impairment: Clinical characterization and outcome. *Archives of Neurology, 56,* 303–308.

Pfeffer, R., Kurosaki, T., Harrah, C., Chance, J., & Filos, S. (1982). Measurement of functional activities in older adults in the community. *Journal of Gerontology, 37,* 323–329.

Radloff, L. (1977). The CES–D scale: A self-report depression scale for research in the general population. *Applied Psychological Measurement, 1,* 385–401.

Rubinstein, J., Meyer, D., & Evans, J. (2001). Executive control of cognitive processes in task switching. *Journal of Experimental Psychology: Human Perception and Performance, 27,* 763–797.

Ruitenberg, A., van Swieten, J. C., Witteman, J. C., Mehta, K. M., van Duijn, C. M., Hofman, A., et al. (2002). Alcohol consumption and the risk of dementia: The Rotterdam Study. *The Lancet, 359,* 281–286.

Saczynski, J., Willis, S., & Schaie, K. (2002). Strategy use in reasoning training with older adults. *Aging, Neuropsychology, and Cognition, 9,* 48–60.

Salthouse, T. (1992). Why do adult age differences increase with task complexity. *Developmental Psychology, 28,* 905–918.

Salthouse, T. (1994). The aging of working memory. *Neuropsychology, 8,* 535–543.

Salthouse, T. (1996). The processing speed theory of adult age differences in cognition. *Psychological Review, 103,* 403–428.

Salthouse, T. (2000). Aging and measures of processing speed. *Biological Psychology, 54,* 35–54.

Salthouse, T. (2004). What and when of cognitive aging. *Current Directions in Psychological Science, 13,* 140–144.

Schacter, D. (1996). *Searching for memory: The brain, the mind, and the past.* New York: Basic Books.

Schaie, K. (1988). Variability in cognitive function in the elderly. *Basic Life Science, 43,* 191–211.

Schaie, K. W. (1998). The Seattle Longitudinal Studies of Adult Intelligence. In M. P. Lawton & T. Salthouse (Eds.), *Essential papers on the psychology of aging* (pp. 263–271). New York: New York University Press.

Schaie, K. W. (2004). Cognitive aging. In R. Pew & S. Van Hemel (Eds.), *National Research Council: Technology for adaptive aging* (pp. 41–63). Washington, DC: National Academy Press.

Schaie, K., & Willis, S. (1986). Can decline in adult intellectual functioning be reversed? *Developmental Psychology, 2,* 223–232.

Schaie, K., & Willis, S. (1991). Adult personality and psychomotor performance: Cross sectional and longitudinal analysis. *Journal of Gerontology, 46,* P275–P284.

Scogin, F., & Prohaska, M. (1993). *Aiding older adults with memory complaints.* Sarasota, FL: Professional Resource Press.

Selkoe, D. (1999). Translating cell biology into therapeutic advances in Alzheimer's disease. *Nature, 399,* A23–A31.

Sharit, J., & Czaja, S. (1994). Aging, computer based task performance, and stress: Issues and challenges. *Ergonomics, 37,* 559–577.

Sherwin, B. (2000). Mild cognitive impairment: Potential pharmacological treatment options. *Journal of the American Geriatrics Society, 48,* 431–441.

Shors, T. (2001). Stress and sex effects on associative learning: For better or for worse. *Neuroscientist, 4,* 353–364.

Siegel, J. (2001). The REM sleep–memory consolidation hypothesis. *Science, 294,* 1058–1063.

Silver, M., Jilinskaia, E., & Perls, T. (2001). Cognitive functional status of age-confirmed centenarians in a population-based study. *Journal of Gerontology, 56,* P134–P140.

Small, S., Tsai, W., DeLaPaz, R., Mayeux, R., & Stern, Y. (2002). Imaging hippocampal function across the human life span: Is memory decline normal or not? *Annals of Neurology, 51,* 290–295.

Spiegel, K., Leproult, R., & Van Cauter, E. (1999). Impact of sleep debt on metabolic and endocrine function. *The Lancet, 354,* 1435–1439.

Tabert, M., Albert, S., Borukkhova-Milov, L., Camacho, Y., Pelton, G., Liu, X., et al. (2002). Functional deficits in patients with mild cognitive impairment: Prediction of Alzheimer's disease. *Neurology, 58,* 758–763.

Terry, R., & Katzman, R. (2001). Life span and synapses: Will there be a primary senile dementia? *Neurobiology of Aging, 22,* 347–348, 353–354.

Tombaugh, T. N., & McIntyre, N. J. (1992). The Mini-Mental State Examination: A comprehensive review. *Journal of the American Geriatrics Society, 40,* 922–935.

Toole, J., & Jack, C. (2002). Food (and vitamins) for thought. *Neurology, 58,* 1449–1450.

Tulving, E. (2000). Introduction to memory. In M. Gazzaniga (Ed.), *The new cognitive neurosciences* (2nd ed., pp. 727–732). Cambridge, MA: MIT Press.

Verhaeghen, P., Marcoen, M., & Goossens, L. (1993). Improving memory performance in the aged through mnemonic training: A meta-analytic study. *Psychology and Aging, 7,* 242–251.

Wahl, H., & Heyl, V. (2003). Connections between vision, hearing, and cognitive function in old age. *Generations, 27,* 39–45.

Waldstein, S. (2003). Health effects on cognitive aging. In P. Stern & L. Carstensen (Eds.), *The aging mind: Opportunities for cognitive research.* Washington, DC: National Academy Press.

Wang, H., Wahlin, A., Basun, H., Fastbom, J., Winblad, B., & Fratiglioni, L. (2001). Vitamin B(12) and folate in relation to the development of Alzheimer's disease. *Neurology, 56,* 1188–1194.

West, R. (1999). Age differences in lapses of intention in the Stroop task. *Journal of Gerontology, 54B,* P34–P43.

Whiting, W., & Smith, A. (1997). Differential age-related processing limitations in recall and recognition tasks. *Psychology and Aging, 12,* 216–224.

Wilder, D., Gurland, B., Chen, J., Lantigua, R., Encarnacion, P., & Katz, S. (1994). Interpreting subject and informant reports of function in screening for dementia. *International Journal of Geriatric Psychiatry, 9,* 887–896.

Willis, S., & Nesselroade, C. (1990). Long term effects of fluid ability training in old-old age. *Developmental Psychology, 26,* 905–910.

Willis, S., & Schaie, K. (1986). Training the elderly on the ability factors of spatial orientation and inductive reasoning. *Psychology and Aging, 1,* 239–247.

Yesavage, J., Brink, T., Rose, T., Lum, O., Huang, V., Adey, M., & Leirer, V. (1983). Development and validation of a geriatric depression screening scale: A preliminary report. *Journal of Psychiatric Research, 17,* 37–49.

Zacks, R., & Hasher, L. (1997). Cognitive gerontology and attentional inhibition: A reply to Burke and McDowd. *Journal of Gerontology, 52,* P274–P283.

APPENDIX 13.1. MINI-MENTAL STATE EXAMINATION

Maximum Score	Score	
		Orientation
5	_____	What is the (year) (season) (date) (day) (month)?
5	_____	Where are we: (state) (county) (town) (hospital) (floor)?
		Registration
3	_____	Name 3 objects: 1 second to say each. Then ask the patient all 3 after you have said them. Give 1 point for each correct answer. Then repeat them until he learns all 3. Count trials and record. Trials:
		Attention and Calculation
5	_____	Serial 7s. 1 point for each correct. Stop after 5 answers. Alternatively spell "world" backward.
		Recall
3	_____	Ask for the 3 objects repeated above. Give 1 point for each correct.
		Language
9	_____	Name a pencil and watch *(2 points)*.
	_____	Repeat the following "No ifs, ands, or buts" *(1 point)*.
		Follow a 3-stage command:
	_____	"Take a paper in your right hand, fold it in half, and put it on the floor" *(3 points)*.
		Read and obey the following:
	_____	Close your eyes *(1 point)*.
	_____	Write a sentence *(1 point)*.
	_____	Copy design *(1 point)*.

30   **Total Score**   _____

Assess level of consciousness along a continuum   Alert   Drowsy   Stupor   Coma

INSTRUCTIONS FOR ADMINISTRATION OF MINI-MENTAL STATE EXAMINATION

Orientation

(1) Ask for the date. Then ask specifically for parts omitted, e.g., "Can you also tell me what season it is?" 1 point for each correct.

(2) Ask in turn "Can you tell me the name of this hospital?" (town, county, etc.). 1 point for each correct.

Registration

Ask the patient if you may test his memory. Then say the names of 3 unrelated objects, clearly and slowly, about 1 second for each. After you have said all three, ask him to repeat them. This first repetition determines his score (0–3), but keep saying them until he can repeat all 3, up to 6 trials. If he does not eventually learn all 3, recall cannot be meaningfully tested.

Attention and Calculation

Ask the patient to begin with 100 and count backward by 7. Stop after 5 subtractions (93, 86, 79, 72, 65). Score the total number of correct answers.

If the patient cannot or will not perform this task, ask him to spell the word "world" backward. The score is the number of letters in correct order, e.g., dlrow = 5, dlorw = 3.

Recall

Ask the patient if he can recall the 3 words you previously asked him to remember. Score 0–3.

Language

Naming: Show the patient a wrist watch and ask him what it is. Repeat for pencil. Score 0–3.

Repetition: Ask the patient to repeat the sentence after you. Allow only one trial. Score 0 or 1.

3-Stage Command: Give the patient a piece of plain blank paper and repeat the command. Score 1 point for each part correctly executed.

Reading: On a blank piece of paper print the sentence "Close your eyes," in letters large enough for the patient to see clearly. Ask him to read it and do what it says. Score 1 point only if he actually closes his eyes.

Writing: Give the patient a blank piece of paper and ask him to write a sentence. Do not dictate a sentence; it is to be written spontaneously. It must contain a subject and verb and be sensible. Correct grammar and punctuation are not necessary.

Copying: On a clean piece of paper, draw intersecting pentagons, each side about 1 in., and ask him to copy it exactly as it is.

Estimate the patient's level of sensorium along a continuum, from alert on the left to coma on the right.

(continued)

APPENDIX 13.1.   MINI-MENTAL STATE EXAMINATION *(Continued)*

Median Mini-Mental State Examination Score by Age and Education Level

	Education				
	0–4y	5–8y	9–12y	≥12y	Total
18–24	23	28	29	30	29
25–29	25	27	29	30	29
30–34	26	26	29	30	29
35–39	23	27	29	30	29
40–44	23	27	29	30	29
45–49	23	27	29	30	29
50–54	22	27	29	30	29
55–59	22	27	29	29	29
60–64	22	27	28	29	28
65–69	22	27	28	29	28
70–74	21	26	28	29	27
75–79	21	26	27	28	26
80–84	19	25	26	28	25
≥85	20	24	26	28	25
Total	22	26	29	29	29

Note. From Agency for Health Care Policy and Research. (November 1996). *Recognition and initial assessment of Alzheimer's disease and related dementias: Clinical practice guideline No. 19.* Rockville, MD: U.S. Department of Health and Human Services, Public Health Service, Agency for Health Care Policy and Research. AHCPR Pub. No. 97-0702.

14

Linda L. Levy, MA, OTR/L, FAOTA
Theressa Burns, OTR

Cognitive Disabilities Reconsidered

Rehabilitation of Older Adults With Dementia

LEARNING OBJECTIVES

By the end of this chapter, readers will

1. Recognize the information-processing dimensions of cognitive impairment in dementia
2. Identify memory systems that are spared and impaired at different stages of dementia
3. Recognize the significance of environmental recognition cues in the rehabilitation of older adults with dementia
4. Recognize the significance of procedural memories in rehabilitation of older adults with dementia
5. Recognize the relationship between principles of cognitive information processing and those that are fundamental to the reconsidered cognitive disability model introduced here
6. Define information-processing characteristics of each of the six cognitive disability levels as related to dementia
7. State various assessment tools and the benefits associated with each one
8. State how a screening assessment and a full assessment are different and how to apply these scores
9. Describe the Cognitive Performance Test as an activities of daily living–based executive-function measure
10. Assess a person with dementia to provide a meaningful care plan that will focus on retained abilities and enhanced function
11. Recognize the importance of caregiver assessment in developing effective treatment plans
12. Design effective treatment plans, including caregiver training
13. Describe the development and significance of cognitive impairment on outcome, work function, skills acquisition, and executive functioning in older adults with dementia.

Dementing illness is common in older adults. Prevalence studies across racial groups suggest that, among individuals older than 65 years, 6% to 8% have dementia, a *syndrome* of memory and other cognitive impairments that significantly interferes with daily function. Prevalence increases with advancing age, and among individuals older than 85 years, the prevalence rate is more than 30% (Bachman et al., 1992; "Canadian Study of Health and Aging," 1994; Evans et al., 1989; Graves et al., 1996; Hendrie et al., 1995). By the next decade, the prevalence of dementias is expected to quadruple, given the dramatic increase in the older adult population.

Although more than 70 distinct causes of dementia have been identified, Alzheimer's disease (AD) accounts for nearly two-thirds of the dementia syndromes. Less common syndromes include dementia with cerebrovascular disease, Lewy body dementia (a variant of Parkinson disease), frontotemporal dementia, the rapidly progressive dementias, primary progressive aphasias, and craniocerebral trauma (traumatic brain injury). Because most individuals with dementias have long survival times (i.e., the median survival from diagnosis to death is more than 6 years and can range from 2 to 20 years), the prevalence rate of dementias greatly exceeds its incidence rate (Fillenbaum et al., 1998; Heyman, Peterson, Fillenbaum, & Pieper, 1996; Jagger et al., 2000). Most dementias are progressive and eventually lead to total disability and 24-hr care. However, in contrast to a decade ago, this care is more often delivered in the home or in alternative, less institutionally based, long-term care settings (e.g., assisted living).

DIAGNOSIS OF DEMENTIA

No laboratory markers currently exist for presymptomatic testing to identify the pathology that begins in early AD and other dementias years before the behavioral symptoms occur. Therefore, physicians must wait to make a diagnosis until after individuals become symptomatic, in a clinical assessment that integrates information from the client's medical history, the assessment of functional status, the mental status examination, and the neurological examination. The diagnosis of dementia is based on changes in behavior and the performance of daily activities *and* on the presence of cognitive dysfunction on mental status examinations or neurological assessments that identify patterns of impairments particular to specific syndromes and disease processes. Likewise, patterns of impairments in daily activities are identified, with changes and problems seen in instrumental activities of daily living (IADLs) in the early stages of the disease and the changes in basic activities of daily living (ADLs) seen with further progression.

Laboratory assessments are part of the diagnostic workup. Computerized tomography or magnetic resonance imaging may be used to eliminate brain structural lesions, including tumors or vascular changes, as the cause of dysfunction. Similarly, bloodwork is focused on the common medical problems in the elderly and identifies potential causes of

347

dysfunction, such as a metabolic disorder, or reversible causes, as in medication toxicity or infection. At present, AD and most other dementias can be confirmed only at autopsy, with microscopic inspection. However, the clinical diagnosis of dementias has been shown to be accurate (Knopman, Bradley, & Peterson, 2003). Laboratory markers for the diagnosis of AD and the other major subtypes of dementia are currently under development.

Many individuals with dementias are not recognized or referred for diagnosis (Knopman et al., 2003). Elderly persons often have comorbid conditions that limit their occupations and obscure emerging cognitive decline. Likewise, relationships and families are diverse, with circumstances that can decrease the sensitivity of family informants for recognizing decline and interference with usual activities. Functional assessment by interview with an informant, typically a spouse or adult child, is an integral part of the diagnostic evaluation because two key principles underlie the concept of dementia: (a) The affected person has experienced a decline from some previously higher level of functioning and (b) the dementia significantly interferes with work or usual complex or social activities. A knowledgeable informant is interviewed because genuine problems with daily activities are most evident to those who are close to the person.

Functional assessment through an informant is considered to be more objective than interviewing the person, because an altered sense of self-awareness occurs frequently as part of the dementia syndrome. Some individuals with incipient memory loss are aware of their declining abilities, but many individuals with progressing dementias seem to be unaware of their deficits or decline; some may be aware but unable to acknowledge that they have dysfunction (Grut et al., 1993; Tabert et al., 2002). For example, persons with AD often have intact immediate awareness of memory dysfunction but may fail to incorporate incidents of memory failure into more generalized self-belief systems (Duke, Seltzer, Seltzer, & Vasterling, 2002).

As we discuss more fully later in this chapter, self-awareness and the awareness of deficit is a complex cognitive ability involving cognitive processes that deteriorate as the disease progresses. Apathy, impaired awareness, and impairments in executive functions are often prominent features already in the early stages of disease and have been associated with disruption in frontal and prefrontal–subcortical circuits (Collette, Van der Linden, Bechet, & Salmon, 1999; Ready, Ott, Grace, & Cahn-Weiner, 2003; Seltzer, Vasterling, Mathias, & Brennan, 2001). These behaviors are proposed to occur after suffi-

cient damage to the frontal lobes and other cortical areas and may involve frontal and right hemisphere cortical and subcortical connections. For example, studies demonstrate that neuropsychological measures of executive and visuospatial functions correlate with both measures of deficit awareness (Boyle et al., 2003; Mangone et al., 1991; Ott et al., 1996) and IADL and ADL functions (Glosser et al., 2002; Perry & Hodges, 2000; Stout, Wyman, Johnson, Peavy, & Salmon, 2003).

As we also explain in the discussion to follow, changes in the performance of daily occupations and the person's impaired awareness of the changes can be predicted by specific cognitive impairments and behavioral symptoms. Specifically, impairments in executive functions and the problematic symptoms of apathy have been shown to be elevated in mild to moderate AD as well as in severe AD. However, there are qualitative differences in these symptoms, depending on the severity of disease. Apathy in early stages may be linked to impaired insight into the impact of memory changes, or errors in judgment, whereas apathy in later stages is more associated with impairments in the ability to initiate required tasks. In addition, apathy has been shown to have a greater association with later changes that emerge in ADLs, whereas impairments more related to executive functions (e.g., reasoning, judgment) are related to the earlier impairments in IADLs (Tekin, Fairbanks, O'Connor, Rosenberg, & Cummings, 2001).

Many caregivers may perceive the apathy and lack of initiation of essential daily activities as willful, describing the person as lazy, unmotivated, refusing to do things, or sitting all day. The rehabilitation program we describe here aims to help caregivers to perceive these behaviors as caused by the disease process rather than as the intent of the person. As will also be seen, this model provides for the development of effective rehabilitative strategies to assist the person, through knowledge of the specific nature of the cognitive impairments that cause the behavioral symptoms, insight into the meanings of problematic behaviors, recommendations for person-centered management strategies, and means for the accurate assessment of remaining strengths and abilities.

We would like to make one final point before proceeding: As was discussed in Chapter 12, early detection of AD is an important public health issue. In addition, older adults are concerned about having AD. Publicity about the disease has produced an increased awareness of memory problems, and older adults are presenting to physicians with their concerns and with early-stage disease. A large intermediate zone is now recognized between a normally aging adult and one with clear dementia. The intermediate zone is referred to as mild cognitive impairment (MCI; Peterson et al., 1999). The MCI category includes individuals who do not score in normal ranges relative to their age because of deficits in at least one cognitive domain (usually recent memory) but who appear to function independently in daily affairs. The problem is that the likelihood of individuals with MCI developing dementia is 5 to 10 times that of cognitively healthy individuals, and the more impaired a person with MCI is, the more likely he or she is to develop AD (Albert, Moss, Tanzi, & Jones, 2001; Peterson et al., 1999).

Yet, the failure to diagnose dementia early in the course of the disease has not resulted in the withholding of preventive therapies, because no such therapies currently exist. Nonetheless, the personal and public health consequences of unrecognized dementias are real. Behind the forgetfulness that appears benign may be important serious mistakes, such as traffic violations or accidents with driving, improperly taken medications, forgotten bills, and malnutrition. The safety and health risks and the costs of health care increase even more for those with co-morbid conditions, because individuals with dementia are eventually not able to manage, for example, their diabetes or cardiovascular disease (Gutterman, Markowitz, Lewis, & Fillit, 1999). The focus is projected to shift in the next decade to earlier diagnosis and identification of individuals at risk for AD or other dementing illnesses. In addition, the highly likely development of effective preventive or arrestive drug therapies in the next 20 years will substantially increase the need for early, accurate clinical diagnosis (Knopman et al., 2003).

REFERRAL TO OCCUPATIONAL THERAPY

In acute-care settings, clients with undiagnosed, suspected, and diagnosed dementias are referred to both occupational therapy psychiatric and physical rehabilitation clinics for functional assessment and recommendations regarding competency issues. Noncompliance with medication regimens; missed medical appointments; memory impairment; and concerns about driving, living alone, and weight loss are common reasons for referral. Requests for family and caregiver education and recommendations concerning placement issues and appropriate living environments may be included in the referral and may involve clients who are admitted to a medical or psychiatric inpatient unit during a crisis.

Referrals for baseline and serial assessments are a growing area of practice (Stringer, 2003; Ward & Kuskowski,

1999). Objective performance assessment is used for baseline and serial adjustments in the person's daily activities and level of care and for making care decisions for those who live alone, with no available informant. Performance assessment is also used in research protocols and may prove to have future utility in the early diagnostic assessment of function in MCI and in early-stage disease (Burns, McCarten, Adler, Bauer, & Kuskowski, 2004; Burns, Mortimer, & Merchek, 1994; Maddox & Burns, 1997; Ostwald, Hepburn, Caron, Burns, & Mantell, 1999).

Occupational therapists who provide rehabilitative services in acute and sub-acute settings consider the client's ability to learn and carry over treatment as well as the capabilities of family and other caregivers to assist with the discharge plan. Cognitive impairment is a client factor that affects performance in all areas of occupation, and in dementia it significantly interferes with the ability to learn. Dementia is often a secondary or concurrent diagnosis for clients who are referred for rehabilitation services. For example, dementia with parkinsonism or the onset of dementia subsequent to a stroke or surgical intervention such as hip replacement are common diagnoses seen in rehabilitation clinics. Rehabilitation services increasingly include the assessment of clients' ability to safely return to independent living or to return home with caregivers.

The model we describe in this chapter provides a reliable theoretical basis for functional assessment and the design of rehabilitative and compensatory behavioral programs that promote safety and the highest level of function and quality of life throughout the course of the disease. It is applied to practice in the growing markets of community-residing older adults, assisted living and specialty homes, and in traditional nursing homes.

COGNITIVE DISABILITIES RECONSIDERED MODEL

In the remaining sections of this chapter we reformulate the cognitive disabilities model for rehabilitation in dementia using the information-processing framework described in previous chapters (see also Levy, 1999). The cognitive disability model has been particularly useful to occupational therapists because it has provided an ordinal scale of functional performance capabilities and limitations that coincides with the trajectory of dementing diseases (Health Care Financing Administration, 1989). It has also long provided clinicians with intervention guidelines that address the consequences of functional performance limitations that emerge (Allen, 1985; Levy, 1974, 1986a, 1989, 1999). The model we introduce here expands on Allen's original work (Allen, 1985, 1987; Allen & Blue, 1998; Allen, Earhart, & Blue, 1992, 1995) to provide consistency with newly emerging theory and concepts from the cognitive neuroscience and neuropsychological literature. It provides a theoretical scaffolding for the cognitive-level scale and provides a means of more specifically delineating the complex relationships between neurocognitive deficits and functional capacities. The "reconsidered" model also provides framework for more accurate assessment of the impact of cognitive impairment on occupational performance as well as intervention guidelines that can more reliably be generalized to the functional performance capabilities of people with dementias.

We begin our discussion with a synthesis of knowledge on the specific nature of cognitive impairments that underlie the functional limitations experienced by people with dementias, in light of information-processing concepts introduced previously. Understanding patterns of impaired and preserved cognitive functions provides the requisite groundwork for understanding the impact of these impairments on functional performance; these are addressed in the reconsidered cognitive disability model that is the focus of this chapter.

INFORMATION-PROCESSING IMPAIRMENTS AND DEMENTIA

Each component of the refined information-processing model (i.e., sensory–perceptual memory, working memory, and long-term memory) is examined here to identify the patterns of information-processing capacities and impairments that occur as dementias progress. It would be impossible to review the specific nature of neuropathologies and cognitive impairments of all types of dementia syndromes in one chapter; thus, the scope of this discussion is limited to AD, the most common of the cortical dementias. Nevertheless, there are essential similarities in the neuropathological abnormalities and patterns of impairment seen in AD and other dementia-producing diseases. It would be helpful to review concepts introduced in previous chapters (including Figure 13.1) prior to this discussion.

Sensory–Perceptual Memory

Recall that sensory–perceptual memory is the large-capacity store of information specific to sensory modality. A perceived stimulus is retained in sensory memory for a matter of milliseconds before fading. Nonetheless, the integrity of this stage of memory input is essential for longer term storage, and impairment at this level will undermine efforts to rehabilitate and compensate for memory difficulties at other stages.

Dementia researchers have found decrements in the sensory–perceptual-memory store (Craik & Jennings, 1992; Mendez, Mendez, Martin, Smyth, & Whitehouse, 1990), although they have been considered to be of limited practical significance. However, recent studies (Tetewsky & Duffy, 1999) have found that an impairment of the visual sensation known as *optic flow* in patients with dementias interferes with the perception and storage of visual cues that may contribute to well-documented deficits in visuospatial abilities that are individually varied but characteristic of all stages of the disease.

At the same time, it is important to recognize that because the sensory–perceptual-memory store represents pure visual or auditory input, it will significantly be affected by sensory impairments that are all too common in the aging population (recall that the majority of people with dementias become affected after the age of 70). The vision or hearing difficulties experienced by most older adults restricts information processing by slowing, limiting, or distorting the sensory–perceptual information that the individual receives. It becomes more difficult to perceive the cues necessary either to pass relevant new information into short-term memory or to retrieve relevant cued information from long-term-memory stores. For example, an older adult with a hearing impairment may not have heard the cue intended to activate relevant associations; what might be interpreted as confusion may simply be the result of never having received reliable information in the first place. An appropriate referral is clearly essential if a sensory deficit is suspected. Often, a new pair of eyeglasses or a hearing aid can have a remarkable effect on the capacity to produce functional behavioral responses. At the same time, sensory deficits (particularly hearing and vision impairments) are related to the severe perceptual distortions of hallucinations or delusions in older people with dementias. Hence, it is essential to test the individual's vision and hearing prior to pharmacological intervention (Leiter & Cummings, 1999).

Nevertheless, it is important to routinely present environmental cues using methods that compensate for the probable sensory problems of all older adults, especially those with dementias (e.g., increased lighting intensity that is glare free, large-print visual cues, use of color contrast, lowered voice pitch; see Levy, 1986b, 1996b, for a full discussion). To reiterate, if the sensory system is impaired, little reliable sensory–perceptual information will either be passed into short-term (working) memory or will provide dependable cues to activate relevant long-term (including visual–perceptual) memories.

Short-Term Working Memory

Recall that working memory is one of the most important concepts in understanding information processing; it is also exceedingly complex. Working memory enables us to combine information retrieved from long-term-memory with information that arrives from the environment. In addition, it both coordinates and constrains the activities of a vast array of neural structures, a process governed by the frontal lobes. In essence, the central role of working memory is to release the individual from reliance on fixed repertoires and reactions (automatic actions) and to allow the mental representation of alternatives (Goldberg, 2001). Thus, working memory is capable of taking an overall view of all of the other functions of the brain (attention, perception, language, long-term-memory stores) and coordinating them. It is a critical factor in determining the ability to focus one's conscious attention; to concentrate; to override automatic reactions when warranted; to move from concrete data to abstract concepts; to understand language; to set goals and to adjust behavior in relation to external circumstances; to engage in planning; to solve problems; and to engage in decision making, reasoning, creativity, judgment, and in the service of all other higher order executive functions, including the ability to carry out IADLs. As currently conceived, it is more of a process, or a state of activation, than a storage system. It is composed of the limited amount information that is in one's immediate awareness.

The neuropathology of AD (Esiri, Lee, & Trojanowski, 2004) involves progressive atrophy and loss of synaptic connectivity within areas of the brain responsible for working memory to carry out its complex work of focusing attention and activating and retrieving relevant knowledge from long-term-memory stores. The hippocampal complex (in the temporal lobes), the primary site for initiating the process of evolving new memories, is the first site of deterioration; here, the person experiences memory loss and difficulty with reading comprehension and writing or complex visual patterns, such as faces. The hippocampal complex is gradually destroyed by the disease. However, as the disease advances, damage tends to spread from the temporal lobes to the frontal and prefrontal regions—as indicated, the sites primarily responsible for activating and synthesizing relevant information for working memory and executive functions.

A person experiencing this deterioration may develop apathy, disorganization, and problems concentrating and may begin to exhibit behavior inappropriate to context. The damage then spreads to the parietal lobes, the areas responsible for spatial orientation; recognition of familiar objects; and body information, including touch (e.g., stereognosis). The occipital lobes, responsible for the visuospatial components of long-term memories (e.g., pattern recognition, shape, form, color, and awareness of visual information) are less affected but are not entirely spared (as indicated above). In contrast, the cerebellum, basal ganglia, and associated structures (sites of procedural and other implicit memories) are generally spared by AD.

The consequences of these neuropathological changes on functional performance capabilities are profound. Hippocampal deterioration induces deficits that are especially severe in the attentional components of working memory (Small et al., 1997), including the capacity for focusing attention, inhibiting distractions, and restraining automatic actions. When combined with deterioration of the frontal lobes (areas responsible for activating and synthesizing relevant knowledge stores and producing thoughtful responses), AD progressively erodes working-memory functions of goal-directed behavior, decision-making capacity, problem-solving ability, reasoning, self-awareness, and all other executive functions.

As the disease progresses, it becomes increasingly difficult to retain information long enough for organization and transfer to long-term memory. Hence, the capacity for acquiring new (i.e., episodic) memory and learning steadily deteriorates until it becomes negligible. For a person with advanced dementia, every day becomes a new day (and eventually, every moment a new moment), completely disconnected to any referents to what occurred in the immediate past. (Nevertheless, it does not require the hippocampus to recall old memories; people may be able to tell accurate stories from childhood, high school, and mid-life.) At the same time, it becomes increasingly difficult to activate relevant information from long-term stores (characteristics of deterioration in these stores are addressed later). Caregivers often report "mindless" actions, such as taking dirty dishes to the bedroom instead of the kitchen or opening the refrigerator looking for gloves. These behaviors reflect early breakdowns of working memory's ability to select and activate task-relevant information and to inhibit automatic reactions (e.g., opening doors) even related to the most mundane kinds of actions; these breakdowns become progressively more severe as the disease progresses (Goldberg, 2001).

Because individuals with dementia eventually experience no new learning capacity, their conscious awareness (activated working memory) becomes progressively limited to familiar working-memory processing alone (addressed in the next section). Concurrently, working memory itself becomes progressively limited in terms of *capacity, processing speed,* and *content.*

In terms of capacity, AD progressively reduces the number of bits of information that can be held in mind. This reduced capacity amounts to roughly three or four units at the middle stage of the disease, as evidenced in the digit span assessment in most mental status examinations. Note also that working-memory capacity is further reduced by progressive deterioration in the ability to focus and control attention by actively inhibiting attention to distracting information and by inhibiting automatic responses when encountering a novel situation (a.k.a. *response inhibition* and *executive control;* Hasher, Tonev, Lustig, & Zacks, 2001; Hasher & Zacks, 1988). As a result, there is progressively less working memory for information that needs to be processed. Note that with all neurocognitive disorders there is a need to reduce environmental distractions that clutter the limited capacity of working memory; one can dramatically improve the person's ability to attend by limiting the amount of information that is registered.

In terms of processing speed, we know that the speed of information processing declines with advancing age (see Chapter 12 for a full discussion); concurrently, the rate at which information is processed in working memory progressively deteriorates, further worsening the capacity of working memory to carry out its complex functions. This deceleration of information-processing speed is significantly amplified in dementia and other neurocognitive disorders (Salthouse & Babcock, 1991), such that limited information is available to working memory to assist in processing, and information is encoded and retrieved far more slowly. (Note again that, with all cognitive disorders, there is need to slow one's rate of speech and to provide the individual with additional response time.)

In terms of content, working memory becomes progressively limited to well-established memories activated and retrieved by whatever cues strike the individual. These can originate either from internally generated thought processes (e.g., whatever one happens to be thinking about at the time) or those that are cued from the environment. Long-term memories accessible for potential activation and retrieval (e.g., language based, visuospatial, visual–perceptual, procedural, and other implicit memories) deteriorate, in reversed ontogenetic order (Reisberg, Franssen, Souren, Auer, & Kenowlsky, 1998; Reisberg, Kenowsky, Franssen, Auer, & Souren, 1999; Reisberg et al., 2002; Levy, 1974, 1986a, 1986b), a process that was recently termed *retrogenesis* (Reisberg et al., 1998). Hence, the most recent memories are most vulnerable to decay, and earliest memories persist until the later stages of the disease. (As was discussed in Chapter. 12, this pattern appears to be based on the fact that early memories are more established and represent the foundation for subsequent memories. Thus, once the foundational memories are established, old memories may be recalled, but more recent memories may remain inaccessible; Haist, Gore, & Mao, 2001; Lopez, 2000.) In like manner, potential memories accessible for activation and retrieval progressively deteriorate from those that consider abstract meanings to those limited to the concrete (Piaget, 1970) and from abstract or complex visual images to those that are simple (Nelson, 1995; Piaget, 1970). Decision making, problem solving, reasoning abilities, and executive functioning follow a similar course. Note that, although these principles of retrogenesis have been recently established (Reisberg et al., 1998, 1999, 2002), they echo theoretical tenets of *reversed ontogenesis* that were developed much earlier in the occupational therapy literature (Allen, 1985; Levy, 1974, 1986a, 1986b).

Long-Term Memory

Recall that long-term memory comprises *explicit* and *implicit* stores. There are two explicit-memory stores, identified as *episodic* and *semantic,* and at least three kinds of implicit-memory stores: (a) *procedural,* (b) *perceptual priming,* and (c) *conditioning. Explicit memory* involves the conscious recollection of information, whereas *implicit memory* refers to information that can be accessed automatically or unconsciously.

Episodic memory is the long-term store most severely affected in the disease (note that these deficits are believed to reflect neuropathological changes in the hippocampal complex). Even in the earliest stages of AD, individuals have difficulty learning new information and retaining it more than momentarily (Duchek, Cheney, Ferraro, & Storandt, 1991); in addition, the inability to recall newly presented information after even a brief delay is typically one of the earliest and most diagnostic symptoms of the disease. People experience increasing difficulty in areas such as making a chronology of events in their lives (e.g., the previous night's activities), remembering personal information (e.g., where they put the hairbrush or where they parked the car), or remembering recent conversations.

Semantic memory is more stable; it shows a lesser rate of decline throughout the course of the disease (note that these deficits are believed to result from neuropathological changes in cortical association areas). As a consequence, people are able to retain conceptual knowledge about the world, visuospatial information (i.e., memory of geometric designs, shapes, and figures; facial features), and syntactical and phonological knowledge about language (i.e., grammar and pronunciation) until later stages (Nebes, 1989, 1992); note that they also maintain the ability to read aloud into the advanced stages of the disease (see our subsequent discussion of procedural memory), even when the ability to understand written material is lost. There is also evidence that information stored in semantic networks is organized in propositional networks and hierarchies from specific (concrete) to general (abstract; Rapp & Caramazza, 1989) and, consistent with retrogenesis, that more recently acquired information is the most vulnerable to decay (Reisberg et al., 1998, 1999, 2002; Rubin, 1998). Initial declines in semantic memory are evidenced most visibly in word retrieval problems (semantic recall), such as remembering names of common objects, even as the form of language (i.e., grammar and pronunciation) remains intact; they are also evidenced in experiences of spatial disorientation (e.g., getting lost in familiar places). As the disease continues, individuals experience greater difficulty recalling nouns and verbs (Hodges, Patterson, Oxbury, & Funnell, 1992) and eventually even the names of their closest loved ones. Language vocabulary becomes progressively limited, and there is little cohesion between sentences. As decrements in semantic memory increase, meaningful content in language decreases (language increasingly contains empty phrases and bizarre content; Tomoeda, Bayles, Trosset, Azuma, & McGeagh, 1996). At the end stage of the disease, language itself is profoundly impaired or absent.

Procedural Memory

Recall that *procedural memory* involves the constellation of motor, perceptual, and cognitive skills associated with movement- or skill-based information. It is the most durable form of memory, and it deteriorates at a significantly slower rate than episodic and semantic memory throughout the course of the disease. Schacter (1983) described an avid lifelong golfer in the moderate stage of the disease. He had no idea what day it was, where he was, by whom he was accompanied, where he placed his tee shots (all episodic memories), or what game was being played (semantic memory). Yet, when shown a golf bag, he chose an appropriate club, and his swing evidenced his former elegant style (procedural memory). Similarly, although people with dementia may have difficulty remembering the name of their third-grade teacher (episodic knowledge), they are likely to remember the cursive writing skills learned from that teacher (LaBarge, Smith, Dick, & Storandt, 1992). Just as the most basic sensory and motor abilities are preserved by the disease process (at least until the later stages), it appears that remembering *how* to perform familiar skilled motor behavior is likewise preserved.

There is also growing evidence even severely impaired AD patients can learn and retain procedural tasks for at least 1 month (Camp, Foss, O'Hanlon, & Stevens, 1996; Dick et al., 1996). Investigators have found that when procedural memories are cued (and thereby activated) for retrieval under constant practice conditions, procedural skills can be "relearned" by reactivating the relevant synapses in the brain. The act of retrieval appears to have a mnemonic effect: A successful recall increases the chance of subsequent recall. In addition, this spared memory capacity is enhanced by the repetition priming effect, which occurs when task performance is facilitated by previous exposure to task cues. Note that this learning capacity is task oriented and situation specific; capacity for generalization is limited.

Nevertheless, the literature is beginning to document that procedural memory based retraining (or perhaps, re-"activating") programs are worthwhile and have the potential to produce lasting changes. This body of research provides occupational therapy practitioners with empirical support for intervention strategies that have long been used to enable cognitively impaired adults to "relearn" or retrieve specific ADLs (e.g., eating, bathing, dressing, toileting) as well as to benefit from cognitive training in the safe use of adaptive equipment, by means of priming, cued recognition, and repetition of procedural memories within a distraction-free environment (Allen, 1982, 1985; Allen, Earhart, & Blue, 1992; Levy, 1986a, 1986b, 1998). Indeed, what Tulving (1985) described as *procedural memory* was recognized as an area of preserved cognitive capacity much earlier in the occupational therapy literature (Levy, 1974), and it remains an essential source of cognitive capacity that is capitalized on in the cognitive disabilities model.

Recall vs. Recognition

Finally, retrieval strategies are essential elements of information processing in dementia. As might be expected, both recall and recognition of information from episodic-, semantic-, and procedural-memory stores are significantly affected in dementia although, as indicated, deterioration within each of these stores proceeds at different rates as the disease progresses. At the same time, recall deficits occur very much prior to recognition deficits within each store, because recall is a far more demanding working-memory task; as was detailed in Chapter 12, *recall* entails an internal process of search and retrieval for relevant information from long-term-memory stores, whereas with recognition, information in storage is matched with an externally provided associational cue, and the associational cue activates the relevant memories with which it is linked.

It also needs to be recognized that connected neurons (or "memories") remain inactive until some cue acts as a reminder and causes them to be reactivated. This, in turn, activates other memories with which they are linked, such that the information is retrieved. As a result, information stored in long-term memory is oftentimes retrievable, if the individual is provided with environmental cues. These cues, however, must be appropriate to the memory stores spared at each stage of the disease.

As has been observed (Levy, 1996a, 1998, 1999), recognition memory is an area of reserved cognitive capacity that is fundamental to the cognitive disability model. In essence, clinicians have been capitalizing on the potential of environmental cues to activate stored memories. The cognitive disability model has identified varying qualities of environmental cues (e.g., language based, visuospatial, tactile, and kinesthetic) that activate relevant memories at different levels of cognitive impairment. The reformulated model expands these concepts and identifies how environmental cues are used to compensate for the progressive capacity of working memory to activate and retrieve information from episodic-, semantic-, and procedural-memory stores. Here, environmental cues are conceived as those that clinicians use to activate relevant networks of stored memories to enable the individual to function to the best of his or her capacities. The overall goal is to create prosthetic environmental contexts in which individuals can optimize occupational performance capabilities by accessing the cognitive capacities that remain. As we discuss later, this is accomplished by reducing demands on progressively impaired working- and explicit-memory systems (episodic and semantic recall) and capitalizing on procedural (implicit) and cued recognition

capacities (episodic and semantic) within the stores that remain. In this way, occupational performance capabilities are optimized within each stage of the disease.

RECONSIDERED COGNITIVE DISABILITY MODEL

The following provides a synthesis of the application of the cognitive information-processing concepts addressed above to reformulation of the cognitive disabilities model. Figure 14.1 is a schematic representation of essential terms and dimensions used in the reconsidered model, as adapted from refinements to the cognitive information-processing model detailed in Chapter 12 (Figure 12.1).

The primary concern of cognitive disability theory is to identify the cognitive capacities that determine whether an individual can perform an activity safely and successfully and the specific nature of the cognitive impairments that need to be compensated for in the event of cognitive limitations. To this end, the cognitive disability model (Allen, 1982, 1985, 1987) proposed a hierarchy of six cognitive levels that theorized components of information processed in pursuing normal life activities and qualitative differences in functional capacities and limitations. This model viewed the following as components of an information-processing system considered at each of the hierarchical cognitive levels: attention (input), sensorimotor associations (throughput), and behavioral responses (output).

Although there are parallels, Allen's information-processing system (Allen, 1987; Allen & Blue, 1998; Allen, Blue, & Earhart, 1995) is not analogous to the cognitive information-processing model used as the theoretical base of the model detailed in this chapter. Allen's original information-processing components are reframed as depicted in Figure 14.1. In the reformulated model, key dimensions of short-term working memory are considered at each of the cognitive levels. Although these dimensions are invariably intertwined (see Chapter 12 for a complete discussion), they are separated here for discussion and to assist in activity analysis. The three dimensions are (a) attentional processes, (b) working-memory processes, and (c) occupational behavioral responses.

Attentional Processes

This dimension has as its primary focus the attentional component of working memory, including both the quantity and quality of information that can be held in mind prior to further processing (i.e., primary memory). Recall that a central principle in attention theory is that inhibitory

FIGURE 14.1. Cognitive disability "reconsidered."

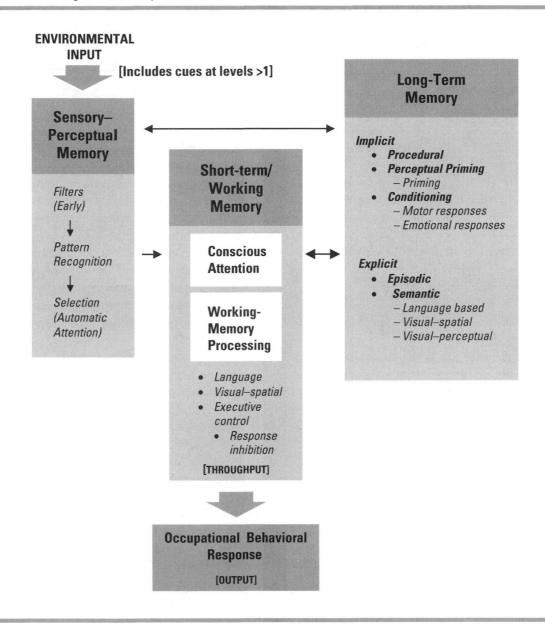

processes act together with activating processes to control the contents of working memory. Recall also that in working memory, *attention* refers to the limited amount of information that is in one's immediate awareness (*controlled attention*). In addition, we have only a limited capacity for conscious attention: hence, we need means and resources to actively screen out that to which we need not attend.

All information processing begins with the ability to attend to relevant information from both the environment (i.e., external cues) and self-activated thoughts (i.e., internal cues), while simultaneously inhibiting attention to

irrelevant distractions and automatic reactions inappropriate to the circumstances. The relevance of information to be attended to is determined, in large part, as it relates to preformulated purposes for action or thought. Cues (both internal and external) are typically used to activate relevant neuronal connections to memories that will eventually lead to the consolidation of new memories; as will be seen, they are also used to activate relevant connections to previously stored memories, to elicit productive behavioral responses—particularly in the event of cognitive impairment.

One problem to be recognized is that cognitive impairment produces significant limitations in the working memory's capacity to activate and attend to the normal *quantity* of information (i.e., approximately 7 ± 2 bits of information). In large part, this is related to progressive declines in information-processing speed. Declines in speed reduce the space in working memory and thereby the amount of relevant information that might otherwise be available to work with; in addition, declines progressively reduce the attentional controls required to inhibit attention to irrelevant information and to restrain automatic reactions that are inappropriate to the context. As a result, people with dementia experience increasing difficulty not only in screening out irrelevant information but also in focusing on the relevant information that would otherwise be necessary to complete a task or achieve a goal. Speed of processing impairments clearly significantly affects the capacity and efficiency of working memory.

Another problem to be recognized is that cognitive impairment produces significant limitations in one's normal capacity to attend to an unlimited variety of cues. With intact cognitive processing, individuals are able attend to the broad variations in environmental and internal cues required to process new information. However, at decreasing cognitive levels the person's capacity to attend to a broad range of cues progressively deteriorates. Consequently, individuals early on in the disease process experience significant limitations in the capacity to form new memories (specifically, episodic and some procedural). They also experience progressive deterioration in the ability to use environmental or self-generated associational cues to activate relevant previously stored memories (episodic, semantic, and procedural). Thus, the quality of long-term memories available for working memory to activate and with which to work progressively declines.

Episodic (and, thereby, semantic) new memory capacities decay first, followed by episodic recall (from self-initiated cues) activation/retrieval capacities, and then episodic recognition (environmentally cued) activation/retrieval capacities; these losses are succeeded by progressive impairments in semantic recall activation/retrieval capacities (from self-initiated cues) and then semantic recognition (environmentally cued) activation/retrieval capacities. Finally, procedural new memory impairments surface, followed by procedural recognition (environmentally cued) activation/retrieval impairments at the latest stages of the disease. As a result, individuals become increasingly reliant on environmental recognition activation/retrieval cues to access spared memory stores as the disease progresses.

In the reformulated model, environmental "recognition" activation cues are ordered as appropriate to each stage of the disease. At the highest (intact) cognitive level, the entire range of possible cues carry the potential to activate attentional processes, including complex abstract cues (e.g., written and graphic cues and verbal hypothetical cues, as well as internally generated ideas, concepts, and images) and environmental cues (e.g., language based, visuospatial, tactile, and kinesthetic) to enable processing of new episodic and semantic memories. At decreasing cognitive levels, attentional processes are activated by a progressively limited range of cues. Consistent with retrogenesis, these limitations emerge in reversed ontogenetic sequence and lead to stagelike changes in the ability to process information. Eventually, environmental cues are able to activate familiar episodic, semantic, or procedural recognition memories (or, less typically, to generate "new" procedural memories—i.e., given extensive demonstration, repetition, and practice). At the lowest cognitive level, attention is limited solely to internal cues, that is, generated by physiological and affective states such as proprioceptive sensations, hunger, and fear; these activate procedural recognition responses (automatic reactions) alone.

To optimize occupational performance capabilities, clinicians adapt activities, occupations, and roles to capitalize on the environmental cues that capture the individual's attention at any given level and that activate spared memories relevant to functional behavior; at the same time, activities and occupations are adapted to limit exposure to those that require attention to cues associated with impaired-memory stores. The goal of intervention is to present the just-right kinds of environmental cues to match the individual's limited attentional capacities and to promote accessibility to memory stores that might not otherwise be retrieved.

Working-Memory Processes

This dimension places emphasis on the processing component of working memory. Recall that *working memory* refers to the set of attention, concentration, goal formulation, and mental representational processes (i.e., verbal and visuospatial, episodic and semantic) that are available to the individual. It requires deciding what information is useful to attend to at the given moment, in light of a previously established goal for action, and then selecting and bringing online only task-relevant information out of the totality of all knowledge available. It also requires sufficient attentional controls (a.k.a. *executive control*) to maintain relevant information in an activated state long enough to be worked with, while inhibiting automatic actions that are unwarranted to the situation. These processes work together to assist in activities such as decision making, planning, problem solving, comprehension, judgment, and reasoning and in the service of all executive functions. The hierarchical arrangement of these cognitive elements is depicted in Figure 14.2.

The problem to be recognized here is that cognitive impairment first produces progressive limitations in the capacity (i.e., quantity and quality) of working memory to process and draw inferences from new information (as discussed above) and thereafter produces limitations in the capacity to process and draw inferences from information self-cued for retrieval from progressively deteriorating memory stores. As a result, goal formulation, planning, problem solving, reasoning, and executive-functioning capacities deteriorate, in reversed ontogenetic sequence.

Recall the sequence of events required for working memory to elicit higher order purposeful behaviors (Goldberg, 2001). First, the behavior must be initiated, in response to a perceived need. Second, the objective must be identified, and the goal of action formulated. Third, a plan of action must be conceptualized according to the goal. Fourth, the means by which the plan can be accomplished must be selected in proper sequence. Fifth, the various steps of the plan must be executed in an appro-

priate order with a smooth transition from step to step. Finally, a comparison must be made between the objective and the outcome of action, to monitor and judge the consequences to see that all is accomplished as intended. In essence, these are the functions that working memory routinely executes in the service of executive functions.

The importance of this intricate constellation of behaviors can be recognized through observation of their deterioration throughout the course of dementing disease. In the initial stages, the person retains (at least to a certain degree) the ability to use a number of cognitive skills in isolation. Basic abilities, such as reading, writing, simple computations, drawing shapes, verbal expression, and familiar movements—that is, the cognitive substrates of performance—remain largely unimpaired. Additionally, and perhaps misleadingly, the person is able to perform well on neuropsychological tests that evaluate these functions in isolation, and yet any synthetic activity requiring the coordination of many cognitive skills into coherent, goal-directed processes becomes progressively impaired. These include all of the complex demands of daily life, including overall occupational and functional performance capabilities, the ability to make decisions in ambiguous real-life situations (a.k.a. *prioritizing alternatives* and "disambiguating" the situation), the ability to make plans and then follow those plans to guide behavior, IADLs and, eventually, ADLs. In essence, the ability to stay on track relative to a preformulated goal (i.e., to maintain a mental image of the purpose) becomes lost early on in the disease, and the person becomes progressively more reliant on incidental distractions (both internal and external) and fixed repertoires and reactions—in lieu of deliberate thought—for behavioral responses.

This ability to stay on track relative to a preformulated goal (i.e., working memory and executive functions) involves performance capabilities in (at least) five major areas (Goldberg, 2001; Lezak, 1995; Luria, 1966), each of which progressively deteriorates as the disease advances: (a) response inhibition, (b) initiation (volition), (c) planning (sustaining action), (d) mental flexibility (shifting), and (e) self-awareness.

Practitioners should note that disorders in these areas can be observed in all occupational behaviors as well as in IADLs and ADLs (Duran & Fisher, 1999; Giovannetti, Libon, Buxbaum, & Schwartz, 2002; Schwartz, 1995; Schwartz, Mayer, Fitzpatrick-DeSalme, & Montgomery, 1993), as we discussed more fully in the discussion of assessment and intervention that follows.

The first area of executive function to be addressed is *response inhibition,* the basic function that enables the

FIGURE 14.2. Cognitive hierarchy.

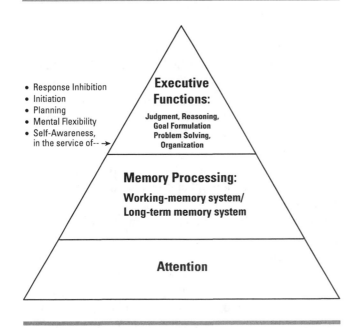

person to "transcend the default mode" (Mesulam, 2002) and to delay automatic responses to external stimuli, thoughts, and changes in the environment. Response inhibition is also crucial to working memory in providing the initial delay in the automatic response to the event during which working memory can be activated. Initially, response inhibition allows the individual an instant to anticipate consequences before acting, in order to avoid mistakes and faulty decisions (a.k.a. *judgment*). However, early on, people demonstrate an inability to anticipate the consequences of their actions and, later, to inhibit the urge for immediate gratification of simple impulses. As the disease advances, people become progressively more reliant on automatic reactions, that is, wandering into other patients' rooms, simply because the doors are there to walk through; picking up and drinking from empty cups, simply because the cup is there; and putting on a jacket that belongs to someone else, simply because the jacket is there—even though these actions have no objective relationship to a self-perceived need or goal. Working memory and executive functions also allow the individual to inhibit primitive reflexes that were inherited as part of primitive brain structures including, for example, the grasp reflex and sucking reflexes. As a result, at the latest stage of the disease this inhibition is removed, and the reflexes return (Reisberg et al., 2002).

The next area is *initiation* (or *volition*), that is, initiating activities or tasks in response to independently generated thoughts (or goals). Difficulties here can be observed in behavior such as delayed response or an inability to respond without prompting. It can also be observed when individuals become increasingly reactive to merely "what's out there" as the disease advances, as opposed to stepping back and thinking through and choosing from a range of alternatives before acting. Cognitively, this represents an increasingly concrete and stimulus-driven (a.k.a. *field-dependent*) approach to the environment wherein behaviors are essentially driven or guided by cues available in the physical and social environments.

The third area is *planning,* that is, the ability to make plans and follow them through in light of preformulated goals. Early on, individuals lose the ability to maintain an image of the "big picture" over time (the pre-established goal) and thereby become progressively unable to conceptualize the sequential steps required to attain the goal, or become absorbed in one or more of the steps required to carry out the plan (i.e., the details), or both.

The fourth area is *mental flexibility.* This involves the flexible shifting of both attention and actions to meet task demands, that is, the ability to not only maintain attention to the task but also to smoothly shift and adjust actions or behavior in relationship to outside circumstances, if necessary (i.e., shifting from Agenda A to Agenda B). For example, understanding that the presence of smoke means possible danger and acting accordingly is critical for judgment and survival. Morbidity and mortality risks are often high in people with dementia as a result of judgment impairments related to this kind of executive function. Note also that mental flexibility involves the ability to bring task-relevant information into focus as needed and then go on to the next bit of task-relevant information smoothly and effortlessly. These transitions become progressively more difficult for individuals as the disease advances. Their minds become "stuck" within one thought or activity; similarly, they experience increasing difficulty tolerating changes in routines and the environment.

The last area to be addressed is *self-awareness,* that is, insight into one's own cognitive world (also called *anosognosia;* Heilman & Valenstein, 1993). People with dementia often lose insight into their impairments. This is likely because early on, they are no longer able to compare the outcomes of their actions with their intentions (a preformulated plan; Goldberg, 2001). Eventually, all sense of intentionality is lost.

Consistent with the above, Levy (1974) recognized early on that the implicit goals that are conceptualized by a person with a cognitive impairment performing a selected activity may not be consistent with more traditionally conceptualized goals associated with that activity. People pursue activities with varying goals in mind, ranging, for example, from an investment in producing a high-quality end product (i.e., having been able to imagine what might be produced and staying on track to produce it), to an interest in the effects of actions on objects (i.e., having used more basic delayed procedural recall capacities related to concrete cause-and-effect relationships), to an investment in the simple awareness of movement (drawing on procedural-recognition capacities alone). Hence, at lower cognitive levels an individual is limited to conceptualizing the goal and meaning of activity based solely on the more primitive memory structures (e.g., automatic repertoires and reactions) that continue at later stages of the disease.

For example, the sight of a vacuum cleaner may activate an automatic procedural recognition response: the motion of pushing the vacuum cleaner back and forth. This person would not be able to conceptualize the more conventional goal of the activity, as would be expected with an individual with more intact working-memory processing capacities—namely, a clean rug. Consequently, at lower cognitive levels, unintentional results, by conventional standards, are commonplace. Thus, it is important to recognize that the inability to comply with the traditional expectations of goals of an activity reflect working-memory and executive impairments that are beyond the individual's control. At the same time, caregivers need to recognize the significant impact that the inability to assess multiple sources of information, to formulate traditional goals, to anticipate consequences of actions, and to stay on track has on the ability carry out occupations and activities with safety. Practitioners can educate caregivers regarding the information-processing deficits produced by the disease and teach them to compensate for this impairment by adjusting conventional expectations for activity performance; at the same time, it needs to be recognized that these people will need environmental modification, supervision, and support to compensate for their inability to maintain their own safety as well.

Occupational Behavioral Responses

Working-memory processes elicit two types of occupational behavioral responses: (a) spontaneous (self-initiated) and (b) cued (here, interpersonally). This dimension of working memory describes qualitative differences in spontaneous responses at any given level and highlights how these responses are enhanced by the provision of the interpersonal elements of environmental recognition cues. At the highest cognitive level, productive behavioral responses are self-initiated; people use attentional controls and have broad access to conceptual information (activated from intact episodic and semantic memories) to initiate actions, formulate goals, and produce solutions to everyday problems. They are able to participate freely in a broad range of roles and occupations. At decreasing cognitive levels, however, productive spontaneous responses become progressively less accessible, and yet these responses can be enhanced by provision of recognition cues to activate contextually appropriate associations and responses appropriate to the cognitive level. These cues range from language based (verbal), to visual–spatial (written, illustrated, or by demonstration), to kinesthetic (provided by simultaneous imitation of the therapist), and tactile (hand over hand).

Consistent with all occupational therapy approaches, the reformulated model relies on activity analysis as a primary means of intervention. It also provides means for analyzing the relative difficulty of any desired activity in terms of requisite working information-processing demands. Environmental factors that facilitate access to remaining memory stores and optimize occupational behaviors are identified at each level. Intervention strategies are derived from conceptualizing how environmental factors associated with the information-processing dimensions cited above might best be adapted within the structure of a desired activity to capitalize on remaining cognitive capacities and to compensate for cognitive limitations. Hence, clinicians modify the structure of a desired activity to capitalize on and compensate for the following:

- The *quantity and quality of environmental and interpersonal cues* that the person is able to attend to at any given level (i.e., those presented in distraction-free environments to activate spared procedural and semantic recognition capabilities into working memory, and circumvent working and episodic/semantic deficits)
- The *quality of working-memory processing* that the person is able to comprehend and the goal (purpose, and meaning) of activity that the individual is able to conceptualize at any given level. This includes consideration of related requirements for environmental structure and support provided by the caregiver to optimize occupational performance and to compensate for the person's inability to maintain his or her own safety.

The overall intent is to enable people with dementia to optimize occupational performance by creating environmental contexts that place desired activities and occupations within their range of comprehension and control.

Application to Cognitive Disability

Regardless of the level of cognitive function, cognitive processes are maximized, and behavioral responses more effectively organized, when environmental cues are presented to the impaired individual in a manner that matches his or her level of cognitive functioning. To conceptualize rehabilitative intervention, the practitioner must identify first the individual's cognitive capacities and limitations and then must identify the environmental factors that can be modified to enable successful participation in desired occupations.

In the discussion that follows we provide an overview of the information-processing dimensions revealed at each level and the environmental factors that are associated with each information-processing dimension. Guidelines are presented for conceptualizing strategies that capitalize on cognitive capacities and that compensate for cognitive limitations at each of the cognitive levels as well as rehabilitation priorities. We must make one point of clarification before proceeding: As indicated, Allen's (1982, 1985, 1987) original scale comprised six cognitive levels of assessment and intervention. In 1992, a decimal system termed *Modes of Performance* was added to provide for more sensitive measures of cognitive disability and for more nuanced strategies for intervention. Initially, this system comprised a 52-point scale that sought to distinguish among 10 modes of performance within each of the cognitive levels, and associated intervention implications (e.g., 1.0, 1.1, 1.2, 1.3, 1.4, etc., ranging from 0.8 to 6.0). In more recent works (Allen & Blue, 1998), the 52-point scale was collapsed to a 26-point scale comprised solely of even numbers along with associated implications for intervention (e.g., 1.0, 1.2, 1.4, 1.6, etc.), and 26 hierarchical "information-processing systems" were proposed to be observed at each of the modes of cognitive performance (Allen & Blue, 1998).

As we detail in the section titled "Evaluation and Assessment Processes and Instruments," we are committed to a system of assessment that is closer to the 52-point decimal scale that was originally proposed, because it retains the advantages of serial assessment, offers better sensitivity for evaluating disease progression and change in function, and has demonstrated empirical support for assessment in dementia (Burns et al., 1994, 2004; Heying, 1985; Holm et al., 1999; Kehrberg, Kuskowski, Mortimer, & Shoberg, 1992). However, for intervention purposes, we present guidelines for each of the six levels and the half-level correlates in Levels 3 and 4 (e.g., 3.5, and 4.5). These guidelines are meant to be individualized further by the practitioner. These adaptations are essential given the specific nature of the client's behavioral responses to the disease and the broad range of personal characteristics that have defined and given meaning to individuals' lives, such as preferred activities and environments, family ties, hobbies and leisure interests, professional accomplishments, and expressions of faith. It is essential that such knowledge be sought from others familiar to the individual prior to the disease to ensure that the individual's interests, values, and wishes are respected in intervention programs, even when he or she can no longer express those preferences.

Finally, Global Deterioration Stages (GDSs; Reisberg, Ferris, Leon, & Cook, 1982) and Medicare assistance codes (Health Care Financing Administration, 1989) are identified for each level. The GDS follows the ontogenetic progression of the disease, forming an inverse relationship to the cognitive levels. Knowledge of the two scales provides a common language between occupational therapists and other professionals. The Medicare assistance codes provide therapists with a means to document levels of cognitive assistance required to maximize functional performance capabilities throughout the course of the disease. It should be noted that, with the likely development of more effective treatments to arrest progression of the disease, therapists may be able to use Medicare codes to document improvements in behavior and abilities (see also Holm et al., 1999). The information-processing capabilities and activity analysis implications at each of the cognitive levels, as described below, are summarized in Table 14.1.

COGNITIVE LEVEL 6: PLANNED ACTIONS

Attentional and Working-Memory Processes

At Level 6 (Medicare assistance code: independent; GDS 1), there is controlled and selective attention for multiple cues and abstract symbolic concepts. The goal of performance is to use abstract reasoning and executive skills to plan action sequences, to speculate about outcomes, and to anticipate errors. Attention is focused with inhibition of irrelevant cues. Episodic-, semantic-, and procedural-memory capacities are intact. Relevant information can be activated and retrieved or called back to working memory to be consciously considered, elaborated on, and used purposefully to carry out complex activities with accuracy and safety. Theoretically, this level represents the absence of cognitive disability. It is the only level at which planning, problem solving, and learning do not depend on overt visuospatial activity, concrete external cues, or both.

Occupational Behavioral Responses

Behavioral responses are self-initiated. Conceptual information is activated from intact episodic and semantic memories to initiate actions, formulate goals, and produce solutions to everyday problems. The person is capable of IADLs and new and complex activity, including managing finances; meals; medications; competitive employment; independent living; and, usually, reading, writing, and calculating. The needs of others are considered through subtle abstract and episodic and semantic recall cues and, likewise, consequences of actions are considered; the person is able to monitor and direct his or her own behavior. Note that a person can have Level 6 information-processing capacities even though his or her test performance and other complex activity performance can be skewed by low education and illiteracy.

TABLE 14.1. Activity Analysis Chart

Level	Attentional Processes	Working-Memory Processes	Occupational Behavioral Responses	Rehabilitation Potential
Level 6	Controlled and selective attention for multiple cues/concepts, inhibition of irrelevant cues, self-activated thoughts.	Focused attention, activation and retrieval of relevant knowledge.	IADLs; new and complex activity; considers needs of others and consequences of actions (self-awareness).	Learns complex procedures, new activity, and safety precautions through written and verbal methods; teach the client.
Level 5	Controlled attention for multiple cues/concepts, but may be slowed; inhibition of irrelevant cues; self-activated thoughts may be skewed by awareness of disability deficit.	Episodic and semantic recall impairments limit or slow the performance of complex tasks.	IADLs with error if complex or new; may not be able to consider the needs of others or consequences of actions/judgments.	Learns through hands-on teaching and verbal discussion of methods/safety precautions; teach the client and teach the caregiver to monitor for errors and needs.
Level 4	Concrete external cues and visual attention; familiar concepts and activity; impaired/slowed simultaneous attention for multiple cues/details; impaired inhibition of irrelevant cues; self-activated thoughts skewed by attention and awareness deficits; highly distractible; generally focused on external events.	Significant episodic and semantic recall impairments limit executive control and prevent the accurate/safe performance of complex and hazardous tasks and the frequency of performance in daily basic tasks; visual and environmental recognition cues facilitate performance.	Concrete parts of IADLs; ADLs but may need setup and reminders; often not able to understand changes in abilities, something new, activity restrictions, or the needs of others.	Learns concrete task steps through much repetition, performance may not generalize to a different setting, safety awareness inconsistent; provide task-specific training for the client and teach the caregiver to provide setup, eliminate hazards, and to expect inconsistency.
Level 3	Minimal attention skills; familiar objects and environments and associated actions; implicit procedural cues; self-awareness significantly impaired.	Severe impairments in explicit memory stores; implicit stores for task procedures are accessed to perform familiar/repetitive actions; minimal evidence of encoding or storage.	Parts of ADLs and repetitive use of objects; often confused about time, place, person; catastrophic reactions common.	Uses familiar objects in familiar ways; poor safety awareness; teach the caregiver to provide setup/step-by-step help with simple verbal plus tactile cues to complete tasks; eliminate hazards.
Level 2	External movements, touch, sounds; internal cues/sensations.	Severe impairments in explicit memory stores; implicit memory stores are accessed to respond to stimuli.	Needs total care; may be able to move to assist caregivers; reflex responses; fear and rejection reaction responses common.	May be able to move or ambulate to assist (or resist) caregivers, may feed self; teach the caregiver total care and feeding techniques.
Level 1	Internal cues/sensations.	Implicit memory stores are accessed to respond to stimuli.	Needs total care; automatic/reflexive responses.	Teach the caregiver total care and comfort care techniques.

Note. IADL = instrumental activities of daily living; ADL = activities of daily living.

Rehabilitation Potential

The client can learn complex procedures, new activities, and safety precautions through written and verbal methods. Occupational therapy intervention aims to teach the client, for example, use of a splint after hand surgery, or transfer techniques.

COGNITIVE LEVEL 5: EXPLORATORY ACTIONS

Attentional and Working-Memory Processes

In Level 5 (Medicare assistance code: stand-by/supervision cognitive assistance; GDS 2), there are beginning deficits in executive thought processes and the processing of abstract complex cues (deficits in working memory and self-activation of explicit stores). Episodic and semantic recall impairments limit or slow the performance of complex tasks. The person begins to have difficulty with simultaneous attention to complex and multiple cues, such as nonvisual or hypothetical concepts, written cues, numbers, and other symbolic or interpretive cues. Problems are observed with short-term or working memory, judgment, reasoning, and planning ahead. The most prominent symptom is episodic recall impairment, followed by less explicit impairments in visuospatial functioning (semantic recall), language (semantic recall), and concentration (short-term memory). Because response inhibition is slowed, there are problems with the anticipation of consequences before acting. Individuals are able to reason by means of direct, concrete, visible cues; however, without executive control they may make faulty plans or need caregiver assistance to evaluate the utility of a plan.

Occupational Behavioral Responses

Behavioral responses are self-initiated. The goal of initiation is to perform as usual according to independently generated thoughts and goals but, with respect to complex tasks, actions may be inefficient and appear exploratory, or may be performed with error. Occupational performance is typified by inefficiency and error when there are many details or subtle cues to consider.

The ability to formulate plans and follow them through is hampered by beginning deficits in the flexible shifting of attention and actions in the face of competing stimuli. As a result, IADLs are difficult in daily life if these are at a complex level. For example, a person who records blood sugar and adjusts his or her insulin is more likely to have problems than someone who only takes a daily pill. Likewise, a person who manages business and financial affairs is more likely to have problems than someone who only pays routine bills. However, earlier diagnosis has led to practice with persons who function in the higher modes of Level 5 and who may not make significant performance errors. Furthermore, older adults are often retired and have less complexity in their daily activities or have simplified lifestyles. Therefore, executive-skill deficits in planning and problem solving may not manifest in their daily affairs. Performance errors in IADLs are more likely to be seen at lower modes in Level 5 and in people who continue to work and lead complex lifestyles.

Rehabilitation Potential

Client and caregiver education programs address any necessary adjustments or compensations in IADLs and occupational roles, the need for replacement activities and community resources, and the need for support during adjustment to the diagnosis of the disease. When a diagnosis of dementia is made at this cognitive level, the person can participate in plans for the future. Early legal, financial, and health care planning will permit the person to have his or her estate and care managed in a manner consistent with his or her wishes. To plan and sign legal documents one must be deemed competent, or in the earlier stages of the disease.

Caregiver education may involve alerting the caregiver to potential safety issues and IADL needs as well as teaching activity simplification or the need to monitor for accuracy and errors. Independent living is usually possible at Level 5. Having someone who can watch for signs of anxiety and frustration and begin to step in to advise or assist with complicated problems and activity errors may be all that is needed. Monitoring the management of medications, driving, and finances may be needed. These activities involve reading, writing, and calculating and the ability to make decisions, keep track of details, and use good judgment. Potential problem behaviors and actions are discussed and explained within the context of the associated attention and working-memory deficits, and strategies to compensate through caregiver approach and environmental modifications are offered.

Rehabilitation programs that involve new learning, such as hip precautions after surgery, circumvent episodic-memory deficits with hands-on teaching techniques. Other programs will involve primarily the assessment for capacity and safety, for example, with driving. The ability to pass a rehabilitation driving exam is inconsistent at Level 5, because problems with driving may or may not manifest and may depend on the extent of the individual client's episodic and semantic recall impairments. Occupational therapists also provide programs for serial assessment (as we detail later) to assist in measuring functional stability or change in response to disease progression and pharmacologic or environmental interventions.

COGNITIVE LEVEL 4.5: GOAL-DIRECTED ACTIVITY

Attentional and Working-Memory Processes

At Level 4.5 (Medicare assistance code: minimum cognitive assistance; GDS 3), significant episodic and semantic recall impairments limit executive (frontal) control; attention becomes progressively limited to working memory alone. In this middle stage of the disease there is a reduced capacity for the number of bits of information that can be held in mind. Working-memory capacity is further reduced by progressive deterioration in the ability to focus attention by actively reducing attention to distracting information; the person is impaired in his or her ability to inhibit irrelevant cues. As a result, there is less working memory to devote to information that needs to be processed. Because information is retrieved far more slowly from long-term memory, working memory becomes progressively limited in content to well-established long-term memories activated and retrieved by recognition cues.

Occupational Behavioral Responses

The person has visible impairment in executive thought processes and simultaneous attention for complex and multiple cues. The ability to shift attention and actions between multiple cues or in the face of competing stimuli is significantly impaired. Executive functions, including explicit memory, judgment, reasoning, and planning ahead show obvious impairment. As a result, complex tasks are performed with inconsistency, difficulty, or error. The goal of performance continues to be the completion of familiar tasks, but with respect to IADLs and other complex tasks, the person struggles to manage the details. Basic daily tasks such as dressing and grooming also begin to show some change or decline, in particular, with respect to initiation and frequency. Self-activated thoughts are skewed by attention and awareness deficits that often results in task initiation deficits, apathy, self-centered behavior, or the inability to consider the needs of others or the extent of one's own disability.

As cognitive abilities decline, coping becomes more difficult; the person continues by using very rigid, familiar routines for carrying out daily activities. The person is often not receptive to activity changes or assistance because he or she cannot comprehend something different or initiate new endeavors. When executive control is declining, the person loses the ability to cope or figure out how to solve problems. This lack of control leaves the person feeling dependent or like he or she is at the mercy of others. People react to frustration in different ways. Some become cautious and hesitant and withdraw or seek advice and assistance from others. A person in a loving, trusting relationship may be able to rely on others and even express awareness and appreciation. Others deny problems and begin to act impulsively, refusing direction or help. With impaired ability in reasoning and judgment,

the person is unable to plan or consider consequences. It is often hard for family members to know whether the person is "covering up" or has lost insight. The person may or may not be aware of the changes, but by Level 4.5 the ability to objectively evaluate situations is impaired. Although the person may be adamant about what he or she wants to do, the determination is based on what is wanted at the time, not on logical reasoning or consideration of the pros and cons of the choices or consequences of the actions in question.

Obvious changes in behavior often begin at Level 4.5. Understanding the deficits described above can help caregivers realize how the impaired thinking affects the person's behavior. Every person will also have emotional responses to the changes taking place in his or her thinking. The emotional reactions may be similar to the person's prior way of coping with problems, or they may seem to be very different from behaviors of the past.

Rehabilitation Potential

Independent living at this level is possible but poses many risks and requires frequent support from others. As a result, many individuals move to an assisted-living facility where services and supervision are available. Independent living, IADLs, and safety hazards need to be assessed and monitored and restricted through environmental and caregiver strategies and approaches. Caregiving during Level 4.5 is usually a difficult period of adjustment for most families. It is a time of uncertainty and ambivalence. There are definite signs of problems, so the caregiver worries, but at other times the person performs well and seems perfectly normal. Families may still be reluctant to believe the diagnosis or to actually make changes until they have to. This stress will build as they wait for a crisis to occur.

Safety issues are discussed in terms of the risks associated with the cognitive-processing limitations. Safety capacity is related to executive control and the ability to process abstract and subtle cues under different circumstances and environments. People who function in Level 6—and, to a lesser degree, in Level 5—have these abilities. This capacity is significantly diminished in Level 4, and errors in the performance of hazardous tasks or evidence of unsafe behavior is commonly reported. For example, medication errors and noncompliance are common reasons for an occupational therapy referral. Caregivers are taught to monitor the overall use of medications and often to set them up, provide daily reminders, or both. A routine medication regime—for example, setting the pills out with breakfast—is important. For people who live alone, weekly visits from a public health nurse or family member is often necessary. The mismanagement of finances and concerns about driving or the capacity for these activities are other common reasons for a rehabilitation referral.

Driving errors are commonly seen at Level 4.5 and include becoming lost, driving too slowly or too fast, and failure to use directional signs and signals. Caregivers often report that they help the person to navigate his or her driving; some may admit their safety concerns. The person is not safe to drive because significant impairments in attention and working memory, and he or she would fail a rehabilitation driving examination for these same reasons. Nevertheless, the person may not be able to see that he or she is presenting a safety risk and may refuse to stop driving. Likewise, family members may minimize the risk, if they rely on the person for transportation or are unable to interpret the risks associated with the errors they see and the assistance they give. Moreover, procedural-memory stores for how to drive or move the car remain intact and can skew both the person's as well as others' perceptions of the person's driving abilities. Discussing the difference between operating (moving) the car and the ability to pay attention and to respond to unusual demands and implications for safety is needed.

Education and support programs address the common behaviors of task inconsistency and the person's misinterpretations of his or her abilities. Structured day programs and concrete replacement activities need to be investigated and can offer the person meaningful occupation within his or her range of ability. Clinicians circumvent deficits in working memory by breaking down complex procedures into fewer concrete steps. Clients who are seen for traditional rehabilitative services may not do well with learning home programs, necessitating caregiver education in providing for safety and implementation of the program.

COGNITIVE LEVEL 4.0: GOAL-DIRECTED ACTIVITY

Attentional and Working-Memory Processing

At Level 4.0 (Medicare assistance code: minimum or moderate cognitive assistance; GDS 4), episodic and semantic capacities are significantly impaired (i.e., both recall and recognition; procedural-memory capacities are less impaired). Individuals may be disoriented to time or place (episodic recall and recognition). They retain conceptual information about the world (e.g., what a potato peeler is; who President Roosevelt was; a relatively intact

vocabulary), although these semantic recall and recognition capacities can mask the severity of their disability. The person is able to use what he or she sees in the environment for cues as to what to do but is not able to process the new information required to perceive safety hazards. Executive thought processes, including the ability to inhibit irrelevant cues, are very impaired. Attention is directed toward visible and tactile cues and is sustained throughout short-term familiar activities.

Occupational Behavioral Responses

The goal in initiating actions is to perceive a concrete cause-and-effect relationship between a visible cue and a desired outcome. Functional responses are limited to the ability to follow highly familiar motor processes. This is an asset when tasks are straightforward and appropriate supplies are readily seen; however, when tasks require too much interpretation, novelty, or effort to figure things out, performance is faulty because decisions are based on superficial, visual, and limited information; problem-solving skills are relatively absent.

The amount of assistance or supervision necessary for the individual's safety increases significantly at this level. Although the person might live alone, with a very structured support system, there are many risks involved, and it is not recommended. If the person is living with family, this is the stage at which questions are raised concerning how long he or she may be left alone at home or how independent he or she can be in getting around the neighborhood or community. The person has significant difficulty with organizing complex activities. He or she may no longer be able to initiate plans or activities, but this must not be mistaken for disinterest or lack of motivation. Family members need to provide daily structure, the same routine, assistance, and reminders. Simple changes in the environment, in approach, and in expectations for performance can help the person to continue to be successful with simple activities. Environmental changes, such as removal of clutter or hazardous equipment, are also important.

Familiar ADLs and concrete tasks, such as dressing and grooming, are remembered, but the quality of performance shows decline. The person cannot manage to take care of himself or herself independently. Although these basic tasks may be done just fine much of the time, abilities are very inconsistent and usually depend on some help from others. The person may know what he or she is trying to do but may have difficulty getting started or keeping on track to finish a task. Thinking appears to be guided by visual information and verbal direction from others. When alone, the person loses track of time, may not know what to do, and may become very anxious.

By Level 4.0, the person does not have the ability to understand complex situations and problems or to make safe decisions. He or she becomes easily confused and frustrated when he or she does not understand the environment. At this level, there are many misperceptions about what is happening. There is confusion about time, space, people, and events. These misunderstandings often lead to suspiciousness, paranoia, and delusional ideas about things that happen. Behavior problems often develop at this stage, if the person has inadequate support and is left to struggle with problems on his or her own.

Changes in an individual depend on the specific areas of the brain affected by the disease. Some may become impulsive or uninhibited, embarrassing family members or causing concern for their safety. Others may retain an awareness of the changes, maintain social graces, or become very inactive. One person may have great difficulty expressing himself, unable to find words to talk to others; another person may seem to carry on quite a normal conversation. However, this conversation is usually superficial and very repetitive. Personality changes or self-centered behavior may become more pronounced, as the person's ability to reason or think about the needs of others is diminished by the disease.

Rehabilitation Potential

Independent living, IADLs, and safety hazards need to be assessed and restricted through environmental modifications and caregiver strategies and approaches. People at this level are not safe to drive. Although they would fail a driving examination, they may continue to drive unless restricted. Other transportation must be available to replace the loss of driving. Family members can take over the driving, community resources need to be investigated, and enlisting the help of neighbors or agencies may be needed. In general, independence in the community needs to be restricted, and care must be taken to recognize the point at which the person requires an escort. Falls are often an issue for people with physical impairments or precarious balance, as judgment in regard to following safety and preventive measures is limited.

Medication management should be closely supervised. The role of the caregiver is to ensure medication compliance and to provide the necessary safety, structure, and assistance. This includes monitoring all general health needs and any special condition, such as diabetes or heart disease. Likewise, money management activities need to be restricted. Most individuals at this level have obvious inability with money management, including paying bills, writing checks, and making cash transactions; family members usually have taken over the person's affairs by this level. However, the person may still be aware of his or her previous role in money matters and attempt to be involved. Family members may need to learn to be subtle about taking control and allow the person to participate on some level, such as continuing to carry a wallet or purse with a limited amount of cash.

Clinicians circumvent deficits in working memory by breaking down complex procedures into fewer concrete steps. Here, the task and materials themselves also provide the recognition cues necessary for optimal performance. Strategies decrease the need to keep several thoughts in mind, thereby decreasing demands on working memory. Procedural memories are used spontaneously, as individuals produce the correct overt responses to environmental cues.

People at this level rely heavily on what they see and can touch to "tell" them what to do. When clothes are laid out for them when they get up in the morning or step out of the shower, they will know to get dressed and what to wear. Without someone to get them started, they may not think of changing clothes or may resist bathing and changing. Without someone to prepare and put food out for them, they may not think of eating and be unable to prepare anything that requires mixing items together or cooking. Malnutrition or failure to thrive may be a reason for rehabilitation referral for those who live alone.

As in the higher modes of Level 4, intervention programs address the common task performance errors and inconsistencies in this level and often the associated misinterpretations of the client's abilities. The major goal of intervention is to provide safety and day-to-day structure. The person becomes increasingly dependent on others to initiate and organize activities. Feelings of trust and the security that come with routine, structured activities are very important to a person who is confused and aware of losing control. Ignoring the person's needs for structure can lead to out-of-control behaviors.

Concrete replacement activities and structured day programs need to be investigated. Other resources, such as companion and home health services and caregiver support services, may be needed. As stated above, clients who are seen for rehabilitative services may not do well with home learning programs. Caregivers are taught to implement home programs and are specifically taught the difference between the person's ability to do the task procedures versus the ability to perform with safety, consistency, and without error.

COGNITIVE LEVEL 3.5: MANUAL ACTIONS

Attentional and Working-Memory Responses

Between Levels 4 and 3 (Medicare assistance code: moderate cognitive assistance; GDS 5), the person loses the awareness of goals and the outcomes of activities. Episodic capacities are negligible, semantic capacities are severely impaired, and procedural-memory capacities are moderately impaired. Individuals may forget the fact that they have children (semantic recognition and recall) or even their own names (usually considered an automatic procedural memory). Intentional actions are limited to tactile exploration of the kinds of effects one's actions have on the environment. These chance actions are neither planned nor goal directed; however, they are typically repeated to verify that similar results occur. Consequently, perseverative and apraxic actions are common. Familiar objects that can be seen and touched are usually perceived or identified accurately, but the use is often incomplete or incorrect.

Activities are caregiver intensive. To elicit functional behavioral actions, the caregiver must initiate, sequence, and sustain the individual's procedural actions; the provision of procedural cues enables the individual to retrieve memories relevant to the context. Procedural-memory processes are also cued by environments structured to mimic the individual's familiar routines as much as possible.

Occupational Behavioral Responses

The person is very dependent and is not able to live alone. Furthermore, because of the poor orientation, lack of awareness of hazards, and inability to solve problems, it is risky to leave the person alone. These individuals' actions are unpredictable, and anxiety increases when they are unsure of what to do in a situation. Recognizing problems or hazards becomes difficult, and complicated situations may be frightening or misconstrued. Actions are often based on what can be seen with no consistent awareness of important environmental cues (e.g., danger signs). Others must perform all IADLs and complex activities. Medications need to be given and their access restricted.

The person can no longer pay attention to health needs or be expected to accurately express pain and discomfort. The caregiver must monitor and care for general health needs and any comorbid condition. Sudden changes in behavior may be the result of infection or pain or another medical problem that needs attention.

Self-care ADLs now require the setup of task supplies within arm's reach and ongoing prompting or direction during the task or to finish the task. Objects need to be limited to a few at a time and may need to be handed and procedures demonstrated to provide recognition cues. Confused dressing behaviors are common at this level, such as layering clothes, rummaging, and disrobing inappropriately. Toileting problems, such as incomplete wiping or accidents, may appear at this time; the person may use receptacles such as the wastebasket. Toileting schedules and incontinence briefs are often started at this level. Resisting bathing and changing clothes are other common ADL behaviors that require subtle caregiver approaches that access the person's implicit rather than explicit-memory stores.

Ambulation and movement often change at this level. People may have difficulty positioning their bodies in space, as in knowing how to sit down in a chair. Extra time and cues, such as pushing the chair up to the person, are needed. Falls may be a problem, especially if the person uses a walking aid or if there is trouble with balance. The ability to judge depth or recognize and avoid hazards while walking is diminished. If the person becomes disabled at this level and requires an aid such as a walker, learning to use it safely may not be possible and will require close supervision.

Independence in eating is maintained longer than in any other activity. Nevertheless, at cognitive Level 3.5 the person may need the food placed on the plate and simplified (peeled, cut, uncovered), with reminders given to begin/finish eating each item. The person may not be able to maintain appropriate social eating behaviors, and good nutrition needs to be the responsibility of others.

Sleep disruption is common by Level 3.5. It is felt that the sleep center in the brain is affected by the disease process, causing the natural rhythm to be disturbed. It is common for people with dementia to insist on going to bed earlier and earlier in the evening, often wanting to retire immediately after the evening meal. However, the person may then be up frequently during the night and possibly fall asleep easily during the daytime. Increased confusion often occurs when the person is awake during the evening and night. Possibly awakened to go to the bathroom, the person may become distracted to any number of other endeavors unless directed quickly back to bed. Although some people may become inactive and sleep a great deal of the time, others become quite anxious and restless. Pacing, searching for something, and "wanting to go home" are common and reflect the inability to independently engage in activity.

Awareness of time, people, and place is considerably diminished and inconsistent. The person may be confused in familiar as well as unfamiliar settings. Orientation may fluctuate—the person may sometimes know he or she is in his or her own home; at other times, he or she becomes lost in the house or asks to go home. These people confuse past with present events, often insisting that people they have been thinking about were actually with them. Likewise, family, familiar friends, or even the primary caregiver may not be recognized or may be accused of being an impostor. Intangible components of tasks or situations are often confusing and may be ignored or rejected. For example, even if the person can read the time on a clock, he or she is not able to comprehend the passage of time. Caregivers must provide simple reminders and help the person to follow daily schedules. There may be great anxiety about time—where the person is going or when he or she needs to be somewhere. The person may also experience separation anxiety when away from the primary caregiver.

Rehabilitation Potential

The person is apraxic to greater or lesser degrees. In testing, occupational therapists observe the inability to initiate and sequence activity; on interview, caregivers report giving direct assistance with ADLs. Institutional placement is common during this level, although many individuals remain in their own homes. Both professional and family caregivers require education concerning the person's function, safety, and individual behaviors, as well as help to interpret behaviors and specific strategies for giving care.

Occupational therapists can address the risk of falls associated with apraxic gross motor movements, difficulty with eating associated with poor attention as well as apraxia, and beginning incontinence, for the same reasons. Programs at this level include fall prevention and home or environmental safety measures, simplified meals and all ADLs, and behavior management programs. Problem solving is the basic strategy that needs to be used for designing care plans that address behaviors. The caregiver is asked about the actions and behaviors of the person, the causes of problems are analyzed, and plans are made for what to change that may help the situation. The person cannot make the changes, but as the disease progresses, the changes made in approach and in the environment become more and more important to the function and security of the impaired person.

Intervention programs also address the design of meaningful, repetitive activity to reduce problematic behaviors, promote function, and the maintenance of procedural skills.

COGNITIVE LEVEL 3.0: MANUAL ACTIONS

Attentional and Working-Memory Processes

Although procedural memory is now very impaired at this level (Medicare assistance code: moderate or maximum cognitive assistance; GDS 6), attention remains directed toward using the hands to explore objects; the goal of action is limited to tactile exploration and simple touch. Objects that can be touched or are handed provide recognition cues for what to do and trigger procedural memories. More difficulty is seen with understanding verbal information or what is heard; visual cues may or may not capture attention. Intangible components of tasks or situations are usually ignored, as episodic and semantic memory are severely impaired. Complex activities and situations cause frustration and rejection and are often the cause of catastrophic reactions.

Awareness of time, place, and people is severely impaired. People are confused in even familiar settings such as their own homes. Recognition of even the primary caregiver may fluctuate. The person's spouse or others may be accused of being impostors. Those who begin new activities or programs frequently resist and will need time to adjust and become familiar with the environment and routines. However, those who have become quite anxious in their own homes may settle more easily into the structured environment of a secure nursing home. Awareness of the progression of time is lost. There still may be great anxiety about time, particularly in relation to insecurity and dependence when away from the primary caregiver. Caregivers are needed to provide simple reminders that help the person to understand what is happening at that time. Obsession about time, place, or person is often a sign that more structure, direction, and simple objects to focus attention are needed.

Occupational Behavioral Responses

Functional behavioral actions are limited to the physical qualities of objects, but there is often little use; misuse; or repetitive, purposeless use, with no awareness of what an action is doing. Task objects often need to be handed to get an action started, and demonstration may be necessary for the person to perform the desired movements. Consequently, caregivers may find it easier to do things for, or to, the person at this cognitive level. However, learning techniques to involve the person can make the daily care and activities more satisfying for both the person with dementia and for the caregiver.

All medications need to be given and monitored for possible side effects. Caregivers must also be alert to the need for pain medication and the possible need for medication for disruptive behaviors. The person can no longer pay attention to health needs or accurately express pain and discomfort. As above, sudden changes in behavior are often the result of infection or pain or another medical problem that needs attention.

The person is very dependent on others to initiate and carry out self-care tasks. Ongoing prompting may be needed for each step, as well as supervision to prevent accidents and achieve intended results (scrub here, shave here). More time is needed for ADLs, and often the performance and quality are so diminished that caregivers provide total care. It may be helpful to determine which basic activities—for example, eating—are appropriate for some participation and those that are too confusing or agitating to expect participation. For those activities that the caregiver does to or for the person, developing an efficient and routine way of giving the care is needed (i.e., have all supplies ready for getting dressed; always start and end the same way, such as pants first, then move to the upper body, or vice versa). The person may do better with accepting care when given something to hold.

Eating abilities are maintained longer than in any other activity. Nevertheless, at Level 3.0 the person will need the food placed onto the plate, ready to eat (peeled, cut, uncovered), with cues to start, keep going, and finish. It may be easier for the person to manage if only one or two foods are presented at a time and if silverware is limited to a spoon. Finger foods may be enjoyed and can be offered frequently during the day as well as at mealtime. If the person has trouble remaining at the table and paces frequently, extra calories may be needed in the diet. Caregivers must be alert to the need for fluids and offer these during and between meals.

Rehabilitation Potential

Total care is required. Occupational therapy intervention can include education and training for professional and family caregivers in efficient comfort-care routines because resistance to ADL care is common; in fall prevention programs, feeding programs with risk for dysphasia, positioning and movement programs; and in other sensory programs that involve objects, touch, and sound. Agitated behaviors may be alleviated with individualized sensory programs or sensory input from designed sensory environments.

Activities that make use of habitual, spontaneous motions may be performed by the individual if objects are positioned within arm's reach or placed in the hands. Caregivers can try repetitive activities, but actions are often carried out in a rather automatic fashion, with little awareness of what is actually being done. However, the person can be engaged with objects to handle and manipulate. Objects can be offered to divert the person from undesirable pursuits and with the hope that a continuous wanderer will sit to rest for a short time.

As much as possible, the freedom to move about unrestricted needs to be allowed. This means that clutter and environmental hazards must be eliminated, including cluttered floors, loose rugs, uneven surfaces, and steps or furniture over which the person might stumble. Sturdy chairs are needed, as well as a bed that will not roll or move. Electrical outlets, cords, and appliances need to be restricted, as do cleaning solutions, medications, and unsafe items from cupboards. The water heater should be turned down to a safe temperature. Unsafe areas can be blocked so the person can't wander into trouble. Safety devices can be added to the bathroom. Caregivers are taught to be prepared for what to do in case of emergencies (e.g., choking, falls, seizures).

The person is not able to organize or carry out even basic daily activities. The environment must be made simple and safe. Approaches must be consistently calm and reassuring. Someone must be attending to the person's basic needs for care as well as managing changing behaviors. The strategies for care require constant supervision and careful attention to the person's responses. One caregiver cannot meet all the person's needs without help from others. Special care units of nursing homes are specifically designed to meet the needs of people at this level. Day care programs can accommodate the needs of people at this level and are an important resource for families who continue to have the person at home. Home care agencies can provide nursing services and personal care, homemaking services, and short-term respite care. Families who continue to care for the person at home can learn some basic techniques for moving, dressing, and bathing and learn to seek ideas and support from others about managing the common behavioral changes.

COGNITIVE LEVEL 2: POSTURAL ACTIONS

Attentional and Working-Memory Processes

In Level 2 (Medicare assistance code: maximum cognitive assistance; GDS 7), attention has shifted from external cues to a reliance on internal cues and proprioceptive cues from muscles and joints that are elicited by one's own familiar body movements. The goal in initiating action is for the effect on the body alone (i.e., on one's sense of position and balance, to relieve pressure or pain). Functional behavioral actions are limited to spontaneous and imitated gross motor actions. The individual is severely apraxic and agnosiac and pays little attention to objects; he or she seems to have lost the meaning of objects. Because objects no longer serve as recognition cues for what to do, they are unable to use most objects in any meaningful way. Planning and organizing even simple activities (e.g., brushing teeth) is not possible. Episodic- and semantic-memory capacities are negligible. Procedural-memory capacities are severely impaired such that the individual no longer remembers how to eat, dress, toilet, and often even to speak. Attention appears to be focused on movement, touch (or what comes in contact with the body), and sounds in the environment.

Occupational Behavioral Responses

The neurological changes affect both physical and cognitive function during this late stage of dementia. Most behavior seems to be purposeless movement. There is very little intentional action, but there is automatic response to sounds, movement, and touch. Agitated behavior occurs in response to unpleasant or confusing things in the environment. However, because the person is no longer so intent on doing things, and the attention span is very short, it is much easier to divert and redirect attention from one thing to another.

Other people must meet all of the person's basic needs, including hygiene, nutrition and elimination, care of illnesses, safety, and emotional needs. One person cannot manage all of the care needs for increased supervision, bathing, feeding, and lifting. Caregivers must learn to work as a team to give efficient care. Family members can alert professionals to the person's preferences and to particular approaches that seem to be calming. The home care nurse or facility staff can teach family caregivers techniques for carrying out tasks.

The ability to express physical discomfort or pain is lost or distorted. It is difficult to monitor how the person is doing because he or she can no longer express pain or discomfort. As stated above, any sudden change in behavior may be a sign of illness; caregivers learn from experience what to watch for. In the late stage of illness, the person may become more restless; refuse to eat; or begin to yell, hit, or grab.

Restlessness or agitation may be due to discomfort. Angry remarks, screaming, or yelling are often an indication that the person is confused and does not understand what is being said or being done to him or her. Interpreting these vague communication attempts is a difficult responsibility of Level 2 caregiving. The profound confusion frequently leads to resistance or even anger. To minimize confusion, simple, clear, brief statements (e.g., "Eat the toast") should be used, with extra time to allow the person to respond. In all activities, caregivers need to be alert for overstimulation and provide ample rest periods.

Visual information may or may not capture attention. Freedom to move about is important, but safety awareness is severely impaired. Caregivers must remove all dangerous items from the environment (see examples above). Balance becomes impaired, and obstacles may be overlooked. Touch may be interpreted as pleasurable or may cause fear and reactions such as hitting or resisting. Even simple tasks, such as moving to a different room, may cause frustration and rejection. Directions must be given one step at a time (e.g., ask the person to come with you first, then tell him or her to sit, then give him or her the spoon and help with the dish of food).

People at Level 2 may begin to move more slowly, but they are not cautious. Although they are still able to walk, they seem to move about without purpose, sometimes even sitting without thinking about whether there is a chair behind them. Their feet are farther apart as they walk, and their balance is unstable. They may seem to move constantly—investigating things, climbing, turning knobs, shuffling through things. Some put inedible things into their mouths.

Rehabilitation Potential

Total care is required. Occupational therapy intervention can include education and hands-on training for professional and family caregivers in efficient comfort-care routines as resistance to ADLs and other care is common, in feeding programs with risk for dysphasia, in fall prevention, in positioning and movement programs, and in other sensory and behavior management programs. Safety and the risk of falls become more of an issue as the person loses awareness of the environment and has difficulty keeping his or her balance when walking; there is no conscious awareness of danger. Safety-proofing the home is important for people who remain at home.

When the person is distressed or bored, he or she can be distracted by using sensory activities. When activities are found that are enjoyed, they can be used over and over. Rather than being bored with repetition, the familiarity seems to foster comfort and security. Music, poetry, dancing or movement, simple exercises, and rocking chairs can be tried. Music may be enjoyed, and the person may hum or sing tunes when he or she has very little other speech. Provide color and texture in items the person can carry, or use soft sweaters or blankets, stuffed animals or dolls, and wall hangings; apply lotion and give massages. Frequent nutritious snacks and liquids can be offered as a routine activity.

Activities need to be done for, or to, the person and are adapted to capitalize on the capacity to use visual, tactile, kinesthetic, and proprioceptive recognition cues for comfort and relatively passive participation. Negative behaviors need to be evaluated and are assessed by how the person reacts to the things going on in the surroundings. Changes are made in the environment or approaches by adding or taking away things surrounding the person. The need for medication needs to be addressed. Each situation takes analysis and a bit of trial and error and creativity.

Family members experience many emotions as they face the changes and must make decisions about care. Often the person with dementia is otherwise quite healthy. Although the physical status has declined, there may be no medical illnesses. Families and the professional caregivers are faced with difficult decisions regarding the treatment during illnesses. The person's prior wishes for care and a careful assessment of the current awareness of his or her surroundings need to be considered in deciding how much treatment is appropriate. The person's response to comfort measures is an important way to gauge what care is important for him or her.

As others take on more of the care, it is important for the caregivers to pay attention to their own health and needs, discuss their concerns with others, and seek spiritual guidance and support to cope with their own emotions. Some find satisfaction in helping other caregivers by offering advice learned from their experiences.

COGNITIVE LEVEL 1: AUTOMATIC ACTIONS

Attentional and Working-Memory Responses

In Level 1 (Medicare assistance code: total cognitive assistance; GDS 7), attention is limited to subliminal internal cues, such as hunger, taste, and smell. Individuals, although conscious, appear to stare and are largely unresponsive to external stimuli. Actions are in response to comfort or discomfort or to follow near-reflexive one-word directives (e.g., sip, turn). Episodic-, semantic-, and procedural-memory capacities are negligible. Complications at this stage (e.g., aspiration pneumonia, malnutrition, sepsis from decubiti, urinary tract infections) lead to death. The person responds less and less to the surroundings. Short attention appears to focus on movement in the environment and on things that come in direct contact with the body (e.g., washcloth, clothing, touching).

Occupational Behavioral Responses

Basic abilities, such as walking and eating, are lost during this level. Speech is infrequent and consists of repetition of words or syllables. Resisting care may still occur, possibly because the person is startled or is reacting to discomfort. As the physical condition declines as well, the person needs increasing nursing care. During this last stage of illness the decisions about care are based on the person's comfort. Treatments and medications may make little difference in the condition and may cause additional pain or agitation. Decisions about the care must be based on what will allow the most comfort for the person.

The person has only vague awareness of the surroundings. There may be interest in one-to-one attention, voices, and music. There may be negative responses, such as yelling or hitting out, when there is too much noise or activity. The person may focus only on objects placed directly in front of him or her and later may notice only things that move. Touch may be interpreted as pleasurable or may cause fear and reactions such as hitting or resisting.

Rehabilitation Potential

All personal care activities (bathing, grooming, dressing, toileting, positioning, and feeding) need to be done for the person. Because the person understands little of what is being done, it is important for caregivers to be as efficient as possible. Dietary and fluid adjustments are needed to help maintain regularity and good nutrition as long as possible. Strategies to deal with feeding problems are considered before tube feedings. A medical evaluation of the person's ability to swallow may be needed. Careful positioning, thickened liquids, pureed foods, use of straws, and techniques to stimulate chewing and swallowing can help for a time. The person's alertness and other abilities at the time need to be considered as well as his or her level of general comfort and interest in the surroundings.

With regard to AD and other progressive dementias, the issues in Level 1 concern the end stage of the disease. Occupational therapists can provide ADLs, behavior management, and sensory and positioning programs. The person may respond positively and seem to relax with soothing and comforting measures that provide a secure feeling, such as soothing music or poetry. Wrapping the person in soft blankets and providing stuffed animals or old favorite objects may help. Passive exercises and massage are very important for maintaining circulation and skin health and can also ease discomfort and facilitate relaxation. Family caregivers require assistance and support with end-of-life decisions. Hospice care may be utilized and reimbursed by Medicare in Level 1.

EVALUATION AND ASSESSMENT PROCESSES AND INSTRUMENTS

Functional assessment in dementia emerged in the 1960s, and numerous questionnaire and observational measures have been developed since. A decade ago it was estimated that 40 such instruments existed (Kluger & Ferris, 1991). A similar trend is observed with quality-of-life scales (MacKeigan & Pathak, 1992). The multiplicity of scales that are being used for assessment reflects the lack of universally accepted measures for these constructs.

The source of most functional assessments originates from the conceptualizations by the Benjamin Rose Hospital staff (1959) and Katz et al. (1963), who identified several specific functional abilities important for treatment effectiveness. Subsequent researchers have used physical activities of daily living (e.g., bathing, dressing, eating, toileting, transferring, ambulating) as the basic set of functional domains to examine. In 1969, Lawton and Brody identified IADLs (e.g., shopping, phoning, doing laundry) to expand on measurement of disability by including more complex everyday tasks. Most current assessment schemes use the ADL/IADL framework with some variations.

Functional ability and occupational performance are affected during the first stages of dementing disease when cognitive deficits become apparent. Both IADLs and ADLs are almost inevitably influenced (McKeith, Cummings, Lovestone, Harvey, & Wilkinson, 1999). Because meaningful and purposeful activity is central to

overall function and health (F. Clark et al., 1997; Cohen-Mansfield, Lipson, Brenneman, & Pawlson, 2001; Wilcock, 1998), an important goal of treatment is to maintain independent function (Mayeux & Sano, 1999). Functional disability is closely related to quality of life, and the importance of assessing both outcomes is increasingly recognized (Gauthier, Gelinas, & Gauthier, 1997; Stern, Hesdorffer, Sano, & Mayeux, 1990).

Current practice guidelines in occupational therapy provide frameworks to help understand the factors that influence function, including person, environment, and occupation factors (Christiansen & Baum, 1997). Although different models are used to depict the relationships, all acknowledge that function is influenced by attributes of the person (e.g., physical, social, and affective components); the occupation, task, or activity being undertaken; and the environment (e.g., physical, social, cultural) in which the occupation is taking place (Letts, Baum, & Perlmutter, 2003). The *International Classification of Functioning, Disability, and Health* (World Health Organization, 2001) also supports the notion of considering person and environment when understanding the complexity of function and activity participation. For example, functional decline does not necessarily occur linearly, as several factors are likely to influence an individual's independence and safety in performing activities (World Health Organization, 1980). Indeed, self-care and performance in productive or leisure activities are determined by the interaction among the affective, spiritual, cognitive, and physical characteristics of any individual in interaction with his or her environment.

Dementia is often characterized by a change in adaptation to the environment. Thus, quality-of-life measures complement functional scales and are used to gather data on the impact of dementia on day-to-day life. These measures tend to combine the biologic aspects of the disease with their social and functional consequences in an overall appraisal (Demers, Oremus, Perrault, & Wolfson, 2000). Although the importance of measuring clients' individual responses to the disease and circumstances such as caregiver support cannot be overlooked, occupational performance is an important starting point for assessment.

The ADL/IADL framework has been useful in broad descriptions of disability. These measures typically assess functional performance over a broad range of dementia severity and assess progression over time. Typically with these scales, individual scores for specific activities are summed for a global functional score. Many dementia researchers agree that the measurement of functional performance on a continuum from independence to dependence is insufficient and suggest consideration of functioning from multiple dimensions (Baltes, 1995; Willis & Schaie, 1994).

The conceptual issue of measuring global versus component abilities is also a measurement issue. Some assessments are skill specific (e.g., check writing, use of the stove), and the extent to which data obtained on one skill or set of skills are equivalent for different abilities (e.g., managing finances, meal preparation) remains unknown. Because occupational therapists also use skill-specific assessment techniques, the ability to generalize the client's performance to his or her global function is an important consideration.

One of the problems with the simple ADL/IADL framework is the lack of attention to contextual elements that affect functional performance (Weiner, Hanley, Clarke, & Van Norstrand, 1990). Beck and Frank (1997) organized contextual elements into three categories: (a) intrapersonal, (b) interpersonal, and (c) environmental. *Intrapersonal elements* refers to the individual's cognitive and physical abilities. *Interpersonal elements* refers to interactions with caregivers during task performance. *Environmental elements* include the physical layout of the environment. All three elements interact to create the context in which to consider functioning.

The cause of occupational performance impairment in dementia likely originates in the disease-related processes, particularly cognitive impairment. However, examination of the relationships between cognitive impairment and the monolithic construct known as *function* is inadequate, because multiple pathways can lead to the same outcome of impaired performance. For example, an individual may be unable to dress him- or herself because of ideational apraxia; arranging the clothes in the proper sequence can lead to task completion. The same outcome, inability to dress, may stem from ideomotor apraxia, which requires physical guidance from another in order to complete the task. Although the type and degree of cognitive disability may explain observed functional deficits, the multiple dimensions of function and the role of contextual factors are needed to reach a comprehensive understanding of the person's abilities.

Occupational therapists have historically tended to assess isolated cognitive components to identify distinct problems related to initiation, planning, problem solving, or other executive functions, but the occupational therapist's primary concern should relate to the ways executive function disorders affect functional performance (Duran & Fisher, 1999; Fisher, 1997). Therefore, it is more useful and efficient to assess executive abilities through direct observation of occupational performance, and there has been a move toward naturalistic assessment of executive abilities (Giovannetti et al., 2002; Schwartz et al., 1993; Shallice & Burgess, 1991). For example, Schwartz and colleagues (1995) stressed the advantages of implementing systematic analyses of a person's ADL task performances and asserted that executive-function disorders can be observed in routine, overlearned activities of daily living; task novelty is not required. In addition to noting the limitations of neuropsychological (cognitive) testing, Schwartz et al. (1993) noted that, "because the focus is on ADL, such an analysis has more immediate relevance for treatment goals and procedures" (p. 65). Moreover, Shallice and Burgess (1991) noted that direct observation of ADL task performance involves observing a person perform complex daily life tasks, that is, "open-ended multiple sub goal situations" (p. 728). They also pointed to the need "to develop quantifiable analogues of the open-ended multiple subgoal situations" (p. 728) when the problems with executive functions become manifest as decreased executive abilities. (See Chapter 1 for more discussion of executive functions and instruments.)

We recommend the CPT (Allen, Kehrberg, & Burns, 1992; Burns 1991, 2002, 2004; Burns et al., 1994) as the most viable approach to assessing occupational performance in the reconsidered cognitive disability model. It is also in the mainstream of current discourse in the area of functional assessment (Beck & Frank, 1997). The intent is to discover the unique nature of the information-processing components underlying functional performance deficits, in lieu of strategies aimed toward identifying isolated neuropsychological functions, or developing generalized task lists, to predict the extent of impairment. The primary focus is the degree to which specifically defined deficits in information-processing capabilities compromise performance in daily occupations. Hence, the manner in which the individual responds to functional task demands of varying complexity is the primary concern. This approach to assessment also differs markedly from occupational therapy assessments that measure the absolute ability versus inability to perform specific ADL/IADL tasks (e.g., Kohlman Evaluation of Living Skills, Kohlman-Thomson, 1992; Robnett Home Safety Screen Program, Robnett, 1995), or the amount of assistance given to complete a specific task (Functional Independence Measure; Granger, Hamilton, Keith, Zielezny, & Sherwin, 1986).

Nevertheless, several tools have been developed to measure the cognitive levels associated with the cognitive disability model. Occupational therapists should understand how these methods of measurement differ and the clinical applications of each tool. The most frequently used tool is the Allen Cognitive Level Screen, a standardized leather-lacing task intended for use as a tool to screen for the cognitive level (Allen, 1990). The numerical scoring is based on the complexity of the lacing stitch that the person is able to imitate, which also represents his or her cognitive level and mode. The Large Allen Cognitive Level Screen was developed to compensate for the visual and fine motor demands of the lacing task (Kehrberg et al., 1992). Studies have demonstrated significant moderate correlations between lacing screen scores and indicators of cognitive and functional skills in individuals with dementia (see Allen, Earhart, & Blue, 1992, for a review). However, because of the brevity of a screening assessment, false-positive and false-negative scores will more often occur. Therefore, the lacing screen alone should not be used as a basis for determining function and care plans. Instead, screening tools are more appropriately used as indicators for possible dysfunction and estimation of severity, clinical pathways, or change (with serial assessment), as in repeated measures to track drug effects. Furthermore, the use of a leather-lacing assessment does not consider the essential contextual factors of function as described above.

Other tools developed to measure the cognitive levels include the Routine Task Inventory (RTI) observation/interview scales (Allen, Earhart, & Blue, 1992) and the Allen Diagnostic Module craft projects (Earhart, Allen, & Blue, 1993). The Allen Diagnostic Module craft projects use the even-mode numerical scores described earlier; to date, however, no validity data exist for these assessments.

The CPT is a standardized ADL-based performance measure of the cognitive levels. The test uses common ADL/IADL tasks (e.g., medbox, shop, toast, phone, wash, dress, travel) for which the information-processing requirements can be systematically varied to assess ordinal levels. It differs markedly from the more common approach to occupational therapy ADL assessment of measuring components of specific tasks (e.g., as used in the Kohlman Evaluation of Living Skills or in kitchen task assessments). Although these assessments may measure impairments and task assistance needs, they do not generate profiles that demonstrate the causes for functional performance deficits; neither are they grounded in a conceptual framework for research and intervention. Thus, rather than focusing on the ability to perform specific tasks included in the test, the CPT places emphasis on the degree to which impairments in executive functions compromise performance in salient activities. And because task performance is interpreted within the context of solid theoretical framework, the average performance across

CPT tasks is meant to be generalized in order to predict and explain function within a wide variety of ADLs, IADLs, and overall occupational performance.

Administration of the CPT is based on the principles of task analysis and gradation used within the reformulated frame of reference and involves the sequential inclusion or elimination of environmental recall and recognition cues as difficulty with performance is observed. For example, in administering the phone task, if difficulty is observed with locating a phone number (which requires use of selective attention to multiple symbolic cues), the phone book is removed, and the number is printed in bold on a notecard. If difficulty initiating the action of dialing follows (use of procedural memory related to complex visual cues), the printed number is removed, and nonspecific dialing is demonstrated to elicit imitation (provision of procedural recognition cues). It should also be noted that the occupational therapist must be able to determine whether performance difficulties are due to impairments in executive functions or may be due to other factors, such as low education, cultural bias of the selected task, or physical impairments. Overall, the focus of the CPT is on the degree to which particular deficits in information processing compromise performance in salient activities and, although the specific tasks that comprise the test have face validity, they are less important than the manner in which clients respond to the information-processing demands of decreasing complexity.

The CPT is similar in conception to the RTI in that it conceives of ADL performance patterns in a hierarchy. However, it differs from the RTI in that it operationalizes common activities in order to detect underlying causes for observable difficulties in impairments in executive functions. In addition, the RTI is used to detect and describe actual performance of specific ADLs/IADLs as observed by caregivers, clients, or therapists, and although this is essential information, day-to-day performance is significantly affected by factors other than cognition (e.g., physical limitations, motivation, environmental and caregiver supports), and informant reports may not tap maximum function or true abilities and disabilities; this can skew assistance and safety needs.

Nonetheless, the RTI scales were adapted from the original Lawton and Brody (1969) scales, which also look at activity performance in the form of a hierarchy and continue to be used in research today. In the assessment of function, these scales provide a method for caregiver interview that matches the trajectory of decline in dementing diseases. Yet caregivers may or may not be reliable informants, as their assessment of the person involves the interpretation of behavior and therefore may involve bias. For example, it is well documented that, in general, caregivers overestimate abilities just as individuals with the disease overestimate their competence to function.

Nevertheless, the caregiver's description of the person's actual day-to-day performance is a useful indicator of where the person may function on the cognitive-level scale. Occupational therapists who understand the scale are able to review records and interview those who know the person to estimate cognitive level based on caregiver descriptions of problematic behaviors and their experiences with strategies for providing assistance. The value of the actual performance test is that it helps to identify discrepancy or agreement between the person's actual versus maximum function and helps to explain "why" the person does what he or she does and how best to manage those behaviors. For example, problems demonstrated in performing day-to-day tasks are directly related to the types of environmental cues to which the person is able and not able to attend during the test. Furthermore, the performance test provides a means for systematic documentation.

As indicated, the CPT uses common tasks for which the information-processing requirements can be systematically varied to assess ordinal levels of functional capacity. Six tasks, titled *Dress, Shop, Toast, Phone, Wash,* and *Travel,* comprise the original test; a new Medbox subtest has been validated against the other subtasks and added (Burns, 2002). For each of the seven subtasks, standard equipment, setup, and methods of administration are required (Burns, 1991, 2002, in press; Allen, Kehrberg, & Burns, 1992). A gross level score is determined for each task; these scores are then added for a total score and averaged (divided by the number of tasks administered) to determine the cognitive level and mode.

Subtasks were selected on the basis of common ADLs and IADLs performed by normal adults and are meant to be familiar in concept but not necessarily familiar by specific experience. For example, an American auto mechanic who rarely cooked would be expected to be able to make toast, because normal adult cognitive abilities would allow for generalization of what to do with the toaster, plug, outlet, bread and butter, and so on, when given these contextual cues. Nonetheless, people who have no concept of a given subtask could earn a skewed score. For example, toast is not culturally common in Israel. Hence, the toast portion of the CPT was changed to making coffee and then validated against the same administration and scoring criteria (Bar-Yosef, Weinblatt, & Katz, 1999).

Performance of the CPT requires working memory and the orchestration of complex cognitive resources, such as attention, perception, language, and memory, to achieve stated and implied goals. Multiple subgoal situations are used to detect and objectively measure and quantify executive function. As discussed previously, these cognitive abilities require intricate neural computations, which are guided by the frontal and prefrontal lobes. Problems with working memory are reflected in performance errors with comprehension/memory of verbal and written cues in decision making, problem solving, and subgoal initiation. In dementia, these difficulties are due to the inability to keep track of all of the relevant information imposed during the test while inhibiting distractions or irrelevant cues (i.e., distracter props), in other words, one's executive (or attentional) control. The CPT imposes written, verbal, and contextual multiple-step task performance requirements, and patterns of performance are observed that relate to each cognitive level. For example, in Level 5, people are able to process multiple written, verbal, and contextual cues, although they may be slow or make overt errors that they correct, as episodic-memory stores are impaired. In Level 4, the deficits in executive control manifest in testing, as the person cannot act on multiple task details and contextual directions without cues. Although the person retains the main goal of each task, he or she is not able to simultaneously pay attention to the details (e.g., the different sizes and prices of the belts in the Shop task) and therefore require step-by-step help. In Level 3, explicit-memory stores are severely impaired, as is task initiation with respect to achieving the main goal; the person relies on implicit-procedural-memory stores to use the objects used in the test (e.g., can try on the belt or perform automatic actions). In Level 2, the person touches or holds the props but cannot perform the associated actions.

The CPT was designed for clinical administration, in an unfamiliar environment, although the tasks themselves are meant to be familiar. Familiar environments and objects can skew perceptions of capacity, as overlearned routines and familiar belongings increase capabilities. Although this is an important consideration for interventions, the assessment may be more objective in the clinic, where the person is asked to generalize his or her performance in a different context. Hence, the effects of a familiar environment are minimized when the CPT is administered in a clinic or within an altered home environment with props that do not belong to the person.

Craft projects have been suggested as the tools of choice for evaluation of higher functioning clients because it may be easier to observe new learning with them, whereas ADLs and the objects used in them are considered to be familiar, such that one can be easily misled into thinking the person is functioning better than he or she actually is (Allen & Blue, 1998). However, we contend that CPT tasks do involve sufficient novelty and complexity within the context of common everyday tasks to provide the more valuable measures of degrees of impairment in executive functions. Moreover, as Salthouse (2004) observed, much of what we typically do may be more dependent on successful access and retrieval of what we already know rather than our ability to solve novel problems or reason with unfamiliar material.

Studies of the CPT were initiated in 1991 at the Minneapolis Veterans Affairs Geriatric Research, Education and Clinical Center (GRECC) as part of a National Institute of Aging longitudinal study of AD (Burns et al., 1994). Seventy-seven community-residing older adults diagnosed with mild to moderate AD were studied. The participants were mostly white and included 56 male and 21 female participants and 15 neurologically normal elderly control participants (8 men, 7 women). The average age of participants was 67.8 years, and the average age of the control participants was 65.2 years. Subsets of the AD participants were assessed again at 4 weeks and at 1, 2, and 3 years after the initial evaluation. Internal consistency of the CPT estimated by alpha was .84. The intraclass correlation for interrater reliability was .91, and for test–retest reliability at 4 weeks, it was .89. CPT scores were significantly correlated with scores on the Mini Mental Status Exam (MMSE; Folstein, Folstein, & McHugh, 1975; $r = .67$) and Lawton and Brody's (1969) measures of caregiver-rated ADL (Instrumental Activities of Daily Living, $r = .64$; Physical Self-Maintenance Scale, $r = .49$). Longitudinal testing ($N = 64$) demonstrated significant decline in mean CPT scores with disease progression and, in contrast to the MMSE, initial CPT scores predicted the risk of institutionalization over the 4-year follow-up period. All participants with an initial CPT score of 4.2 or less were institutionalized within 3.6 years of the baseline assessment, whereas 40% of participants whose initial scores were above 4.2 remained in the community.

Thralow and Rueter (1993) also studied the predictive validity of the CPT and found a correlation of .78 between CPT total scores and the Self-Care Performance Test, an observational tool used by nurses to record the abilities and needs of demented patients in performing self-care tasks.

Bares (1998) studied the neuropsychological and functional status of AD patients and corresponding psychometric properties of the CPT. This retrospective study of AD patients who were evaluated in the Minneapolis GRECC found significant relationships between performance on the CPT and on neuropsychological measures. The sample included 100 mostly male, white patients aged 59 or older with mild- to moderate-stage disease. The average age was 74.9 years. In a hierarchical regression analysis of neuropsychological variables predicting function as measured by the CPT, significant predictors were neuropsychological measures that involved psychomotor skill with a planning, sequencing, and attentional component, whereas measures of episodic memory, language, background variables, and comorbidity were not predictive of CPT function. Bares characterized the neuropsychological predictors of performance on the CPT under the rubric of executive function.

Other analyses showed that CPT tasks were highly related to each other. Pearson correlations among the six tasks ranged from .20 (Travel and Dress tasks) to .51 (Travel and Phone tasks). Burns et al. (1994) found slightly larger correlations among the six tasks, ranging from .36 (Travel and Dress tasks) to .68 (Wash and Toast tasks). The CPT was found to have high internal consistency reliability ($\alpha = .76$), which is comparable to, although somewhat lower than, the previous finding of .84. From these data, Bares (1998) found no evidence to suggest that any of the six tasks assess a distinct functional ability, such as the ability to shop or to cook. Factor analyses of the six CPT subtests supported Burns et al.'s (1994) conclusion that the tasks are nonspecific. Bares's findings support the conclusion that the CPT total score, not the individual tasks, should be used.

Burns et al. (1994) examined Spearman correlations between CPT tasks and caregiver rated IADLs. Correlations between similar items (e.g., shopping, food preparation [making toast], and telephone use) on the two scales were only slightly higher on the average than correlations of items addressing different ADL activities. For example, with caregiver-rated food preparation, a stronger relationship was seen with the CPT Phone and Shop tasks than with the CPT Toast task, a food preparation activity. Findings from these studies suggest that CPT tasks reflect a single construct characterized as global functional status rather than discrete functional living skills.

Jennings-Pikey (2001) conducted similar studies of the relationship between neuropsychometrics and the CPT. One hundred eleven inpatient records from an inpatient psychiatric hospital in the upper Midwest were accessed for study through archival records. The sample was mostly white, 81% female ($N = 91$) and 19% male ($N = 20$), 58 years of age and older. The average age was 79.6 years. Sixty-four and a half percent ($N = 71$) of the participants received a primary diagnosis of dementia or memory loss. There was a significant difference on the CPT between the means of the group that was given a memory loss diagnosis and those who did not receive this diagnosis, demonstrating that people with a memory loss diagnosis functioned at a lower level on the CPT. The difference was not only statistically significant, $t(108) = -5.87, p < .001$, but also clinically meaningful. The magnitude of the effect size was .86 (Cohen's d), which indicates that the differences between the dementia-related memory loss group and the no memory loss group are clinically meaningful.

The validity of the CPT was supported to the extent that the test showed strong positive correlations with measures known to be sensitive to cognitive functioning in older adults (Wechsler Adult Intelligence Subtests; Wechsler, 1997). Convergent validity was also found when correlating the CPT with the MMSE. Burns and colleagues (1994) found a correlation of .67 when administering both the CPT and the MMSE to AD participants ($N = 77$). Jennings-Pikey (2001) found a more robust correlation of .74 with a more heterogeneous population ($N = 71$) of psychiatric inpatients. This suggests that the MMSE, which is a reliable measure for moderate to severe cognitive decline, and the CPT both measure cognitive decline.

Convergent validity was also demonstrated by a positive, significant correlation between the examinee's Global Assessment of Functioning (*Diagnostic and Statistical Manual of Mental Disorders;* American Psychiatric Association, 1994) at hospital discharge and CPT total scores ($r = .49, p < .01$). Jennings-Pikey (2001) concluded that the CPT is a strongly homogeneous measure supported by a Cronbach's alpha of .86, which is comparable to Burns et al.'s (1994) finding of .84 and upheld the CPT as an internally consistent measure of competency to carry out independent-living skills.

As mentioned above, the CPT was adapted and studied in Israel, including translation of the test manual into Hebrew (Bar-Yosef et al., 1999). Study results showed the CPT to be valid and reliable. Participants included 30 elderly people with dementia and a group of 30 age- and gender-matched control participants. High interrater reliability ($r = .98$) and internal consistency ($\alpha = .95$) were demonstrated. Concurrent validity was established by high correlations of the CPT and RTI–II (Allen, Kerhberg, & Burns, 1992) therapist, and moderate high with RTI–II caregiver, in both the study and control groups. CPT scores correlated significantly with the MMSE (study group; $r = .88$; control group; $r = .76$), further supporting concurrent validity of the CPT (Bar-Yosef et al., 1999).

Recently, Wachtel-Spector (2003) used the CPT to examine the relationship between awareness of functional cognitive level among elderly people living in the community following stroke and agreement with caregivers.

Participants included 30 elderly individuals (18 men, 12 women) without severe cognitive decline (MMSE score >23) who attended a senior day care center in the center of Israel. Instruments to assess cognitive functional level included the RTI–II subject, the RTI–II caregiver, and the CPT, with awareness questions administered before and after. Significant correlations were found between the participants' and the caregivers' reports in the basic and instrumental scales and part of the communication scale on the RTI–II assessment showing adequate awareness, but not for safety. Significant correlations were also found between the participants' and caregivers' reports on the RTI–II assessment and selected CPT subtasks (e.g., Dress, Wash, Phone, Coffee). However, a low anticipatory awareness of functional level was found.

Additional functional assessment instruments for use in dementia are numerous and varied. Many tools have been designed to assess the prevalence and to stage the functional impairment of dementia (e.g., Lawton & Brody's [1969] ADL/IADL scales; the Alzheimer's Disease Cooperative Study/Activities of Daily Living scale [Galasko et al., 1997]). Many staging tools use indicators of both cognitive and functional disability (e.g., the Global Deterioration Scale [Reisberg et al., 1982] and corresponding Functional Assessment Staging Instrument [Scalen & Reisberg, 1992] and the Clinical Dementia Rating Scale [Hughes, Berg, Danziger, Coben, & Martin, 1982]).

Other instruments were designed to measure the cognitive dimension of functional performance rather than stage of disease by rating specific cognitive skills and behavior in daily tasks (Functional Activities Questionnaire [Pfeffer, 1995; Pfeffer, Kurosaki, Harrah, Chance, & Filos, 1982]; Kitchen Task Assessment [Baum & Edwards, 1993]; Disability Assessment for Dementia [Gelinas, Gauthier, McIntyre, & Gautheir, 1999]).

As with craft assessments, the limitations with the above-mentioned instruments concern the ability to generalize the findings. For example, scores may not reflect the impact of cognitive impairments on the person's overall functioning and well-being and may not predict the person's functioning and participation in different contexts and situations. Additionally, intervention can only be implemented on the basis of an individual's level of functioning and the range of activities that may or may not be performed (Ustun, Chatterji, Bickenbach, Kostanjsek, & Schneider, 2003).

Individuals with dementias usually progress from normal abilities at Level 6; to early dementia at Level 5; and through the moderate and late stages of Levels 4, 3, 2, and 1. The CPT assessment provides a functional profile to design task gradation approaches that match abilities with desired occupations and roles.

INTERVENTION PROGRAMS

Individual Programs

People with dementia are increasingly being referred to occupational therapy psychiatric and physical rehabilitation clinics. Therapists assess occupational performance and teach caregivers how to grade the information-processing demands of occupations and modify their interactions to enable the person to still meet activity demands, despite the significant deficits that exist. By teaching home and institutional caregivers how to grade desired occupations and to provide for safety, therapists optimize the individual's remaining capacities and assist both the individual and his or her caregivers to retain a sense of competence, comprehension, and control throughout the course of the disease. Education programs direct family and professional caregivers to implement strategies consistent with the person's cognitive level.

In Appendix 14.1, the case study of Mr. B. illustrates the assessment and caregiver education process. Note that the occupational therapist educates both the family and the medical staff. Mr. B. was seen several times over the course of 2 years for IADL competency assessments, including driving, and later for institutional placement issues. The latter issue addressed an environment in which he could smoke and the assessment of safety with this activity. Note how the behaviors reported by his son and the medical staff, as well as the client's self-reports, are indicative of his assessed cognitive level or CPT score. Note also how the screen scores (e.g., MMSE, Large Allen Cognitive Level Screen) are less valid or indicative of his function with decline. Reports are written in the traditional Subjective, Objective, Assessment, Plan (SOAP) format and represent the actual occupational therapy notes and physician's orders from Mr. B.'s medical chart.

Mr. B. was initially an outpatient who was referred for functional assessment and then, after a fall, an inpatient who was receiving rehabilitation services. Occupational therapy services were focused on identifying capacities and assistance needs. Although Mr. B.'s capacities to remain living with his son were of concern, for Mr. B., the ability to continue smoking was the primary concern, thus the focus on this in the assessment process.

Furthermore, multiple hip dislocations necessitated fall prevention (i.e., environmental) strategies as opposed to teaching these directly. In rehabilitation, therapists teach strategies but must realize when caregivers are needed to implement the plan.

Individuals with dementia experience progressive working-memory limitations as well as progressive impairments in semantic, episodic, and procedural memory. The most effective rehabilitative strategies to enhance functional capabilities are those that reduce demands on the memory systems that are progressively impaired and that access memory systems that remain throughout the course of the disease. This is accomplished by creating occupational environments that minimize demands on the progressively impaired working- and declarative-memory systems (episodic and semantic) and capitalize on procedural and semantic recognition memory capacities that remain.

Adapted Work Programs

The above principles of the reconsidered cognitive disability model were applied in the GRECC Adapted Work Program (AWP; Burns & Buell, 1990; Burns et al., 2004; Ebbitt, Burns, & Christiansen, 1989), a sheltered workshop program for community-residing veterans with early- to middle-stage disease. Work tasks with minimal safety risk were selected by the AWP occupational therapist from available routine opportunities within the medical center and were screened for information-processing demands. Tasks that required more than minimal reading, writing, and alphabetizing or that consisted of numerous steps were considered too complex in terms of working-memory and recall demands and were eliminated, leaving repetitive tasks that included packaging, shredding, folding laundry, crushing cans, stapling, stamping, and labeling.

Task adaptations for individual workers were based on their CPT scores and followed the model of care. The job of shredding provides an example: Level 5 workers needed no adaptations, as they can learn to operate the finger-guarded shredder, including the on/off and reverse buttons, and can think about checking and changing the bin beneath when full. Workers in mid- to low Level 4 were monitored and assisted with these components, which involved problem solving and recall, and workers in Level 3 accessed procedural memories and recognition cues to spontaneously or with demonstration put the paper in; allowances were made for their function that resulted in slow, stop-and-go performance with no need to change a bin that didn't fill. Strategies are described fully elsewhere

(Burns & Buell, 1990; Ebbitt et al., 1989; Trafton, 2002), along with the early studies of the program. These studies demonstrated the feasibility of the program and worker productivity and satisfaction. Depression was significantly reduced in depressed people who entered the program, as compared to a control group (Ebbitt et al., 1989).

Fiscal decisions in regard to budget deficits and resources resulted in closing the AWP and transferring within a few weeks the former workers to the hospital's traditional Adult Day Health Care (ADHC) program, located adjacent to the AWP. Although some work activities were incorporated into the ADHC program, they were no longer adapted to the capabilities of the worker. However, the majority of the day was spent participating in the large-group leisure and verbal activities, such as bingo and current events. The former workers were assessed 4 months after the move (Burns et al., 2004).

For all 7 workers, observed scores were significantly lower than expected scores on both the MMSE and the CPT. In a paired-samples test, the mean difference between expected and observed MMSE scores was 4.9, with an expected mean of 17.7 and an observed mean of 12.9. MMSE score is expected to decline only 2 to 4 points a year in a person with AD (C. M. Clark et al., 1999; Han, Cole, Bellavance, McCusker, & Primeau, 2000).

The mean difference between expected and observed CPT was 0.64, with an expected mean of 4.7 and an observed mean of 4.0. Compared with a historical control group, the 7 workers declined at a significantly faster rate. Annual mean slope in CPT was −0.07 (0.32) for the former AWP workers compared with −0.40 (0.25) in a control group with longitudinal scores over a 4-year follow-up period ($N = 52$; Burns et al., 1994).

In this study (Burns et al., 2004), all participants declined rapidly in function after changing from the AWP to the ADHC. All spouse–caregivers reported ADL declines and an increase in their efforts at home. An ADL disability at a CPT score of 4.7 is associated with the initiation and organization of tasks, as in not knowing when to bathe or when or what clothes to change, as opposed to the inability to sequence the main components or steps of the task. Basic self-care activities are mildly impaired at 4.7, as sequencing skills and procedural memory for concrete familiar activity are intact. The observed CPT mean score after the move was 4.0, a level at which ADL performance shows not only the problems with initiation and organization but also the additional problems with attending to and sequencing the steps of these tasks. As a result, caregivers need to directly assist the person during the task. Thus, the difference in ADL ability between a score

of 4.7 and a score of 4.0 ranges from a decline in performance frequency necessitating reminders or prior setup, to the need for one-to-one care.

In the AWP, jobs were adapted by controlling for the types of cues involved according to each worker's cognitive level. This allowed workers to perform their jobs with relative ease or with repetitive, continuous performance. Continuous repetition of several task steps, within a variety of activities, allowed for the practice of procedural skills; practice may have translated into abilities in sequencing self-care activities at home.

As was mentioned earlier, evidence is growing that even severely impaired AD patients can learn and retain procedural tasks for at least 1 month when procedural memories are cued (and thereby activated) for retrieval under conditions of constant practice (Camp et al., 1996; Dick et al., 1996). The act of retrieval appears to have a mnemonic effect: A successful recall increases the chance of subsequent recall. Hence, the literature is beginning to document that procedural-memory-based retraining (or re-"activating") programs are worthwhile and have the potential to produce lasting changes. This body of research provides occupational therapy practitioners with empirical support for intervention strategies that have long been used to enable cognitively impaired older adults to relearn or retrieve basic ADLs (e.g., eating, bathing, dressing, toileting), or repetitive work and leisure tasks, by means of cued recognition and repetition of procedural memories within a controlled environment.

LONG-TERM CARE

Sevier and Gorek (2000) implemented the model of CPT assessment-driven care in a long-term care facility with dementia-specific secured units. Most individuals who reside in dementia specialty care are functioning in the moderate to severe stages of disease, where the caregiving and supervision needs become enormous. Cognitive Level 3 is associated with the moderate to severe stages of the disease, and although many individuals in later stages remain at home with family, Cognitive Level 3 is perhaps the most common level in which secured, institutional placement occurs. Thus, on any given unit the population of residents is proposed to be functioning primarily in Level 3, with some individuals admitted already in Level 4 and others admitted in or regressed to Level 2. Many facilities move individuals functioning in Level 1 to other units or to hospice care.

Caregiver assistance with ADL in Level 3 is one-to-one care, as the person uses mainly implicit-memory stores to

Table 14.2. Caregiver Education Chart

Allen Level	Normal Function	Difficulties	Caregiver Assistance
Level 6	Plans actions; anticipates effects; uses symbols and abstract ideas.	Independent.	None.
Level 5	Has poor short-term memory; problems with planning and judgment; may be hesitant or impulsive, may be anxious or depressed.	Difficulty with complex tasks, abstract thoughts, seeing the whole picture.	Encourage independence, watch for anxiety; simplify tasks; provide printed information; help plan ahead; point out consequences; help family to understand and support the person.
Level 4	Shows decline in many areas of thinking (orientation, perception, attention, concentration, language, coordination); is goal directed for familiar activity; needs visual cues; uses trial and error.	Increasing confusion and errors; inability to perform complex tasks accurately or safely; may have delusions, catastrophic reactions; needs supervision for hazardous activities; needs assistance with ADLs.	Set up items for each task; remove extra items from site; give simple and concrete directions; maintain simple daily routines; remind and help person to keep on track; monitor for safety and errors.
Level 3	Demonstrates generalized confusion; manual actions only (needs tactile cues); grasps and uses objects but is not aware of goal; may perseverate or misuse; often enjoys 1–1 social contact as a means to focus attention.	Profound confusion; may have restlessness, sleep disruption, psychotic ideation, agitation, and aggression in response to stress; reacts to many stresses; balance may show decline and increased risk for falls.	Simplify environment and approaches and interactions; give step-by-step help for basic tasks; hand items to the person (demonstrate, use simple nouns and verbs; remind when to go and stop); keep dangerous objects out of reach; provide object-centered repetitive leisure activity; monitor all activity.
Level 2	Exhibits posture actions only (little use of objects); slow reflexes; focuses attention on touch, movement, and sound, and things that come in contact with the body; may cooperate or resist care.	Needs total care; a risk for falls; may exhibit repetitive verbalization; grasping, pinching, or hitting others.	Learn efficient total care techniques for all ADLs, including dressing, bathing, toileting; may offer one food item and utensil at a time or finger foods and monitor for swallowing difficulties; provide stimuli in the environment (comforting textures, massage, range of motion, colorful or moving objects, music).
Level 1	Shows continual decline, uses reflex actions only (responds to internal stimuli), may respond to touch or being moved.	Needs total care: monitoring and comfort; increased risk of skin breakdown, aspiration, and infections; needs late-stage decisions regarding life-sustaining measures.	Comfort care; family support.

Note. ADL = activities of daily living.

function. Occupational therapists can aim to teach caregivers assistance techniques that allow the person to access these remaining abilities. Although procedural memories—for example, how to put the shirt on—can be accessed, working-memory and explicit stores are severely impaired, resulting in the person not knowing when to put the shirt on or take it off or how to use it within the context of the entire dressing task. This results in "confused" dressing behaviors, as in clothes put on inside out, fasteners left unadjusted, or clothing layered. Although some caregivers want to learn to facilitate functional abilities, as in handing the person one clothing item at a time,

for many it is often easier and faster for the caregiver to do the task for the person. Intervention plans consider the abilities of the caregiver as well as the needs of the person.

Caregiver education priorities are delineated in Table 14.2. Often, understanding the function and typical behaviors at each level is the priority, rather than teaching the caregiver to implement strategies that he or she finds to be time consuming. In long-term care, the lack of time is simply a reality. In this table, the function at each level is described as normal, with the difficulties at each level described as behavioral manifestations at that level.

Sevier and Gorek (2000) were concerned more about recreational programming than ADL programs. Although strategies for ADL intervention were incorporated, the focus was on changing the available activities throughout the day. Because most residents functioned in Level 3, activities were shifted to repetitive procedures, such as sorting and folding activities. Group activities, including verbal discussions and games, were mostly eliminated, as they involve explicit-memory stores. As a result, behavioral problems such as agitation were reportedly reduced with implementation of the new activity program.

SUMMARY

In this chapter we have reformulated theoretical tenets of the cognitive disability model in light of recent findings from the cognitive neuroscience and cognitive psychology literature. A theoretically sound conceptual model is essential for practitioners and caregivers in rehabilitation of dementias because it provides guidance for detecting the causes of cognitive impairments and behavioral symptoms, for understanding the meanings of behaviors, for developing effective assessment protocols, and for developing useful intervention strategies to maximize quality of life throughout the course of the disease. Strengthening the theoretical base of the model also enhances incentives for the research community to conduct research wherein multiple studies build on one another to create strong bodies of evidence for the profession.

Newly emerging findings from cognitive neuroscience and cognitive psychology expand the theoretical base of the cognitive disability model and provide an exciting opportunity to further our understanding of relationships between the information processes that underlie cognitive disabilities and the occupational limitations experienced by people with dementia. Development of the best possible management strategies for the cognitive and behavioral symptoms in dementia is as important for the quality of life of individuals with dementia as is management of pain for individuals with cancer (Volicer & Hurley, 2003).

REVIEW QUESTIONS

1. Describe how each of the three information-processing stages of cognition is affected by dementia.
2. Name three forms of long-term memory and describe how each is affected by dementia.
3. What is the focus of the reconsidered cognitive disability approach to the treatment of dementia?
4. How are activities analyzed in reconsidered cognitive disability theory?
5. How is the activity of driving analyzed; what is the difference between safe driving and operating the car?
6. Your client is at mid-Level 4. Describe the typical IADL errors and concerns associated with independent living at this cognitive level. Give some examples of compensations to promote remaining abilities and safety.
7. At which cognitive level can activities that use two- or three-step familiar motor actions with predictable visible results be accomplished successfully? How would this person's performance of IADLs be characterized?
8. Your client is at mid-Level 3. Describe the characteristics of appropriate activities, and give some examples. How would this person's performance of ADLs be characterized?
9. At which cognitive level would you use activities with one-step motor actions with highly familiar near-reflexive gross motor patterns that can be imitated? How would a person at this level of cognition perform ADLs?
10. How is an individual's cognitive level determined?
11. How does the CPT measure the progression from executive control to reliance on procedural-memory stores?
12. What are some indicators of the CPT's reliability and validity for different populations?

REFERENCES

Albert, M. S., Moss, M. B., Tanzi, R., & Jones, K. (2001). Preclinical prediction of AD using neuropsychological tests. *Journal of International Neuropsychology and Sociology, 7,* 631–639.

Allen, C. K. (1982). Independence through activity: The practice of occupational therapy (psychiatry). *American Journal of Occupational Therapy, 36,* 731–739.

Allen, C. K. (1985). *Occupational therapy for psychiatric diseases: Measurement and management of cognitive disabilities.* Boston: Little, Brown.

Allen, C. K. (1987). Activity: Occupational therapy's treatment method. *American Journal of Occupational Therapy, 41,* 563–575.

Allen, C. K. (1990). *Allen Cognitive Level (ACL) test manual.* Colchester, CT: S&S Worldwide.

Allen, C., & Blue, T. (1998). Cognitive disabilities model: How to make clinical judgments. In N. Katz (Ed.), *Cognition and occupation in rehabilitation: Cognitive models for interven-*

tion in occupational therapy (pp. 225–279). Rockville, MD: American Occupational Therapy Association.

Allen, C. K., Blue, T., & Earhart, C. A. (1995). *Understanding cognitive performance modes.* Ormond Beach, FL: Allen Conferences.

Allen, C. K., Earhart, C. A., & Blue, T. (1992). *Occupational therapy treatment goals for the physically and cognitively disabled.* Rockville, MD: American Occupational Therapy Association.

Allen C. K., Kehrberg, K., & Burns, T. (1992). Evaluation instruments. In C. K. Allen, C. A. Earhart, & T. Blue (Eds.) *Occupational therapy treatment goals for the physically and cognitively disabled* (pp. 46–50, 69–84). Rockville, MD: American Occupational Therapy Association.

American Psychiatric Association. (1994). *Diagnostic and statistical manual of mental disorders* (4th ed.). Washington, DC: Author.

Bachman, D. L., Wolf, P. A., Linn, R., Knoefel, J. E., Cobb, J., Belanger, A., et al. (1992). Prevalence of dementia and probable senile dementia of the Alzheimer type in the Framingham Study. *Neurology, 42,* 115–119.

Baltes, M. M. (1995). Dependency in old age: gains and losses. *Current Disability Psychology Science, 4,* 14–19.

Bares, K. (1998). *Neuropsychological predictors of functional level in Alzheimer's disease.* Unpublished doctoral dissertation, University of Minnesota.

Bar-Yosef, C., Weinblatt, N., & Katz, N. (1999). Reliability and validity of the Cognitive Performance Test (CPT) in an elderly population in Israel. *Physical & Occupational Therapy in Geriatrics, 17,* 65–79.

Baum, C. M., & Edwards, D. F. (1993). Cognitive performance in senile dementia of the Alzheimer's type: The Kitchen Task Assessment. *American Journal of Occupational Therapy, 47,* 431–436.

Beck, C. K., & Frank, L. B. (1997). Assessing functioning and self care abilities in Alzheimer's disease. *Alzheimer's Disease and Associated Disorders, 11* (Suppl. 6), 73–80.

Benjamin Rose Hospital Staff. (1959). Multidisciplinary studies of illness in aged persons: A new classification of functional status in activities of daily living. *Journal of Chronic Illness, 9,* 55–62.

Boyle, P. A., Malloy, P. F., Salloway, S., Cahn-Weiner, D. A., Cohen, R., & Cummings, J. L. (2003). Executive dysfunction and apathy predict functional impairment in Alzheimer disease. *American Journal of Geriatric Psychiatry, 11,* 214–221.

Burns, T. (1991). *Cognitive Performance Test (CPT): A measure of cognitive capacity for the performance of routine tasks.* Minneapolis: Geriatric Research, Education and Clinical Center, Minneapolis Veterans Affairs Medical Center.

Burns, T. (2002). *Cognitive Performance Test (CPT).* Minneapolis: Geriatric Research, Education and Clinical Center, Minneapolis Veterans Affairs Medical Center.

Burns, T. (in press). *Cognitive Performance Test (CPT).* Pequannock, NJ: Ableware, Maddak Inc.

Burns, T., & Buell, J. (1990). The effectiveness of work programming with an Alzheimer population. *Occupational Therapy Practice, 1,* 64–73.

Burns, T., McCarten, J. R., Adler, G., Bauer, M., & Kuskowski, M. A. (2004). Effects of repetitive work on maintaining function in Alzheimer's disease patients. *American Journal of Alzheimer's Disease and Other Dementias, 19,* 39–44.

Burns, T., Mortimer, J. A., & Merchek, P. (1994). Cognitive Performance Test: A new approach to functional assessment in Alzheimer's disease. *Journal of Geriatric Psychiatry and Neurology, 7,* 46–54.

Camp, C., Foss, J., O'Hanlon, A., & Stevens, A. (1996). Memory interventions for persons with dementia. *Applied Cognitive Psychology, 10,* 193–210.

Canadian Study of Health and Aging: Study methods and prevalence of dementia. (1994). *Canadian Medical Association Journal, 150,* 899–913.

Christiansen, C., & Baum, C. M. (1997). Person–environment occupational performance: A conceptual model for practice. In C. Christiansen & C. M. Baum (Eds.), *Occupational therapy: Enabling function and well-being* (2nd ed., pp. 46–71) Thorofare, NJ: Slack.

Clark, C. M, Sheppard, L., Fillenbaum, G. G., Galasko, D., Morris, J. C., Koss, E., et al. (1999). Variability in annual Mini-Mental State Examination score in patients with probable Alzheimer disease: A clinical perspective of data from the Consortium to Establish a Registry for Alzheimer's Disease. *Archives of Neurology, 56,* 857–862.

Clark, F., Azen, S. P., Zemke, R., Jackson, J., Carlson, M., Mandel, D., et al. (1997). Occupational therapy for independent-living older adults: A randomized controlled trial. *Journal of the American Medical Association, 278,* 1321–1326.

Cohen-Mansfield, J., Lipson, S., Brenneman, K. S., & Pawlson, L. G. (2001). Health status of participants in adult day care centers. *Journal of Health and Social Policy, 14,* 71–89.

Collette, F., Van der Linden, M., Bechet, S., & Salmon, E. (1999). Phonological loop and central executive functioning in Alzheimer's disease. *Neuropsychologia, 37,* 905–918.

Craik, F. I., & Jennings, J. (1992). Human memory. In F. Craik & T. Salthouse (Eds.), *Handbook of memory disorders* (pp. 51–110). New York: Wiley.

Demers, L., Oremus, M., Perrault, A., & Wolfson, C. (2000). Review of outcome measurement instruments in drug trials: Introduction. *Journal of Geriatric Psychiatry and Neurology, 13,* 161–169.

Dick, M., Shankle, R., Bet, R., Dick-Muehlke, C., Cotman, C., & Kean, M. (1996). Acquisition and long-term retention of a gross motor skill in Alzheimer's disease patients under constant and varied practice conditions. *Journal of Gerontology, 51B,* P103–P111.

Duchek, J. M., Cheney, M., Ferraro, F. R., & Storandt, M. (1991). Paired associate learning in senile dementia of the Alzheimer type. *Archives of Neurology, 48,* 1038–1040.

Duke, L. M., Seltzer, B., Seltzer, J. E., & Vasterling, J. J. (2002). Cognitive components of deficit awareness in Alzheimer's disease. *Neuropsychology, 16,* 359–369.

Duran, L., & Fisher, A. (1999). Evaluation and intervention with executive functions impairment. In C. Unsworth (Ed.), *Cognitive and perceptual dysfunction: A clinical reasoning approach to evaluation and intervention* (pp. 209–255). Philadelphia: F. A. Davis.

Earhart, C. A., Allen, C. K., & Blue, T. (1993). *Allen Diagnostic Module: Instruction manual.* Colchester, CT: S&S Worldwide.

Ebbitt, B., Burns, T, & Christiansen, R. (1989). Work therapy: Intervention for community-based Alzheimer's patients. *American Journal of Alzheimer's Care and Related Disorders & Research, 4,* 7–15.

Esiri, M., Lee, V., & Trojanowski, J. (2004). *The neuropathology of dementia* (2nd ed.). New York: Cambridge University Press.

Evans, D. A., Funkenstein, H. H., Albert, M. S., Scherr, P. A., Cook, N. R., Chown, M. J., et al. (1989). Prevalence of Alzheimer's disease in a community population of older persons: Higher than previously reported. *Journal of the American Medical Association, 262,* 2551–2556.

Fillenbaum, G. G., Heyman, A., Huber, M. S., Woodbury, M. A., Leiss, J., Schmader, K. E., et al. (1998). The prevalence and 3-year incidence of dementia in older Black and White community residents. *Journal of Clinical Epidemiology, 51,* 587–595.

Fisher, A. G. (1997). An expanded rehabilitative model of practice. In A. G. Fisher (Ed.), *Assessment of motor and process skills* (2nd ed., pp. 73–85). Fort Collins, CO: Three Star Press.

Folstein, M. F., Folstein, S. E., & McHugh, P. R. (1975). Mini-Mental State: A practical method for grading the cognitive state of patients for the clinician. *Journal of Psychiatric Research, 12,* 189–198.

Galasko, D., Bennett, D., Sano, M., Ernesto, C., Thomas, R., Grundman, M., et al. (1997). An inventory to assess the activities of daily living for clinical trials in Alzheimer's disease. *Alzheimer's Disease and Associated Disorders, 11,* 533–539.

Gauthier, S., Gelinas, I., & Gauthier, L. (1997). Functional disability in Alzheimer's disease. *International Psychogeriatrics, 9*(Suppl. 1), 163–165.

Gelinas, I., Gauthier, L., McIntyre, M., & Gauthier, S. (1999). Development of a functional measure for persons with Alzheimer's disease: The Disability Assessment for Dementia. *American Journal of Occupational Therapy, 53,* 471–481.

Giovannetti, T., Libon, D., Buxbaum, L., & Schwartz, M. (2002). Naturalistic action impairments in dementia. *Neuropsychologia, 40,* 1220–32.

Glosser, G., Gallo, J., Duda, N., de Vries, J. J., Clark, C. M., & Grossman, M. (2002). Visual perceptual functions predict instrumental activities of daily living in patients with dementia. *Neuropsychiatry and Neuropsychological Behavioral Neurology, 15,* 198–206.

Goldberg, E. (2001). *The executive brain: Frontal lobes and the civilized mind.* New York: Oxford University Press.

Granger, C. V., Hamilton, B. B., Keith, R. A., Zielezny, M., & Sherwin, F. S. (1986). Advances in functional assessment for medical rehabilitation. *Topics in Geriatric Rehabilitation, 1,* 59–74.

Graves, A. B., Larson, E. B., Edlund, S. D., Bowen, J. D., McCormick, W. C., McCurry, S. M., et al. (1996). Prevalence of dementia and its subtypes in the Japanese American population of King County, Washington state: The Kame Project. *American Journal of Epidemiology, 144,* 760–771.

Grut, M., Jorm, A. F., Fratiglioni, L., Forsell, Y., Viitanen, M., & Winblad, B. (1993). Memory complaints of elderly people in a population survey: Variation according to dementia stage and depression. *Journal of the American Geriatric Society, 41,* 1295–1300.

Gutterman, E. M., Markowitz, J. S., Lewis, B., & Fillit, H. (1999). Cost of Alzheimer's disease and related dementia in managed-Medicare. *Journal of the American Geriatric Society, 47,* 1065–1071.

Haist, F., Gore, J., & Mao, H. (2001). Consolidation of human memory over decades revealed by functional magnetic resonance imaging. *Nature Neuroscience, 4,* 1139–1145.

Han, L., Cole, M., Bellavance, F., McCusker, J., & Primeau, F. (2000). Tracking cognitive decline in Alzheimer's disease using the Mini-Mental State Examination: A meta-analysis. *International Psychogeriatrics, 12,* 231–247.

Hasher, L., Tonev, S., Lustig, C., & Zacks, R. (2001). Inhibitory control, environmental support, and self-initiated processing in aging. In M. Naveh-Benjamin, M. Moscovitch, & R. L. Roedinger (Eds.), *Perspectives on human memory and cognitive aging: Essays in honour of Fergus Craik* (pp. 286–297). East Sussex, England: Psychology Press.

Hasher, L., & Zacks, R. (1988). Working memory comprehension and aging: A review and new view. In G. Bower (Ed.), *The psychology of learning and motivation: Advances in research and theory* (Vol. 22, pp. 193–225). New York: Academic Press.

Health Care Financing Administration. (1989). *Outpatient occupational therapy Medicare Part B guidelines* (DHHS Transmittal No. 55). In *Health Insurance Manual* (pp. 71–83). Baltimore: Author.

Heilman, K., & Valenstein, E. (Eds.). (1993). *Clinical neuropsychology.* New York: Oxford University Press.

Hendrie, H. C., Osuntokun, B. O., Hall, K. S., Ogunniyi, A. O., Hui, S. L., Unverzagt, F. W., et al. (1995). Prevalence of Alzheimer's disease and dementia in two communities: Nigerian Africans and African Americans. *American Journal of Psychiatry, 152,* 1485–1492.

Heying, L. M. (1985). Research with subjects having senile dementia. In C. K. Allen (Ed.), *Occupational therapy for psychiatric diseases: Measurement and management of cognitive disabilities* (pp. 339–362). Boston: Little, Brown.

Heyman, A., Peterson, B., Fillenbaum, G., & Pieper, C. (1996). The Consortium to Establish a Registry for Alzheimer's Disease (CERAD), Part XIV: Demographic and clinical predictors of survival in patients with Alzheimer's disease. *Neurology, 46,* 656–660.

Hodges, J. R., Patterson, K., Oxbury, S., & Funnell, E. (1992). Semantic dementia: Progressive fluent aphasia with temporal lobe atrophy. *Brain, 115,* 1783–1806.

Holm, A., Michel, M., Stern, G. A., Hung, T. M., Klein, T., Flaherty, L., Michel, S., & Maletta, G. (1999). The outcomes of an inpatient treatment program for geriatric patients with dementia and dysfunctional behaviors. *The Gerontologist, 39,* 668–676.

Hughes, C., Berg, L., Danzinger, W., Coben, L., & Martin, R. (1982). A new clinical scale for the staging of dementia. *British Journal of Psychiatry, 140,* 566–572.

Jagger, C., Anderson, K., Breteler, M. M., Copeland, J. R., Helmer, C., Baldereschi, M., et al. (2000). Prognosis with dementia in Europe: A collaborative study of population-based cohorts. *Neurology, 54*(11, Suppl. 5), S16–S20.

Jennings-Pikey, M. (2001). *A validation study of the Cognitive Performance Test.* Unpublished doctoral dissertation, Wheaton College.

Katz, S., Ford, A. B., Moskowitz, R. W., Jackson, B. A., & Jaffee, M. W. (1963). Studies of illness in the aged. *Journal of the American Medical Association, 185,* 914–919.

Kehrberg, K. L., Kuskowski, M. A., Mortimer, J. A., & Shoberg, T. D. (1992). Validating the use of an enlarged, easier-to-see Allen Cognitive Level Test in geriatrics. *Physical & Occupational Therapy in Geriatrics, 10,* 1–14.

Kluger, A., & Ferris, S. (1991). Scales for the assessment of Alzheimer's disease. *Psychiatric Clinics of North America, 14,* 309–326.

Knopman, D. S., Bradley, F. B., & Peterson, R. C. (2003). Essentials of the proper diagnoses of mild cognitive impairment, dementia, and major subtypes of dementia. *Mayo Clinic Practice, 78,* 1290–1308.

Kohlman-Thomson, L. (1992). *Kohlman Evaluation of Living Skills.* Bethesda: American Occupational Therapy Association.

LaBarge, E., Smith, D. S., Dick, L., & Storandt, M. (1992). Agraphia in dementia of the Alzheimer type. *Archives of Neurology, 49,* 1151–1156.

Lawton, M. P., & Brody, E. (1969). Assessment of older people: Self-maintaining and instrumental activities of daily living. *The Gerontologist, 9,* 179–186.

Leiter, F., & Cummings, J. (1999). Pharmacological interventions in Alzheimer's disease. In D. Stuss, G. Winicur, & I. Robertson (Eds.), *Cognitive neurorehabilitation* (pp. 153–173). New York: Cambridge University Press.

Letts, L., Baum, C. M., & Perlmutter, M. (2003, June 2). Person–environment–occupation assessment with older adults. *OT Practice, 8*(10), 27–33.

Levy, L. (1974). Movement therapy for psychiatric patients. *American Journal of Occupational Therapy, 28,* 354–357.

Levy, L. L. (1986a). Cognitive treatment. In L. J. Davis & M. Kirkland (Eds.), *Role of occupational therapy with the elderly* (pp. 289–324). Bethesda, MD: American Occupational Therapy Association.

Levy, L. L. (1986b). A practical guide to the care of the Alzheimer's disease victim: The cognitive disability perspective. *Topics in Geriatric Rehabilitation, 1,* 16–26.

Levy, L. L. (1989). Activity adaptation in rehabilitation of the physically and cognitively disabled aged. *Topics in Geriatric Rehabilitation, 4,* 53–66.

Levy, L. L. (1996a). Cognitive integration and cognitive components. In K. O. Larson, R. Stevens-Ratchford, L. Pedretti, & J. Crabtree (Eds.), *The role of occupational therapy with the elderly (ROTE)* (2nd ed., pp. 573–598). Rockville, MD: American Occupational Therapy Association.

Levy, L. L. (1996b). Health and impairment: The performance context. In K. O. Larson, R. Stevens-Ratchford, L. Pedretti, & J. Crabtree (Eds.), *The role of occupational therapy with the elderly (ROTE)* (2nd ed., pp. 169–198). Rockville, MD: American Occupational Therapy Association.

Levy, L. L. (1998). Cognitive disabilities model in rehabilitation of older adults with dementia. In N. Katz (Ed.), *Cognition and occupation in rehabilitation: Cognitive models for intervention in occupational therapy* (pp. 195–221). Rockville, MD: American Occupational Therapy Association.

Levy, L. L. (1999, Nov 8). Memory: An overview for cognitive rehabilitation intervention. *OT Practice, 4*(9), CE1–CE8.

Lezak, M. (1995). *Neurological assessment.* New York: Oxford University Press.

Lopez, J. (2000). Shaky memories in indelible ink. *Nature Reviews Neuroscience, 1,* 6–7.

Luria, A. (1966). *Higher cortical functions in man.* New York: Basic Books.

MacKeigan, L. D., & Pathak, D. S. (1992). Overview of health-related quality-of-life measures. *American Journal of Hospital Pharmacology, 49,* 2236–2245.

Maddox, M. K., & Burns, T. (1997). Positive approaches to dementia care in the home. *Geriatrics, 52*(Suppl. 2), 54–58.

Mangone, C. A., Hier, D. B., Gorelick, P. B., Ganellen, R. J., Langenberg, P., Boarman, R., & Dollear, W. C. (1991). Impaired insight in Alzheimer's disease. *Journal of Geriatric Psychiatry and Neurology, 4,* 189–193.

Mayeux, R., & Sano, M. (1999). Treatment of Alzheimer's disease. *New England Journal of Medicine, 341,* 1670–1679.

McKeith, I. G., Cummings, J. L., Lovestone, S., Harvey, R. J., & Wilkinson, D. J. (Eds.). (1999). *Outcome measures in Alzheimer's disease.* London: Martin Dunitz.

Mendez, M. F., Mendez M. A., Martin, R., Smyth, K. A., & Whitehouse, P. J. (1990). Complex visual disturbances in Alzheimer's disease. *Neurology, 40,* 439–443.

Mesulam, M. (2002). The human frontal lobes: Transcending the default mode through contingent encoding. In D. Stuss & R. Knight (Eds.), *Principles of frontal lobe function* (pp. 8–30). New York: Oxford University Press.

Nebes, R. D. (1992). Cognitive dysfunction in Alzheimer's disease. In F. Craik & T. Salthouse (Eds.), *The handbook of aging and cognition* (p. 373–445). Hillsdale, NJ: Erlbaum.

Nelson, C. (1995). The ontogeny of human memory: A cognitive neuroscience perspective. *Developmental Psychology, 31,* 723–738.

Ostwald, S. K., Hepburn, K. W., Caron, W., Burns, T., & Mantell, R. (1999). Reducing caregiver burden: A randomized psychoeducational intervention for caregivers for persons with dementia. *The Gerontologist, 39,* 299–309.

Ott, B. R., Lafleche, G., Whelihan, W. M., Buongiorno, G. W., Albert, M. S., & Fogel, B. S. (1996). Impaired awareness of deficits in Alzheimer disease. *Alzheimer Disease and Associated Disorders, 10,* 68–76.

Perry, R. J., & Hodges, J. R. (2000). Relationship between functional and neuropsychological performance in early Alzheimer disease. *Alzheimer Disease and Associated Disorders, 14,* 1–10.

Peterson, R. C., Smith, G. E., Waring, S. C., Ivnik, R. J., Tangalos, E. G., & Kokmen, E. (1999). Mild cognitive impairment: Clinical characterization and outcome. *Archives of Neurology, 56,* 303–308.

Pfeffer, R. (1995). A social function measure in the staging and study of dementia. In M. Bergener, J. Brocklehurst, & S. Finkel (Eds.), *Aging, health and healing* (p. 618). New York: Springer.

Pfeffer, R., Kurosaki, T., Harrah, C., Chance, J., & Filos, S. (1982). Measurement of functional activities in older adults in the community. *Journal of Gerontology, 37,* 323–329.

Piaget, J. (1970). Piaget's theory. In P. H. Mussen (Ed.), *Carmichael's manual of child psychology* (pp. 703–732). New York: Wiley.

Rapp, B., & Caramazza, A. (1989). General to specific access to word meaning: A claim re-examined. *Cognitive Neuropsychology, 6,* 251–272.

Ready, R. E, Ott, B. R., Grace, J., & Cahn-Weiner, D. A. (2003). Apathy and executive dysfunction in mild cognitive impairment and Alzheimer disease. *American Journal of Psychiatry, 11,* 222–228.

Reisberg, B., Ferris, S., Leon, M., & Cook, T. (1982). The global deterioration scale for the assessment of primary degenerative dementia. *American Journal of Occupational Therapy, 139,* 1136–1139.

Reisberg, B., Franssen, E., Souren, L., Auer, S., Akram, I., & Kenowsky, S. (2002). Evidence and mechanisms of retrogenesis in Alzheimer's and other dementias: Management and treatment import. *American Journal of Alzheimers and Other Dementias, 17,* 160–174.

Reisberg, B., Franssen, E., Souren, L., Auer, S., & Kenowskky, S. (1998). Progression of Alzheimer's disease: Variability and consistency: Ontogenic models, their applicability and relevance. *Journal of Neural Transmission, 54,* 9–20.

Reisberg, B., Kenowsky, S., Franssen, E., Auer, S., & Souren, L. (1999). Toward a science of Alzheimer's disease management: A model based upon current knowledge of retrogenesis. *International Psychogeriatrics, 11,* 7–23.

Robnett, R. (1995, June 8). Is your client safe at home? *OT Week,* 22–23.

Rubin, D. (1998). Things learned early in adulthood are remembered best. *Memory & Cognition, 26,* 3–19.

Salthouse, T. (2004). What and when of cognitive aging. *Current directions in psychological science, 13,* 140–144.

Salthouse, T., & Babcock, R. (1991). Decomposing adult age differences in working memory. *Developmental Psychology, 27,* 763–776.

Scalen, S., & Reisberg, B. (1992). Functional Assessment Staging (FAST) in Alzheimer's disease: Reliability, validity, ordinality. *International Psychogeriatrics, 4,* 66–69.

Schacter, D. (1983). Amnesia observed: Remembering and forgetting in a natural environment. *Journal of Abnormal Psychology, 92,* 236–242.

Schwartz, M. (1995). Re-examining the role of executive functions in routine action production. In J. Grafman, K. Holyoak, & F. Boller (Eds.), *Annals of the New York Academy of Sciences: Vol. 769. Structure and function of the human prefrontal cortex* (pp. 321–335). New York: New York Academy of Sciences.

Schwartz, M., Mayer, N., Fitzpatrik-DeSalme, E., & Montgomery, M. (1993). Cognitive theory and the study of everyday action disorders after brain damage. *Journal of Head Trauma Rehabilitation, 8,* 59–72.

Seltzer, B., Vasterling, J. J., Mathias, C. W., & Brennan, A. (2001). Clinical and neuropsychological correlates of impaired awareness of deficits in Alzheimer disease and Parkinson disease: A comparative study. *Neuropsychiatry and Neuropsychology Behavioral Neurology, 14,* 122–129.

Sevier, S., & Gorek, B. (2000). Cognitive evaluation in care planning for people with Alzheimer disease and related dementias. *Geriatric Nursing, 21,* 92–97.

Shallice, T., & Burgess, P. W. (1991). Deficits in strategy application following frontal lobe damage in man. *Brain, 114,* 727–741.

Small, G., Rabins, P., Barry, P., Buckholtz, N., DeKosky, S., Ferris, S., et. al. (1997). Diagnosis and treatment of Alzheimer's disease and related disorders: Consensus statement. *Journal of the American Medical Association, 278,* 1363–1371.

Stern, Y., Hesdorffer, D., Sano, M., & Mayeux, R. (1990). Measurement and prediction of functional capacity in Alzheimer's disease. *Neurology, 40,* 8–14.

Stout, J. C., Wyman, M. F., Johnson, S. A., Peavy, G. M., & Salmon, D. P. (2003). Frontal behavioral syndromes and functional status in probable Alzheimer disease. *American Journal of Geriatric Psychiatry, 11,* 683–686.

Stringer, A. Y. (2003). Cognitive rehabilitation practice patterns: A survey of American Hospital Association rehabilitation programs. *Clinical Psychologist, 17,* 34–44.

Tabert, M. H., Albert, S. M., Borukhova-Milov, L., Camacho, Y., Pelton, G., Liu, X., et al. (2002). Functional deficits in patients with mild cognitive impairment: Prediction of AD. *Neurology, 58,* 758–764.

Tekin, S., Fairbanks, L. A., O'Connor, S., Rosenberg, S., & Cummings, J. L. (2001). Activities of daily living in Alzheimer's disease: Neuropsychiatric, cognitive, and medical illness influences. *American Journal of Geriatric Psychiatry, 9,* 81–86.

Tetewsky, S., & Duffy, C. (1999). Visual loss and getting lost in Alzheimer's disease. *Neurology, 52,* 958–965.

Thralow, J. U., & Rueter, M. S. (1993). Activities of daily living and cognitive levels of function in dementia. *American Journal of Alzheimer's Care and Related Disorders & Research, 8,* 14–19.

Tomoeda, C., Bayles, K., Trosset, M., Azuma, T., & McGeagh, A. (1996). Cross sectional analysis of Alzheimer's disease effects on oral discourse in a picture description task. *Alzheimer's Disease and Associated Disorders, 10,* 204–215.

Trafton, E. (2002). The Adapted Work Program and its application in VA hospitals and other facilities: An interview with Theressa Burns. *Activities Directors' Quarterly for Alzheimer's and Other Dementia Patients, 3,* 4–10.

Tulving, E. (1985). How many memory systems are there? *American Psychologist, 40,* 385–398.

Ustun, T. B., Chatterji, S., Bickenbach, J., Kostanjsek, N., & Schneider, M. (2003). The International Classification of Functioning, Disability and Health: A new tool for understanding disability and health. *Disability and Rehabilitation, 25,* 565–571.

Volicer, L., & Hurley, A. (2003). Management of behavioral symptoms in progressive degenerative dementias. *Journal of Gerontology, 58,* M837–M845.

Wachtel-Spector, N. (2003). Examining awareness to functional cognitive level among elderly living in the community following stroke. Unpublished master's thesis, Hebrew University of Jerusalem.

Ward, S. W., & Kuskowski, M. A. (1999). *Usage patterns in practice: The Cognitive Performance Test in VA medical centers and Minnesota health care facilities* (Minneapolis Geriatric Research, Education and Clinical Center annual report). Minneapolis: Publisher.

Wechsler, D. (1997). *Wechsler Adult Intelligence Scale* (3rd ed.). San Antonio, Psychological Corporation.

Wiener, J. M., Hanley, R. J., Clarke, C., & Van Norstrand, J. F. (1990). Measuring the activities of daily living: Comparisons across national surveys. *Journal of Gerontology, 45,* S229–S237.

Wilcock, A. A. (1998). Reflections on doing, being and becoming. *La revue Canadienne d'ergothérapie, 65,* 248.

Willis, S. L., & Schaie, K. W. (1994). Assessing everyday competence in the elderly. In C. B. Fischer & R. M. Lerner (Eds.), *Applied developmental psychology* (p. 62). New York: McGraw-Hill.

World Health Organization. (1980). *International classification of impairments, disabilities, and handicaps: A manual of classification relating to the consequences of disease.* Geneva, Switzerland: Author.

World Health Organization. (2001). *International Classification of Functioning, Disability and Health.* Geneva, Switzerland: Author.

APPENDIX 14.1. CASE EXAMPLE: MR. B.

JUNE 2002

REASON FOR REQUEST: (complaints and findings)

76 y. o. man with MCI has a MMSE of 27/30. Please evaluate functional status.

PROVISIONAL DIAGNOSIS: Mild Cognitive Impairment

TITLE: GRECC Consult

SUBJECT: Cognitive–Functional Evaluation

Mr. B. was evaluated for 60 minutes with the Large Allen Cognitive Level Screen (LACLS) and Cognitive Performance Test (CPT). He reports problems with his memory but denies any impact on function or IADL. His son, who he has been staying with while he receives treatment at the hospital, reports occasional mistakes in the Pt.'s set-up of medications and reports assisting him with refills. Son also reports monitoring Pt.'s bills due to errors including overpayments. Pt. may go back to his home in Texas where he drives and has access to a gun. Concern about impulsive behavior with the gun was expressed by his son.

CPT Scores

Medbox: 4.5/6—Made errors in following new label directions on 3 of 4 bottles; not able to correct the box when cued to specific errors.
Shop: 5.0/6—Able to select and pay with inefficiency and error; able to correct with cue.
Wash: 5.0/5—Completed concrete task.
Toast: 4.0/5—Completed task with cue to operate toaster.
Phone: 5.0/6—Able to locate #, and obtain partial info requested.
Dress: 4.0/5—Completed task; selection was not the best choice for hypothetical conditions.
Travel: 6.0/6—Followed simple map to destination.

TOTAL: 33.5/39 = 4.8/5.6   LACLS (lacing screen): 4.8/5.8

Mr. B.'s performance indicates an Allen Cognitive Level of 4.8/6. Persons who function at 4.8 demonstrate mild to moderate deficits in task planning and problem solving abilities, depending on the complexity/familiarity of the task. These deficits interfere with efficient and error-free performance of complex and hazardous tasks. Discussed IADL errors noticed by son as typical for this level of function. Discussed needs for assistance with managing medications and finances. Discussed risks associated with hazardous activities and independent living in Texas. Discussed assisted living options with son or the MN Veterans Home. Issued Caregiving Guidance Handout 5.0. Recommend a Driver's evaluation.

JUNE 2002

REASON FOR REQUEST: (complaints and findings)
Please evaluate ability to safely operate a motor vehicle.

PROVISIONAL DIAGNOSIS: Mild Cognitive Impairment

TITLE: Driver Training Consult

SUBJECT: Mr. B. was seen for 120 minutes of driving evaluation

Background Information: Pt. lives in Texas and reports that he drives 3 times a week. He drives 6 to 7 blocks on relatively busy streets to get to the grocery store and gas station. He reports that he does not drive at night. Son reports concerns about Pt.'s driving because Pt. tends to be impulsive and he drives on busy streets. Pt. has no family in Texas and one neighbor with whom he does things occasionally.

Vision: Pt.'s vision was evaluated with the Bausch & Lomb Occupation Vision Test. Pt. scored in the normal range for far lateral and vertical phoria, and near acuity in both eyes. Pt. scored below standard range for far acuity in both eyes, and depth perception in right eye.

Reaction Time: Pt.'s reaction time was tested using a simulator. Pt. scored 68.5 feet. A normal and safe reaction time is 60 feet or less which is the distance a vehicle travels before one is able to get the foot to the brake when a stimuli to do an emergency stop is presented. Pt.'s reaction time is slightly delayed.

Written Examination: Pt. was given a test of 24 multiple-choice questions of the knowledge of the rules of the road. Pt. scored 14/24 correct which gives him a score of 58%. A score of 80% is needed to pass the state written examination in Minnesota.

Behind-the-Wheel Examination: Pt. was taken to a low traffic area where the speed limit does not exceed 35 mph. No stoplights are present, nor highway or freeway driving. During the evaluation, Pt.'s performance was as follows:

Gas and brake coordination:	Good
Signaling:	Poor; Pt. did not use signals at all throughout the evaluation
Right turns:	Poor; made turns too wide and too fast
Left turns:	Fair; made turns too fast

(continued)

APPENDIX 14.1. CASE EXAMPLE: MR. B. *(Continued)*

Identify changing conditions:	Fair; needed cueing to slow down for ruts in the road
Scanning techniques:	Fair
Regulation of speed:	Poor; drove faster than posted speeds on occasions, did not slow down soon enough for turns
Keep car on straightaway:	Good
Stops:	Poor; did not stop behind signs and occasionally did not come to a complete stop
Lane change:	Poor; did not check mirrors or blind spots, did not signal
Parallel park:	Fair; did not signal, hit curb
U-turn:	Good
Backing up:	Fair; drove too fast, needed to be told 2–3 times when to stop

Behavior/Attitude: Pt. was generally pleasant throughout the testing but did not understand why he had to drive in Minnesota because he never drives here. When Pt. was informed that he did not use the signals on the road test, he insisted that he had.

Assessment: Based on this evaluation, Pt. presents with cognitive impairments particularly in the areas of judgment, awareness, impulsivity, and executive functioning that greatly impact his ability to safely operate a motor vehicle. Based on this evaluation, Pt. did not pass a written test or a road test.

Plan: It is recommended that the Pt. not drive. The results of the evaluation were discussed with Pt. and son. No further driving evaluation or training at the VA is indicated.

MAY 2003

REASON FOR REQUEST (complaints and findings)
77 y. o. with progressive dementia here s/p hip revision due to multiple dislocations (x6) since 6/01. Patient has been more difficult to manage at home due to increased dementia. Son would like testing to evaluate appropriate level of care needed. Will need input for short and long term placement plan.

PROVISIONAL DIAGNOSIS: Alzheimer's disease

TITLE: GRECC Consult

SUBJECT: Cognitive–Functional Evaluation

Mr. B. was evaluated for 60 minutes with the Large Allen Cognitive Level Screen (LACLS), Cognitive Performance Test (CPT), and MMSE. He was alone. Previous scores are available for comparison. Pt. reports that he stays with his son to be close to the Minneapolis VA. He reports that he spends 90% of his time in the hospital due to a hip replacement. He reports that he rents his home in Texas to relatives who pay for the upkeep of the home and his car. He reports that his memory is "not worth a damn" since (skin) cancer operations on his head and brain. He reports that his son works a lot and that he is often home alone. He reports that he makes oatmeal for breakfast and prepares frozen dinners. Per chart review, his son reports that he prepares meals and uses the microwave less often now. Pt. reports that his son sets up his medications, which he takes several times a day from a pillbox. He describes his daily routine to include smoking on the porch as his son does not allow it in the house, and reading western magazines.

CPT Scores:

Medbox: 4.5/6—made errors in following new label directions on 2 of 4 bottles; not able to correct the box when cued to specific errors.
Shop: 4.0/6—needed step-by-step assist to select and pay; not able to attend to multiple details simultaneously.
Wash: 5.0/5—completed concrete task.
Toast: 5.0/5—completed concrete task.
Phone: 4.0/6—not able to locate # in the phone book; when given #, able to dial and obtain info.
Dress: 4.0/5—completed task; selection was not the best choice for hypothetical conditions.
Travel: 5.0/6—followed simple map with error and self-correction to destination.

TOTAL: 31.5/39 = 4.5/5.6   LACLS: 4.8 today and 5/02.   CPT from 5/02: 4.8/5.6   MMSE: 26/30 today vs. 27/30 in 5/02.

Mr. B.'s performance indicates an Allen Cognitive Level of 4.5/6, and represents decline from 4.8 in 5/02. Persons who function at 4.5 demonstrate moderate deficits in task planning, judgment, problem solving, and new learning abilities. These deficits interfere with or prevent safe and accurate performance of complex tasks. Following safety precautions at 4.5 will be inconsistent, as learning abilities for safety procedures do not generalize or are impaired.

Fall prevention strategies need to be implemented since Pt. will not consistently use safety precautions (night light, clear floors, sturdy shoes, grab bars, easy access to and monitoring use of his walker for safety and consistency).

Meal preparation at 4.5 becomes difficult as the person experiences planning errors with food preparations, or may not think to eat or follow schedules. May want to consider MOW or leaving prepared food out in a visible place.

Compliance with following medication regimes even with a set-up is often inconsistent or with some error at 4.5.

Persons at this level of function are good candidates for assisted living environments. Home alone poses risks for safety and inconsistent follow through with meals and medications.   *(continued)*

APPENDIX 14.1. CASE EXAMPLE: MR. B. *(Continued)*

MAY 13, 2003

REASON FOR REQUEST: (complaints and findings) Looking at AL vs NH placement. Would ask that you work with Pt. for pathfinding and memory regarding being able to get himself to smoker and back. AL possibility has outside smoking and Pt. would need to remember to only smoke outside, get himself outside and back in successfully. This AL provides all meals, cleaning, laundry, activities, etc. Please recommend how to assess and/or achieve this goal.

PROVISIONAL DIAGNOSIS: Dementia, hip dislocation

PRECAUTIONS/RESTRICTIONS: Patient is on wandergaurd and yellow vest programs. Also has had unpredictable behavior in past (agitation, i.e. when son took him out on pass recently, he would not get out of the car to return to VAMC at first)

TITLE: GRECC Consult

SUBJECT: AL vs NH placement; pathfinding capacity

Mr. B. was recently evaluated for cognitive–functional abilities and limitations according to the Allen scale; see GRECC OT note dated 5/1/03. The Allen cognitive levels range from normal at level 6, to profound disability at level 1. Mr. B. scored 4.5 on this scale. Persons who function at 4.5 demonstrate moderate deficits in task planning, problem-solving, and learning capabilities. Therefore, training needs to be in context or done at the actual site of the activity; learning does not generalize well at this level of function. Pathfinding along simple routes is feasible at 4.5, with much repetition needed to learn the route.

Recommend that staff at the AL provide repetitive drills, and supervise Pt. initially; training could take several weeks. Pt is already in the habit of smoking outside only while living with his son. Care must be taken to note when smoking is no longer safe, with further disease progression. By level 3, persons are apraxic and access to hazardous objects needs to be restricted, as does independent trips to the smoker.

Pt.'s feelings or response to moving to the AL can serve as an indicator of flight risk; for example, if he does not want to live there or thinks that he will be going back to his son's home, this increases the risk of him leaving the facility. Recommend that Pt. visit the facility and assess his response. In general, persons who function at 4.5 are good candidates for AL. With further disease progression, a more restricted environment will be necessary.

While Pt. is here, staff could allow him to try and direct (point) the way out to the smoker, using the exact route each time.

NURSING PROGRESS NOTES

5-14-03 15:00

Pathfinding for smoking has gone well per physical therapy. Patient is approved for trial independent smoking. Plan will be for Pt. to sign in/out and leave gold vest at the desk while he is outside. Son supports this plan.

5-14-03 22:58

Patient went out to smoke ×3. Pt. did walk down to 1f ward first and staff from 1f brought Pt. back to see if he could be off ward. Pt. did return to ward on own. Signed out with some instruction and signed back in upon return. Will continue to monitor.

5-15-03 07:06

Patient awake for 0500 IV and oral meds. Has not requested to leave ward this shift. Out at nurses desk area at 0630, talking with other pts. Telling pts that he can now go off ward to smoke and will go after breakfast.

5-17-03 14:00

Patient compliant with new smoking policy. Does request 1 cigarette with lighter and removes yellow vest before going to smoke. Returns to ward after smoking with minimal time. Ambulates with walker on and off ward with slow steady gait.

Note. y.o. = years old; MCI = mild cognitive impairment; MMSE = Mini-Mental Status Exam; GRECC = Geriatric Research, Education, and Clinical Center; Pt. = patient; IADL = instrumental activity of daily living; VA = Veterans Affairs; AL = assisted living; NH = nursing home; VAMC = Veterans Affairs Medical Center; OT = occupational therapy.

PART

All Populations

15

Naomi Hadas-Lidor, PhD, OTR
Penina Weiss, MSc, OTR

Dynamic Cognitive Intervention

Application in Occupational Therapy

In the first part of this chapter, we present the theoretical base of the *dynamic cognitive intervention* (DCI) approach for cognitive modifiability in the evaluation and treatment of cognition. Vygotsky's (1978) concept of higher mental processes and Feuerstein's (1979, 1980) theory of structured cognitive modifiability (SCM), mediated learning experience (MLE), and applied systems deriving from the theory are the basis for the development of Hadas-Lidor's DCI approach for health care professionals, with a specific focus on the role of occupational therapists.

The principles and guidelines developed by Hadas-Lidor are presented in the second part of this chapter. These include clinical applications of the principles, the effect they have on the therapist, and their resulting impact on the therapeutic interaction. The third part of this chapter is dedicated to clinical and research implications for the future.

THEORETICAL BASIS

The concept of cognition as a dynamic entity shaped by human mediation was introduced by Vygotsky in the 1920s and 1930s. His contribution was in presenting human cognition as a sociocultural phenomenon rather than a natural property of an individual. Vygotsky (1978) distinguished between *lower* cognitive processes, whose development is governed by the forces of maturation and direct experience, and *higher* cognitive functions, whose development depends on

mediation provided by the society through cultural and linguistic artifacts (e.g., speech, writing, pictures) and sociocultural activities. Vygotsky was one of the first who suggested that static assessment tests do not provide an adequate picture of the dynamics of cognitive development. He proposed making a distinction between the child's *zone of actual development*, which reflects functions that are fully mastered by the child, and the *zone of proximal development*, which reflects functions that the child can master only through mediation provided by an adult or a more competent peer.

Working in the same theoretical direction, Feuerstein (1980) formulated his concept of SCM, which presented the human being as an open system that can be modified regardless of age and disability status. In general, Feuerstein's approach is concerned first with the cognitive prerequisites of human learning and problem-solving abilities; second, with examining why these abilities fail to develop during early childhood in the absence of human mediation; third, with focusing on systematic learning mediated by a caring adult; and fourth, with how much later than generally thought possible, identified cognitive deficits can be remediated by a formal instructional program. This formal program is based on a deductive style of training and teaching. Hadas-Lidor's contribution to the field of dynamic cognition is in her approach being therapeutically based while including a rehabilitative approach and putting a direct emphasis on emotional-related issues and the way they affect cognitive development.

Populations Exposed to Structural Cognitive Modifiability

This method of intervention started in the 1950s with the evaluation and treatment of adolescents experiencing cultural deprivation (Feuerstein, 1979). Since then, many diverse populations with special needs, experiencing activity limitations and participation restrictions, have been exposed to the intervention techniques developed by Feuerstein; these populations include new immigrants; student with learning disabilities; children with hearing and vision impairments; children with genetic syndromes, brain injuries, autism, and other disorders; and elderly individuals with mental retardation (Lidz & Elliott, 2000; Kozulin, 1997; Kozulin & Rand, 2000). In addition, high-functioning populations in industrial settings, especially in France (Avanzini, 1990), benefited from exposure to the principles of MLE and instructional enrichment (IE),

as did populations that are considered to have above-average intelligence, such as Israeli Air Force pilots. The fact that Feuerstein's techniques have been used on these very diverse populations incorporates one of the unique aspects of Feuerstein's theory: the belief that cognitive modifiability can be induced and developed at all ages, in all types of disabilities and functional limitations. Furthermore, everyone can benefit from structured cognitive dynamic intervention, leading to better management strategies in real-life situations, especially those involving high levels of stress and quick decision making.

Populations Exposed to Dynamic Cognitive Intervention

The following list is a partial description of different populations that have been exposed to DCI. Figure 15.1 includes references to these populations and illustrates the diverse applications of the approach: high-functioning populations, including gifted children; affected family members (usually parents) of people with limited occupation participation; caregivers; professionals and multi-

FIGURE 15.1. DCI in occupational therapy.

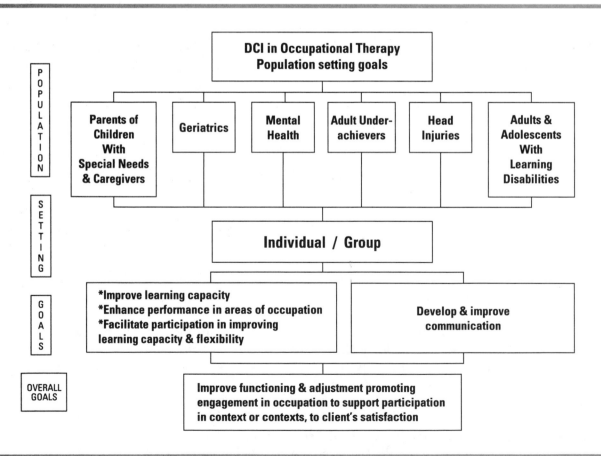

disciplinary staff members; the general public, through forum Internet exposure; populations with participation restrictions and activity limitations, such as adult under-achievers, geriatric populations, mental health populations, people with head injuries, and adults and adolescents with learning disabilities.

As can be seen in Figure 15.1, the DCI intervention approach has been made applicable to a diverse range of populations. Despite the differences in the makeup of the populations described in the figure, they all share some common attributes:

- They all have delayed or inhibited participation in life tasks and actions that deter them from achieving wholesome self-actualization of their desires and abilities. For example, parents of children with mental disabilities often pay a social price because of their total absorption with their child's life and needs, guilt, embarrassment, and fear. They limit themselves to social contact with people who are dealing with similar life situations.
- In spite of the differences between them, members of these populations have in common their need for and willingness to receive help. For example, an older adult dealing with many age-related health problems can decide to voluntarily seek cognitive intervention because of age-related memory impairments to improve his or her quality of life.

Researchers and educators in the field of cognitive psychology and cognitive education in many countries, such as England, Brazil, Chile, the United States, and Israel, are working on development and implementation of applied programs based on SCM theory (Kozulin & Rand, 2000).

PHILOSOPHY AND CONCEPT OF COGNITIVE MODIFIABILITY

The individual is regarded as an open system because modifiability is considered to be the basic condition of human beings. The individual's manifest level of performance at any given point in his or her development cannot be regarded as fixed or immutable, much less a reliable indication of future performance. This viewpoint has been expressed through the rejection of IQ scores as a reflection of a stable or permanent level of functioning. Instead, and in accordance with the open-system approach, intelligence is considered a dynamic, self-regulating process that is responsive to external environmental intervention. The view of the human being as an open system is used in various occupational therapy theoretical approaches, most obviously in the model of human occupation (Kielhofner, 1985, 1995).

The belief that intervention causes structural change is similar to sensory integration theory in occupational therapy, whereby changes are assumed to occur within the central nervous system causing adaptive responses to the environment (Ayers, 2000; Fisher, Murray, & Bundy, 1992). Toglia (1989, 1991, 1998) has presented a dynamic interactional model of cognitive rehabilitation that is based on the conceptualization of cognition as a dynamic interaction among the individual, the task, and the environment. In people with cognitive dysfunction, treatment within the multicontextual approach aims at systematically changing task and environment variables to enhance cognitive function that is embodied in the person's ability to process, monitor, and use information. Tapping a person's potential for learning, strengthening underlying strategies, and awareness comprise the focus of this intervention approach, which is influenced by Feuerstein's theoretical foundations (Feuerstein, 1979). In contrast, *cognitive disabilities theory* (Allen, 1985; Allen & Blue, 1998; Allen, Earhart, & Blue, 1992) is based on the assumption that occupational therapy intervention centers on the client's current capabilities, providing the just-right challenge and adapting the task and the environment to the individual. This direction also agrees with current approaches in rehabilitation (Anthony, Cohen, & Farber, 1990; Neff, 1985).

Current trends in research, together with the exponential growth in new technology, show the brain to be a far more plastic organ than previously thought (Sohlberg & Mateer, 2001). After injury, the brain is capable of considerable reorganization that forms the basis for functional recovery (Sohlberg & Mateer, 2001). The fact that specific alterations in behavior are reflected in characteristic functional changes in the brain is currently accepted by biologists (Kandel, 1998). Thus, the ideas related to cognitive modifiability expressed by Feuerstein (Feuerstein, 1979, 1980), pertaining to structural cognitive changes, are being found to be not just theoretical but are in the process of becoming scientifically based.

THEORY OF MEDIATED LEARNING EXPERIENCE

The theory of MLE is the underlying basis for the concept of cognitive modifiability. The basic assumption in this theory is that the major factor causing cognitive differences among people is the MLE. Deficit or lack of MLE is a stronger explanation than any etiologic differences.

Feuerstein conceives the development of cognitive structures in the organism as a product of two interactions between the organism and its environment: (a) direct exposure to sources of stimuli and (b) mediated learning (Feuerstein & Feuerstein, 1991). The first and the most universal modality is the organism's direct exposure to all sources of stimulation that it receives from the very earliest stage of development. This exposure changes the organism by affecting its behavioral repertoire and its cognitive orientation. These changes in turn affect its interaction with the environment, even when the environment itself remains constant and stable. Direct exposure to stimuli continues to affect the learning of the organism throughout its life span, to the extent that the stimuli present are varied and novel.

The second modality, which is far less universal and is characteristic of human beings, is MLE, a quality of interaction that explains the universal phenomenon of SCM and is considered the proximal factor that determines the flexibility and plasticity of the human mind that then leads to SCM (Feuerstein, Feuerstein, & Schur, 1997). It is conceived as a contextual environmental facilitator, determining the way in which stimuli emitted by the environment are transformed by a *mediating agent* (e.g., a parent, teacher, or therapist). This mediating agent, guided by his or her intentions, culture, and emotional investment, selects and organizes the world of the stimuli for the client (i.e., student). The mediator selects stimuli that are most appropriate and then frames, filters, and schedules them. He or she determines when certain stimuli appear or disappear and ignores others. Through this process of mediation, the cognitive structures of the client are affected. The client acquires behavior patterns and learning sets, which in turn become important ingredients of his or her capacity to become modified through direct exposure to stimuli. Because direct exposure to stimuli over time constitutes the greatest source of the individual's experience, the individual's cognitive development is influenced significantly by whether he or she has sets of strategies and repertoire that permit him or her to efficiently use this exposure.

The relationship between MLE and direct exposure to stimuli, the two modalities for the development of cognitive structures, can be set forth as follows: The more often and the earlier an individual is subjected to MLE, the greater will be his or her capacity to efficiently use and be affected by direct exposure to sources of stimuli. On the other hand, the less MLE the developing individual is offered, in terms of both quantity and quality, the lower his or her capacity will be to be affected and modified by direct exposure to stimuli. Feuerstein and Feuerstein (1991) outlined 12 parameters that describe the quality of the MLE. The three crucial parameters of the MLE are (a) *reciprocity,* (b) *transcendence,* and (c) *mediation of meaning.*

1. ***Intentionality and reciprocity:*** MLE requires a degree of intentionality on the part of the mediator. The voluntary nature of the mediated interaction is evident in certain well-defined instances. The purpose is to increase the intentionality of the recipient and raise his or her awareness of the ways he or she acts.

2. ***Transcendence:*** An interaction that provides mediated learning must be also directed toward transcending the immediate needs or concerns of the client by venturing beyond the here and now, in space and time. The premise of the approach is that working on transcendence is an integral part of the process of intervention. Transcendence, in terms of the ability to make generalizations, is done according to MLE during the process of intervention.

3. ***Mediation of meaning:*** In contrast to the first two parameters, mediation of learning deals mainly with the energetic dimensions of the interaction (i.e., with why things happen or are done). It raises the individual's awareness and understanding and makes explicit the implicit reasons and motivations for doing things. Mediation of meaning focuses on the interaction of the individual with the environment and aims to increase his or her ability to make choices.

The remaining nine parameters, unlike the first three, are not universal but contextual (Feuerstein & Feuerstein, 1991). The quality of mediation may sometimes be achieved without them. In certain contexts, however, these parameters become crucial. One such additional parameter has been adopted by Hadas-Lidor (1996) as being crucial to the success of the MLE because the latest research in the field of recovery has shown that a feeling of competence is a dominant feature of the recovery process. The therapist plays a crucial role in establishing this feeling in the client (Lachman & Roe, 2003).

4. ***Mediation of competence:*** This parameter deals with the way the mediator helps the individual feel a sense of competence and ability, in relation to him- or herself and to the task he or she undertakes.

The intentionality of the mediator and the transcendent (i.e., generalization) nature of mediative interaction is directed toward building new cognitive structures and broadening the individual's system of needs for functioning. Thus, MLE can take place in any interaction that is goal oriented, between human beings, depending on the parameters of the specific interaction, whether between parent and child, employer and employee, shopkeeper and client, teacher and student, therapist and client, and so on.

In Feuerstein's MLE model (Feuerstein & Feuerstein, 1991), a human being is the agent that mediates between stimuli and organism. The DCI pyramidal multidimensional model (see Figure 15.2) developed by Hadas-Lidor and Weiss (2004) expands the model developed by Feuerstein (Feuerstein & Feuerstein, 1991) by specifically including detailed factors that are pertinent to MLE from a health perspective, according to current *International Classification of Functioning, Disability, and Health (ICF)* terminology (World Health Organization, 2001), also adopted by occupational therapists (American Occupational Therapy Association, 2000). The expert mediator—for the purposes of this chapter, an occupational therapist—plays a crucial role in bonding and synchronizing in mediating among the client, environment, activity, and participation.

Occupational therapists are constantly redefining their interactional approach with the clients they treat (Hahn-Markowitz & Roitman, 2000), as can be seen in the client-centered approach that guides evaluation and intervention, for example, the development of measurement tools such as the Canadian Occupational Performance Measure (Law et al., 1998), which emphasizes the mutual

responsibility of the therapist and client to the intervention goals and procedures (Law, Baum, & Baptiste, 2002). Thus, the role of the mediator is in some ways similar conceptually to the role of the occupational therapist as a facilitator.

An individual may lack MLE because of the following two main reasons: (a) the nature of his or her environment (i.e., poverty, cultural deprivation, and disturbed families) and (b) his or her condition at a given point in development (i.e., learning disabilities, brain injuries, emotional disturbances, and mental retardation). According to Feuerstein and Feuerstein (1991), a lack of MLE has greater implications on functional outcomes in comparison to other causes or diagnoses. The goal of any intervention based on MLE is always to restore a normal pattern of development. The purpose of MLE, as reflected in the IE program and in DCI, is never to train the individual merely to master a set of specific skills that will enable him or her to function only in a limited way but to change the cognitive structures of the low performer and to transform him or her into an autonomous, independent thinker capable of initiating and elaborating actions. Thus, the focus is not on a functional approach but more on a cognitive remediation approach (Neistadt, 1990). Within the intervention process, the therapist works directly on helping the individual mediate structural generalizations.

In short, according to the theory of MLE, the goal set for cognitively low performers is adaptation to a normal environment, as opposed to adapting the environment to meet the specific needs of these performers.

FIGURE 15.2. DCI pyramid multidimensional model.

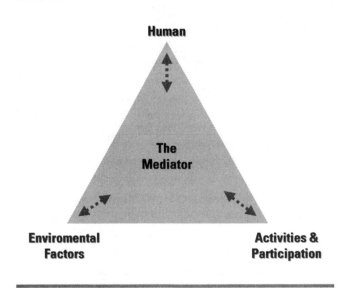

Applications of the Mediated Learning Experience in Dynamic Cognitive Intervention Approach

The applications described in this chapter refer to six aspects of the influence and change brought about by exposure to MLE:

1. On the individual being treated
2. On peers
3. On caregivers (usually represented by parents)
4. On the therapist
5. Online Internet-based application of MLE
6. On multidisciplinary staff members.

Influence of the Mediated Learning Experience on the Individual Client

Moreno (1996) described the treatment process of a 20-year-old man who had experienced the effects of a brain injury for 3 years. The treatment followed all 12 MLE components and adapted the principles to the special needs of the client and his physical difficulties. As a result of this intervention, the client became increasingly cooperative, less impulsive, and more independent and, together with his family, viewed the future with optimism.

Tzuriel and Eiboshitz (1992) investigated the efficacy of the Structural Program of Visual–Motor Intervention (SP–VMI) with preschool disadvantaged and special education children. The SP–VMI is based on the theoretical perspectives that emphasize developmental principles and needs for mastery of perceptual–motor skills in relation to writing and reading skills (i.e., Gesell and Montessori) and on the MLE theory that stresses mediation of meta-cognitive strategies and an active–modificational approach. The major findings of Tzuriel and Eiboshitz's study show that children in the experimental group significantly improved their performance from pre- to postintervention on perceptual–motor tests, measures of cognitive modifiability, and adjustment categories. The improvement on the dynamic test of the Rey Complex Figure (Feuerstein, Rand, Haywood, Hoffman, & Jensen, 1983) was significantly higher for the disadvantaged children in the experimental group as compared to the parallel subgroups among the control group. The findings, in general, confirm the efficacy of the SP–VMI and support the integration of MLE processes with perceptual–motor training.

Occupational therapists in the field of pediatrics have also begun to embrace a more cognitive, top-down approach, based on MLE, as a means to guide children into discovering repertoires of cognitive strategies to solve problems that they encounter with daily occupational performance (Missiuna, Malloy-Miller, & Mandich, 1998).

Influence of the Mediated Learning Experience on Peers

A study conducted by Kaufman and Burden (in press) aimed to use the sociocultural perspective for elucidating the process and outcome of peer learning interactions between young adults with serious learning disabilities. A heterogeneous group of 10 young adults between the ages of 18 and 27 participated in a year-long cognitive program based on the principles of Feuerstein's (1979, 1980) mediated learning and IE. Six of the participants had Down syndrome, and the others had various disabilities, including brain damage and cerebral palsy. The program included 178 hr of IE cognitive intervention. The peer mediation process was supplemented by an additional emphasis on collaborative group discussion at the end of every

session. A post-positivist research design similar to the *design experiment* of Russian Vygotskians was used to evaluate both the process and the outcomes of the intervention program. The results show that after 1 year the participants' learning self-concepts were above average. Moreover, their reflections about how they had changed as a result of their involvement in the program and their descriptions of what was required to provide effective mediation demonstrated deep levels of cognitive, emotional, and social development.

Influence of the Mediated Learning Environment on Caregivers

Kushnir (1996) discussed the preventive intervention program that she carried out with healthy mothers, native to the Caucasus, who immigrated to Israel. She described the unique characteristics of this ethnic group and the crisis and changes they experienced in Israel. The aim of the intervention program, according to Feuerstein's (1979) theory, was to improve both the adjustment of the mothers to the new cultural environment and the quality of the mother–infant interaction. This in turn would enable an MLE that would improve the children's cognitive modifiability.

A unique group model named KESHET (Advancement, Participation, and Communication), based on the principles of MLE, was developed by clinicians in the field of dynamic cognitive therapy, headed by Naomi Hadas-Lidor. Each group includes 15 participants who are parents and caregivers of people from populations with special needs. The KESHET model has two rationales: The first is to enforce the therapeutic gains made by the client through the limited amount of therapy received while in treatment in the Israeli health service system, which is usually short and inadequate because of strict and limited budgets. The second rationale is to provide caregivers with the skills and knowledge they feel they lack in order to understand, encourage, advance, and communicate with the family member who has functional impairment. The first group of parents completed an attitude questionnaire relating to beliefs, knowledge, and actions in relation to their children, at the onset and conclusion of the group sessions. Analysis of the questionnaires demonstrated significant statistical differences between attitudes before and after group participation in the areas of perception of knowledge, perception of personal behavior, and action style toward others. Combining the average scores for all three parameters before and after group participation revealed a statistical significant difference, with higher scores on all three parameters. All participants (45 to date) conveyed satisfaction from the exposure to the MLE principles (Hadas-Lidor & Chasdai, 2004). Figure 15.3 depicts the DCI model as applied in the intervention with parents and exemplifies the process of the involved parent developing skills in mediation with the guidance of an expert mediator.

The following is an account of one of the parents who participated in the first KESHET group. Aside from being a parent to a child with special needs, Dan works in a community-based mental health service that is managed by an occupational therapist. His role is to accompany and coach people with mental health disabilities who reside in community dwellings.

Case Study

Dan is a coach to Adrian, a 45-year-old bachelor who resides with his brother and sister-in-law. Adrian has been diagnosed with chronic schizophrenia and has very low self-esteem and confidence. He spends his time straightening up his room and does not participate in other household activities; his only income is from a governmental disability stipend. Adrian's daily schedule consists of waking up at noontime, reading the newspaper, and watching television until late hours. His family ties are superficial and evolve around the payment of household bills. In recent years, his living space has become restricted to the square mile around his residence because he fears coming across problems he won't be able to overcome. When Adrian first met Dan, he asked him, "Do you have experience with people like me who are unsuccessful, unhappy, and are fed up with it all?" Dan replied, "This difficult situation you're in, that you're sick and tired of, is a situation that we can change together" (this response is *reciprocal mediation*). Following this exchange, Adrian gave his consent to participate in the community setting rehabilitation attempt. In their initial meeting Adrian described his major difficulties that led to severe activity restrictions: boredom, fear of movement outside home, work, fear of intimate relationships, and lack of a purpose in life.

Dan uses a number of principles in his coaching. These principles are based on DCI and Anthony, Cohen, Farkas, and Gagne's (2002) rehabilitation theory.

- He views the rehabilitation process as a dynamic one that has pitfalls and setbacks along the way.
- The process has to be partaken by a multidisciplinary staff team because the disability affects different aspects of a person's life (physical, emotional, mental, social, vocational, and economical).

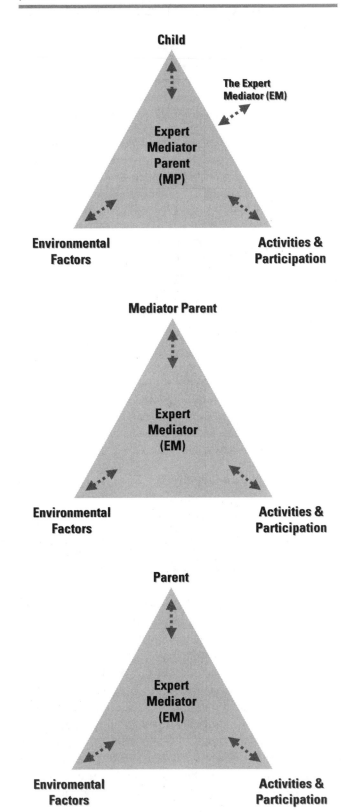

FIGURE 15.3. DCI process model—Mediation to parents.

- Staff must maintain the belief in optimal participation and not necessarily maximum participation.
- The process is approached while relating to a person's natural environment or habitat.
- A person's satisfaction is the measure of the rehabilitation process' progress and outcome.
- The hope and belief of the mediator and the client in the success of the rehabilitation outcome influence the realization of goals and belief in change.

The rehabilitation is regarded not only as a change-evolving process but also as a broad and far-reaching vision of the mediator that is tuned to inclusive multi-dimensional sides of the client that can be seen in two aspects of the process:

1. *Choice:* The ability of a person to choose determines the quality of his or her life. The value of choice is the belief that a person should determine as much as possible his or her lifestyle.
2. *Empowerment:* Whereas *choice* is the ability of a person to determine how he or she lives, *empowerment* is the ability to act according to the choices made. Empowerment is a value that implies that a person has awareness of choices and the opportunity and independence to act according to choices he or she has made. *Self-control* and *self-definition* are terms within empowerment, and their character determines the measure of empowerment that an individual experiences.

At the end of their first meeting, Dan and Adrian made a mutual decision regarding the first goal they set out to accomplish: trying to expand Adrian's access to the physical environmental space surrounding his home. They started out with a 20-min walk to a public park, where Adrian commented that he had never had such a sense of freedom.

At this point, when Adrian was filled with a sense of competence, Dan gave Adrian in-depth feedback and emphasized his ability to make a meaningful step forward, that he is capable of much more than he believed himself to be. This meeting was terminated by setting up a schedule for the next set of meetings, which were to take place three times a week, for 90 min each, for 3 months. During the next meetings, Dan and Adrian walked farther and farther, in different directions, and then started to try to exercise Adrian's newfound abilities on bus rides. At first Adrian was afraid to pay the bus driver, but after two trips he was able to determine his destination, find out about ticket prices, and prepare the sum to be paid in advance. Adrian's feeling of competence grew until he was able to travel independently by bus from one city to another, with Dan waiting at the final destination (mediation of transcendence and anticipation).

At each stage, Dan stressed Adrian's successful experiences. As the days passed, Adrian was less restricted, fearless, and capable of traveling daily to different destinations independently, with less and less preparation suited to his specific needs.

At this point, Dan held a meeting with Adrian's family, in which Adrian shared his successful experiences with them. Dan raised, with Adrian's prior consent, the issue of the need to broaden Adrian's rehabilitation program to include sheltered vocational issues. Adrian and Dan held meetings with a psychiatrist and treatment coordinator who found a sheltered vocational setting suitable to Adrian's needs in the vicinity of his home. Adrian expressed fears about his ability to be integrated in the work environment and to be diligent after many years of unemployment.

The following meetings focused on maintaining Adrian's sense of success, based on all he had accomplished so far, and in developing a sense of competence along with mediation of transcendence.

A few days before Adrian was to begin work, Dan accompanied him along the route he would be taking daily to plan a timetable and practice the route. Dan accompanied Adrian on the bus ride on his first day on the job and spent the time discussing his abilities, emphasizing that he was faced with a real-life experience, not a trial. Within days, Adrian was working 5 days a week. During the first week, Dan and Adrian's meetings were spent discussing the meaning of work, getting used to a framework, and focusing on Adrian's ability to prove to himself his ability to successfully manage this central domain in his life.

Now that Adrian was making meaningful changes in his life, his family reciprocated by supporting him in a much more meaningful way. Adrian's sense of belonging and sharing grew with each step. Without prior discussion, Adrian started to actively participate in household chores and went shopping with the family, and his self-esteem and self-image improved drastically.

The next meetings were focused on maintaining all that Adrian had accomplished and stabilizing his success. Emphasis was placed on feedback and on recognizing criteria of successful experiences in different areas of activity: recognition of his own needs and desires, negotiating with family, socializing, planning, and more.

Almost all the meetings between Adrian and Dan took place outside Adrian's home to maintain a sense of reality and make use of situations that arose in the diverse settings they came across.

An important aspect of the meeting was Dan's maintenance of a sense of humor and optimism: receiving Adrian off the bus as if a VIP were arriving, composing songs and stories about his journey, and making a best-employee ceremony after a month at work.

Since then, Adrian has started to learn a foreign language in a structured course; this was also an opportunity for social interaction that was an excellent tool to prove Adrian's transference ability and feeling of competence. Other criteria of mediation that were seen in the process included feelings of belonging; mediated sharing behavior; mediation of goal-seeking, goal-setting, goal-planning, and achieving behavior; mediation of challenge; and the awareness that he is a person who performs changes in his life.

Another example that exemplifies the changes Adrian went through is the following: In the language course, Adrian met a woman who resides in a different city. He expressed his will to start a relationship with the woman. He and Dan spent a few meetings dealing with this new topic. Adrian initiated a meeting with her in a community mental health center in her hometown. The day after they met, he reported to Dan that the meeting went so well that he missed his last bus. He dealt with the situation efficiently by taking the bus to a large city and from there continuing to his hometown. These incidents point out that Adrian has begun to mediate to himself. Within this incident one can identify the four parameters crucial to mediation: (a) intentionality and reciprocity, (b) meaning, (c) transcendence, and (d) competence.

The knowledge and security of Adrian as a person who can make choices and act according to those choices are the result of an ongoing meaningful process. The search for an optimistic alternative has become part of his life, without enabling regressions to shake the stable grounds obtained.

Dan stated that three additional components contributed to Adrian's successful rehabilitation:

1. *Protection component:* The mediator incorporates a protective measure toward the client. The choice of goals is always within the limits the mediator believes the client is capable of obtaining.
2. *Success component:* Every experience is viewed as a successful one, and positive feedback is a part of every experience, thus strengthening the feeling of competence in preparation for the next experience.
3. *Emotional component:* This is the most important component in the process. It is expressed in the com-

radeship, sharing, empathy, sensitivity, encouragement, and a deep feeling of respect on the part of the mediator for the client's awareness that he or she is partaking in a long and tedious voyage toward change and new experiences.

In regard to his perspective on his experience with Adrian and the influence of his participation in the KESHET group on his life, Dan states that, prior to his participation in the group, and his introduction to the DCI principles, he coached in an intuitive way. He could not define or explain what he did or why he chose to intervene in a certain way. He now has a clearer definition of his role as a coach and mediator, and he views himself as a partner of the people with whom he works, constantly adapting himself to his partners' needs. He uses his new-found structured knowledge in diverse situations, the most significant of these being sitting down with his son, who has chronic schizophrenia, and introducing him didactically to the principles that Dan learned in KESHET and used to help guide his son through a successful rehabilitation process.

Influence of the Mediated Learning Experience on the Therapist

Occupational therapists working in the field of physical disabilities who have had exposure to mediation techniques find them an additional meaningful tool for enhancing functional physical treatment goals and thus use cognition not as a treatment goal but as an avenue for intervention. In a single-case study described by Hinda Torchin (personal communication, December 18, 2003), a woman with limited range of motion in her left shoulder from lymphoma, who was treated in physical therapy with limited recovery of function and residual chronic pain, was referred to an occupational therapist who had specialized in the field of DCI techniques. Using MLE parameters, within 3 months the client regained substantial range of motion (before occupational therapy treatment, shoulder abduction was 45 degrees, after treatment it was 140 degrees) that enabled her to independently perform tasks she previously was incapable of doing.

A group of occupational therapists specializing in the field of cognitive dynamic therapy participated in a workshop intended to add an extra dimension to their professional ability, in that it would train them to become instructors for an educational program developed for therapists from diverse health allied professions that would help them become dynamic cognitive therapists. The emphasis was on incorporating, encouraging, and promoting the belief in the ability and commitment to personal change. The workshop was developed on the basis of a model of collaborative learning and was based on the parameters of MLE. Qualitative and quantitative data show that the workshop facilitated changes in the participants' attitudes toward teaching on emotional, cognitive, and practical levels. After the workshop, most participants were integrated as instructors and teachers in the educational program (Hadas-Lidor, Naveh, & Weiss, 2003).

An additional program that bears on the influence of the MLE on the therapist is the diploma program that we describe later in this chapter.

Online Internet-Based Application of the Mediated Learning Experience

A group of dynamic cognitive therapists initiated an online forum for therapists and interested surfers on the Web to be used as a medium for the exchange of ideas and strategies for coping with real-life situations. This medium allows people to deal with real-life situations according to MLE criteria and in relation to the intervention principles of the DCI. The forum also provides a place for the fruitful exchange of ideas among dynamic cognitive therapists. The forum apparently answers a need because the general public uses the forum to better deal with lifetime situations and dilemmas they are working through.

For example, a special education arts teacher presented a question regarding the management of an art class for children with attention-deficit disorder and attention-deficit/hyperactivity disorder who do not respond well to medication (e.g., Ritalin), with most of the time spent in class dealing with problematic behavioral issues.

Suggestions from the therapists included encouraging the motivation of the students by creating in class, together, rules and guidelines for the art class. The rules were to be expressed in a positive, encouraging manner and not as a list of "don'ts" and "nos." The art teacher was advised to copy the selected rules onto a large sheet of paper and have the children decorate and draw around the rules, thus turning the expressed rules into a work of art. The art teacher reported following this advice with success and the interested participation of the children.

As another example, an 18-year-old high school senior presented the forum with his dilemmas regarding his plans after high school. Members of the forum advised him to draw up a table comparing criteria for the different possibilities he was considering. He needed help with structuring the comparison but ended up with a well-put-together table that portrayed a very clear and extensive picture of all the aspects of his dilemma. He attached the table as a document when he thanked the forum, and he stated that the cognitive intervention helped him with defining things more clearly and helped him feel less confused.

Influence of the Mediated Learning Experience on Multidisciplinary Staff Members

For the past 4 consecutive years, courses for managers of rehabilitation units from the field of mental health have been taking place at Tel Aviv University in Israel. The course is based on the principle of on-the-job training and is intended for professionals from various fields: social workers; occupational therapists; educators; and others who manage different types of rehabilitation units, including vocational, home settings, and leisure units. They have different amounts of professional experience and are of diverse ages.

The course is structured around central topics related to rehabilitation: recovery, organization, analysis of managerial incidences with staff, supervision, parents, and so on, with the analysis achieved using MLE parameters.

These applications of MLE suggest that MLE concepts are practical and adaptable to many aspects of the rehabilitation process of people with disabilities and others, while also making a meaningful imprint on the mediator him- or herself.

APPLICATIONS IN OCCUPATIONAL THERAPY BASED ON STRUCTURED COGNITIVE MODIFIABILITY

This section is divided into three parts: (a) evaluation and assessment techniques, (b) treatment principles and methods, and (c) the role of environment as facilitator to treatment.

Therapeutic Dynamic Cognitive Assessment Approach

The dynamic assessment approach was developed to alter the cycle of failure that low performers experience on the classical intelligence tests (i.e., a static assessment approach). The measurement and remeasurement of an individual's existing capacities should be abandoned in favor of first inducing and then assessing the individual's modified performance within the test situation. By assessing modifiability, one must focus on the cognitive functions that are directly responsible for the demonstrated deficiencies. One must also continually remember that these deficiencies experienced by the client at the input and output phases of the mental act may be attributable to motivational components, emotional components, or both and do not necessarily reflect the fact that the individual has a deficient elaboration capacity. Treatment may then be directed at correcting deficiencies, by which the individual will be able to change the course of his or her development. The first dynamic assessment battery that was developed was the Learning Potential Assessment Device (LPAD; Feuerstein, 1979).

According to the intervention approach described in this chapter, the initial intervention is always started with an interview. In this interview, the therapist helps the client to clearly define his or her functional needs and decides which standardized (preferably adapted with dynamic MLE principles) or dynamic tools will guide the therapist to a deeper professional analytical understanding of the client's needs as expressed by the client.

Principle 1[1]

The intervention approach is structured according to individual needs; therefore, the diagnosis or cause in itself is not the central criterion that will define the disability-specific approach to intervention. As a result, the mediation protocols to treatment are flexible and adapted specifically to each individual. This approach differs from other models that supply structured guidelines to dynamic cognitive therapy as exemplified in the work of Feuerstein and Feuerstein (1991) and Toglia (1998). The initial intervention approach to evaluation and assessment is client centered, meaning that the beginning of the evaluation process is guided by defining goals as decided on mutually by the tester and testee. In certain cases when this cannot be accomplished with the testee, the goals are defined with the help of the caregiver.

Case Study

Gary sustained a head injury 1 year ago. He is 27 years old and resides with his parents. His discharge papers and cognitive assessments that he completed while hospitalized describe many cognitive deficits and functional limitations, such as categorization, problem solving, attention

---

[1]These principles are numbered for the benefit of readers and are not to be interpreted as a hierarchical rating.

deficits, and so on. At the beginning of the intervention, Gary expressed his wish to live independently within a year. This need directed the focus and the tools of the assessment to topics related to handling money and time, decision making, problem solving in everyday situations, basic social skills, and so on.

Principle 2

According to the DCI concept of dynamic assessment, principles related to dynamic assessment as laid down by Feuerstein (1979; Feuerstein, Feuerstein, Falik, & Rand, 2002) should be used in diverse evaluation contexts that the therapist encounters and, if possible, applied to standardized static evaluation tools familiar to the clinician.

There are a variety of approaches to dynamic assessment and a growing amount of data support the realization of this type of assessment as a valuable resource for helping to understand people's potential (Grigorenko & Sternberg, 1998). In the professional field of occupational therapy new assessment tools based on principles of dynamic testing have been developed; an example is dynamic interactional assessment, developed by Toglia (1998). Others are researching the use of dynamic assessment techniques on traditional popular assessments that were initially developed using standard static evaluation procedures, as demonstrated by the work of Bartal-Bahat (2001) on the Test of Visual Motor Skills and Bar-Korzen (2003) on the Beery–Buktenica Developmental Test of Visual–Motor Integration. LPAD testing tools and procedures are also the focus of research by clinicians, as was demonstrated in a study that compared the performance of the complex figure drawing test in healthy adults and rehabilitation clients diagnosed with schizophrenia (Weiss, 2001). Original assessment tools are also being developed to cater to specific needs, such as the Puzzle Assessment, developed by Ginton and Gelis (2000), which assesses children's learning ability. The child completing the Puzzle Assessment undergoes a structured learning process of a puzzle construction and then is required to use the strategies he or she learned to construct another, different puzzle. During this process, special emphasis is put on focusing on which cognitive functions the child uses to complete the task and his or her capacity for transference and learning potential after receiving MLE.

In the approach described in this chapter, interview, observation skills, and dynamic and static evaluation tools are used concurrently to obtain a comprehensive picture of the client's functional operative abilities and learning potential.

Dynamic assessment differs essentially from classic assessment. The major components that make up the dynamic assessment are as follows:

- The structure of test instruments (i.e., cognitive tests are analyzed for their components and divided into various graded exercises)
- The test logistics and testing procedures (i.e., first, the relationship of tester–testee is transformed into teacher–student or therapist–client, as described in the MLE, and second, the assessment is not timed— only the length of the whole process is considered)
- Mediation as an integral part of the assessment process, withs goals that are twofold: To analyze and grade the test material in a way that enables the testee to accomplish the task and to enable him or her to identify his or her style of thinking and strategy for dealing with the task at hand (meta-cognition)
- The interpretation of the results (i.e., the focus is on the change process and the individual's investment in it, and the score is not the sole end product taken into account)
- The general orientation of the test (from product to process).

The goals of a dynamic cognitive evaluation are as follows:

- To assess an individual's modifiability when he or she is confronted with conditions that aim at producing a change in him or her
- To assess the extent of the observed modifiability in terms of both the functional levels made accessible to the individual through the process of modification and the significance of the levels he or she attained in the hierarchy of cognitive operations
- To determine how much intervention was necessary to bring about a given amount or type of modification
- To determine how much significance the modification achieved in one area can have for other general areas of functioning
- To search for the individual's preferred modalities that represent areas of relative strength and weakness in terms of both his or her existing inventory of responses and preferred strategies for achieving the desired modification in the most efficient and economical way.

Case Study

During Tom's evaluation, it became apparent that verbal mediation was a preferred mode of MLE for him.

While reproducing the Rey Osterrieth Complex Figure (Feuerstein et al., 1983) from memory, Tom guided himself by verbal instructions, spoken aloud. This behavior was repeated in additional parts of the evaluation, in which he initially expressed insecure and hesitant behavior, with a request for many verbal explanations before any attempted action. These verbal explanations improved his performance. The initial purpose is to strengthen Tom's sense of security; therefore, the treatment process began with the use of IE tools that rely heavily on clear and detailed verbal instruction and tools that emphasize self-perception and a social sense of adequacy.

In using dynamic assessment techniques, the therapist is not interested in passively collecting data about skills the client may or may not possess. Instead, the therapist assesses general learning modifiability by measuring the individual's capacity to acquire a given principle, learning set, skill, or attitude, depending on the specific task at hand. The extent of modifiability and the amount of treatment investment necessary to bring about the change are assessed respectively by

- Measuring the client's capacity first to grasp and then to apply these new skills to a variety of tasks progressively more distant from the one in which the principle was taught
- Measuring the amount of explanation and training investment required to produce the desired result.

The significance of the attained modification is measured by the client's developing patterns of behavior that prove his or her efficiency in areas other than those that were actively modified by the training process. The use of this dynamic approach in assessment assumes that the individual represents an open system that may undergo important modifications through exposure to external stimuli, internal stimuli, or both (Lidz, 1987). However, the degree of the individual's modifiability through direct exposure to various sources of stimulation is considered to be a function of the quantity and quality of mediated learning experience.

An additional tool for assessment, the LPAD—Basic (LPAD–B; Feuerstein et al., 2002), was developed recently to accommodate the special dynamic assessment needs of special populations: children who have not yet developed cognitive functions, adults who have lost their cognitive capacities because of trauma and other acquired conditions and who need to "reacquire" functions to build back to higher levels, and people with severe developmental or behavioral disabilities such as those with Down syndrome or autism. The LPAD–B is a downward extension of the LPAD and, in contrast to the LPAD, it aims not at exposing latent structures but rather at creating them. One of the prominent theoretical features of the LPAD–B is that once new structures are established, the objective is to consolidate them.

The goals of LPAD–B deviate from currently existing preschool evaluations in three ways:

1. Instead of demonstrating samples of performance to place the examinee's performance on a developmental scale, the LPAD–B aims at assessing the examinee's openness to the processes of mediation.
2. The findings from the LPAD–B are not interpreted by an external standard but instead are used to contribute to understanding the examinee's processes of thinking and learning underlying performance.
3. The ultimate goal is the evaluation of the propensity for modifiability and determination of the most appropriate mediational processes.

Tzuriel (2001) developed a preschool dynamic assessment battery, based on Feuerstein's (1979) and Vygotsky's (1978) theories, that encompasses unique characteristics for young children, including adaptation of test materials to developmental requirements, bridging of concrete operations to abstract levels of functioning, assessment of nonintellective factors and their modifiability as integrative components of dynamic assessment, use of transfer problems as a component of testing, and use of mediation phase with transfer problems.

Katz, Parush, and Traub Bar-Ilan (in press) adapted and further developed the Loewenstein Occupational Therapy Cognitive Assessment (LOTCA; Itzkovich, Elazar, Averbuch, & Katz, 2000) into the Dynamic Occupational Therapy Cognitive Assessment for Children for youth ages 6 to 12 years. The battery includes 22 subtests in five areas: (a) orientation, (b) spatial perception, (c) praxis, (d) visuomotor construction (with memory), and (e) thinking operations. Scores on each subtest range from 1 *(low)* to 5 *(maximal performance)*. The test includes a baseline score, a mediation score (on a 5-level cueing system adapted from Togila [1994] with her permission), and a posttest score. A comparison of the performance of children with traumatic brain injuries and children with learning disabilities with control children revealed significant differences on all subtests between each client group and the control children in Israel. All children groups showed improvement, with the dynamic/mediation process enabling evaluation of their potential (Katz et al., in press).

Principle 3

In the presented intervention approach there is no clearly defined border among evaluation, treatment, and follow-up elements. They are continuously intertwined throughout the intervention procedure. As described earlier, the initial assessment is based on the needs and wishes expressed by the client. It is difficult to define exactly when the assessment ends and the treatment process begins. Furthermore, the initial assessment process is accomplished by MLE and therefore, by definition, a process of change has already been put into motion. Additionally, after initial goals have been set, and the therapeutic process has begun in a more focused manner, there is a constant re-evaluation of these goals, which are always related to function.

Case Study

A student with learning disabilities requested strategies to help him summarize academic material. During the initial assessment, he was presented with an exercise of summarizing a newspaper article. This exercise portrayed good comprehension of the material, with expressive difficulties in the correct use of words in general and the use of conjunctions in particular, difficulty differentiating between the central idea expressed and information of secondary importance, and sequencing.

Throughout the intervention process, the student wrote and summarized textbook materials, newspaper articles, poetry, and so on. Analytic perception and illustrations (cartoons), IE tools, were also used, with a focus on non-verbal expressive ability. Thus, a rich variety of self-written material was created. A parallel focus of the intervention was introducing and instructing the student in the use of academic writing structures, use of conjunctions, and how to identify the central idea expressed in written passages. This process enabled the therapist and student to identify, clarify, document, learn, experience, and follow up on the ongoing changes taking place throughout the intervention process.

PRINCIPLES AND INSTRUMENTS

In this chapter, Hadas-Lidor proposes a dynamic therapeutic-based treatment approach that has evolved from Feuerstein's (1979, 1980) dynamic deductive-based approach. We next present a model that describes the place of DCI within a cycle of adjustment difficulties and adaptation because of disability. This is followed by a description of the IE program developed by Feuerstein and an explanation of how it is incorporated into the principles developed in Hadas-Lidor's DCI approach, which also includes a variety of activities (some of which are more familiar to occupational therapists) including reading and writing exercises, analysis of life events and family picture albums, games, and the cognitive map. Last, we illuminate the importance of environment settings in the process of intervention.

DCI is a unique cognitive model that combines remedial and adaptational interventions that directly and simultaneously enhance participation in major life areas (see Figure 15.4). The model presents a circular connection among disability, activity, and participation. A link among these three elements can be a vicious cycle, because it can cause acquired helplessness. This can be explained by the process in which disability causes difficulty in performance and capacity for learning and applying knowledge that can cause low self-esteem, which causes acquired helplessness. These affect motivation, activity, and participation in major life areas. As can be seen in the model, the DCI makes a critical difference by challenging the vicious cycle at a point between the dif-

ficulty in performance and capacity for learning and the limited participation, by improving and expanding learning ability and self-perception through the themes that a person identifies and chooses to focus on during the intervention. It is important to emphasize that DCI sees participation not as an outcome of the intervention but as an accompanying element that simultaneously broadens and expands a person's ability for activity and participation (see also second parameter of MLE: transcendence).

INSTRUMENTAL ENRICHMENT: AN INTERVENTION PROGRAM FOR COGNITIVE MODIFIABILITY

There are two major types of MLE-based intervention programs. Programs of the first type infuse the principles of MLE into educational or treatment programs without introducing specially designed learning materials or tools, such as DCI. Programs of the second type, of which Feuerstein's *Instrumental Enrichment* (Feuerstein, 1980) and Haywood's *Bright Start* (Haywood, Brooks, & Burns, 1992) are representative, are orga-

F I G U R E   1 5 . 4 .   Model of relationship between participation restrictions and DCI.

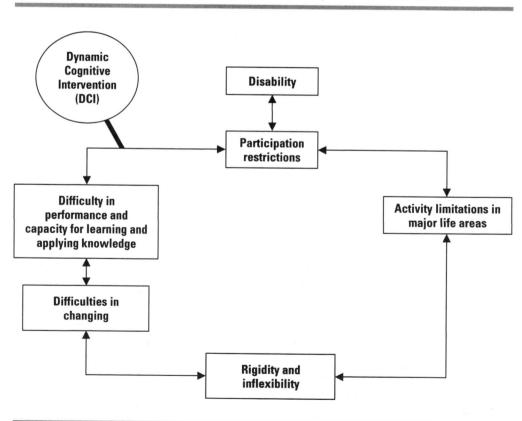

nized around specially designed learning materials that serve as tools for the enhancement of cognitive modifiability. The IE program is used in the DCI approach as a central axis for the redevelopment of cognitive structures in cognitively low performers.

The IE program is designed as a direct and focused approach to those processes that, because of their absence, fragility, or inefficiency, are responsible for poor intellectual performance, irrespective of underlying etiology. The IE program consists of more than 500 working pages of paper-and-pencil exercises, divided into 14 instruments (see Table 15.1). A detailed description of IE tools is described elsewhere (Hadas-Lidor & Katz, 1998). Each part focuses on a specific cognitive deficiency but can also address the acquisition of many other learning prerequisites. This structured approach assists the therapist/teacher in his or her choice of the materials to be taught/used and in their sequence of presentation. By knowing the focus of each section, the therapist/teacher is able to select and match specific material to the needs and deficits of particular clients/students. Intervention is done either individually or in groups and takes place in approximately three to five sessions per week (Feuerstein, 1980).

A new recent expansion in the field of IE, and in conjunction with the development of the LPAD–B, has been the development of seven additional types of exercises catering to the needs of very young children and intended for low-performing populations for whom the traditional IE program imposes a level of complexity above their existing level of comprehension and learning ability (see Table 15.1). The new exercises also directly put emphasis on domains that are subtly addressed in the established IE program, such as identification

of feelings and behavioral regulation (Feuerstein & Feuerstein, 2003).

The major goal of IE is to increase the individual's capacity to be modified through direct exposure to stimuli and experiences that occur throughout life and with formal and informal learning opportunities. To attain this major goal, the following six subgoals should serve as guidelines for the construction of the IE program and its application:

1. Correcting the deficient functions to change the structure of the cognitive behavior.
2. Acquiring basic concepts, labels, vocabulary, operations, and relationships necessary for IE as represented by the content of the materials, which themselves are purposely content free.
3. Developing (producing) intrinsic motivation through habit formation. To verify that whatever is taught will become part of an active repertoire, spontaneously used by the individual, one has to verify that the need for its use will be an intrinsic one rather than a response to an extrinsic system.
4. Producing reflective, insightful processes in the student/client as a result of his or her confrontation with both failing and successful behaviors in the IE tasks.
5. Creating task-intrinsic motivation, which has two aspects, including the enjoyment of a task for its own sake and the social implication of succeeding in a task that is difficult even for independent adults.
6. Providing the cognitively low-performing individual with a self-identity that sees him or her as capable of generating information and ready to function as such, as a result of this self-perception.

A comparison of these subgoals to current themes outlined in the occupational therapy literature and to cognitive psychology reveal that Feuerstein's (1980) approach can be identified in more modern terminology, that is, producing reflective insightful processes that can be termed as developing meta-cognition or self-awareness.

An additional structured intervention program based on Vygotskian theory and Feuerstein's MLE is the Bright Star program. Developed by Haywood (Haywood et al., 1992) for preschoolers and primary-grade children who may have pervasive developmental disorders or a high risk of learning failure, the essence and most distinguishing feature of the program is the mediation of psychological tools in the context of the zone of proximal development. It is a program of cognitive education and remediation aimed at enhancing the development of basic cognitive processes and thinking skills, developing task-intrinsic

TABLE 15.1. IE Materials

IE Materials for Adults	IE Materials for Children
• Organization of dots	• Organization of dots
• Analytic perception	• Orientation in space
• Illustrations (cartoons)	• Tri-Channel Attentional Learning
• Orientation in space 1	• From empathy to action
• Orientation in space 2	• Compare and discover the absurd
• Comparisons	• Identifying emotions
• Family relations	• From single units to grouping
• Numerical progressions	
• Stencil design	
• Categorization	
• Instructions	
• Temporal relations	
• Transitive relations	
• Syllogisms	

Note. IE = instrumental enrichment.

motivation, and increasing learning effectiveness and readiness for school learning. This is accomplished by introducing a mediation teaching style using process-oriented questions rather than content-oriented ones, within seven cognitive instructional units (Gindis, 2003).

DYNAMIC COGNITIVE INTERVENTION IN OCCUPATIONAL THERAPY

The DCI approach uses a person's learning potential as a base for enabling, broadening, and expanding participation in the environment. Occupational therapy, as a profession, encompasses these elements across all target populations, stages of illness, types of disability, and at all stages of the life cycle. Feuerstein's SCM approach and IE program have been used in Israel with adult populations since the 1980s (Katz & Hadas, 1995). At the outset, it was used mainly by occupational therapists who specialized in rehabilitation of adolescent and adult populations with various dysfunctions (physical, cognitive, emotional, behavioral). IE is used in conjunction with evaluation and treatment of daily living skills (activities of daily living), vocational/professional skills, and social skills, as well as during transitions from the hospital to the community.

An independent model of intervention is proposed by Hadas-Lidor in this chapter. The principles of this intervention approach, called *DCI,* are presented throughout this chapter. This approach enables a broader range of populations to be exposed to this type of intervention, and it integrates IE instruments with other tools that are used commonly by occupational therapists as well as introduced new techniques and instruments.

The goals of the occupational therapist in this approach are

- Improvement of independent learning ability;
- Development of awareness, insight, and feelings of competence; and
- Expansion of participation in activities in the person's natural environment according to his or her interests, intentions, and wishes.

ADDITIONAL PRINCIPLES AND GUIDELINES DEVELOPED BY HADAS-LIDOR FOR THERAPISTS

Principle 4

Always focus on the existing, on the positive; emphasize the person's strength and believe in it. Many times we explore and explain the mistakes; rarely do we interpret

and empower success and strength. Spend more time on successful experiences, analyze them, explore them, and explain them; this attitude leads to a growth of future successes.

Principle 5

The treatment stage is commenced using the IE exercises in a horizontal, free-choice, need-specified approach in accordance with the chosen goal of treatment and with the client's consent. A maximum exposure to IE exercises is desirable to enhance development of a wide range of strategies and develop mental flexibility. This approach differs from Feuerstein's (1979) traditional approach to intervention, in which clients/students are given a structured preset sequence of the IE program according to specific cognitive deficiencies.

Principle 6

From the person to the intervention tool to be used, connect the tool that is most meaningful to the client, to his or her ability, culture, desire, and need. The intervention is a constant dialogue.

Principle 7

Motivation is a product of ability. Lack of motivation is a product of low self-esteem and a lack of skills, or strategies, or both.

For example, in prior years, people diagnosed with mental health disorders spent years in psychiatric hospitals, where they had only a bed and a bedside dresser. All of their personal belongings could be contained in a plastic bag. When asked if they were interested in changing anything in their lives, they expressed satisfaction with the way things were, with no need for change. Following the current trend of community-dwelling solutions for this population, these same people, who now have their own rooms, beds, closets, personal possessions, work, or occupations, express additional needs, such as for money, leading a family life, and taking a trip abroad. This can be seen as an expression of increased competence and belief in their ability.

Hadas-Lidor, Katz, Tyano, and Weizman (2001) studied the effect of DCI principles on clients with chronic schizophrenia. One of their assumptions was that the treatment would cause an increase in self-esteem and satisfaction. Surprisingly, the results pointed to a slight decrease in these parameters despite an increase in ability and living status. The central explanation for this is that an increase in ability may cause a decrease in satisfaction and a need for further change and development.

Principle 8

The intervention is an ongoing and interwoven combination process that includes multifaceted sides: cognition, emotions, and function.

Principle 9

The intervention involves a constant reference to metacognition through Feuerstein's (Feuerstein & Rand, 1997) transference mediation criterion of the MLE. The transference is accomplished by relating to life situations and roles (e.g., family, work environment, studies). This is accomplished by an ongoing analysis of what I'm doing (definition of task at hand), how I'm accomplishing the task (process), and why I'm doing it (choosing among strategies). This principle differs from the remedial approach by not assuming that the transfer of skills will happen automatically following cognitive intervention and is similar to Toglia's (1998) approach, which views generalization, establishing criteria for transfer, practice in multiple environments, and meta-cognitive training as crucial aspects of the treatment process. The DCI approach assumes that application of strategies to real life can happen only if treated directly during intervention.

Principle 10

The intervention is multidisciplinary; all professionals and caregivers take part in enhancing intervention goals. To this end, all involved are exposed to MLE principles. This cooperation enables further fulfillment of transcendence from DCI to other areas of the client's life. One way to accomplish this purpose was the development of a study program developed by Hadas-Lidor in the Occupational Therapy Department at Tel Aviv University (described later in this chapter) that is intended for multidisciplinary health professionals.

Principle 11

In DCI, affect and emotional issues that arise and are identified as deterrents to functional ability are dealt with directly and intentionally, through the use of MLE and operating cognitive functions (see Table 15.2).

Another example is the use of family picture albums as stimuli for discussion about relationships, culture, values, emotions, and family difficulties.

An additional benefit of this approach is that, by cognitively analyzing emotional issues, distancing is accomplished and that, in turn, enables coping and accessibility in dealing with sensitive life situations. This is an innovative approach for occupational therapists, who traditionally, with the use of other cognitive approaches, would not directly deal with emotional aspects of an individual during intervention.

Principle 12

The intervention is basically always individualized. Group intervention is not permanent and takes place around an identified issue or problem, such as methods for writing a curriculum vitae to obtain work.

Principle 13

The client is encouraged to maximize independence during the intervention procedure and between intervention sessions. This is accomplished also by giving IE exercises similar to those worked on during the intervention as homework, finishing exercises according to principles worked on during intervention sessions, and analysis of school homework according to criteria of the cognitive map (described further in this chapter).

Principle 14

Addition of tasks to the intervention process, besides IE exercises, are constructed in a similar fashion, used according to the same principles (see Tables 15.2 and 15.3).

COGNITIVE MAP

The cognitive map is a tool constructed by Feuerstein (1979) to construct the IE tools, conceptualizing the relationship between the characteristics of a task and its performance by an individual. The map was adapted by Hadas-Lidor (1997) for different age groups as an invaluable instrument that can be considered a useful tool for occupational therapists because it contributes to activity analyses of therapeutic tasks and enhances the intervention process by being used as a communication device.

The cognitive map was constructed as a tool for defining activity demands. It was adapted by Hadas-Lidor

TABLE 15.2. Writing of Life Events: A Case Study Using Principles of Dynamic Cognitive Therapy

Intervention Process	Writing Task	IE Exercises Intended for Expansion, Variety, and Distancing
Client chooses life event to work on	My mother shut off the television at 11:00 p.m., during my favorite program.	
Unstructured writing of the event	Spontaneous, subjective writing	
Choosing a suitable structure for reporting the event	• Topic • Place where event took place • Time of event • Participants • Order of events	
Inspection of the writing	• Proper structure • Clarity of language • Proper use of conjunctions • Sequencing • Consideration of addressee • Suitable equilibrium among parts: feelings, cognition, and behavior	• Categorization • Analytic perception • Stencil design
Writing of event from mother's perspective	What did mother think, feel, and do.	Orientation in Spaces 1 and 2
Comparison of structure	Examination according to • Proper structure • Clarity of language • Proper use of conjunctions • Sequencing • Consideration of addressee • Suitable equilibrium among parts: feelings, cognition, and behavior	Comparisons
Comparison of content	Compare your story with your mother's story.	Cartoon that depicts a topic from two points of view, such as the mouse and the cheese; Family relations, viewing the same event from different points of view

Note. From "The Dynamic Cognitive Approach—A Means and Not a Goal in Itself," by N. Hadas-Lidor, 2004. Paper presented at "A Journey Towards Myself: Implementations of the Cognitive Dynamic Therapy," Tel Aviv University, Tel Aviv, Israel. Adapted with permission.

TABLE 15.3. Comparing Feuerstein's (1980) Cognitive Map With Hadas-Lidor's Application of the Map as an Intervention Instrument for Children

Feuerstein (1980)	Hadas-Lidor
Content	What is the subject of the exercise?
Modality/language	How is the exercise presented (e.g., words, sentences, numbers, tables, designs, geometric shapes)?
Phase of mental act: Input, elaboration, output (cognitive functions)	How should you think in order to do the exercise? (Collect information, learn new phrases, carefully read instructions, ask for advice, summarize)—Cognitive functions
	What steps should you take in order to do the exercise? (Write, draw, calculate, cut, make draft)—Process
Cognitive operation	What should the end product of the exercise be? (Summary, picture, table, graph)
Level of complexity	How difficult was the exercise for you? (Easy, moderate, difficult)
Level of abstraction	Did the exercise deal with familiar material to you? (Very familiar—things I can see, hear, or touch; familiar—things I know but can't see or touch, e.g., square, circle; not familiar, abstract—love, honor, cognition)
Level of efficiency	How did I accomplish the exercise with minimum of mistakes and at suitable speed?

(1997) for diverse age groups and populations, to be used as an intervention tool to analyze and comprehend the task together with the learner, and to make the task suitable to the individual. DCI goals that are applied to the intervention process with the use of the map include

- Arousing the client's awareness to his or her performance and ability,
- Establishing or restoring the client's belief in his or her ability and in his or her will and need for improvement,
- Creating a contract between therapist and client in regard to the intervention process, and
- Developing the client's ability for self-estimation.

This development of the cognitive map is used directly with clients (for an example in pediatrics, see Table 15.3), DCI therapists, teachers, and parents as tools for making choices and selection of suitable tasks for intervention.

DYNAMIC ENVIRONMENT

Three conditions help to design and transform environments that promote changes in a person. An environment that promotes change is (a) encouraging, (b) obligating, and (c) enabling. The construction stages that help create an environmental context that promote change for the individual are assessment of ability, assessment of pathways to change, and creation of an enabling environment.

Attention must be given to the fact that certain environments by definition are not enabling, such as environments that specifically cater to populations with special needs. If, at the base of the environmental context is the ideology that there is no reason to try to create and encourage change, then environments based on beliefs that were popular in the past, that viewed genetic structure as fixed and unchangeable, lead to the establishment of sheltered environments of work or study, such as special education settings and workshops. A preferable type of environment creates the needs and demands of the individual. If the individual will not adapt him- or herself internally to it, it will be difficult for him or her to be integrated into the environment (Anthony et al., 2002; Feuerstein & Rand, 1997).

Case Study

Stan is a pupil in a class for children with learning disabilities. He has many friends who attend regular classes, and he wants to join them. To accomplish this, he must make behavioral changes, such as sitting through a class without getting up for 45 min. The DCI therapist has to enable, develop, and teach strategies for making this change.

RESEARCH ON INSTRUMENTAL ENRICHMENT

At present, the literature on IE-based research and implementation studies includes several hundreds of items. A selected sample of programs was presented by Kozulin and Rand (2000). The major populations of application are students with learning disabilities; children with special learning disabilities; otherwise-normal, low-achieving students; gifted students; culturally different students and students who are members of ethnic–minority groups; and students with vision and hearing impairments. The program has proved to be rich and flexible enough to be applicable with different populations of learners. All the applications described by Kozulin and Rand are didactically based, in educational settings, with the instruction of IE achieved by specially trained teachers who have been coached in the principles of mediated learning, which emphasizes intentionality of teacher–student interactions, transcendence of the principles discovered in the course of study, mediation of meaning, and a number of other parameters elaborated by Feuerstein and Feuerstein (1991). Conclusions drawn from analysis of the studies conducted point to several important issues: defining the amount of IE teaching that is sufficient for producing desirable results, the importance of exposing students to a wide range of IE instruments, and the importance of monitoring teachers' mediation style by experienced IE counselors. Apparently, different goals require appropriate didactical changes transmitted to IE teachers working with different populations. Furthermore, without evidence of tangible results in areas of content, the educational system rarely accepts pure improvement of cognitive functioning as a valuable outcome (Kozulin & Rand, 2000).

A study based on DCI principles that differs from the studies described above, in that it incorporates therapeutic and rehabilitative aspects, was described by Hadas-Lidor et al. (2001). They investigated the effectiveness of cognitive dynamic treatment through the use of IE with adults with mental illness. The participants included 60 clients who had schizophrenia and required treatment at a rehabilitation day center. The clients were randomly assigned into two groups; one was given IE as treatment, and the other was treated according to traditional methods. Length and scheduling of treatment was equal for both groups. The study had a pre–post quasi-experimental design and lasted for half a year. The following variables were measured before and after treatment: cognitive performance, self-concept, and daily functioning. The results after treatment showed significant differences between the study group and the control group in the areas of cognitive performance and daily functioning, within both the home and work environments. No significant differences were found regarding self-concept. This study, which is the first treatment effectiveness study with adults with schizophrenia, has important implications, as it suggests both that the IE program is effective and that clients with schizophrenia can improve in their cognitive skills as well as everyday functioning.

The theory behind and the practice of the IE program and the LPAD dynamic assessment are still under development, and research is being conducted in many countries worldwide and by different professionals. The dynamic approach has also been recommended for inclusion in the framework of cognitive rehabilitation in populations of adults with brain injuries (Groverman, Brown, & Miller, 1985; Hadas-Lidor, 1996; Toglia, 1989, 1991).

ADDITIONAL ACADEMIC APPLICATIONS

In addition to the development in the fields of treatment, assessment, and research, programs based on SCM theory and DCI are being developed in the academic field, led by prominent occupational therapists.

A postprofessional diploma program in the theory of SCM and DCI and their applications to the health professions has been designed by Naomi Hadas-Lidor, at Tel Aviv University in Israel. The curriculum includes theoretical aspects on brain development and function; learning theories; and applied courses in the fields of assessment, treatment, and mediated learning. An additional unique aspect of the program is concurrent supervision based on group discussion and analysis of events. The program participants come from diverse health-related professions and include occupational therapists, psychologists, speech therapists, nurses, and social workers. Attitude questionnaires given to participants before and after conclusion of studies point to significant changes in beliefs, emotions, and behaviors in relation to their roles as dynamic cognitive therapists and to their belief in their clients' ability to change and develop as a result of the therapeutic intervention and interaction (Hadas-Lidor & Weiss, 2004).

The Israeli Ministry of Health is currently encouraging and participating in a comprehensive program aimed at integrating cognitive dynamic therapy techniques in the field of mental health. Occupational therapists are playing a central role in this project, which includes subcommittees concentrating on different aspects of the endeavor: research, comprehensive models for treatment applications in mental health, and applicability of the program within medical services and privileges granted to populations with special needs.

SUMMARY

In this chapter, we presented the DCI, an applied model of intervention for people with special needs. This approach relies on concepts developed by Feuerstein (1979, 1980) and Vygotsky (1978) and includes evaluation and intervention methods and techniques based on their concepts. We presented 13 unique principles that portray the difference and uniqueness of the approach as compared to other theoreticians and directions.

DCI principles enable one to reach out to populations that previously were not a focus of intervention, for example, underachievers, adults with learning disabilities, families, and caregivers. The DCI approach views cognition, emotion, and function as a simultaneous connection that is the combined focus of all intervention stages.

We also described initial applications of DCI in the field of research and academic and clinical programs. Our aim is to further the development of DCI by encouraging evidence-based research, both on evaluation and treatment aspects of intervention.

REVIEW QUESTIONS

1. In what way are dynamic cognitive interventions preferable to static approaches?
2. Compare Hadas-Lidor's DCI approach to Feuerstein's SCM approach.
3. How does the DCI encompass emotional aspects in the intervention process?
4. To what populations would you apply DCI principles?

REFERENCES

Allen, C. K. (1985). *Occupational therapy for psychiatric diseases: Measurement and management of cognitive disabilities.* Boston: Little, Brown.

Allen, C. K., & Blue, T. (1998). Cognitive disabilities model: How to make clinical judgments. In N. Katz (Ed.), *Cognition and occupation in cognitive models for intervention in occupational therapy* (pp. 225–280). Bethesda, MD: American Occupational Therapy Association.

Allen, C. K., Earhart, C., & Blue, T. (1992). *Occupational therapy treatment goals for the physically and cognitively dis-*

abled. Bethesda, MD: American Occupational Therapy Association.

American Occupational Therapy Association. (2000). Occupational therapy practice framework: Domain and process. *American Journal of Occupational Therapy, 56,* 609–639.

Anthony, W., Cohen, M., & Farber, M. (1990). *Psychiatric rehabilitation.* Boston: Center for Psychiatric Rehabilitation.

Anthony, W., Cohen, M., Farkas, M., & Gagne, C. (2002). *Psychiatric rehabilitation* (2nd ed.). Boston: Sargent College of Health Rehabilitation Sciences.

Avanzini, G. (1990). *Pedagogies de la Mediaton. Autour du PEI programme d'Enrichissement Instrumental du Professeur Reuven Feurerstein* [*Principles of Mediation. Professor Reuven Feuerstein author of Instrumental Enrichment Program*]. Lyon, Depot Legal, France: Chronique Sociale.

Ayers, A. J. (2000). *Sensory integration and the child.* Los Angeles: Western Psychological Services.

Bar-Korzen, S. (2003). *The Beery–Buktenica Developmental Test of Visual–Motor Integration (VMI)—A comparison between standard–static assessment and dynamic assessment (mediated learning experience), between two groups: Low grade achievers and appropriate-high grade achievers.* Unpublished master's thesis, Tel Aviv University, Tel Aviv, Israel.

Bartal-Bahat, E. (2001). *The Test of Visual Motor Skills (TVMS)—A comparison between standard–static assessment and dynamic assessment (mediated learning experience.* Unpublished master's thesis, Tel Aviv University, Tel Aviv, Israel.

Feuerstein, R. (with Rand, Y., & Hoffman, M. B.). (1979). *The dynamic assessment of retarded performers: The Learning Potential Assessment Device: Theory, instruments, and techniques.* Baltimore: University Park Press.

Feuerstein, R. (with Rand, Y., Hoffman, M. B., & Miller, R.). (1980). *Instrumental enrichment: An intervention program for cognitive modifiability.* Baltimore: University Park Press.

Feuerstein, R., & Feuerstein, S. (1991). Mediated learning experience: A theoretical review. In R. Feuerstein, P. S. Klein, & A. J. Tannenbaum (Eds.), *Mediated learning experience (MLE): Theoretical, psychosocial, and learning implications* (pp. 3–51). London: Freund.

Feuerstein, R. S., & Feuerstein, R. (2003). *Instrumental Enrichment for Young Age: IE-Basic.* Jerusalem: International Center for the Enhancement of Learning Potential Press.

Feuerstein, R., Feuerstein, R. S., Falik, L. H., & Rand, Y. (2002). *The dynamic assessment of cognitive modifiability: The Learning Propensity Assessment Device: Theory, instruments, and techniques.* Jerusalem: International Center for the Enhancement of Learning Potential Press.

Feuerstein, R., Feuerstein, R., & Schur, Y. (1997). Process as content in education of exceptional children. In A. Kozulin (Ed.), *The ontogeny of cognitive modifiability: Applied aspects of mediated learning experience and instrumental enrichment* (pp. 1–24). Jerusalem: International Center for the Enhancement of Learning Potential Press.

Feuerstein, R., & Rand, Y. (1997). *Don't accept me as I am—Helping retarded performers excel* (rev. ed.). Jerusalem: International Center for the Enhancement of Learning Potential Press.

Feuerstein, R., Rand, Y., Haywood, C., Hoffman, M., & Jensen, M. (1983). *Learning Potential Assessment Device Manual* (Unpublished). Jerusalem: Haddash-Wizo Research Institute.

Fisher, A. G., Murray, E. A., & Bundy, A. C. (1992). *Sensory integration: Theory and practice.* Philadelphia: F. A. Davis.

Gindis, B. (2003). Remediation through education. In A. Kozulin, B. Gindis, V. S. Ageyev, & S. M. Miller (Eds.), *Vygotsky's educational theory in cultural context* (pp. 200–224). New York: Cambridge University Press.

Ginton, C., & Gelis, M. (2000). *Puzzle assessment.* Retrieved from http://health.tau.ac.il/yedion03_04/occupational/Teuda/takdim/sifrut/articles/diagnosis_by_pazel.htm.

Grigorenko, E. L., & Sternberg, R. J. (1998). Dynamic testing. *Psychological Testing, 124,* 75–111.

Groverman, A. M., Brown, E. W., & Miller, M. H. (1985). Moving toward common ground: Utilizing Feuerstein's model in cognitive rehabilitation. *Cognitive Rehabilitation, 3,* 28–30.

Hadas-Lidor, N. (1996). Feuerstein's theory of cognitive modifiability and its applications to occupational therapy. *Israeli Journal of Occupational Therapy, 5,* E1–E5.

Hadas-Lidor, N. (1997). Dynamic cognitive intervention in a population suffering from schizophrenia. In A. Kozulin (Ed.), *The ontogeny of cognitive modifiability: Applied aspects of mediated learning experience and instrumental enrichment* (pp. 201–215). Jerusalem: ICELP International Center for the Enhancement of Learning Potential.

Hadas-Lidor, N., & Chasdai, A. (2004). *Keshet—Intervention program for parents of children with special needs in mental health.* Manuscript submitted for publication.

Hadas-Lidor, N., & Katz, N. (1998). A dynamic model for cognitive modifiability: Application in occupational therapy. In N. Katz (Ed.), *Cognition and occupation in cognitive models for intervention in occupational therapy* (pp. 281–304). Bethesda, MD: American Occupational Therapy Association.

Hadas-Lidor, N., Katz, N., Tyano, S., & Weizman, A. (2001). Effectiveness of dynamic cognitive intervention in rehabilitation of clients with schizophrenia. *Clinical Rehabilitation, 15,* 349–359.

Hadas-Lidor, N., Naveh, E., & Weiss, P. (2003). ממטפל למורה- [כניסה לתפקיד הוראתי-שלב נוסף בהתפתחות הזהות המקצוצית [From therapist to teacher—Additional stage in the development of professional identity]. *The Israel Journal of Occupational Therapy, 12,* 177–191.

Hadas-Lidor, N., & Weiss, P. (2004). *Change of attitudes and beliefs of students after participation in diploma studies.* Unpublished manuscript.

Hahn-Markowitz, J., & Roitman, D. M. (2000). Literature digest review: The client–therapist relationship in occupational therapy. *The Israel Journal of Occupational Therapy, 9,* 3–11.

Haywood, H. C., Brooks, P. H., & Burns, S. (1992). *Bright start: Cognitive curriculum for young children.* Watertown, MA: Charles Bridge Publishers.

Itzkovitch, M., Elazar, B., Averbuch, S., & Katz, N. (2000). *Loewenstein Occupational Therapy Assessment (LOTCA) battery.* Pequannock, NJ: Maddak.

Kandel, E. R. (1998). A new intellectual framework for psychiatry. *American Journal of Psychiatry, 155,* 457–469.

Katz, N., & Hadas, N. (1995). Cognitive rehabilitation: Occupational therapy models for intervention in psychiatry. *Psychiatric Rehabilitation Journal, 19,* 29–37.

Katz, N., Parush, S., & Traub Bar-Ilan, R. (in press). *Dynamic Occupational Therapy Cognitive Assessment for Children (DOTCA–Ch).* Pequannock, NJ: Maddak.

Kaufman, R., & Burden, R. (in press). Peer tutoring and collaborative learning between young adults with severe and complex learning difficulties: Some effects of mediation training with Feuerstein's instrumental enrichment program. *European Journal of Psychology of Education.*

Kielhofner, G. (Ed.). (1985). *A model of human occupation, theory and application.* Baltimore: Williams & Wilkins.

Kielhofner, G. (Ed.). (1995). *A model of human occupation, theory and application* (2nd ed.). Baltimore: Williams & Wilkins.

Kozulin, A. (Ed.). (1997). *The ontogeny of cognitive modifiability: Applied aspects of mediated learning experience and instrumental enrichment.* Jerusalem: International Center for the Enhancement of Learning Potential.

Kozulin, A., & Rand, Y. (2000). *Experience of mediated learning: An impact of Feuerstein's theory in education and psychology.* New York: Pergamon.

Kushnir A. (1996). Mediated intervention with mothers native to the Caucasus who immigrated to Israel. *Israeli Journal of Occupational Therapy, 5,* E105–E126.

Lachman, M., & Roe, D. (2003). התלמה מסכיזופרניה וממחלות נפש כרוניות [The evolvement of recovery from schizophrenia and chronic mental illness]. *Sichot, 18,* 1.

Law, M., Baptiste, S., Carswell, A., McColl, M. A., Polatojko, H., & Pollok, N. (1998). *Canadian Occupational Performance Measure* (2nd ed. rev.) Ottawa, ON: CAOT Publications.

Law, M., Baum, C., & Baptiste, S. (2002). *Occupational based practice: Fostering health through occupation.* Thorofare, NJ: Slack.

Lidz, C. S. (1987). *Dynamic assessment.* New York: Guilford Press.

Lidz, C., & Elliott, J. (Eds.). (2000). *Dynamic assessment: Prevailing model and applications.* New York: Elsevier.

Missiuna, C., Malloy-Miller, T., & Mandich, A. (1998). Mediational techniques: Origins and application to occupational therapy in pediatrics. *Canadian Journal of Occupational Therapy, 65,* 202–209.

Moreno, C. (1996). Feuerstein's mediated learning and instrumental enrichment: Applications in occupational therapy intervention: A case study. *Israeli Journal of Occupational Therapy, 5,* E152–E158.

Neff, S. W. (1985). *Work and human behavior* (3rd ed.). New York: Aldine.

Neistadt, M. (1990). A critical analysis of occupational therapy approaches for perceptual deficits in adults with brain injury. *American Journal of Occupational Therapy, 44,* 299–304.

Sohlberg, M. M., & Mateer, C. A. (2001). *Cognitive rehabilitation: An integrative neuropsychological approach.* New York: Guilford Press.

Toglia, J. P. (1989). Approaches to cognitive assessment of the brain injured adult: Traditional methods and dynamic investigation. *Occupational Therapy Practice, 1,* 36–37.

Toglia, J. P. (1991). Generalization of treatment: A multicontext approach to cognitive perceptual impairment in adults with brain injury. *American Journal of Occupational Therapy, 45,* 501–516.

Toglia, J. P. (1994). *TCA—The Toglia Category Assessment.* Paquanncock, NJ: Maddak.

Toglia, J. P. (1998). A dynamic interactional model to cognitive rehabilitation. In N. Katz (Ed.), *Cognition and occupation in cognitive models for intervention in occupational therapy* (pp. 5–50). Bethesda, MD: American Occupational Therapy Association.

Tzuriel, D. (2001). *Dynamic assessment of young children.* New York: Plenum.

Tzuriel, D., & Eiboshitz, Y. (1992). Structured Program of Visual–Motor Integration (SP–VMI) for preschool children. *Learning and Individual Differences, 4,* 103–124.

Vygotsky, L. S. (1978). *Mind in society: The development of higher psychological processes.* Cambridge, MA: Harvard University Press.

Weiss, P. (2001). *Comparison of performance on a dynamic assessment of a complex figure in healthy adults with rehabilitation clients suffering from schizophrenia.* Unpublished master's thesis, Tel Aviv University, Tel Aviv, Israel.

World Health Organization. (2001). *International Classification of Functioning, Disability and Health.* Retrieved February 24, 2004, from http://www.who.int/classifiction/icf.

Index